COMPARATIVE VETERINARY HISTOLOGY

WITH CLINICAL CORRELATES

Elizabeth Aughey
BVMS, MRCVS
Department of Veterinary Anatomy
University of Glasgow Veterinary School, UK

Fredric L. Frye
BSc, DVM, MSc, CBiol, FIBiol, FRSM
Fredric L. Frye & Associates
Davis CA, USA

Clinical Correlates by
Fredric L. Frye BSc, DVM, MSc, CBiol, FIBiol, FRSM
Hazel Johnston BVMS, MRCVS

CRC Press
Taylor & Francis Group
Boca Raton London New York

CRC Press is an imprint of the
Taylor & Francis Group, an informa business

CRC Press
Taylor & Francis Group
6000 Broken Sound Parkway NW, Suite 300
Boca Raton, FL 33487-2742

International Standard Book Number-: 978-1-87454-566-8 (Hardback) 978-1-84076-148-1 (Paperback)

Visit the Taylor & Francis Web site at
http://www.taylorandfrancis.com

and the CRC Press Web site at
http://www.crcpress.com

Printed and bound by CPI Group (UK) Ltd, Croydon, CR0 4YY

CONTENTS

Preface 5
Dedications 6
Bibliography 7

1. Introduction 9
Origin of tissues 9
Preparation of tissue sections 10
Staining techniques 14
Microscopy 18
Artefacts induced by histological processing 18
Clinical correlates 20

2. The cell 21
Epithelium 22
Glands 28
Clinical correlates 30

3. Connective tissue 31
Embryonal, mesenchymal and mucoid connective tissues 31
Connective tissue proper 32
Cartilage and bone 40
Clinical correlates 49

4. Blood 51
Blood cells and platelets 51
Clinical correlate 51
Bone marrow: production of blood cells 59
Clinical correlates 61

5. Muscle 65
Muscle types 65
Clinical correlates 70

6. Cardiovascular system 71
Arteries 71
Capillaries and venules 74
Sinusoids 74
Veins 76
Arteriovenous anastomoses 78
Heart 78
Lymphatic vessels 80
Clinical correlates 80

7. Respiratory system 82
Conduction of air 82
Respiration 88
Clinical correlates 92
Avian respiratory system 93
Reptilian, amphibian and fish respiratory systems 95
Clinical correlates 96

8. Digestive system 97
Oral cavity 97
Clinical correlates 105
Alimentary canal 105
Clinical correlates 113
Alimentary system of reptiles and amphibians 117
Clinical correlates 121
Liver 124
Clinical correlates 126
Gall bladder 128
Clinical correlates 128
Pancreas 129
Clinical correlates 130
Reptilian, amphibian and fish pancreas 131
Clinical correlates 132
Avian digestive system 132

9. Urinary system 137
Kidneys 137
Renal pelvis 141
Ureter 141
Urinary bladder 142
Urethra 142
Avian urinary system 143
Reptilian urinary system 144
Amphibian urinary system 145
Fish urinary system 145
Clinical correlates 145

10. **Endocrine system** 149
Endocrine tissue 149
Clinical correlates 149
Hypophysis cerebri (pituitary gland) 150
Clinical correlates 153
Thyroid gland 154
Clinical correlates 155
Parathyroid gland 155
Adrenal gland 156
Clinical correlates 158
Epiphysis cerebri (pineal gland) 159
Avian endocrine system 160
Reptilian, amphibian and fish endocrine system 161
Clinical correlates 165

11. **Male reproductive system** 167
Testis 167
Production of spermatozoa 168
Structure of spermatozoa 169
Tubuli recti rete testis, efferent ducts 169
Epididymis and ductus deferens 170
Urethra 171
Penis 172
Male accessory genital glands 174
Clinical correlates 176
Avian testis 178
Reptilian, amphibian and fish male reproductive system 180
Clinical correlates 182

12. **Female reproductive system** 183
Ovaries 183
Uterine tubes (oviducts) 188
Uterus 189
Vagina 192
Vestibule 194
Vulva, labia and clitoris 194
Mammary glands 194
Placentation 196
Umbilical cord 203
Clinical correlates 204
Avian female reproductive system 208
Reptilian, amphibian and fish female reproductive system 212
Clinical correlates 214

13. **Nervous system** 215
Peripheral nervous system 216
Central nervous system 219
Clinical correlates 226

14. **Special senses** 227
Eye 227
Clinical correlates 236
Avian eye 236
Reptilian, amphibian and fish eyes 237
Clinical correlates 238
Ear 239
Clinical correlates 242
Avian ear 242
Reptilian and amphibian ears 242
Organ of smell (olfactory organ) 243
Other specialized sense organs 244

15. **Lymphatic system** 247
Lymph nodes 247
Spleen 250
Thymus 252
Local aggregations of lymphoid tissue 254
Clinical correlates 256
Avian lymphatic system 258
Reptilian lymphatic system 259
Amphibian lymphatic system 259
Fish lymphatic system 260
Clinical correlates 260
The immune system 261

16. **Integumentary system** 263
Skin 263
Clinical correlates 268
Avian skin 270
Reptilian skin 270
Amphibian skin 274
Fish skin 274
Clinical correlates 274
Specialized integumentary structures 275
Hair 277
Sinus (tactile) hairs (vibrissae) 280
Hooves, horns and claws 280

Appendices 284

Index 289

PREFACE

The objective of this atlas is to stimulate in veterinary undergraduates an appreciation of the relationship between structure and function, which is essential in the context of understanding cell biology. In our long experience of teaching histology we have seen the allotted course time reduced, even though students are expected to have the breadth and depth of knowledge necessary to carry them forward to the expanding fields of cell biology, and to histopathology.

All too often the relevance of histology is not emphasized to students, with the result that students often query the need for so much detail. However, a knowledge of histology is especially relevant today in the wider context of understanding cell function. In the past, it was sufficient to describe the lymphocyte as small or large, with a nucleus and a variable rim of cytoplasm; our present day understanding of the multiple functions of lymphocytes, as demonstrated by immunocytochemistry, in the context of the immune system requires a lecture course on this cell alone to cover all aspects of development, origin, lineage and functions. Such is the diverse nature of histology teaching compared with the more pedantic microscopic anatomy of the past, and this significance is hopefully more stimulating to the student.

Each chapter discusses mammalian aspects of the topic first and foremost. However, reptiles, birds and various other species are kept as pets, and included in the undergraduate curriculum with the common domestic animals. Therefore, some relevant histology is included in the text to highlight evolutionary differences and clinical relevance. More detailed coverage can be found in specialized texts.

Finally, why expect the student to have a working knowledge of normal structure and function? The simple answer is, if you do not know the histology of normal healthy cells and tissues, how can you recognize the abnormal? We have included a series of clinical correlates at the end of each system to demonstrate the changes made by the disease process. In this way we hope to stimulate the student to think about histology as an integral part of biology, with relevance to anatomy, physiology, cell biology, immunology, molecular biology and histopathology.

Elizabeth Aughey
Fredric L. Frye

DEDICATIONS

My introduction to histology began in the Department of Histology and Embryology in the University of Glasgow Veterinary School. The head of the department was Mr Aitken, a dedicated histologist/embryologist with an encylopaedic knowledge of his subject. From him I learned to appreciate that histology was not microscopic anatomy, but a separate discipline: a subject encompassing the origin of the three embryonic germ layers, namely ectoderm, mesoderm and endoderm; the differentiation of these into four basic tissues – epithelium, connective tissue, muscle tissue and nervous tissue; and the complex interaction of these tissues woven together to form the body of the animal. I shall be for ever in his debt.

The preoccupation with cells and cell lines in contemporary research is understandable, but regrettable in that it loses sight of both the whole picture and the very special ability of cells to interact, and it devalues histology as a discipline. I believe that this text affirms my conviction that molecular biology is an impressive research tool, but a small part of the larger canvas of histology.

My thanks go to colleagues in the Department of Veterinary Anatomy and in the University of Glasgow Veterinary School for their help and support, with special appreciation to Allan H. May (Photography). Finally, a tribute goes to my husband and family; without their love and support over the years I would not have been able to devote the time and energy to my chosen subject, histology.

Elizabeth Aughey

To my wife Brucye who, for more than 42 years, has encouraged me and has shared my interest and enjoyment as I have amassed and catalogued the specimens that comprise my portion of this text; to Lorraine, Bice, Erik, Noah and Ian; and to the many comparative histologists and histopathologists who pioneered this discipline to which Elizabeth Aughey and I have been devoted throughout much of our professional careers.

Fredric L. Frye

BIBLIOGRAPHY

Veterinary Anatomy

Dyce KM, Sack WO, Wensing CJG. *Textbook of Veterinary Anatomy*, 2nd edn. 1996; WB Saunders.

Veterinary Embryology

Latshaw WK. *Veterinary Developmental Anatomy*. 1987; BC Decker.

Noden DM, DeLahunta A. *The Embryology of Domestic Animals*. 1985; Williams & Wilkins.

Veterinary Histology

Bacha WJ Jr, Bacha LM. *Color Atlas of Veterinary Histology*, 2nd edn. 2000; Lippincott, Williams & Wilkins.

Dellman HD, Eurell JA. *Veterinary Histology*, 5th edn. 1998; Lippincott, Williams & Wilkins.

Reptilian Histology

Frye FL. *Biomedical and Surgical Aspects of Captive Reptile Husbandry*, 2nd edn. Two volumes. 1991; Krieger Publishing.

General Histology

Bloom W, Fawcett DW. *A Textbook of Histology*, 12th edn. 1993; Chapman & Hall.

Burkitt HG, Young B, Heath JW. *Wheater's Functional Histology*, 3rd edn. 1993; Churchill Livingstone

Carleton HM, Drury RAB. *Histological Technique*. 1967; Oxford University Press.

Kerr JB. *Atlas of Functional Histology*. 1998; CV Mosby.

Stevens A, Lowe J. *Human Histology*, 2nd edn. 1996; CV Mosby.

Placentation

Stevens DH. *Essays in Structure and Function*. 1996; CV Mosby.

Pathology

Carlton WW, McGavin MD. *Thomson's Special Veterinary Pathology*, 2nd edn. 1995; CV Mosby.

1. INTRODUCTION

Anatomy is the science of the shape and structure of organisms and their parts; dissection of dead material is employed to provide information on the gross structure. Early anatomists recognized that an animal's body is made up of different types of tissue, and with the development of the light microscope, histology – the science of tissues – became a new field of study. The new science expanded further when varieties of dyes able to stain dissected material specifically were developed. It became evident that only four basic tissues are present: epithelium, connective tissue, muscle tissue and nervous tissue. All the various parts of the body are derived from these components, and the distinctive appearance of gross anatomical structures depends on which type of tissue is predominant. Each tissue is an assemblage of cells and their derivatives. The balance of cells of different types and these derivatives, and the combination of the different tissues give each part of the body a definitive appearance that can be identified microscopically.

Numerous microscopic techniques are available for studying cells. The most common of these is the examination of living or fixed dead cells (which can be stained with various dyes) under the light microscope. Fixed dead cells can be examined at much higher resolution under the transmission electron microscope, and three-dimensional contours of living and dead cells can be revealed under the scanning electron microscope.

Before the appearance of the various organs of the body systems can be studied, the four basic tissues must be understood, the embryonic origin identified, and the capacity for growth, regeneration and repair assessed.

Veterinary science has changed significantly during the past three decades. The diverse species examined and cared for by veterinarians has increased from traditional domestic animals bred for food, fibre and human companionship to include many 'exotic' animals, such as ornamental fish, amphibians and reptiles. Therefore, the variety of tissues that are illustrated and described in this text reflects the diversity of the animals that are now the responsibility of the veterinary profession.

In order to make this text more pertinent within the current clinical milieu, we have added clinical correlates sections (discussed below) that will facilitate comparing normal tissues with diseased tissues and will help students appreciate why it is so important to study histology. Historically, students have wondered why they must learn the myriad number of names and be able to identify the specialized cells and tissue types, but in order to recognize and understand the often subtle changes in tissues that are induced by disease, it is imperative to know what normal tissues look like. Physiological details of some species and the pathophysiology of various conditions are included so that their influence on form and function can be better comprehended. For example, consider the osmoregulatory stresses imposed on teleost fish, which spawn in hypo-osmotic fresh water and then must migrate and grow to maturity in hyperosmotic seawater, or the enormous and momentous anatomical, metabolic and physiological changes that occur during metamorphosis of amphibian larvae to their adult stage.

It is beyond the scope of this text to cite every abnormal condition known to occur in every organ, in every tissue type and in every species likely to be examined by a veterinary clinician. Rather, examples of those diseases most likely to be encountered in general and specialized veterinary practices are included.

Origin of tissues

The fertilized egg is totipotential, so defined because it gives rise to every cell in the body. The daughter cells arising from the first divisions of this egg are capable, if separated from one another, of becoming new single individuals or identical twins, triplets and quadruplets. If they remain together, however, this totipotentiality is lost: the daughter cells in subsequent divisions follow specific lines of development (differentiation) and gain new attributes, but lose potentiality and develop recognizable characteristics (phenotype). One cell population does not behave in this way, but is segregated in very early embryonic life and retains totipotentiality; these are the germ cells. They migrate to the developing gonads and at puberty become the male and female germ cells. Three basic germ layers, from which all the cells and tissues of the body are derived (see Appendix Table 1), develop in the early embryo at gastrulation: ectoderm (outer layer), mesoderm (middle layer) and endoderm (inner layer).

Preparation of tissue sections

Fixation

For tissue sections to be evaluated, they must have been fixed or preserved so that their cells and architecture do not decompose after cell death. Generally, a 10% neutral buffered formalin solution is employed as a tissue preservative. However, for certain tissues, such as adrenal gland, brain, eyes and a few other structures, special fixative solutions such as Bouin's or Karnovsky's are preferable. Usually, specimens of blood and some body fluids containing cells are fixed onto the glass slide with absolute methanol before staining by one of various dyes. In some cases, such as when supravital staining is used, the stain is applied directly to a specimen without prior fixation.

Small portions (blocks) of tissue, usually less than 0.5 cm in thickness, are removed from the animal as soon as possible after death and immersed in a special preservative fluid, a fixative (**1.1**). Delay for even a minute can lead to serious degenerative changes in the tissue caused by the release of enzymes from the cells. The smaller the sample, the faster the fixative can penetrate the whole block of tissue before degenerative changes occur.

Although many different fixatives are available for different purposes, the most commonly used general-purpose fixative is 10% formol saline. It is important to use adequate volumes of fixative: approximately 50 volumes of fixative to one volume of specimen. Depending on the temperature and size of the specimen and the type of fixative, fixation time is a minimum of 2 days.

Fixation kills the cell quickly, stops the postmortem degenerative processes and preserves the structural integrity of the cellular components of the tissue. Soft specimens, such as brain, are hardened by fixation, which allows easier manipulation. By coagulating proteins, fixation prevents their leakage from the cells and allows their position to be identified *in situ*. Fixation facilitates subsequent staining of the tissue.

Paraffin embedding

Once the specimen is properly fixed it is embedded in paraffin wax to support the tissue during the cutting process without altering the morphology of the specimen. The process begins with the removal of the water-based fixative by immersion in a graded series of alcohols of increasing concentration until the tissue is saturated with 100% ethanol (i.e. dehydrated). The specimen is then infiltrated with a clearing agent, such as xylene, that is miscible with both paraffin wax and alcohol. The specimen is infiltrated with warm paraffin wax to replace the xylene (**1.2**). The wax hardens as it cools, holding the tissue firmly in place (**1.3** and **1.4**). This procedure is usually done automatically in a tissue processor. There are disadvantages in paraffin embedding; it is time consuming and the clearing agents are lipid solvents, so this method cannot be used to demonstrate fats (*see* Freezing).

Excess paraffin is trimmed and the block is ready for cutting on a microtome. The block is clamped onto the cutting frame of the microtome, and is moved toward the blade of the microtome using an adjustable wheel until the face of the block is against the blade. With each revolution thin slices (optimally less than 6 μm thick) of the block are cut into a ribbon and emersed (floated) in a warm water-bath (**1.5**). The sections flatten and are floated onto glass slides (**1.6**). The slides are placed on a warm plate to

1.1

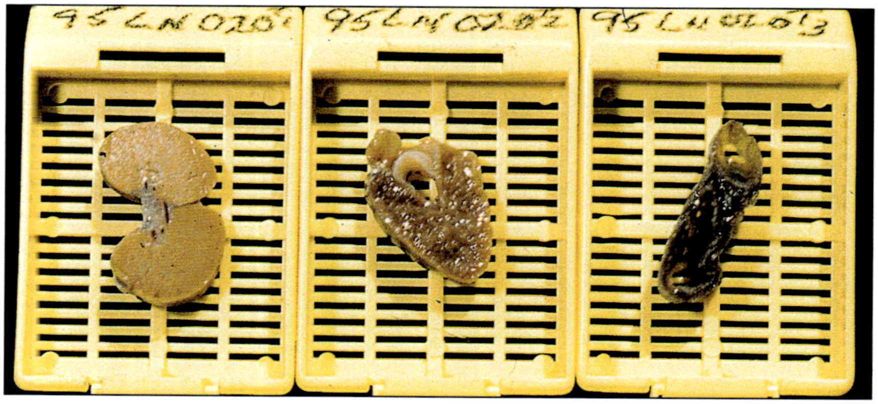

1.1 Specimens of fixed tissues are placed into disposable plastic cassettes that confine and identify each accession during laboratory processing.

1.2a

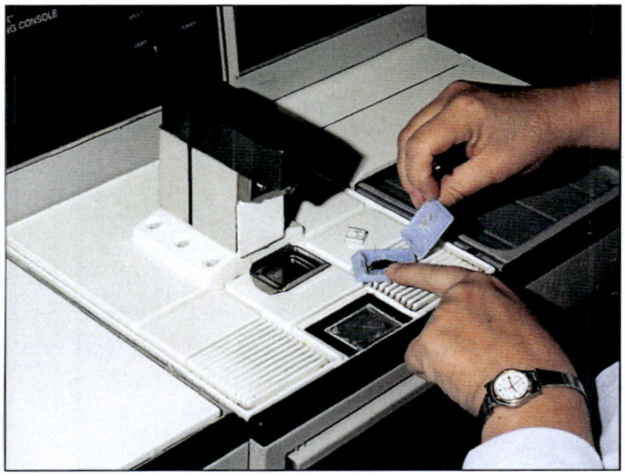

1.2b

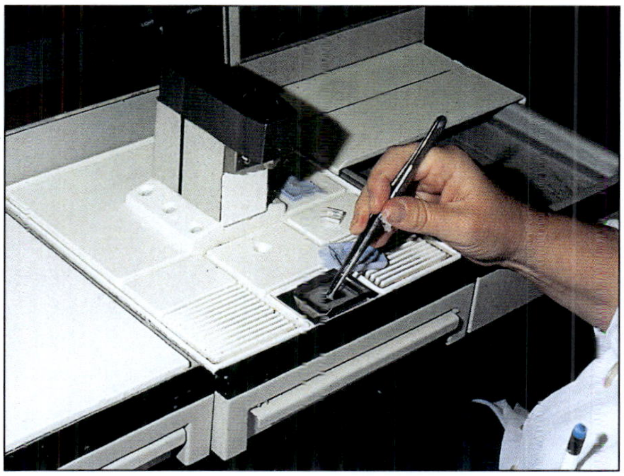

1.2 (a) Once the tissue has dehydrated, (b) a histology laboratory technician embeds it in a melted paraffin wax–plastic polymer compound.

1.3

1.3 A small piece of paper listing special staining requests is embedded on the opposite side of the cassette. In this instance, haematoxylin and eosin (H & E) and periodic acid–Schiff (PAS) stains will be applied to separate duplicate tissue sections.

1.4

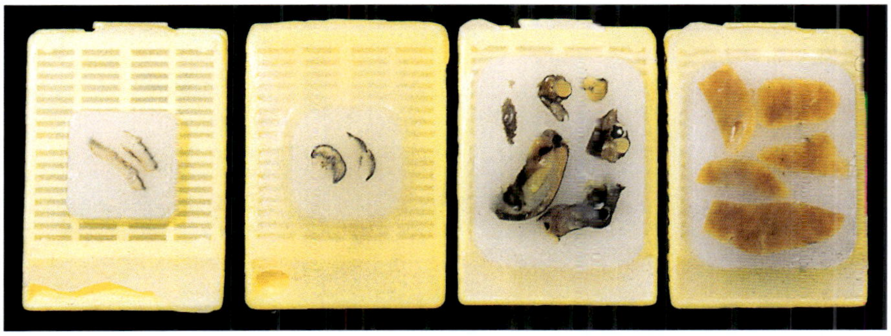

1.4 Four cassettes containing paraffin-embedded tissue ready for sectioning by a microtome.

1.5

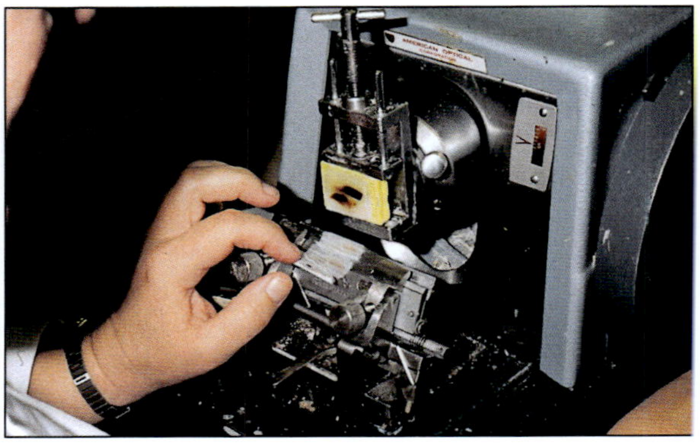

1.5 Using the finely honed microtome blade, the histology technician cuts a thin ribbon of paraffin-embedded tissue.

1.6

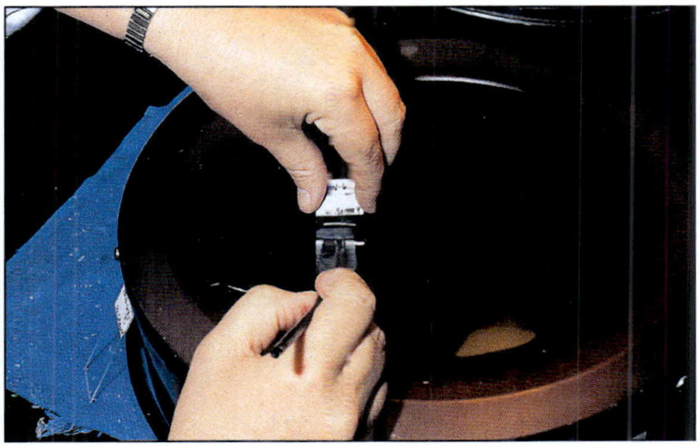

1.6 The tissue section is transferred to a water bath and is floated onto the glass microscope slide with a fine camel's hair brush. Note the matt black finish of the water bath, which facilitates visualizing the nearly transparent tissue section.

dry, and the section adheres to the glass slide (**1.7**). Removal of the paraffin wax by a suitable solvent, such as xylene, and rehydration allows the tissue to be examined unstained; this has no advantage over the direct examination of living cells. It is necessary to stain the component cells and tissues selectively and make a permanent preparation for examination with the light microscope; a selection of these techniques is described later (*see* Staining technique).

Decalcification is necessary for tissue with ossified or calcified components before paraffin embedding, otherwise the hardness of the tissue will result in difficulty in cutting the sections, causing artefacts. Specimens are fixed in formalin or other chemical fixatives, and then transferred to the decalcifying solution to allow removal of the mineral salts. Most of these decalcifying agents contain acids such as formic, malic, glacial acetic, hydrochloric or nitric.

Freezing

A cryostat, a microtome confined to a freezing chamber, is required to cut frozen sections (**1.8**). These may be from fixed or from unfixed tissue. The advantage of this method is that the time between taking the sample and examining it under the microscope is much reduced. A biopsy may be taken and examined while the patient is still in the operating room. Fat-containing cells retain the lipid content and the tissue is often more life-like in appearance than non-frozen sections. The disadvantages of this method are tissue distortion, caused by the freezing and thawing, and thicker sections. Once the sections are cut and mounted on glass slides, conventional staining techniques are used.

Consequence of freezing unfixed tissues

When unfixed tissues are frozen and then thawed before being chemically fixed, their delicate cell membranes may become distorted or ruptured, or both, by the forces induced by the expansion and contraction of the intracellular fluid as it freezes and thaws. Therefore, if tissues are to examined histologically, unfixed specimens must not be frozen. Examples of tissues that were frozen before histological fixation and processing are illustrated in **1.9**.

1.7

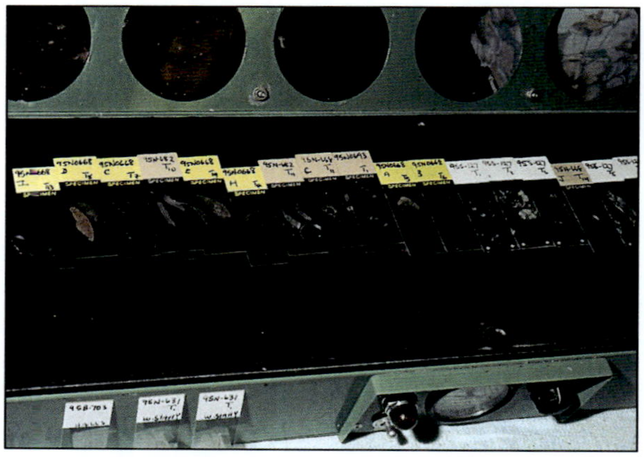

1.7 Slides bearing thin tissue sections are warmed on a thermal table, which causes evaporation and enhances the adhesion of the sections onto the glass surfaces, and smooths out irregularities, which is preparatory to xylene clearing.

1.8

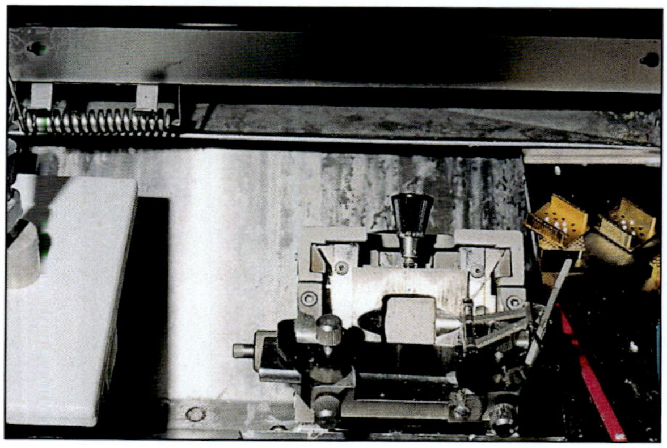

1.8 Frozen tissue sections are created with the use of a cryostat, which is a conventional microtome enclosed within a freezing temperature chamber. Whereas tissue enzymes and some other cellular constituents cannot be detected in paraffin-embedded sections, specially stained frozen tissue sections reveal them. The advantages of frozen tissue sections are that they require less time than paraffin-embedded sections to process, and stained tissue specimens obtained during surgery can be examined and interpreted while the patient is still in the operating room. Fat-containing cells retain their lipid contents because they are not dissolved by xylene.

The rehydrated sections of tissue are now immersed in a solution of one or more stains; any excess stain is removed during this process. The slides are dried again, cleared in xylene, and permanently mounted beneath a glass or plastic coverslip using a mounting medium that is xylene miscible. Sections that require special stains are stained and given individual coverslips, as shown

1.9 Histological sections of (a) myocardium, (b) kidney and (c) liver from a boa constrictor (*Boa C. constrictor*) that were frozen before being fixed in 10% neutral buffered formalin solution. Note the disruption and distortion of the histological architecture, and the loss of all but the erythrocytic nuclei. Such destruction can be prevented if the tissues are fixed before freezing. H & E. a, ×62.5; b, ×62.5; c, ×62.5.

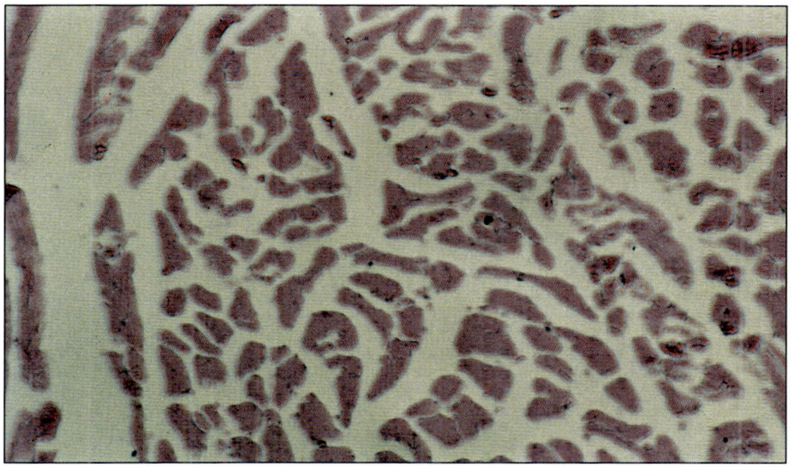

1.9a

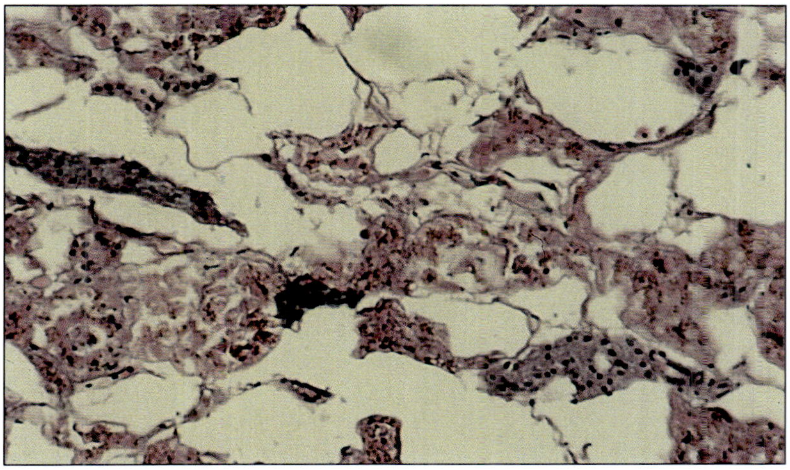

1.9b

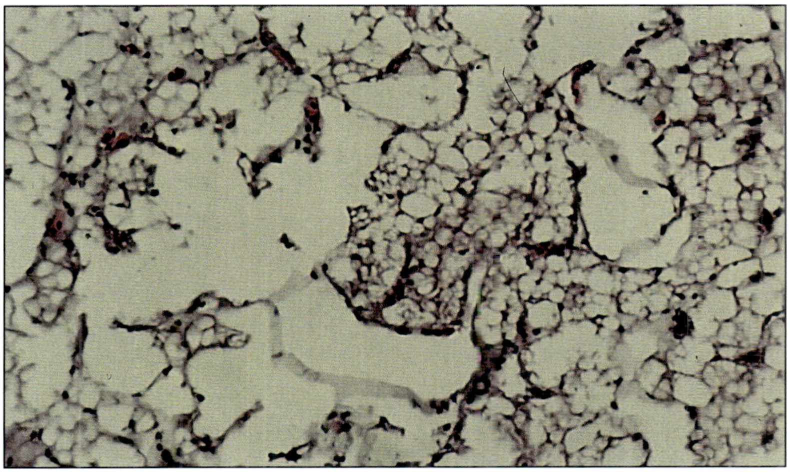

1.9c

in 1.10. Sections requiring standard haematoxylin and eosin (H & E) stain are stained and coverslipped by automated machines that process the tissues and then dispense an appropriate volume of mounting medium, apply a coverslip and compress the finished mounted slide to remove any trapped bubbles of air (1.11). The completed stained microsections are placed onto the surface of a warming table beneath a fume hood, where the xylene in the mounting medium evaporates. This final step fixes the coverslip firmly to the tissue and glass slide, forming a permanent 'sandwich' that can be handled without dislodging any portion of the stained section.

Staining techniques

Numerous different dyes in various combinations are formulated into stains that are used to impart specific and reproducible colouration. Many of these dyes possess positive and negative electrical charges and are attracted or repulsed by electrostatic charges that are characteristic of certain tissue constituents. In order for some dyes to combine with tissue components, a metallic salt, termed a mordant, is required. The combination of a dye with an appropriate mordant forms a 'lake' and carries a positive electrostatic charge. Dye-mordant combinations with positive charges are cationic and are termed

1.10

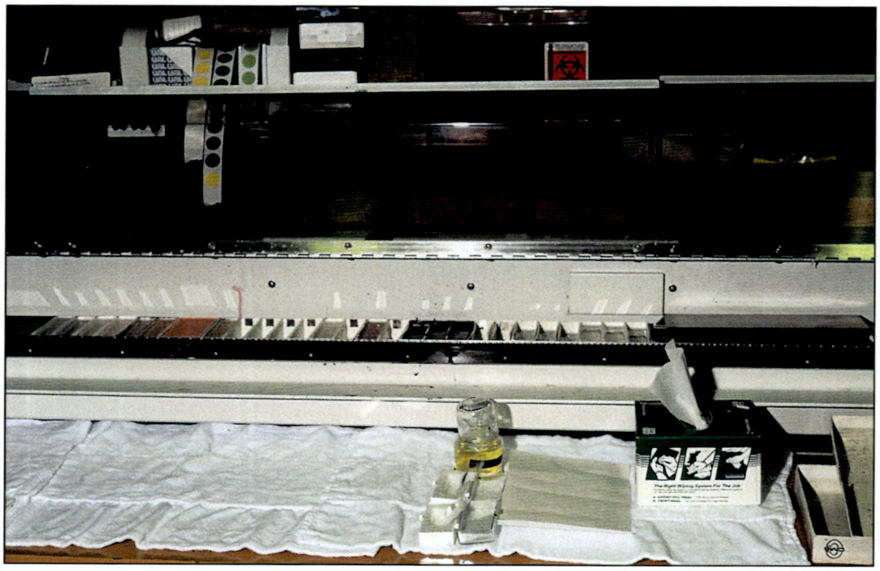

1.10 Slides that have received special staining are coverslipped manually. Exposure of laboratory personnel to potentially toxic xylene vapours is reduced by conducting the coverslipping operations beneath a vacuum fume hood.

1.11

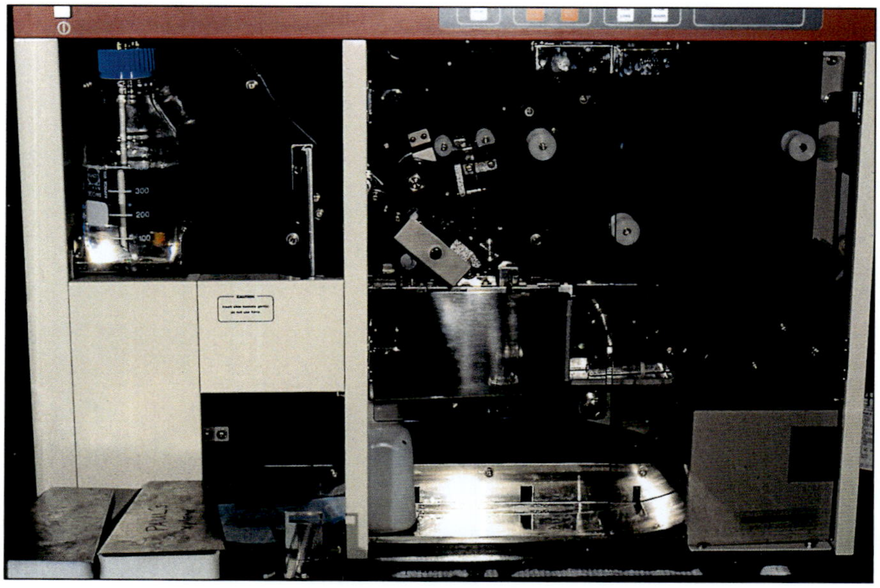

1.11 When large volumes of slides with standard H & E stain must be coverslipped, an automatic coverslipping machine is employed.

'basic' stains. These cationic basic lakes combine electrochemically with negatively charged tissue constituents, such as nuclear chromatin, other nucleoproteins, and phosphate groups. Some dyes are inherently basic without requiring the addition of a mordant; they carry their own positive electrostatic charge. Basic fuchsin, toluidine blue and methylene blue are examples of naturally basic stains. Conversely, anionic or 'acidic' dyes carry a negative or anionic charge, and are called 'acidic' because they are attracted to and combine with tissue constituents that possess a negative electrostatic charge. Eosin is an example of an acidic stain. Differential staining is possible because some tissues may be acidic, basic or amphoteric. Thus, the pH of the extracellular fluid causes their electrostatic charge to vary and, as a result, their acceptance of acidic and basic stains varies.

Many special dye combinations, some requiring rare metallic salts, are used to stain certain tissue types and constituents, micro-organisms, metabolic by-products and so on. Many formularies containing recipe-like staining formulae are available and new staining techniques are continually being developed.

Examination of living cells with the light microscope yields very little information. Therefore, thin sections of tissue, after they have been excised and processed, are stained with special dyes to enable detailed observations to be made on their structure. The most widely used staining technique is H & E. Haematoxylin stains a deep purple colour and acts as a basic stain (basophilic). Eosin is pink to red in colour and acts as an acid stain (acidophilic or eosinophilic). Haematoxylin reacts with deoxyribonucleic acid and ribonucleic acid, and eosin reacts with cytoplasmic proteins and a variety of extracellular structures. Thus, nuclei and rough endoplasmic reticulum stain blue to purple and cytoplasm stains pink to red depending upon the concentration of the basic and acid components of the cell (**1.12**).

Specialized staining methods are used to illustrate particular features. Osmic acid reacts with fat to give a grey–black colour (**1.13**), periodic acid Schiff (PAS)

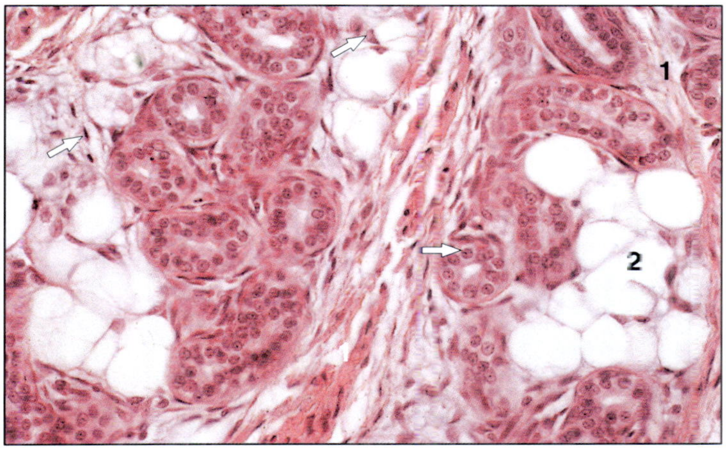

1.12 Digital pad (dog). The nuclei are stained deep blue (arrowed). (1) The cytoplasm and fibres are stained varying shades of pink with eosin. (2) Fat cells are unstained, the fat is lost during processing. H & E. ×160.

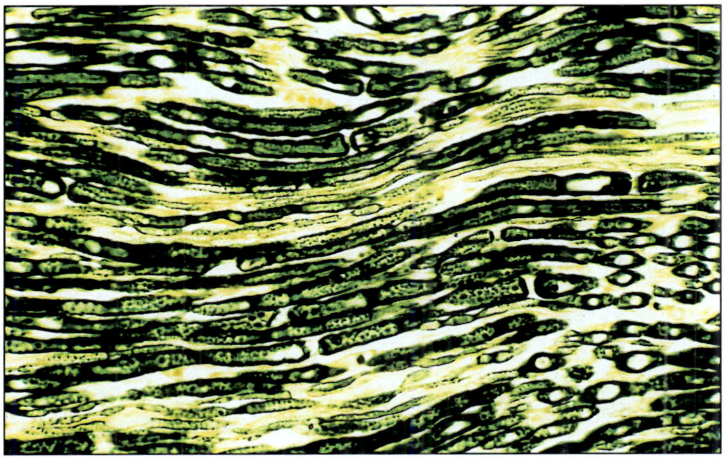

1.13 Longitudinal section (LS nerve (dog). The myelin sheath surrounding the nerve fibre reacts with osmic acid and stains black; the supporting connective tissue is unstained. Osmic acid. ×250.

and alcian blue reveal glycosaminoglycans (**1.14** and **1.15**), silver impregnation displays reticular fibres and some aspects of nervous tissue (**1.16** and **1.17**), and Masson's trichrome differentiates between connective tissue and muscle (**1.18** and **1.19**). Some circumstances require the combination of two or more staining methods to yield the maximum information. There are many other methods available, but only the commonly used ones are mentioned here.

Examination of living material with the electron microscope has necessitated the development of new techniques in preparation procedures to illustrate the arrangement of organelles, membranes and cell contents (**1.20**). It has been further refined to provide a three-dimensional picture without distortion (**1.21**). All of these techniques are now strandard tools in histology and have advanced our understanding.

1.14

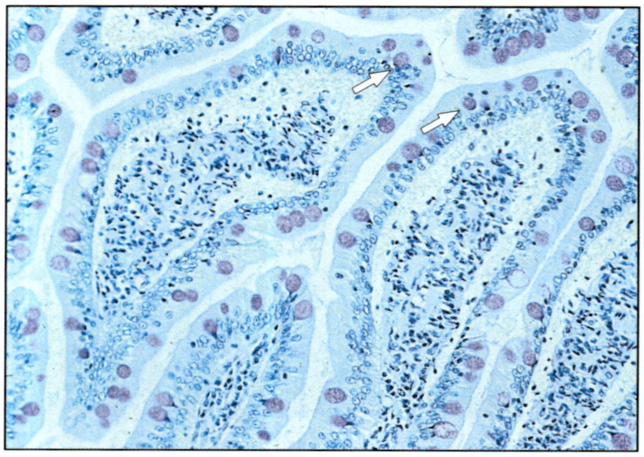

1.14 Duodenum (dog). The mucus-secreting goblet cells react with PAS (arrowed). Haematoxylin/PAS. ×125.

1.15

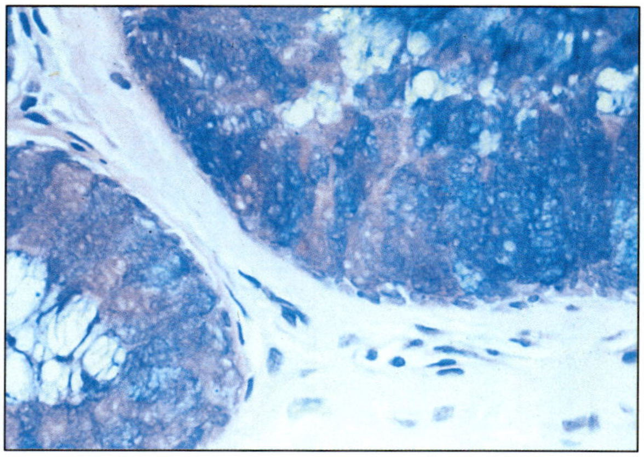

1.15 Cervix (sheep). The epithelial cells lining the cervix react with either alcian blue or PAS, illustrating chemical differences in the types of mucus secreted. Alcian blue/PAS. ×200.

1.16

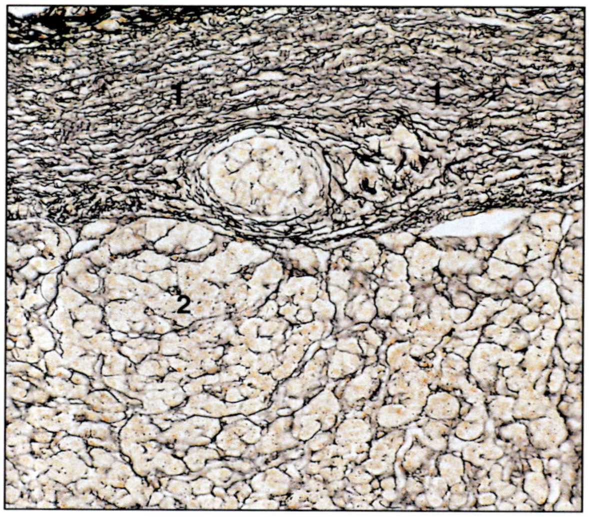

1.16 Adrenal (horse). The reticular fibres form a fine network in (1) the capsule and (2) as a delicate supporting framework for the adrenal secretory cells. The method of Gordon and Sweet for reticular fibres. ×125.

1.17

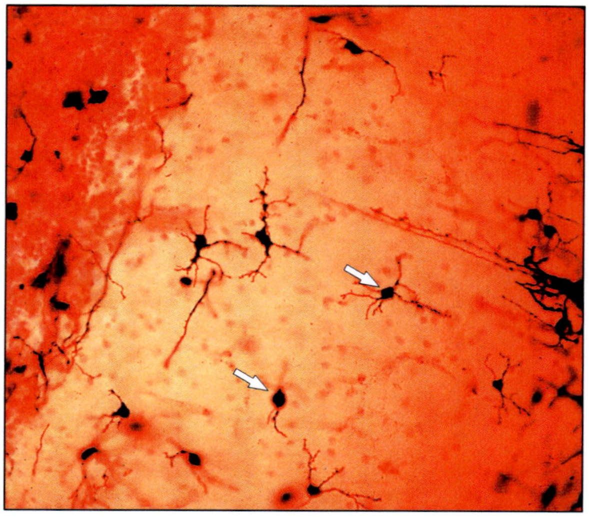

1.17 Stellate cells in the cerebellum (cat). This method is used specifically to illustrate the cytoplasmic processes of the neurons of the central nervous system (arrowed). Cajal's uranium silver. ×250.

1.18

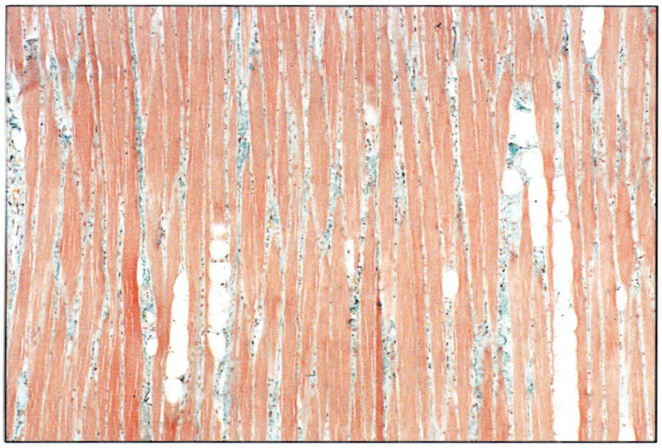

1.18 Tongue (dog). The muscle is stained red and the connective tissue is stained green. Masson's trichrome. ×50.

1.19

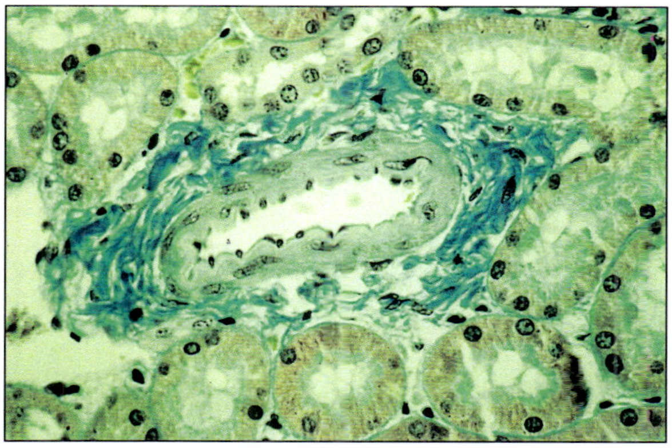

1.19 Kidney (dog). In this trichrome stain the connective tissue is stained a blue/green. Gomori's trichrome. ×125.

1.20 Transmission electron micrograph of a fibroblast (sheep). (1) Nucleus, (2) nuclear membrane, (3) cisternae of rough endoplasmic reticulum (RER), (4) plasmalemma, (5) mitochondria, (6) fat droplet and (7) collagen fibrils. ×8000.

1.20

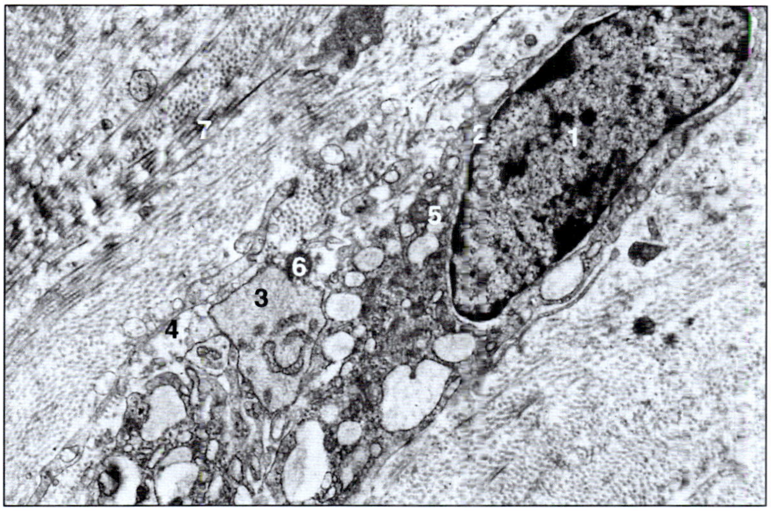

1.21 Scanning electron micrograph of kidney (dog). (1) Renal tubule, (2) interstitial connective tissue, (3) free erythrocyte – a biconcave disc with the typical indentation. ×675.

1.21

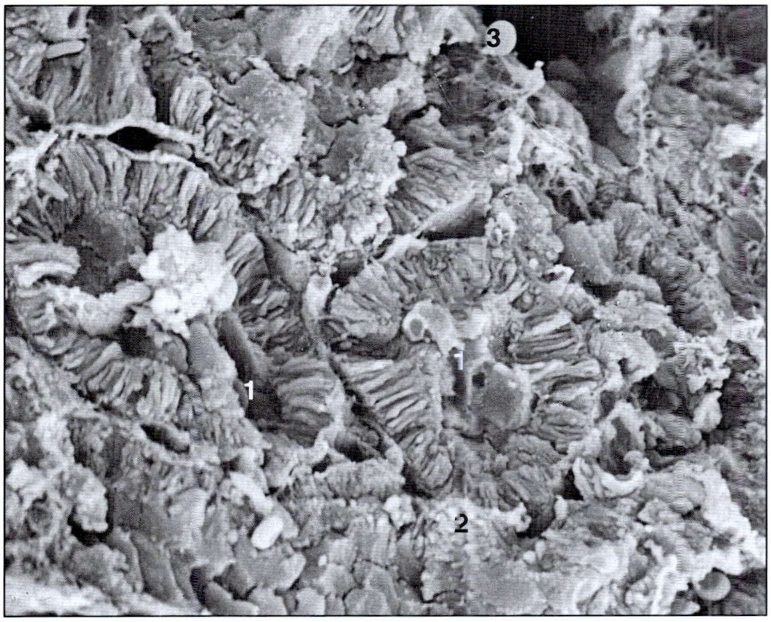

Microscopy

The examination and study of normal cells and tissues by microscopy is called histology or microscopic anatomy. The study of abnormal cells and tissues is histopathology. An understanding of the normal is essential for the recognition of the abnormal. Investigative microscopes range from the simple light microscope to the sophisticated high-resolution electron microscope. In between lie a wide variety of specialized microscopes to meet special needs, such as phase contrast, polarizing and fluorescence microscopes, and the scanning electron microscope.

Units of histological measurement

A micrometre (μm) is equal to a millionth part of a metre and is the unit of measurement of the light microscope; a red blood cell is approximately 8 μm in diameter.

A nanometre (nm) is equal to a billionth part of a metre. The thickness of the basal lamina of an epithelial cell is 70 nm, which can be resolved using the electron microscope.

Light microscopy

The light microscope is the instrument most commonly used for the visualization of cells and tissues. With it magnifications of up to 2000 times are possible. The limit to the size of the structure that can be distinguished with the light microscope is limited by the physical nature of light. The wavelength of visible light ranges from 0.4 to 0.7 μm. Therefore, even with the best optical system available the resolution, or resolving power, of the light microscope is limited to 0.2 μm, and anything smaller than that will not be clearly distinguished.

In order to achieve the best results a few basic preliminary checks must be made.

- Ensure that the glass slide is clean, free from dust and smears.
- Ensure that the microscope condenser, objectives and ocular lenses are clean – take great care to clean the microscope with soft lens tissues.
- Set the microscope up for critical illumination for each objective by:
  (1) closing the iris diaphragm (the substage condenser diaphragm),
  (2) adjusting the condenser until the circular area of illumination has a sharp edge, and
  (3) making sure the condenser is centred by using the adjusting screws.

Always begin with the lowest objective and increase the magnification slowly.

Transmission electron microscopy

This microscope uses an electron beam instead of a light source and allows resolution of structures as small as 1 nm. Small pieces of tissue (cubes not more than 1 mm on a side) are fixed rapidly (to avoid artefacts induced by tissue degradation) in cold glutaraldehyde-based fixative, dehydrated and embedded in epoxy resin. Sections are cut at 0.03–0.05 μm on an ultramicrotome using a glass or a diamond knife, mounted on copper grids and stained with heavy metal solutions such as lead sulphate and uranium nitrate. The vapours of fixatives used for electron microscopy processing are volatile and hazardous to the eyes and mucous membranes, so an exhaust hood or adequate ventilation is essential.

Scanning electron microscopy

Solid pieces of tissue fixed in a glutaraldehyde fixative, are dried, coated with gold and placed in the microscope. The electron beam scans the specimen and a three-dimensional representation of the surface is obtained.

Artefacts induced by histological processing

The preparation of tissue sections involves a number of stages during fixing, dehydrating, paraffin embedding, sectioning, deparaffinizing, rehydrating, staining and coverslipping. Each of these processes necessitates the manipulation of tissue specimens and laboratory reagents, thus providing opportunities for errors to be made. Just one flawed laboratory technique can spoil the final result. Some of the common artefacts are illustrated in **1.22–1.26**.

.22

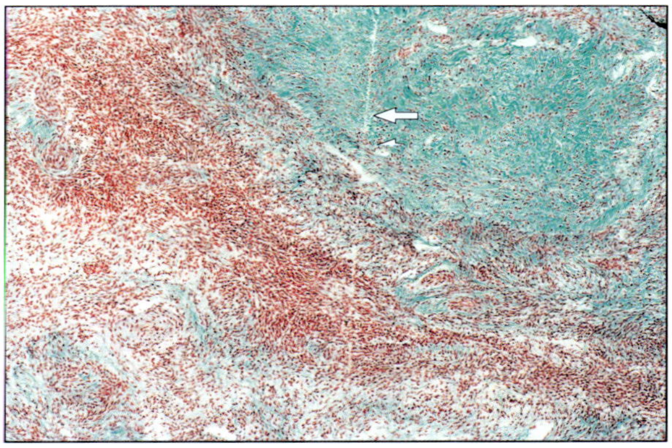

1.22 Ovary (sheep). A knife mark, caused by a nick in the microtome's cutting edge, leaves a straight line across the section (arrowed). Masson's trichrome. ×25.

1.23

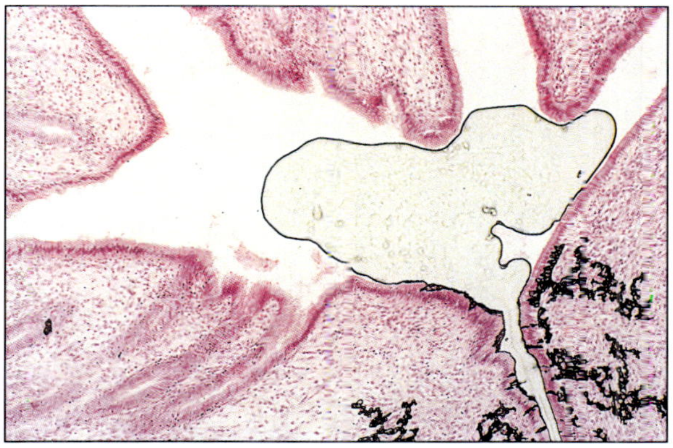

1.23 Uterus (cat). Shrinkage of the adhesive medium used to mount the coverslip to the slide captures air and causes bubbles. H & E. ×65.5.

.24

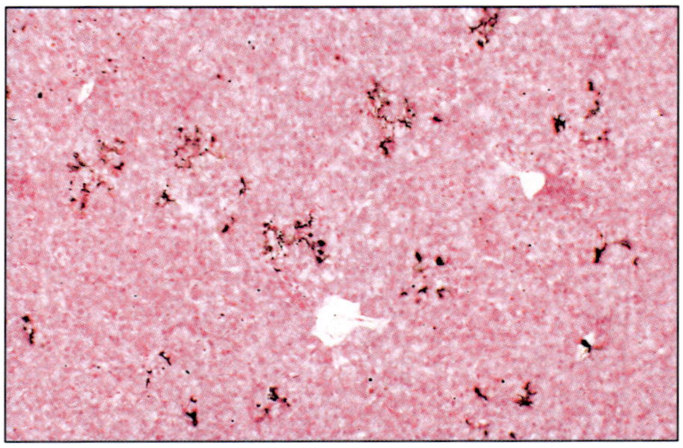

1.24 Spleen (bird). When crystals accumulate in the stain solutions or are not removed during standard processing, stain deposits precipitate onto the surfaces of the tissue section. H & E. ×25.

1.25

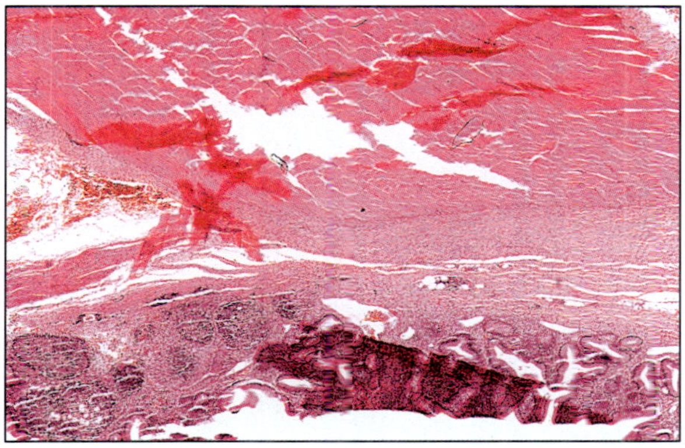

1.25 Cloacal bursa (bird). Raised areas, overlapping folds and cracked and separated tissue are present because it is often difficult to flatten the tissue completely, particularly in very thin sections. H & E. ×25.

1.26 Spleen (dog). Compression of the paraffin-embedded tissue causes parallel 'chatter' marks. H & E. ×25.

1.26

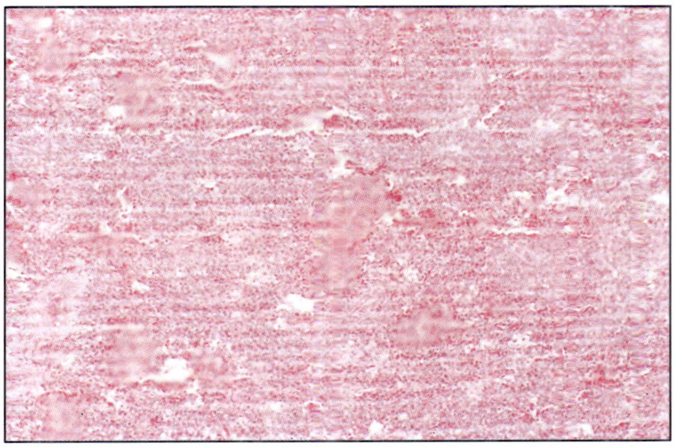

Clinical correlates

In order to appreciate the often subtle alterations that accompany disease or other physical abnormalities, it is useful to compare the characteristic changes by which histopathological diagnoses are made and classified. To that end, clinical correlates sections are inserted throughout this text. It is important to note that in many instances the tissues comprising an organ of one species are similar or even identical to those found in a disparate species.

Generally, there are fewer substantive differences within a phylogenetic group of animals than between different groups of animals. For instance, the livers of sheep, cattle, horses, swine, dogs and cats are relatively quite similar; the liver tissues of many fish resemble the hepatic tissue found in amphibians; and the hepatic tissues of many reptiles resemble those observed in birds. Because of these characteristic similarities and differences, we have selected examples of tissues that are particularly instructive in order to avoid showing repetitively the same tissues for every animal, irrespective of its phylogeny. However, examples from a wide variety of species are included for purposes of comparison.

These correlates are placed where they most readily illustrate specific, clinically significant medical conditions. Recognizing normal tissue facilitates interpreting the often subtle alterations in abnormal tissues. Where appropriate, the physiological attributes or significance, or both, of a particular organ or structure are discussed briefly so that their importance to the survival of the animal becomes apparent.

2. THE CELL

The cell is the basic unit of a living structure, a complex gel of protein, carbohydrate, fat, nucleic acids and inorganic material. Cells are limited by a cell membrane, the plasmalemma. Within the cell lies the membrane-bound nucleus. The nucleus is surrounded by a double membrane, the nuclear membrane or envelope, and sequesters the cell complement of deoxyribonucleic acid (DNA), which consists of two long strands wound together in a double helix. The DNA is organized into chromosomes, which carry the genetic information: the genes. Chromosomes are rarely visible, except during cell replication (**2.1**) and where protein–DNA complexes are seen as chromatin. The small, darkly staining bodies within the nucleus are the nucleoli. Ribonucleic acid (RNA) is present within the nucleoli together with a small amount of DNA. Small amounts of DNA are also present in the cytoplasmic organelle, the mitochondrion. Ribosomal RNA is synthesized in the nucleoli and lines the outer nuclear membrane as it expands into the cytoplasm to become the rough endoplasmic reticulum (RER).

Cytoplasm surrounds the nucleus and is bound by the plasmalemma. The components of the cytoplasm are divided into organelles and inclusions lying in the cytoplasmic matrix (or cytosol). The organelles may be membranous (e.g. the cell membrane, mitochondria, RER and smooth endoplasmic reticulum, Golgi apparatus, secretory vesicles and granules, and lysosomes) or non-membranous (e.g. stored food, fat and glycogen, and a variety of pigments).

2.1

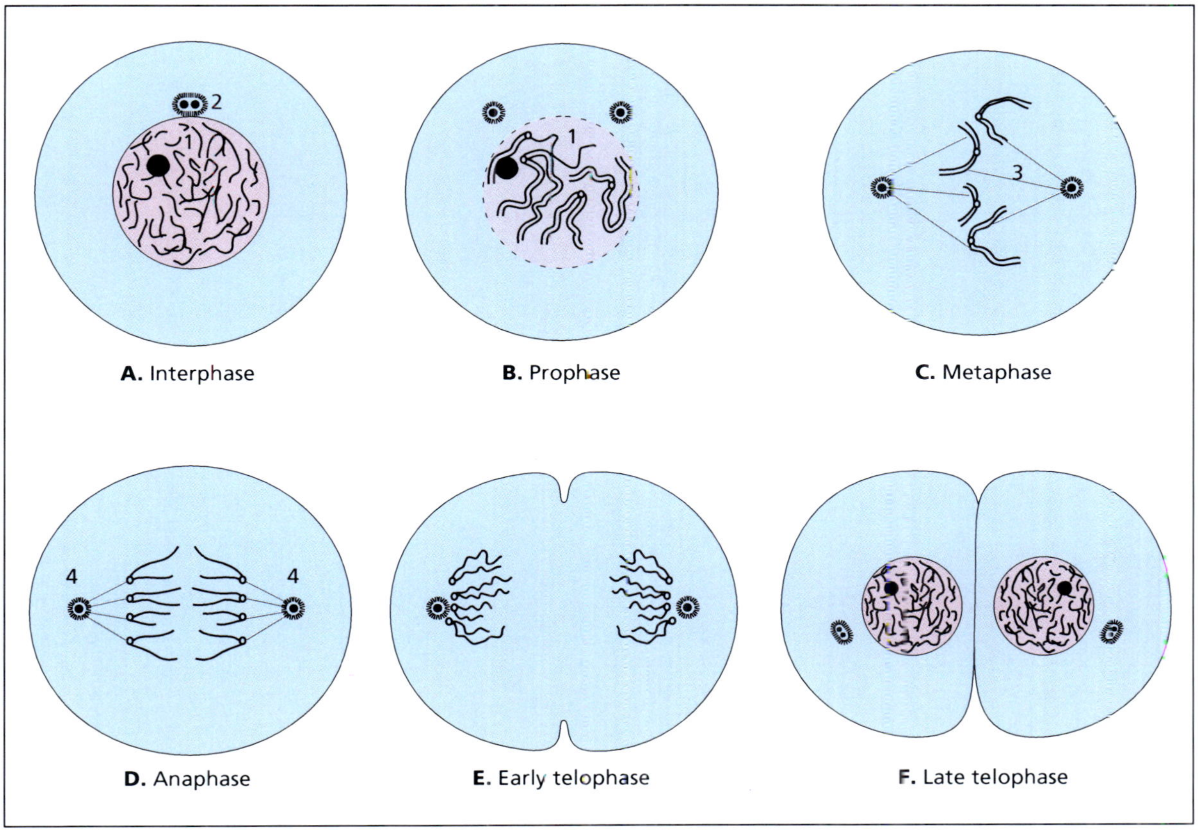

2.1 The stages of mitotic division. **(A) Interphase.** (1) Nucleus. (2) Centromere. **(B) Prophase.** The granular appearance of the nucleus (1) is the early condensation of the nuclear chromatin in preparation for division. **(C) Metaphase.** The short, compact chromosomes are arranged around a central spindle. **(D) Anaphase.** The centromere has divided and two chromatids for each chromosome have separated and moved towards each centromere (4). **(E) Early telophase.** Separation of the daughter chromosomes is complete and the cytoplasm begins to divide. **(F) Late telophase.** The nucleus (1) of each daughter cell is reconstructed with a nuclear membrane and a nucleolus; the chromosomes are no longer visible. The cytoplasm divides.

Epithelium

Epithelium is the term used for all the covering and lining membranes of the body. It is composed of contiguous cells linked by cell junctions and resting on a specialized matrix, the basement membrane. All epithelia are avascular and are supported and nourished by the underlying connective tissue capillary bed. They are derived from all three basic germ layers (ectoderm, endoderm and mesoderm). The ectoderm provides the nervous system, the outer layer of the skin and the epidermis, and the endoderm provides the lining of the respiratory and digestive tracts. Both ectoderm and endoderm grow into the underlying embryonic connective tissue (mesenchyme) and form exocrine and endocrine glands. Exocrine glands secrete onto the surface of the epithelial membrane through a system of ducts. Endocrine glands are ductless; islands of secretory cells embedded in connective tissue secrete into the local capillary bed and thus directly into the blood to be carried to the target organ.

Epithelium of mesodermal origin forms a thin squamous membrane lining the pleural, peritoneal and pericardial cavities of the body. The mesodermally derived epithelium lining the heart, blood and lymphatic vessels is called endothelium.

The urogenital system is derived from mesoderm, and the epithelial membranes of most of the genital system, the kidneys and ureters are of mesodermal origin. All epithelial membranes are capable of regeneration and repair. Damaged and dead cells are replaced by adjoining cells to maintain the cover and the integrity of the membrane.

Epithelium may be either simple, where a single layer of cells is present, or stratified, where a variable number of cell layers are superimposed.

Simple epithelium

Squamous

Simple squamous epithelium is a single continuous layer of flattened cells, which is often so attenuated that it is difficult to identify the boundaries of individual cells using the light microscope. The nucleus bulges from the thickest part of the cell, as in the endothelium lining blood vessels (2.2) and in the mesothelium of the body cavities (2.3).

Cuboidal

Simple cuboidal epithelium is a single layer of cells; each cell is square in cross-section with a central nucleus. Minor variations in proportion may occur to give short cuboidal and tall cuboidal cells. Examples can be found covering the ovary, thyroid gland and mammary gland (2.4–2.6).

Columnar

Simple columnar epithelium is a single continuous layer of tall hexagonal cells with a basal nucleus forming a relatively thick membrane. These cells are often specialized, performing a particular function. In secretory epithelium the cells secrete mucus and have a lubricant and protective function; examples can be found in the stomach and cervical canal (2.7 and 2.8). In the small intestine the luminal surface area is markedly increased by microvillous processes to form a striated border, a functional adaptation designed to increase the surface area for absorption. Adjoining goblet cells secrete mucus, keeping the membrane moist and protecting against digestion by the luminal contents (2.9).

2.2

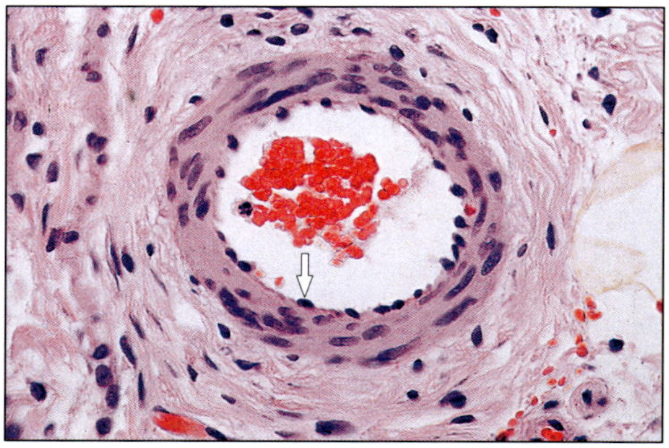

2.2 Simple squamous endothelium. Uterus (cat). Arteriole. Simple attenuated squamous cells line the lumen; the nucleus of one cell is arrowed. H & E. ×250.

2.3

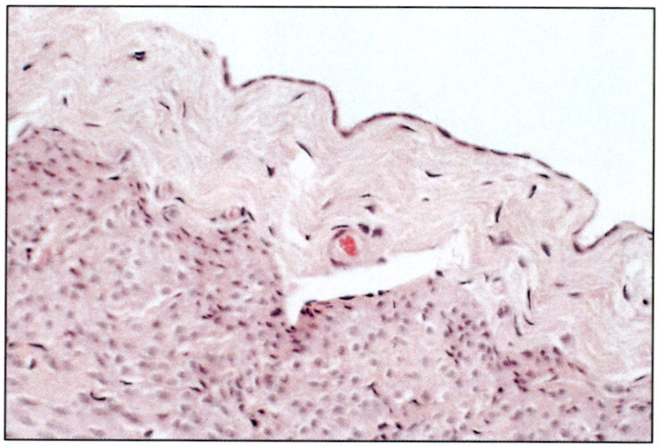

2.3 Simple squamous mesothelium. Uterus (cat). The simple squamous cells are on the free serous surface of the uterus. H & E. ×160.

2.4

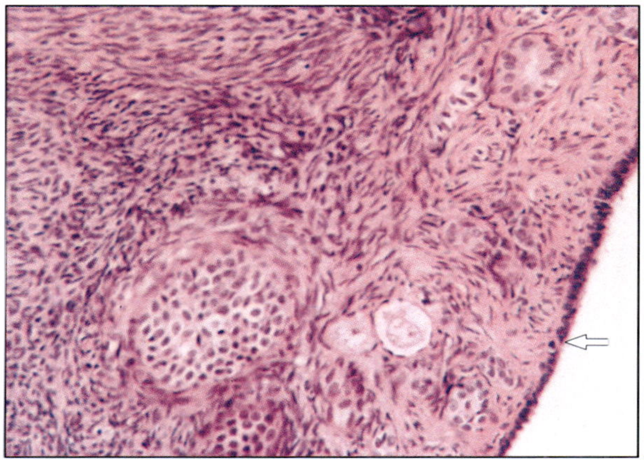

2.4 Simple cuboidal epithelium. Ovary (sheep). The simple cuboidal epithelium on the free surface of the ovary is arrowed. H & E. ×50.

2.5

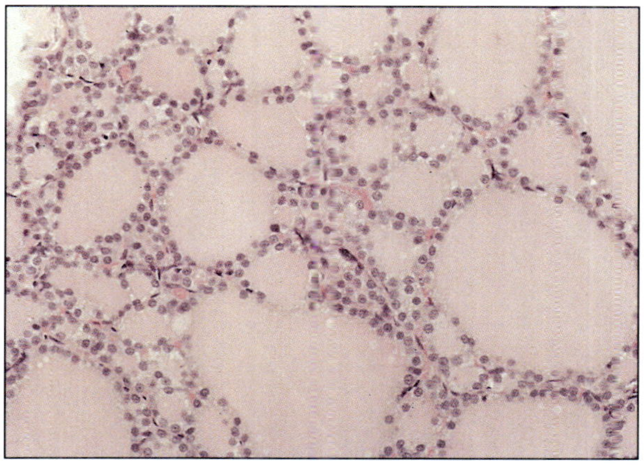

2.5 Simple cuboidal epithelium. Thyroid (dog). The simple cuboidal epithelium lines the colloid filled thyroid follicles. H & E. ×20.

2.6

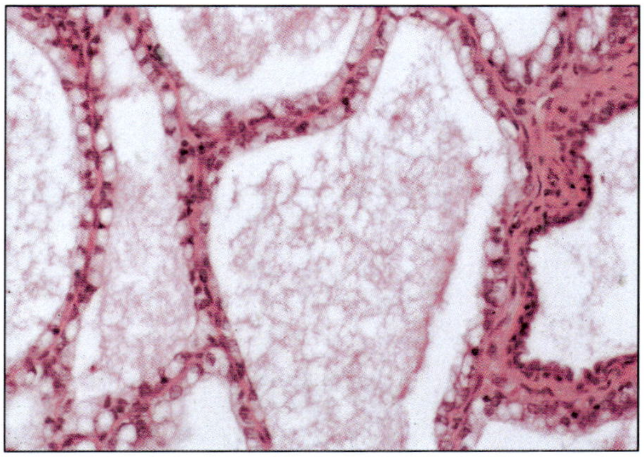

2.6 Simple cuboidal epithelium. Lactating mammary gland (cow). The secretory alveolus of the mammary gland is lined by simple cuboidal cells. H & E. ×125.

2.7

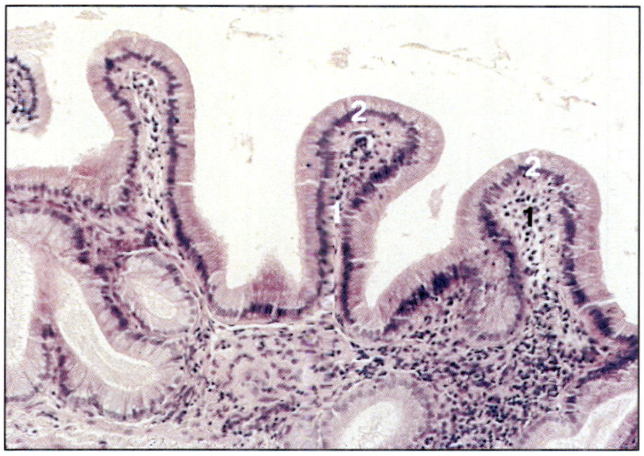

2.7 Simple columnar epithelium. Gall-bladder (dog). (1) Connective core of the lamina propria. (2) Tall hexagonal epithelial cells with a basal nucleus. H & E. ×125.

2.8

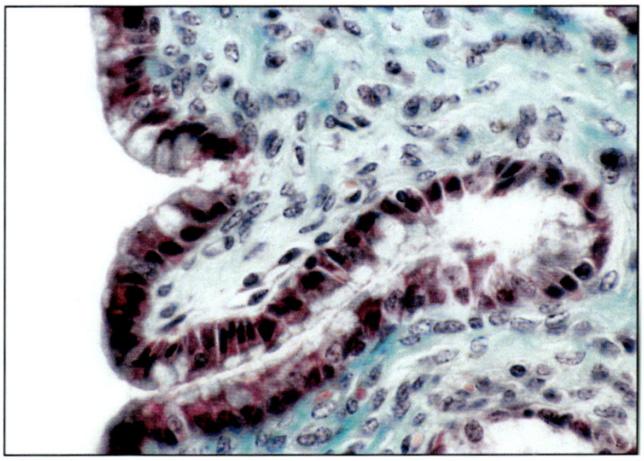

2.8 Simple columnar epithelium. Cervix (sheep). The epithelium lining the cervix secretes mucus, stained green. Masson's trichrome. ×200.

2.9

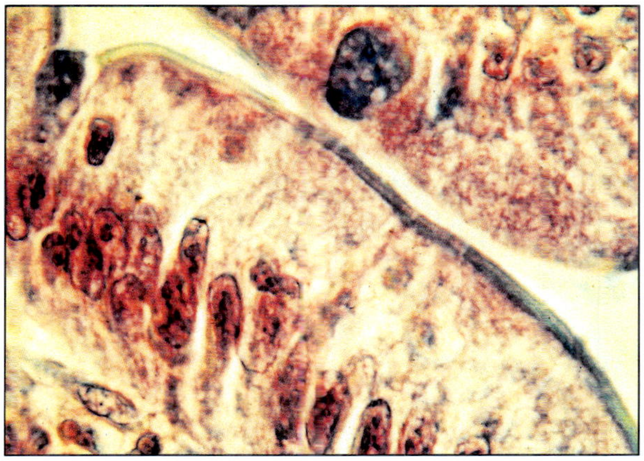

2.9 Simple columnar epithelium. Duodenum (dog). The brush (striated) border appears as a dark line on the luminal surface; the single mucus-secreting goblet cell is stained purple. Haematoxylin/PAS. ×500.

2.10

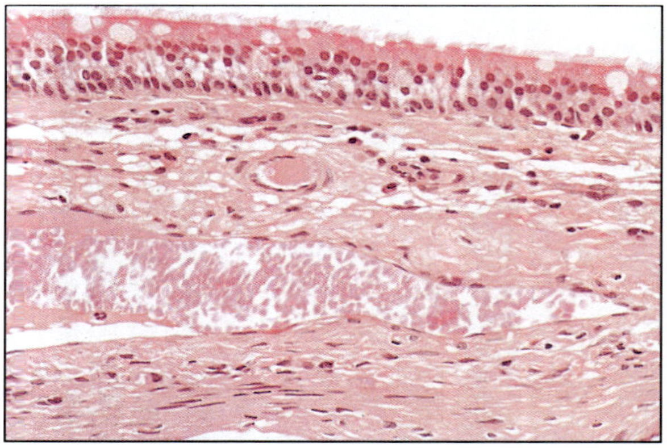

2.10 Pseudostratified columnar ciliated epithelium with goblet cells; respiratory epithelium lining the nares (horse). The cilia appear as a fringe on the free surface, the goblet cells, as clear rounded spaces. There are several layers of nuclei, but all the cells rest on the basement membrane. H & E. ×100.

Pseudostratified

Pseudostratified epithelium appears to consist of more than one layer of cells. All the cells are in contact with the basement membrane, but not every cell reaches the luminal surface. The nuclei lie at different levels, causing the stratified appearance. This type of membrane is seen in the respiratory tract (**2.10–2.12**) and in the genital tract (**2.13**), where cells may be secretory or ciliated.

2.11

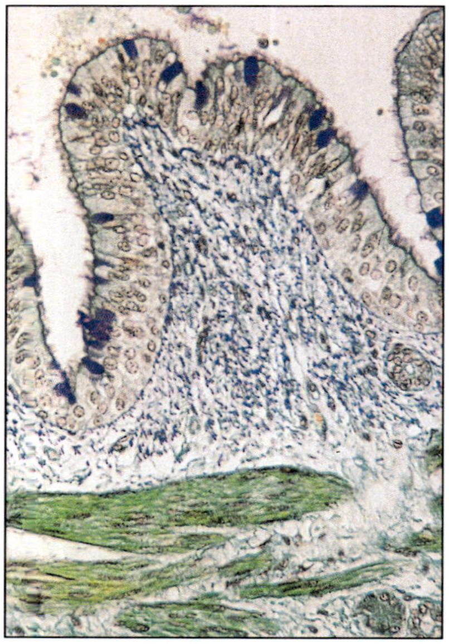

2.11 Respiratory epithelium. Lung (cow). The mucus-secreting goblet cells are individually stained. Gomori/aldehyde fuchsin. ×100.

2.12

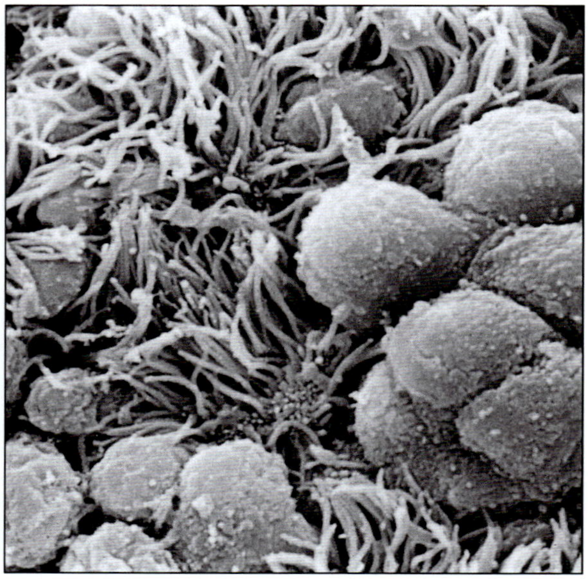

2.12 Respiratory epithelium. Lung (donkey). In this scanning electron micrograph the mucus secretion is a bulbous projection surrounded by cilia. ×2500.

2.13

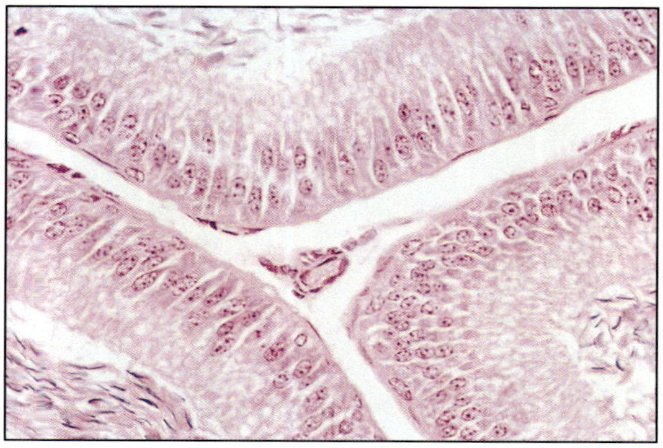

2.13 Pseudostratified epithelium. Epididymis (bull). Several rows of nuclei create the appearance of a stratified epithelium, but all the cells rest on the basement membrane. The stereocilia give a fringe effect to the luminal surface. H & E. ×200.

Stratified epithelium

Designed to withstand wear and tear, stratified epithelia consist of two or more layers of cells with only the basal layer resting on the basement membrane. Stratified columnar and cuboidal epithelia are found lining large gland ducts and the urethra (**2.14** and **2.15**). They are usually not suitable for absorption and require gland secretion to keep the surface moist, but the epithelium lining the rumen is absorptive (see Chapter 8, Digestive System).

Squamous

Stratified squamous epithelium may be keratinized or non-keratinized. The latter is common on surfaces subject to wear and tear, where the secretions necessary to keep the surface wet come from associated glands, and is found lining the oesophagus and vagina (**2.16** and **2.17**). The basal cell layer is mitotically active and the new cells are continually formed and pushed towards the surface, moving away from the nourishing capillary bed beneath the epithelium. These cells are dead or dying by the time the surface

.14

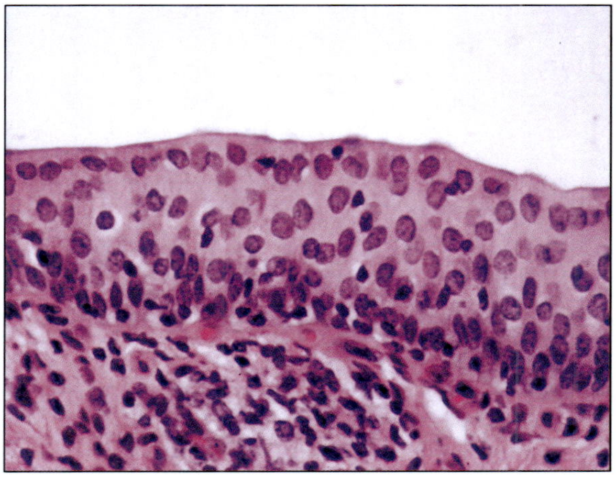

2.14 Stratified columnar epithelium. Penile urethra (horse). The epithelium is several layers deep; the superficial layer is columnar. H & E. ×200.

2.15

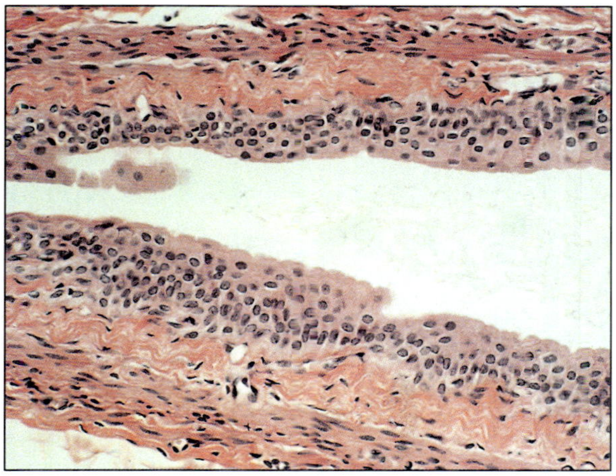

2.15 Stratified cuboidal epithelium. Urethra (bitch). The surface layer of cells is cuboidal. H & E. ×100.

.16

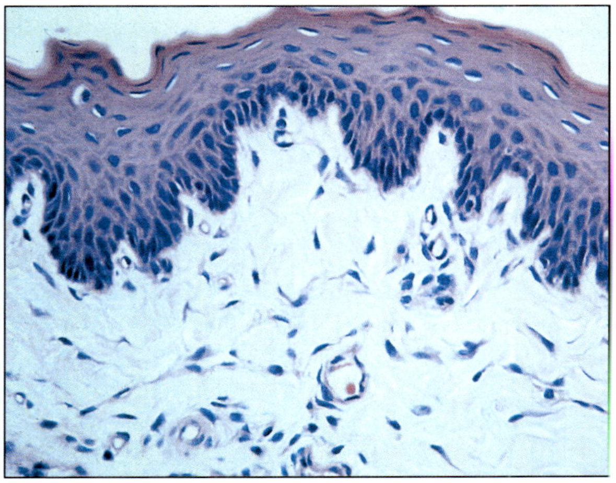

2.16 Stratified squamous non-keratinized epithelium. Oesophagus (cat). The polyhedral cells of the basal layer divide and the daughter cells are pushed towards the surface where the dead squames are shed. H & E. ×125.

2.17

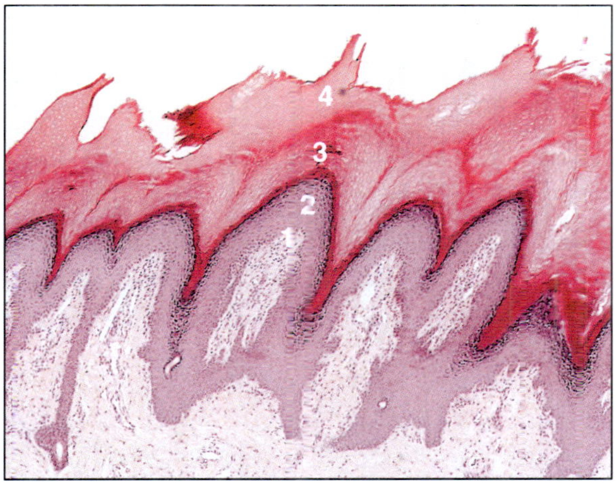

2.17 Stratified squamous keratinized epithelium. Footpad (dog). (1) Stratum germinativum; the basal layer of simple columnar cells. (2) Stratum spinosum; several layers of pear-shaped cells. (3) Stratum granulosum; layer of cells deeply stained containing keratohyalin granules. (4) Stratum corneum; multilayered zone of anucleate squames. H & E. ×100.

is reached. There they lose their nuclei and become detached (desquamate); only on the surface layers are the cells squamous. In some sites, such as the epidermis and the tongue, the cells become keratinized and form a protective waterproof layer on the surface (2.18 and 2.19).

Urethelium (transitional epithelium)

Urethelium lines most of the renal pelvis, the ureters and the urinary bladder, and is designed to allow stretching of the membrane without rupture. It is classified as pseudostratified, because in the relaxed, unstretched state a number of layers of cells are present. The surface cells are rounded (2.20). In the stretched state the appearance is that of stratified squamous epithelium. The cells have the ability to stretch and distort, without pulling apart, and are ideally suited to the demands of the bladder and ureters. The surface is thickened and gives a waterproof coating.

2.18

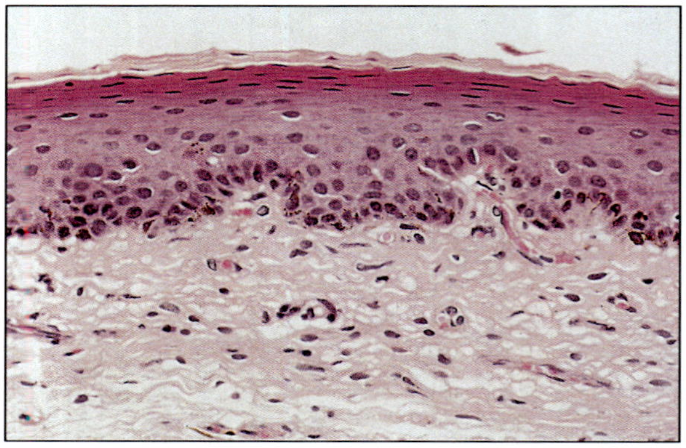

2.18 Stratified squamous keratinized epithelium. Skin (cow). Relatively fewer layers of cells; the surface is covered with keratin. H & E. ×100.

2.19

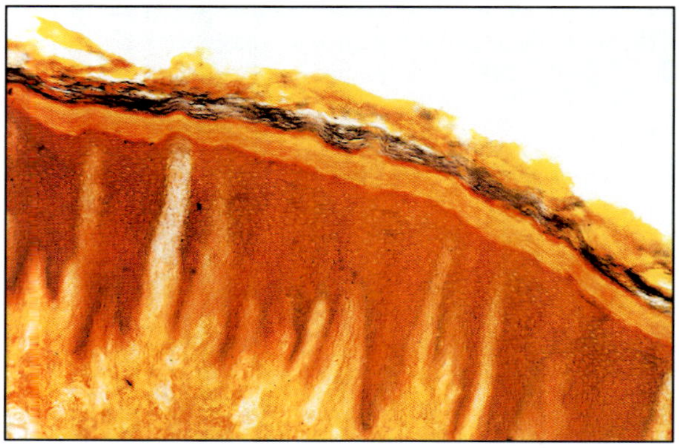

2.19 Stratified squamous epithelium. Teat (cow). The stratum lucidum is present in thick skin as a clear translucent layer. Phosphotungstic acid haemotoxylin. ×100.

2.20

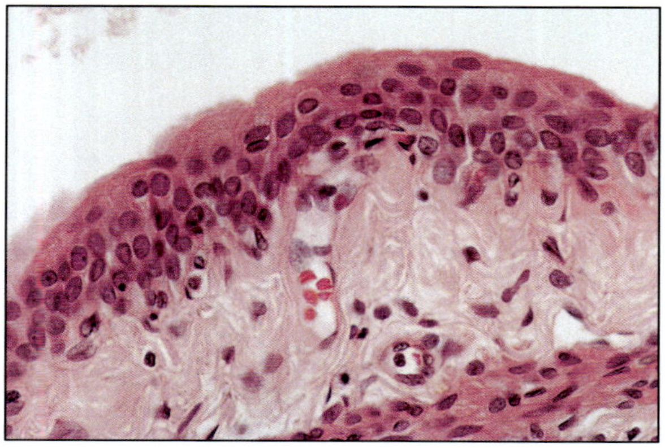

2.20 Urethelium. Bladder (dog). The surface cells have a rounded appearance, the middle layer of cells are pear-shaped and the basal layer is columnar. H & E. ×125.

Myoepithelium

Myoepithelial cells, derived from ectoderm and endoderm, are found in sweat and mammary glands and lie between the secretory epithelial cell and the basement membrane. Myoepithelial cells are also found in the modified salivary (venom) glands and ducts of venomous snakes. The cytoplasm has myofilaments and the cell is capable of contraction, thus assisting the expulsion of the secretions from these structures (2.21–2.23).

2.21

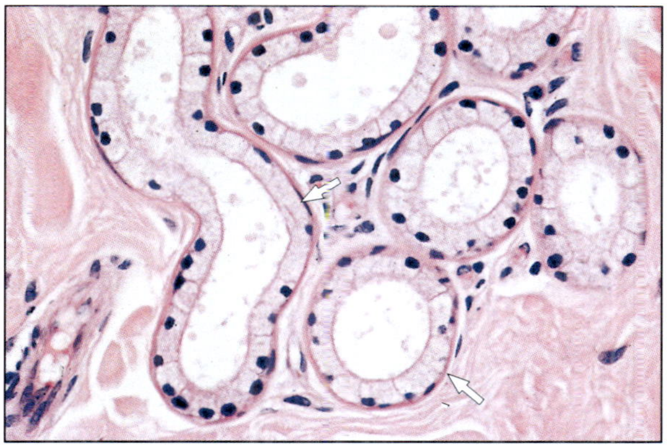

2.21 Sweat gland. Skin (horse). Myoepithelial cells lie between the simple columnar secretory epithelium and the basement membrane, and appear as a deep pink line (arrowed). H & E. ×125.

2.22

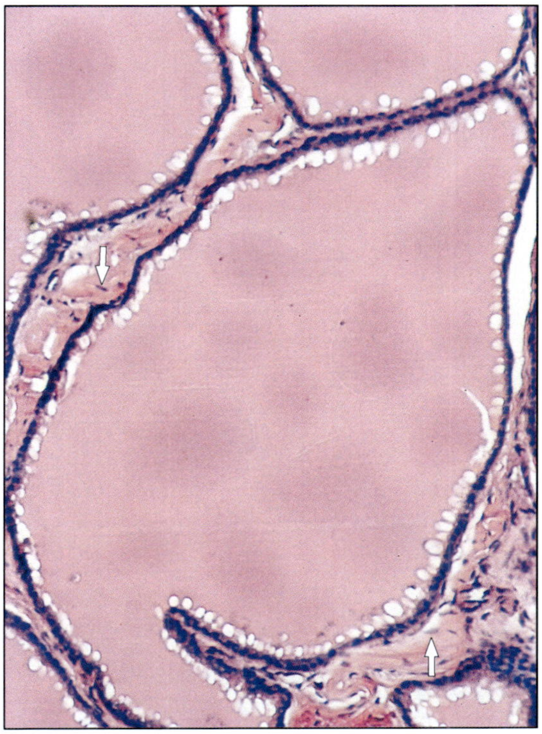

2.22 The paired venom glands of many venomous snakes [and the four pairs in the single genus of venomous lizards (*Heloderma*)] are composed of thin-walled, follicle-like structures lined by a single layer of non-keratinized squamous-to-plump cuboidal epithelial secretory cells. These dilated follicles store the pink staining, protein-rich venom until it is delivered via the duct system and fangs. Contractile myoepithelial cells (arrowed) and skeletal muscle aid in the expression and delivery of venom through the coiled ducts and into the hollow fangs of snakes (and to external grooves in the solid teeth of Helodermatid lizards). Illustrated is a section of the venom gland of a small Mexican rattlesnake (*Crotalus enyo*). H & E. ×85.

2.23

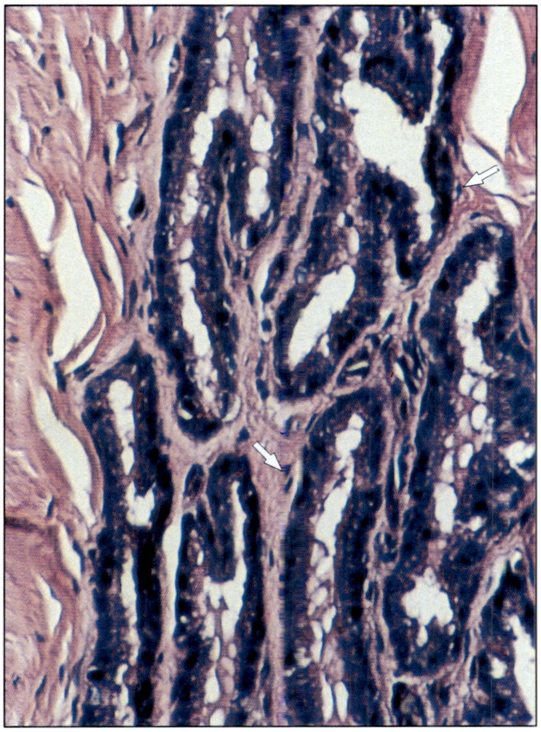

2.23 The much coiled venom duct of this rattlesnake is thin-walled and is lined by low cuboidal cells with dark staining basal nuclei. The coiled sections of the duct are separated from each other by connective tissue in which many myoepithelial cells (arrowed) are embedded. The entire duct is surrounded by the temporal and masseter skeletal muscles which, when they contract, augment the myoepithelial cells in forcing venom to and through the fangs. H & E. ×43.

Glands

All glands are derived from either ectoderm and mesoderm or endoderm and mesoderm. The ectoderm and endoderm form the epithelial secretory cell, the parenchyma. The mesoderm forms the supporting connective tissue framework, the stroma. Where the demand for the secretion is low, a single secretory cell is sufficient. The mucus-secreting goblet cell of the small intestine, for example, is adequate. At the other extreme is the liver, the largest gland in the body, which is required to cope with the food absorbed by the gut.

Exocrine glands

Exocrine glands secrete onto the membrane surface either singly – the unicellular mucus-secreting goblet cell – or by a duct system. The simple tubular gland of the endometrium consists of a single layer of cells secreting into a duct opening into the uterine lumen (2.24). Compound glands have a branched duct system draining a number of secretory units. The connective tissue capsule extends into the gland, carrying blood vessels and nerves, and divides it into lobes and lobules. The secretory units may take the form of acini where the height of the lining cell is greater than the diameter of the lumen, or of alveoli/saccules where the lumen exceeds the height of the lining cell (2.25–2.27).

There are two types of glandular secretion: merocrine and holocrine. In the merocrine gland, the vesicles containing the secretion in the cytoplasm fuse with the cell membrane and release the contents onto the cell surface. In the holocrine gland the cell builds up the secretion in the cytoplasm, migrates away from the basement membrane and the source of nutrient, and dies. The cell debris itself becomes the secretion. The sebaceous glands are holocrine (2.28).

2.24

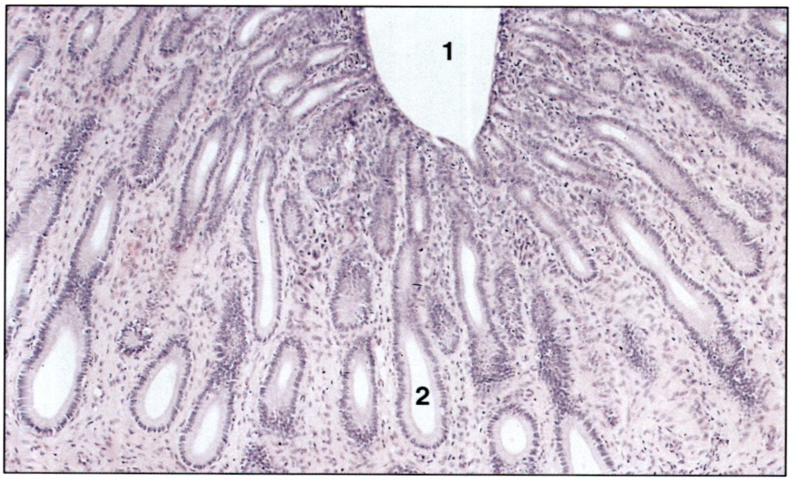

2.24 Simple tubular glands. Uterus (cat). (1) Lumen of the uterus. (2) Simple tubular glands in the endometrium of the uterus. H & E. ×20.

2.25

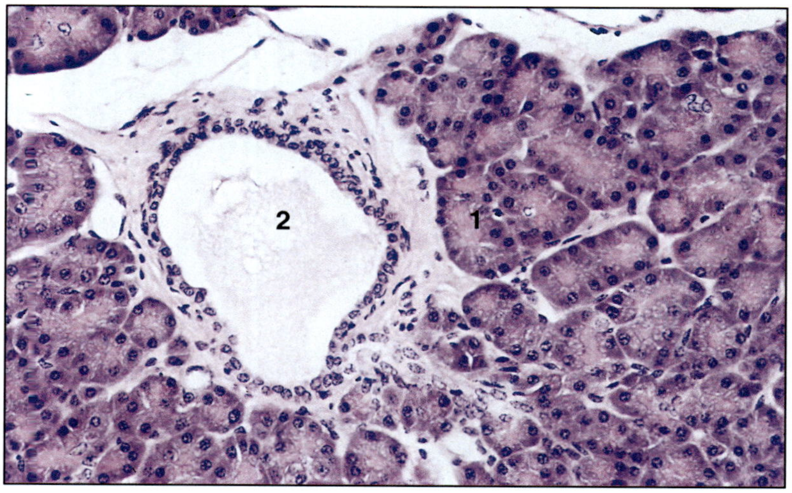

2.25 Compound acinar gland. Pancreas (dog). (1) The acinus is lined by secretory epithelial cells with a basal nucleus. (2) The excretory duct is lined by a stratified cuboidal epithelium. H & E. ×250.

2.26 Alveolar gland. Carpal skin (pig). The secretory alveoli are cut in cross-section; the diameter of the lumen exceeds the height of the lining secretory cells. H & E. ×100. (*See also* mammary gland, Fig. 2.6.)

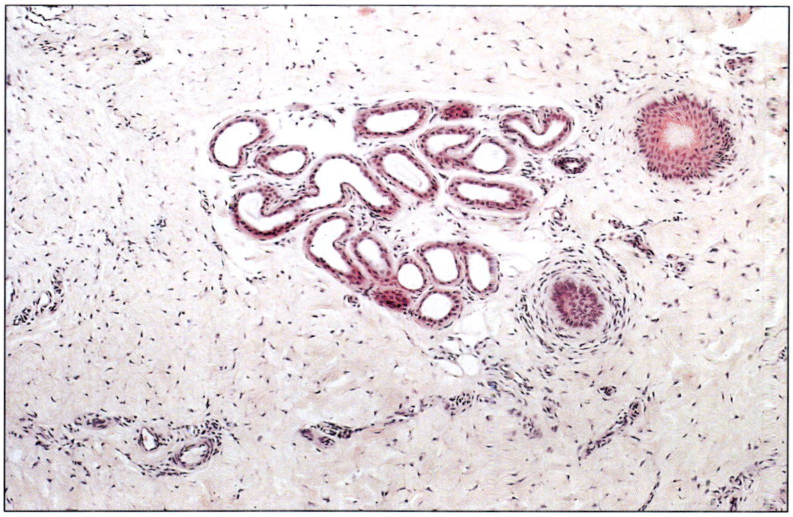

2.26

2.27 Compound tubuloacinar gland. Mixed seromucous salivary gland. The pale staining mucus-secreting cells are filled with secretion and almost obliterate the lumen. The serous cells form a darkly stained demilune around the mucous cells (arrowed). A thick strand of connective tissue with a blood vessel represents the supporting framework of the gland. H & E. ×125.

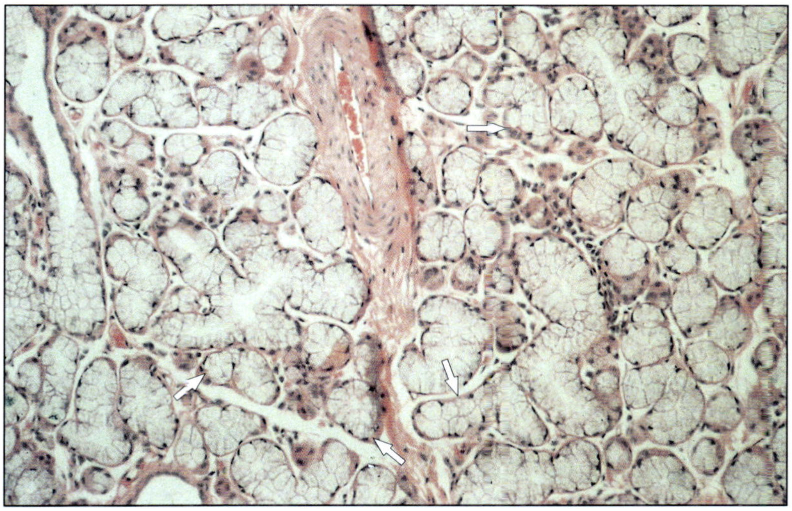

2 27

2.28 Sebaceous gland. Skin (dog). The gland consists of pale staining cells filled with sebum, fatty substance. This forms the secretion, an example of a holocrine gland. Gomori's trichrome. ×125.

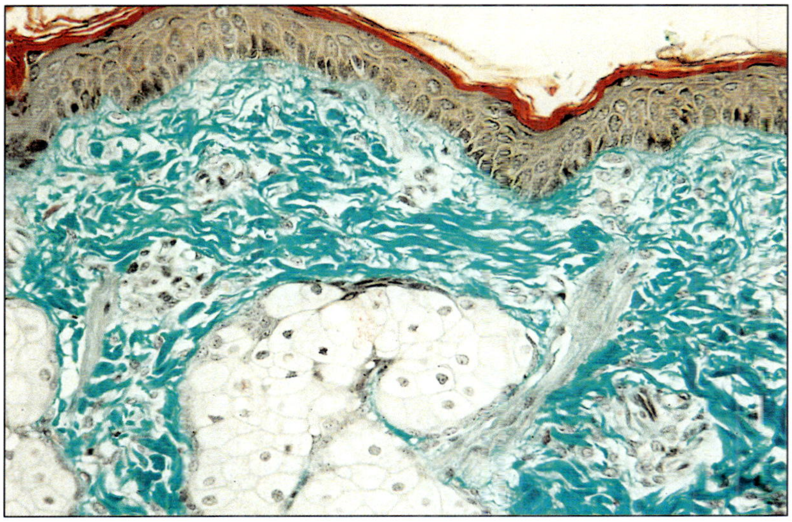

2.28

Endocrine glands

Endocrine glands have no ducts. Small groups of cells secrete hormones, chemical messengers, into the capillary network, lymphatic vessels or tissue fluid for transmission to the target organ a variable distance away (**2.29**). Detailed discussion of these glands can be found in Chapter 10.

2.29

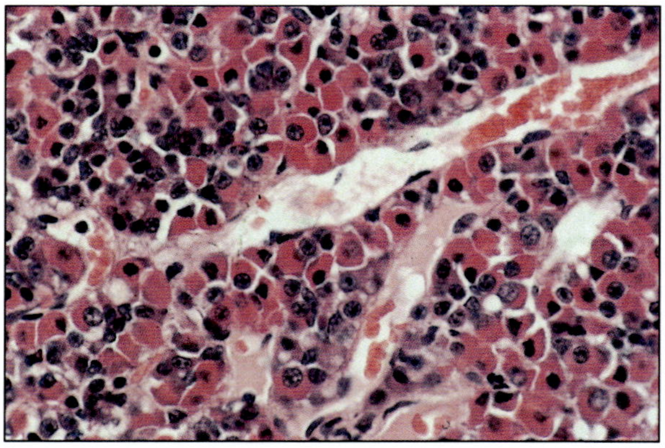

2.29 Pars distalis of the adenohypophysis (pituitary gland; cat). The secretory cells are closely associated with a rich network of blood vessels. H & E. ×200.

Clinical correlates

A large variety of benign and malignant epithelial tumours are recognized in domestic animals. A squamous cell carcinoma, a malignant tumour of squamous epithelium taken from the eyelid of a cow, is shown in **2.30**. The neoplastic cells are large with abundant eosinophilic cytoplasm and form nests where cells differentiate and keratinize towards the centres. There is variation in nuclear and cellular size and mitotic figures can be seen.

Bovine ocular squamous carcinoma is relatively common and of some economic importance. Its occurrence is related to ultraviolet light exposure, particularly in white-faced breeds such as Herefords. The tumour develops through premalignant stages before progressing to carcinoma *in situ* and finally to invasive carcinoma.

A pulmonary adenoma, a benign tumour of glandular origin, is shown in **2.31**. The cells are uniform in size and appearance and arranged in a recognizable papillary pattern. The columnar epithelial cells all rest on a supporting stromal framework. This tumour was an incidental finding at necropsy in an aged cat.

2.30

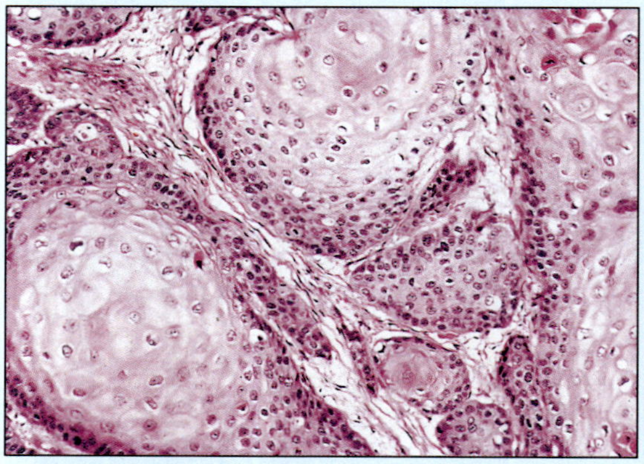

2.30 Squamous cell carcinoma from the eyelid of a cow. H & E. ×200.

2.31

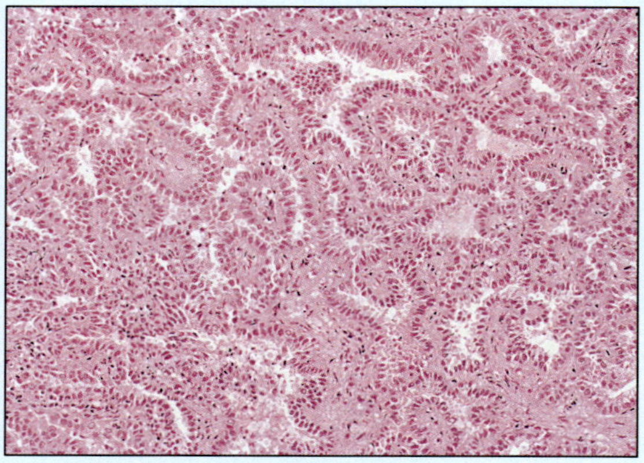

2.31 Pulmonary adenoma in an aged cat. H & E. ×125.

3. CONNECTIVE TISSUE

Connective tissue can be classified as follows:

- Embryonal connective tissues.
- Mesenchyme and mucoid connective tissues.
- Connective tissue proper, including loose (areolar) and dense (regular and irregular) tissues, as well as the special types, reticular, elastic and adipose.
- Cartilage and bone.
- Blood cells and blood-forming tissues.

Embryonal, mesenchymal and mucoid connective tissues

Connective tissue is derived from mesenchyme, the loose embryonic packing tissue of mesodermal origin. Mesenchymal cells have long slender processes and are embedded in an amorphous gelatinous substance, the extracellular matrix (3.1). Mucoid connective tissue is found in the embryo, and also occurs in limited regions in adult animals, the comb and wattle of the chicken, and around a healing wound. There are few cells, which are usually stellate undifferentiated fibroblasts; the ground substance is abundant and gelatinous with very few fibres. This type of tissue stains poorly with haematoxylin and eosin (H & E) (3.2), but stains well with mucin dyes.

3.1

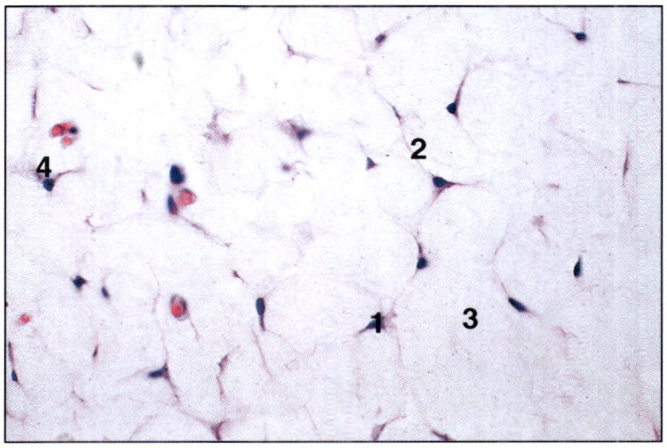

3.1 Umbilical cord (foal). (1) Nucleus of the stellate mesenchymal cell. (2) Long cell processes. (3) Extracellular matrix. (4) Blood vessels. H & E ×125.

3.2

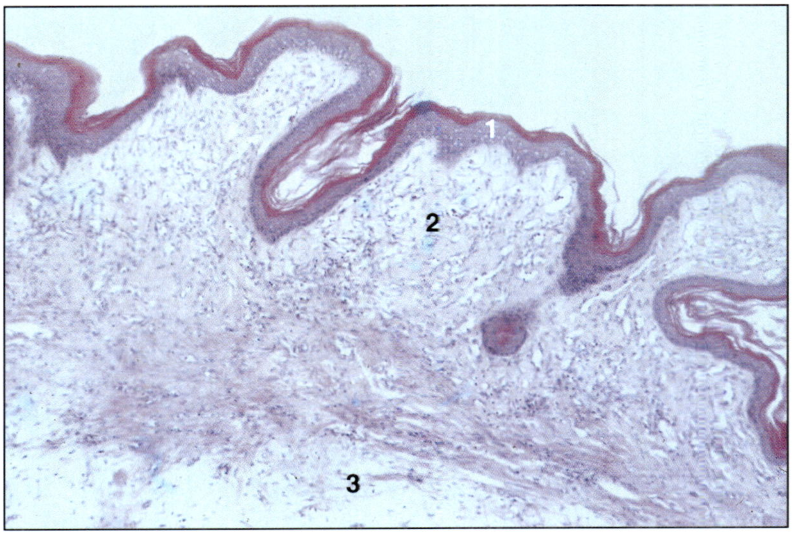

3.2 Mucoid connective tissue. Comb (chicken). (1) Stratified squamous epithelium. (2) Lamina propria. (3) Mucoid connective tissue. H & E. ×50

Connective tissue proper

Connective tissue proper fills the interstices of tissues and organs, and forms a continuous structure that carries blood vessels and nerves throughout the body. The relative proportions of the basic components – fibres, cells and extracellular matrix – determine the functional characteristics of the tissue, giving it tensile strength in ligaments and tendons and mechanical stability in cartilage and bone, and acting as a fluid-transport medium: blood.

Collagen fibres are thick (2–10 μm in diameter) and unbranched; when fresh they are white when unstained and wavy in section. They stain pink with eosin and green with Masson's trichrome, which distinguishes them from muscle fibres (**3.3** and **3.4**). Elastic fibres are relatively thin (about 1 μm in diameter), less wavy than collagen fibres, unbranched and yellow in unstained material. Because they stain poorly with H & E, selective staining is used (**3.5–3.7**). Reticular fibres, narrow bundles of collagen fibrils, are fine and delicate, branching extensively to form a supporting network. These also do not stain with standard methods, so a selective process such as silver impregnation is used (**3.8**).

3.3

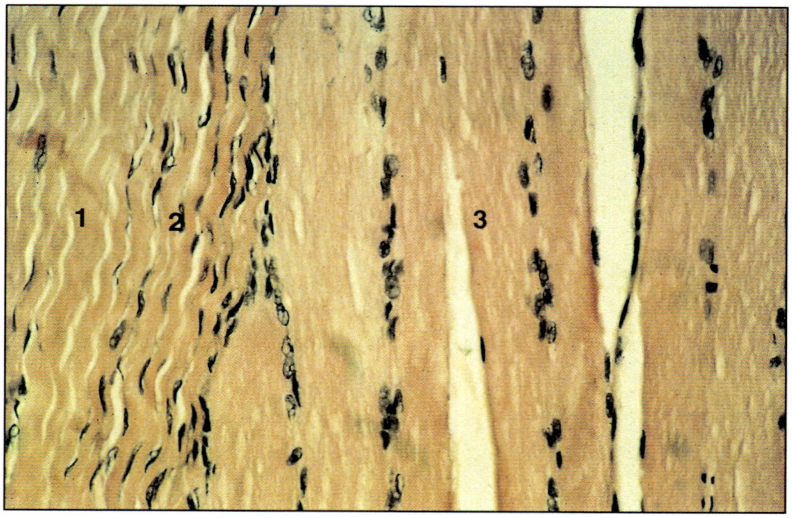

3.3 Tendon/muscle insertion (dog). (1) Collagen fibres; note wavy appearance. (2) Fibrocytes. (3) Striated muscle fibres. H & E. ×200.

3.4

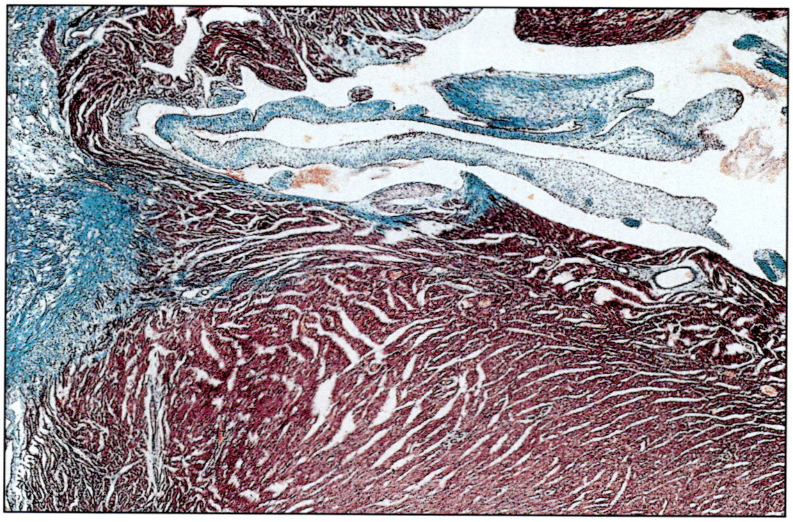

3.4 Heart (kitten). The collagen fibres and valve cusps are stained green and the heart muscle is stained red. Masson's trichrome. ×50.

3.5 Ligamentum nuchae (ox). The elastic fibres are stained red and the collagen fibres are stained blue/green. Gomori's trichrome. ×250.

3.5

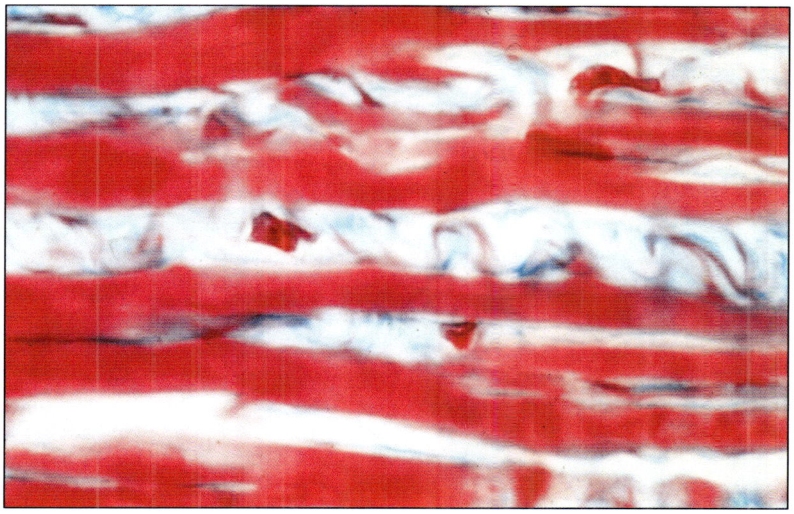

3.6 Elastic artery (horse). The elastic fibres are selectively stained. Weigert's elastin. ×62.5.

3.6

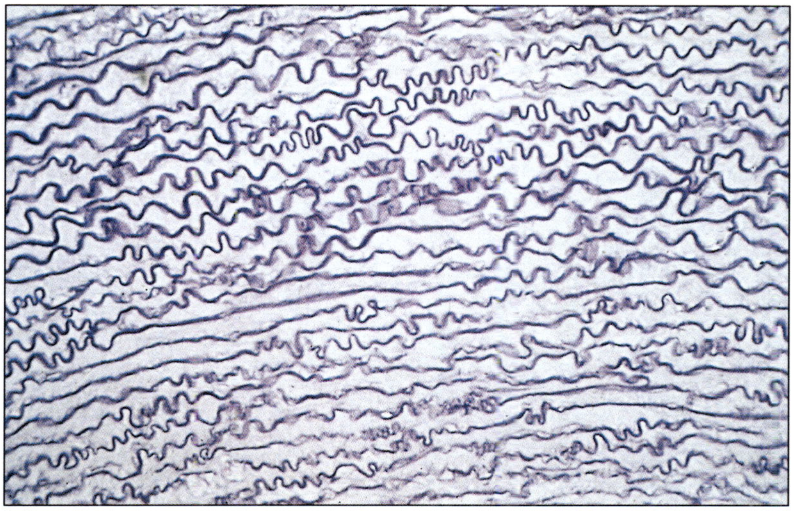

3.7

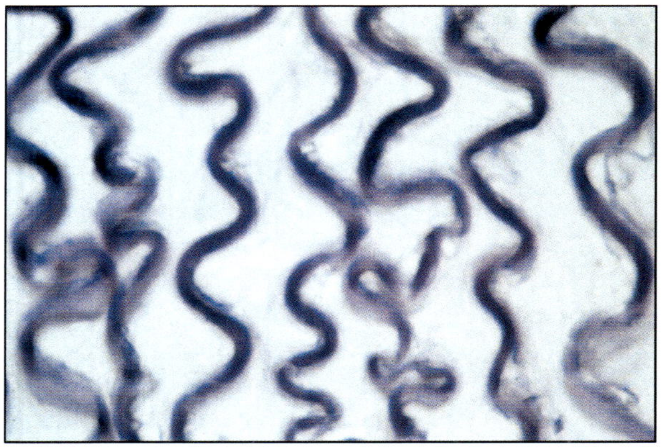

3.7 Elastic artery (horse). The elastic fibres are selectively stained. Weigert's elastin. ×500.

3.8

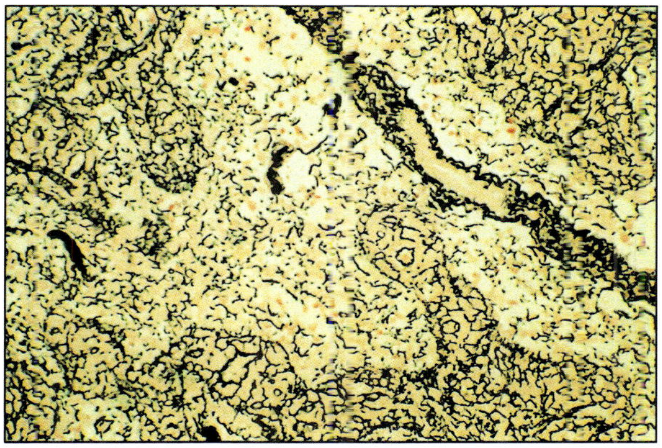

3.8 Lymph node (dog). The reticular fibres are silver plated by this method and appear as black strands. The delicate network of these fibres supports the lymphatic tissue. Gordon and Sweet. ×125.

Cell types

Fibroblasts/fibrocytes are the commonest cell type, synthesizing collagen, elastin and reticular fibres, and the extracellular matrix. The fibroblast is the active form, is elongated and spindle-shaped, and has abundant cytoplasm and an oval- or cigar-shaped nucleus. It is found in sites of active repair or growth. The fibrocyte is the less active stage of the cell, acting in a maintenance capacity. The cytoplasm is reduced in volume and is less reactive to stains. The nucleus is flattened and the chromatin is condensed (**3.9** and **3.10**).

Macrophages, also referred to as histiocytes, are part of the mononuclear phagocyte system. They are large, free, mobile phagocytic cells with a round nucleus. They are part of a large population of scavengers capable of ingesting cell debris, taking an active part in the protection of the body by eliminating some micro-organisms. Identification may be achieved by using the ability of the cell to engulf particulate matter, such as carbon particles injected *in vitro* (**3.11** and **3.12**).

Plasma cells have a basophilic cytoplasm and the nucleus is eccentric with densely clumped chromatin distributed beneath the nuclear membrane to give

3.9

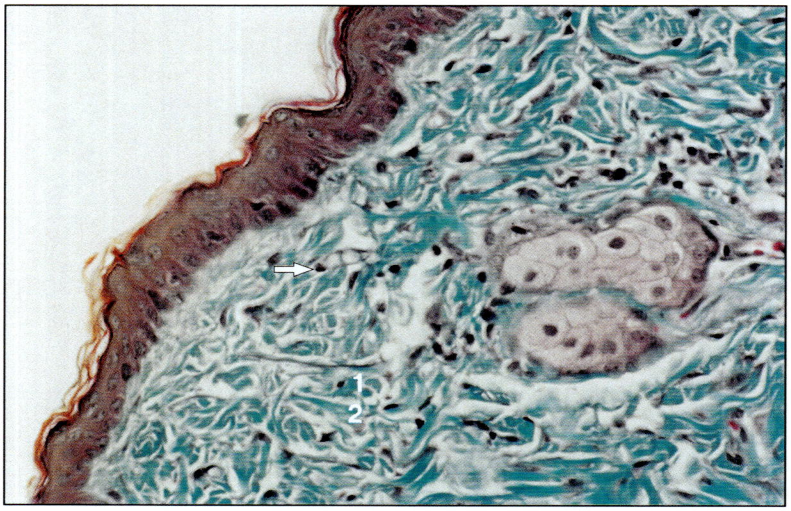

3.9 Dense irregular connective tissue (dog). Nucleus of the fibrocyte (arrowed). (1) Collagen fibres cut in transverse section. (2) Collagen fibres cut in longitudinal section. Masson's trichrome. ×125.

3.10

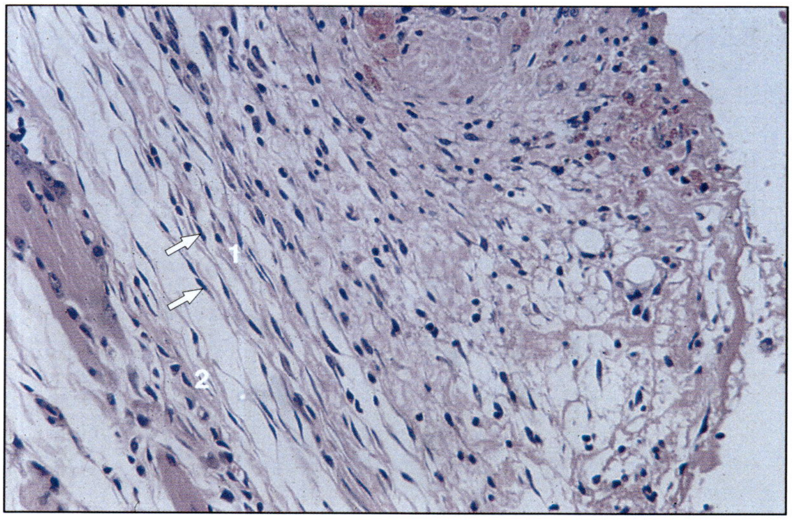

3.10 Fibroblasts in a healing wound (dog). Nucleus (arrowed) of the fibroblast. (1) Cytoplasm of the fibroblast. (2) Collagen fibres. H & E. ×125.

a characteristic clock face appearance. Plasma cells are involved in the body's immune response and represent the cellular source of circulating immunoglobulin (antibody). They are common both to loose connective tissue and to the lymphatic system (**3.13** and **3.14**).

Mast cells are round or ovoid and the nucleus is often obscured by the cytoplasmic granules. They are metachromatic (stain purple with a blue dye such as toluidine blue or Giemsa) and contain heparin and histamine and other mediators of inflammation. Mast cell degranulation causes a local irritant effect caused by the release of histamine (**3.15**).

3.11

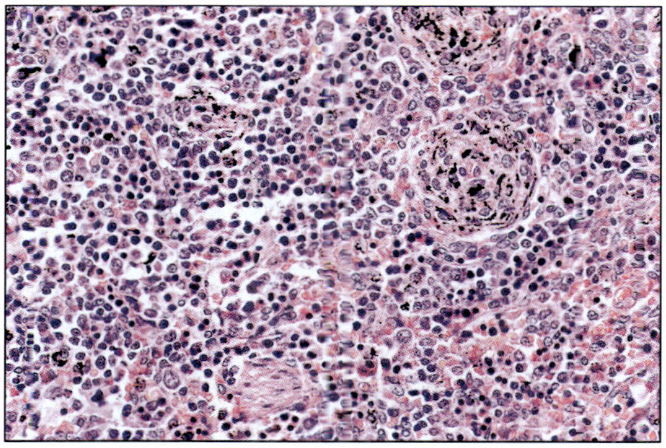

3.11 Spleen (dog). The macrophages have phagocytosed the carbon particles. Carbon injected, with H & E counterstain. ×50.

.12

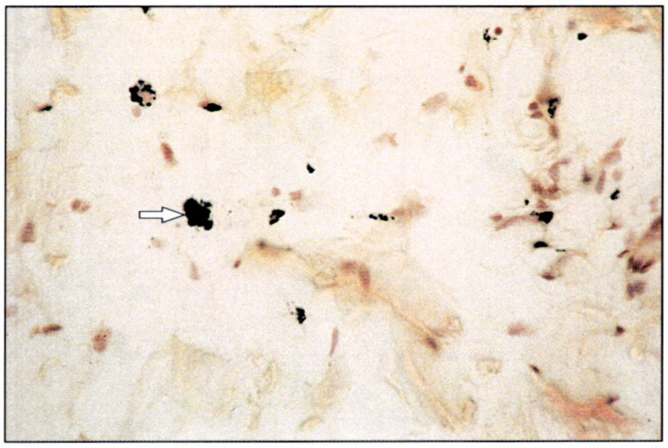

3.12 Loose connective tissue (dog). A tissue macrophage is arrowed. Carbon injected, with H & E counterstain. ×200.

3.13

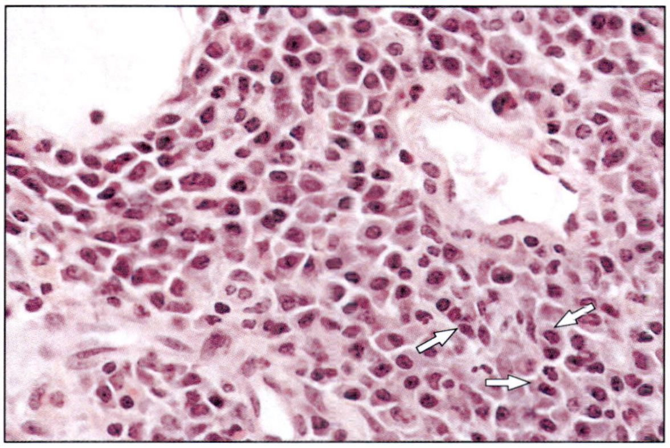

3.13 Plasma cell (dog). Lymph node. Plasma cells are arrowed. H & E. ×200.

.14

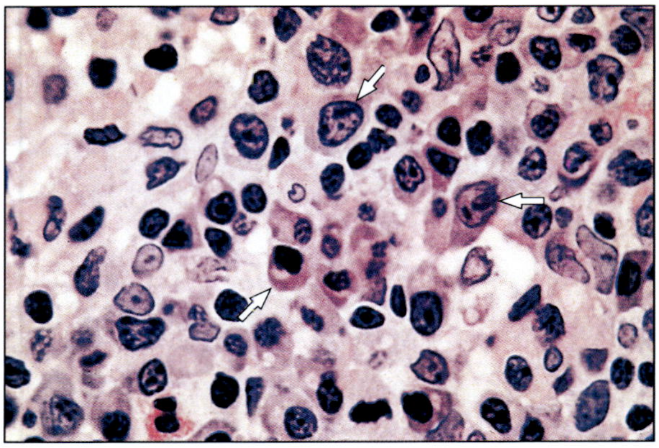

3.14 Plasma cell (dog). Lymph node. Plasma cells are arrowed. H & E. ×500.

3.15

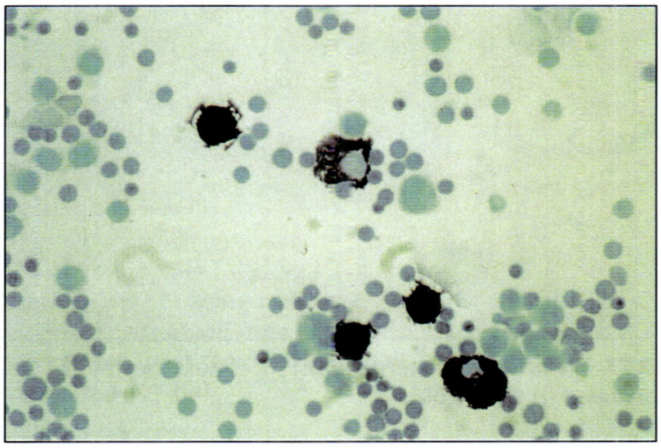

3.15 Mast cell (sheep). The granules stain purple with the blue dye, toluidine blue. Metachromasia. Toluidine blue. ×500.

3.16

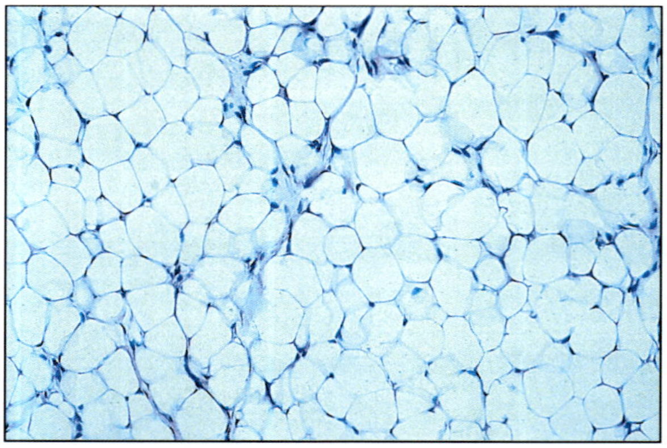

3.16 Adipocytes. Foot pad (dog). The fat has been lost during processing and the lacy network is formed by cytoplasm and cell membranes. H & E. ×50.

Fat cells (adipocytes) arise from pericapillary mesenchymal cells. They accumulate fat in the cytoplasm as lipid droplets that coalesce until the cell is filled with one large droplet. The cytoplasm forms a peripheral rim and the nucleus is displaced to lie immediately beneath the plasma membrane. Fat cells may occur singly or in groups in loose connective tissue to become adipose tissue. Fat may be white, in which each cell has a single large droplet, or brown, in which small individual droplets are scattered throughout the cytoplasm. Processing dissolves the fat and leaves a network of lacy, empty spaces in H & E sections. The cells are usually described as appearing like a signet ring with the nucleus constituting the signet (**3.16**).

Pigment cells are derived from neural crest ectoderm. However, cells carrying pigment granules (melanin, erythrin, xanthin) are often found in connective tissue and are called chromatophores (literally, pigment carriers) and can be macrophages (melanophages, erythrophages, xanthophages; **3.17–3.20**).

Neutrophils (polymorphonuclear leucocytes in mammals; azurophils, see p. 58, in some lower vertebrates), eosinophils, lymphocytes and monocytes are blood cells commonly found in loose connective tissue. They are migratory and move freely between

3.17

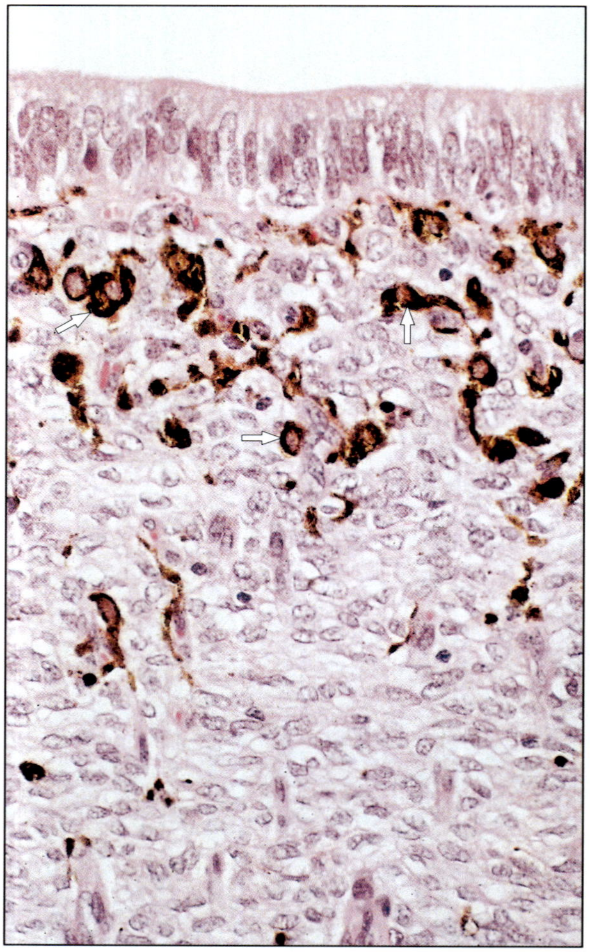

3.17 Melanocytes. Uterus (ewe). The melanocytes are arrowed. H & E. ×200.

3.18

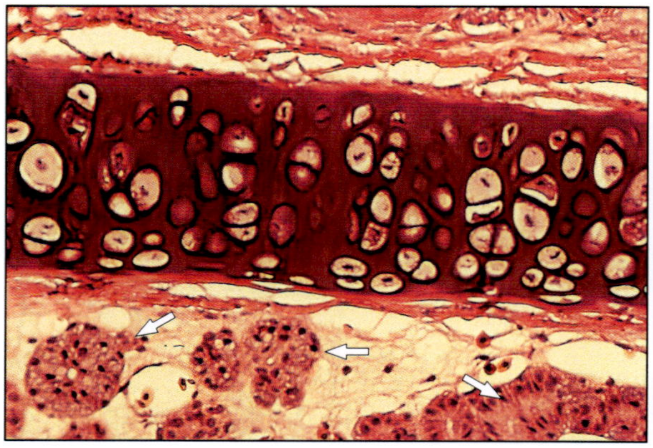

3.18 Nasal septum of green iguana. A supporting sheet of hyaline cartilage is seen in the centre. Immediately beneath are saline-secreting nasal salt glands (arrowed). H & E. ×100.

3.19

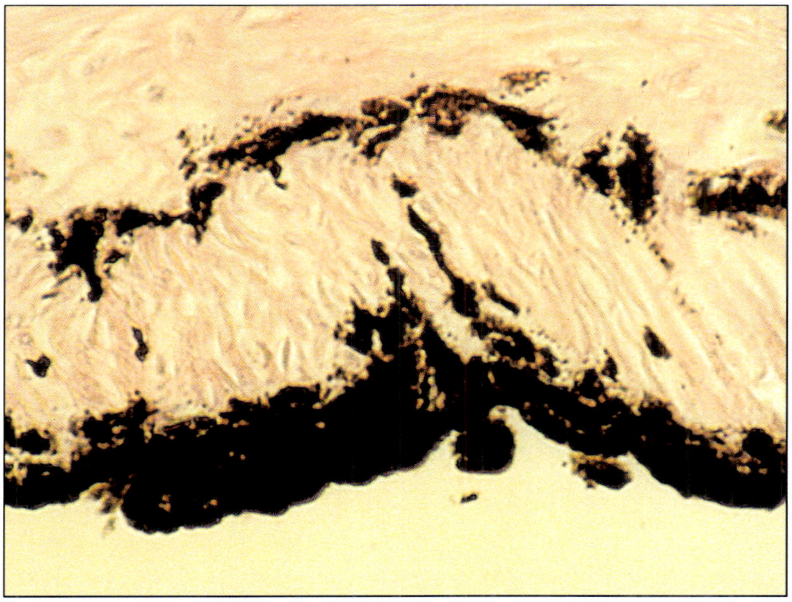

3.19 Serosal surface of chameleon small intestine. Note heavily pigmented coelomic surface and zone between longitudinal and circular muscular layers. H & E. ×50.

3.20

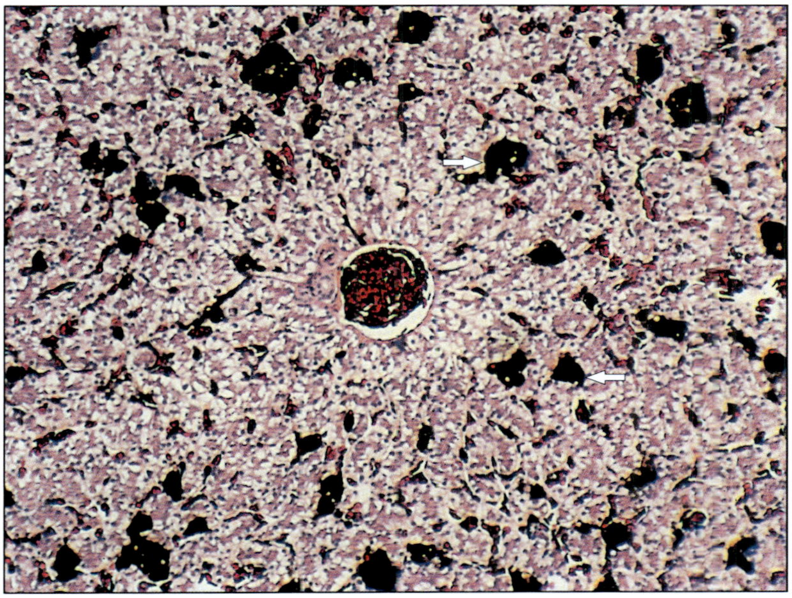

3.20 The hepatic parenchyma of many amphibians and reptiles is characterized by abundant aggregates of melanin pigment contained in melanophages (arrowed). Illustrated is a section of liver from an African clawed frog (*Xenopus laevis*). The hepatocytes are arranged in ray-like cords extending outward from a thin-walled central vein, next to which are small tributaries of the hepatic artery and bile duct. H & E. ×100.

the blood vessels and the surrounding tissue in response to local conditions (3.21–3.23).

Endothelial cells and pericytes form a special cell population in connective tissue, retaining the capacity to divide and to synthesize collagen and the extracellular ground substance. The endothelium is often fenestrated in the capillary bed and it controls the tissue fluid content locally. Pericytes are pale staining, connective tissue cells lying adjacent to the capillary endothelium. They are comparatively undifferentiated and can give rise both to fibroblasts and to smooth muscle cells in areas of tissue repair, as well as assist in the revascularization and repair of damaged blood vessels (3.24).

Loose areolar connective tissue

Loose areolar connective tissue is found as packing material throughout the body and carries the blood vessels and nerves. It contains many scattered cells of various types, blood and lymphatic vessels, and a loose network of fine collagenous, reticular and elastic fibres. It is widespread throughout the body, surrounding vessels and nerves, and is found in serous membranes, the lamina propria of mucous membranes, subcutaneous tissue and the superficial layer of the dermis (3.25). Amorphous ground substance is particularly abundant in loose connective tissue. It is composed of a group of carbohydrates, the glycosaminoglycans, which may be complexed with a protein to form proteoglycans. These substances stain poorly with H & E.

Dense connective tissue

Composed principally of thick collagenous fibres, dense connective tissue contains few cells. Fibrous elements predominate and the commonest cell is the

3.21

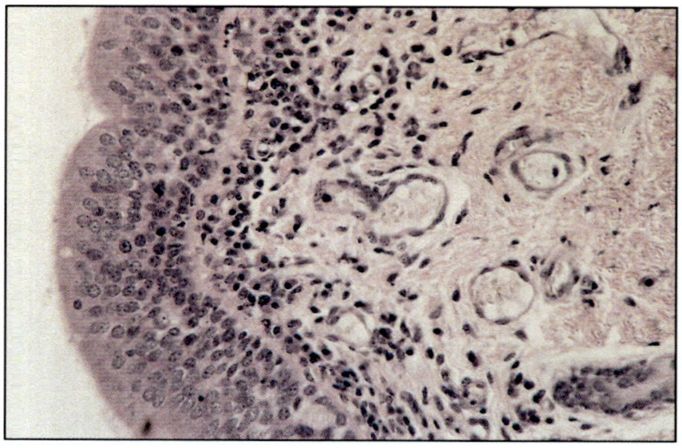

3.21 Polymorphonuclear leucocytes. Bronchus (ox). The polymorphonuclear leucocytes have invaded the connective tissue of the lamina propria in response to infection. H & E. ×125.

3.22

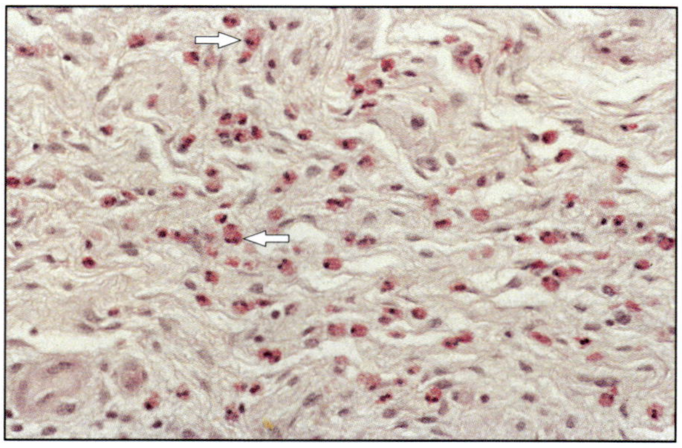

3.22 Eosinophils. Colon (horse). The eosinophils are arrowed. H & E. ×125.

3.23

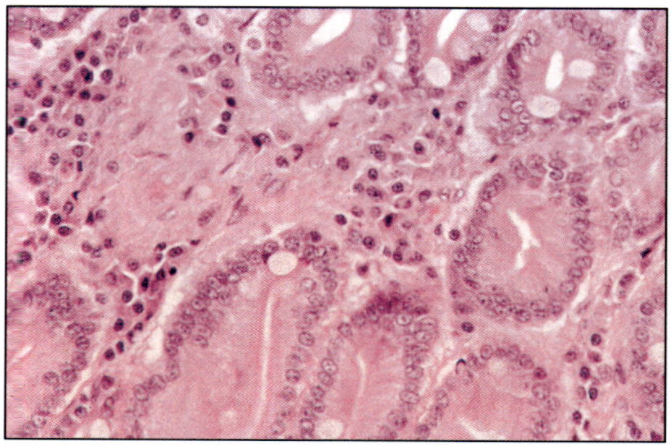

3.23 Lymphocytes. Duodenum (ox). Lymphocytes are present in the lamina propria of the duodenum. H & E. ×125.

3.24

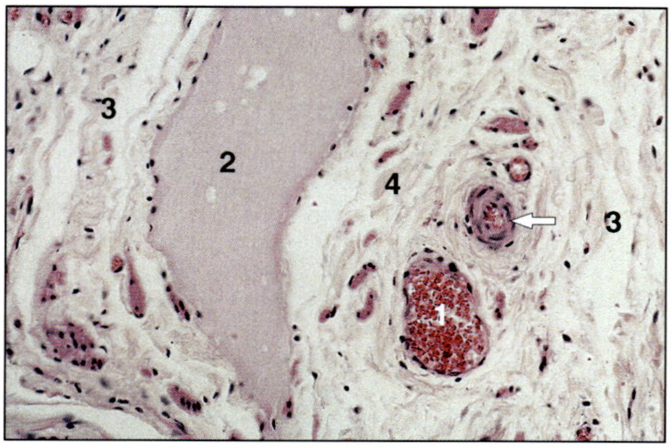

3.24 Pericyte. Loose connective tissue (cat). The pericyte is arrowed in the wall of the arteriole. (1) Vein. (2) Lymphatic vessel. (3) Fibrocyte. (4) Extracellular matrix. H & E. ×100.

fibrocyte. In dense regular connective tissue the fibres may be arranged in rows to provide tensile strength in tendons and ligaments, and as sheets in aponeuroses (*see* 3.3 and 3.4). In dense irregular connective tissue the fibres are arranged in different planes to allow stretching without tearing of the surface membrane, as in the dermis and the vagina (3.26 and 3.27).

3.25 Loose connective tissue (cat). Blood vessels: (1) artery; (2) vein. (3) Nerves. (4) Extracellular matrix. (5) Fibrocytes. (6) Collagen fibres. (7) Smooth muscle of the uterine wall. H & E. ×100.

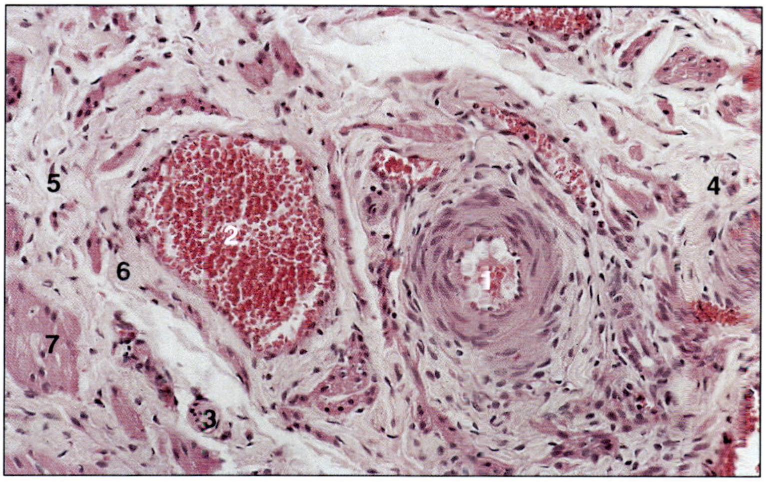

3.25

3.26 Dense connective tissue (dog). Fibrocytes (arrowed). (1) Collagen fibres. (2) Blood vessels. Masson's trichrome. ×100.

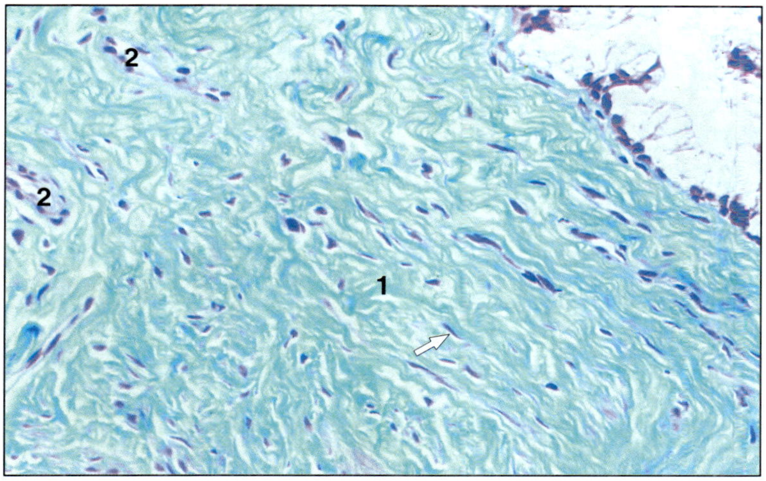

3.26

3.27 Dense connective tissue. Vagina (sheep). The collagen fibres are stained green. Masson's trichrome. ×160.

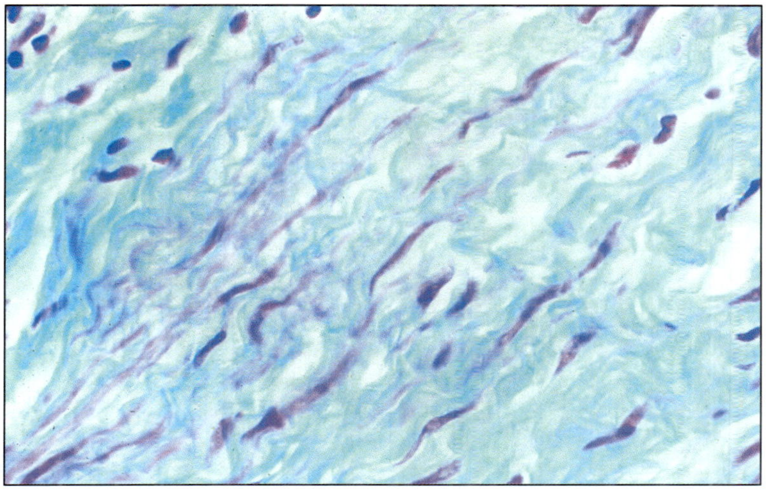

3.27

Special types of connective tissue

Reticular tissue is composed of numerous reticular fibres and stellate reticular cells, forming a supportive network for structures such as the spleen, lymph node, kidney and bone marrow. Elastic tissue, characterized by numerous regularly or irregularly arranged elastic fibres, is exemplified by the ligamentum nuchae and the elastic fascia of the ruminant abdomen. Adipose tissue consists of groups of adipocytes (see above).

Cartilage and bone

Cartilage

Cartilage is a specialized form of connective tissue combining a degree of rigidity with flexibility and strength. There are three types of cartilage: hyaline, elastic and fibrocartilage; differing only in the distribution of the main components: the cells, fibres and matrix.

Hyaline cartilage

This type of cartilage is bluish/white in the fresh state and is the most prevalent form. In the embryo, the precursors of the long bones begin as cartilage models (3.28). As the neonate grows, the cartilaginous template undergoes progressive mineralization. In postnatal life, cartilage is present in the rings of the trachea and in plates in the larynx and nose. With ageing and under certain conditions of hypervitaminosis-D_3 and hypercalcaemia, cartilage may become pathologically mineralized. Cartilage also caps the ends of bones in articulating joints (**3.29**).

At predetermined sites in the embryo, mesenchymal cells round off and differentiate into chondroblasts (cartilage-forming cells) and secrete a matrix consisting of proteoglycans and collagen fibrils. The space occupied by each cell is a lacuna and once the matrix is laid down, the cells are called chondrocytes (cartilage cells; **3.30**). Chondrocytes are capable of dividing and several cells may come to occupy a lacuna; then they are known as an isogenous group or cell nest (**3.31**). Compared with the bulk of the matrix, which stains poorly with H & E, the matrix in the immediate vicinity of the cells stains intensely with metachromatic dyes because of the presence of glycosaminoglycans. Mesenchymal tissue surrounds the developing cartilage and forms a fibrous covering, the perichondrium. The inner layer of the perichondrium is capable of generating new chondroblasts. Cartilage is thus able to grow from the pericardium by appositional growth, and by interstitial growth from within by chondrocyte division and deposition of new matrix. It is avascular – the cells are nourished by diffusion.

3.28

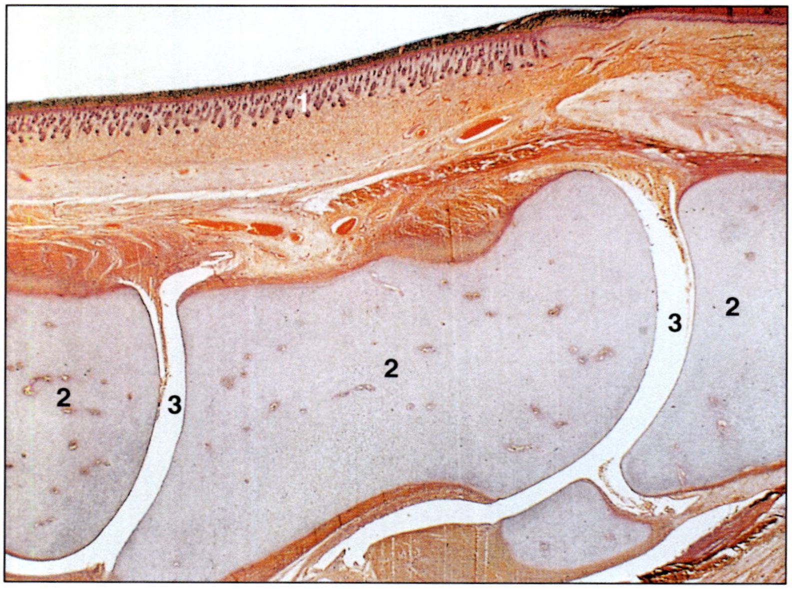

3.28 Developing hoof (foal). (1) Skin. (2) Hyaline cartilage models of the digits. (3) Joint cavity. H & E. ×25.

3.29 Scapulohumeral articulation of a small skink, *Scincella lateralis*. (1) Both the humeral head (lower right) and the scapula (upper left) contain cancellous spaces filled with bone marrow. (2) Articular cartilage. H & E. ×25.

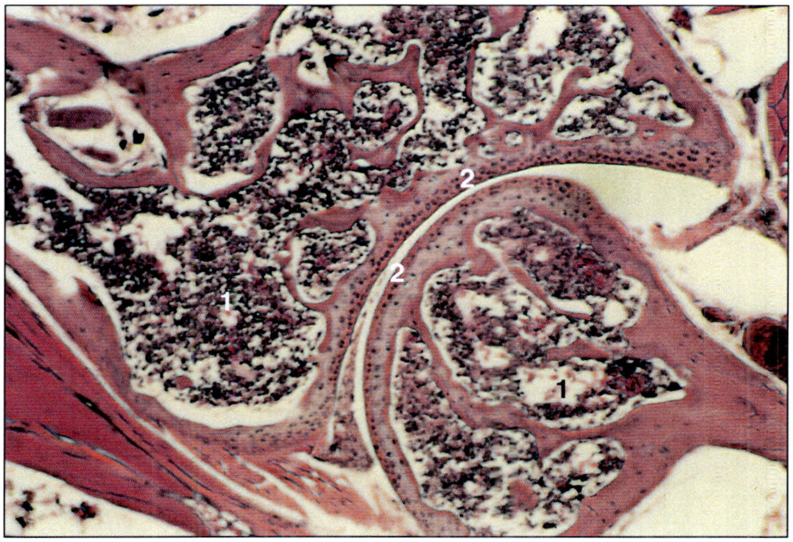

3.29

3.30 Hyaline cartilage. Costal cartilage (dog). (1) Hyaline cartilage. (2) Chondrocytes. (3) Perichondrium. H & E. ×100.

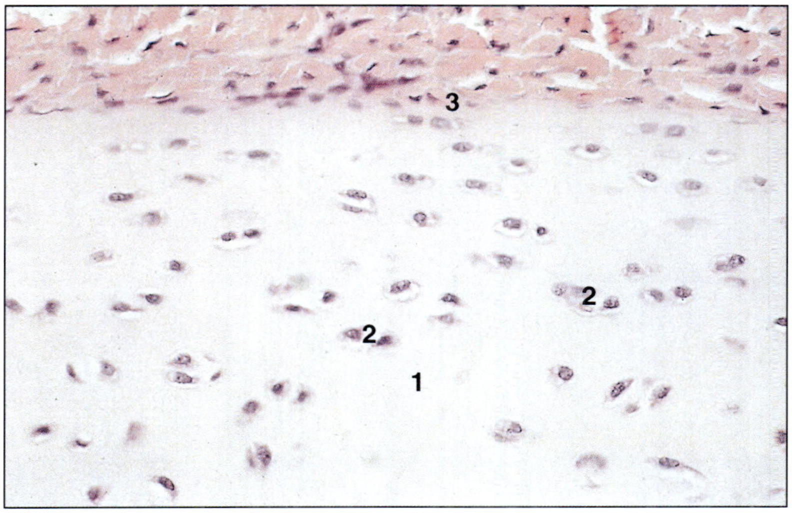

3.30

3.31 Hyaline cartilage. Costal cartilage (dog). (1) Chondrocyte in a lacuna. (2) Extracellular matrix. H & E. ×250.

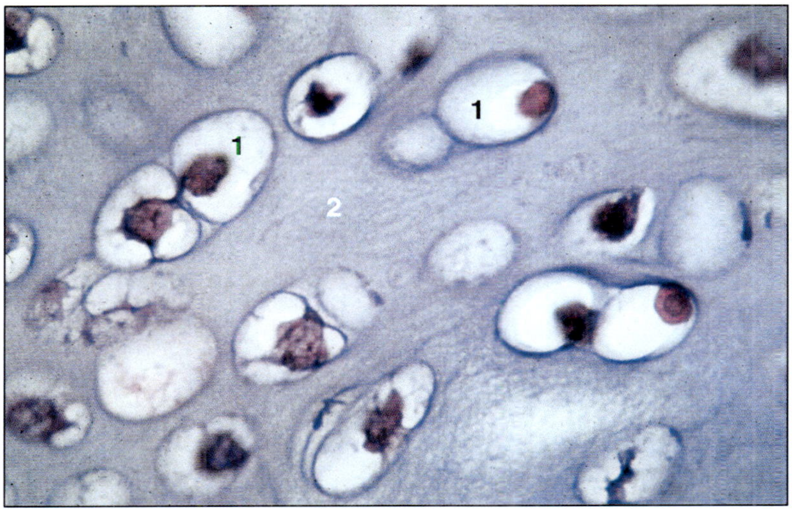

3.31

Elastic cartilage

Elastic cartilage is specially adapted to give resilience and withstand repeated bending. The matrix contains elastic fibres. Examples of elastic cartilage can be found in the epiglottis and the pinna (3.32–3.34).

Fibrocartilage

Fibrocartilage occurs at the site of tendon insertions and in the intervertebral discs, where firm support and tensile strength are necessary. The chondroblasts lie in rows between parallel bundles of collagen fibres and secrete cartilage matrix (3.35–3.37).

3.32

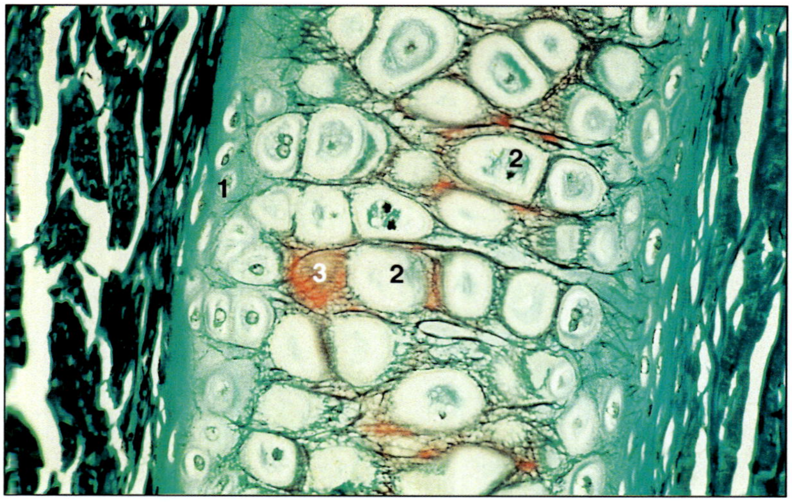

3.32 Elastic cartilage. Pinna (dog). (1) Perichondrium. (2) Chondrocyte in lacuna. (3) Extracellular matrix with red elastic fibres. Masson's trichrome. ×160.

3.33

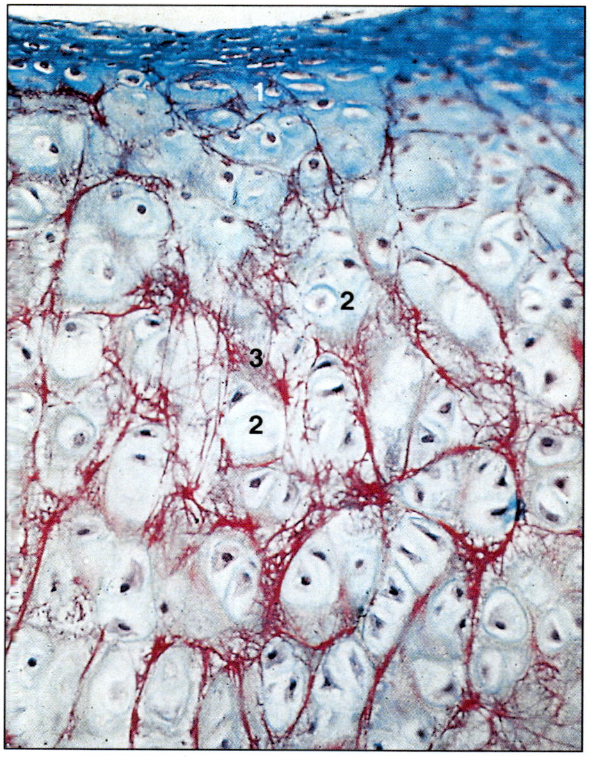

3.33 Elastic cartilage. Pinna (dog). (1) Perichondrium. (2) Chondrocyte in lacuna. (3) Extracellular matrix with red elastic fibres. Gomori's trichrome. ×160.

3.34

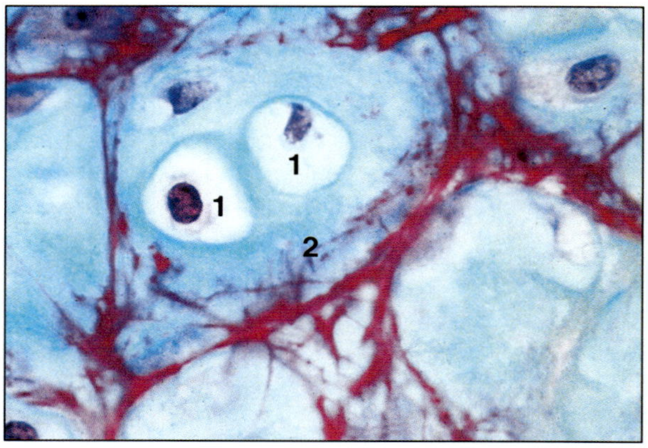

3.34 Elastic cartilage. Pinna (dog). (1) Chondrocyte in lacuna. (2) Extracellular matrix with red elastic fibres. Gomori's trichrome. ×250.

3.35 Fibrocartilage (ox).
(1) Chondrocyte. (2) Collagen fibres arranged as dense regular connective tissue. H & E. ×125.

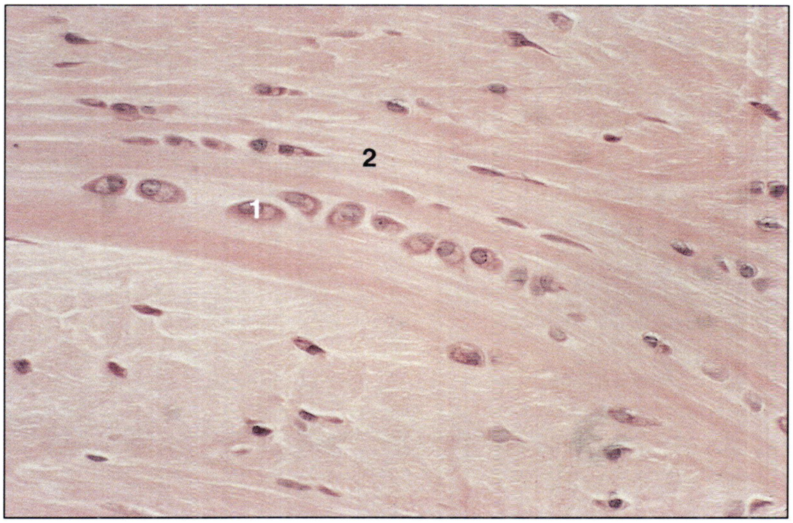

3.35

3.36 Fibrocartilage (ox).
(1) Chondrocyte. (2) Collagen fibres arranged as dense regular connective tissue. Gomori's trichrome. ×160.

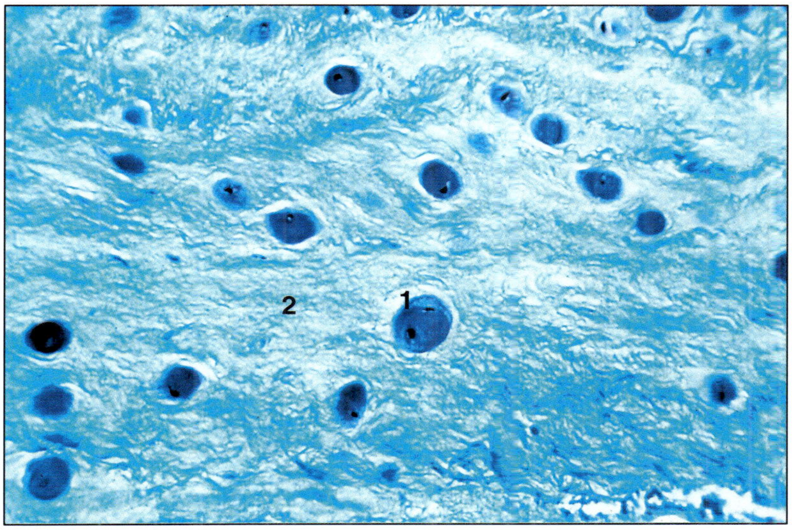

3.36

3.37 Fibrocartilage (ox).
(1) Chondrocyte. (2) Collagen fibres. Gomori's trichrome. ×250.

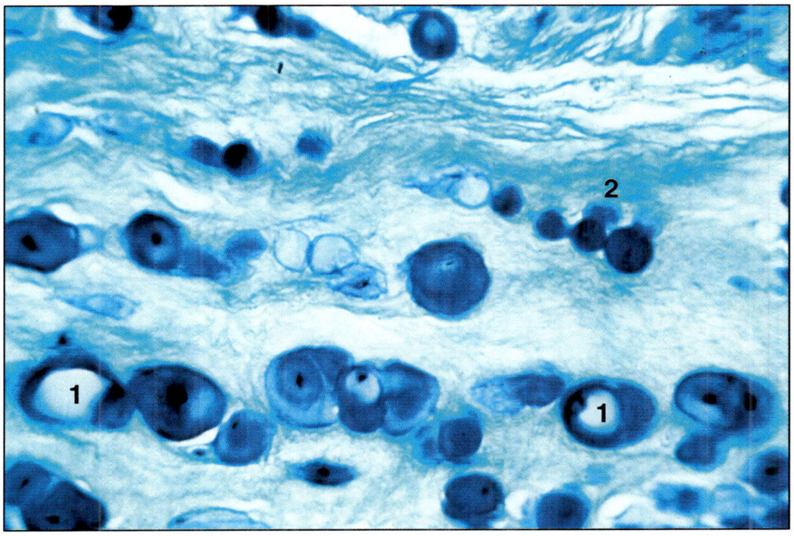

3.37

Bone

Bone is a rigid form of connective tissue composed of cells embedded in an intercellular matrix of collagen fibres, glycosaminoglycans and calcium phosphate deposited as hydroxyapatite crystals. Bone provides the framework of the body and serves as a lever for muscle action, as protection for viscera, as a haemopoietic organ, and as a reservoir of body stores of calcium and phosphorus. Small bones are found in soft tissues to provide extra rigidity – the os penis in the dog and ossa cordis in the ox. Bone is a living tissue that is supplied with blood vessels and nerves, and is constantly changing in response to body stresses and circumstances.

There are two forms of bone: cancellous (spongy, medullary) and compact (cortical, dense). All bones have both cancellous and compact forms of bone deposition. Cancellous bone consists of irregular interconnecting bars, the trabeculae, forming a three-dimensional network of lined spaces filled with bone marrow (3.38 and 3.39). Compact bone is a solid continuous mass in which the spaces are only visible with the aid of a microscope (3.40).

Bones are covered with a specialized connective tissue, the periosteum, the inner layer of which is osteogenic (capable of laying down new bone; 3.40). Spaces in bone, like the marrow cavity (3.38–3.40) and the canal system (3.40–3.42), are lined with a single layer of osteogenic cells, the endosteum. The characteristic feature of all bone tissue is the arrangement of mineralized bone matrix in layers, the lamellae. Small lacunae present in the lamellae are occupied by a single bone cell, the osteocyte. Tubular passages, the canaliculi, radiate from each lacuna and link up with canaliculi from adjacent lacunae to create an extensive system of interconnecting canals. This arrangement is clearly defined in compact bone where the lamellae are arranged concentrically around a longitudinal canal to form an osteon (Haversian System; 3.41–3.43). The central canal of the osteon carries blood vessels,

3.38

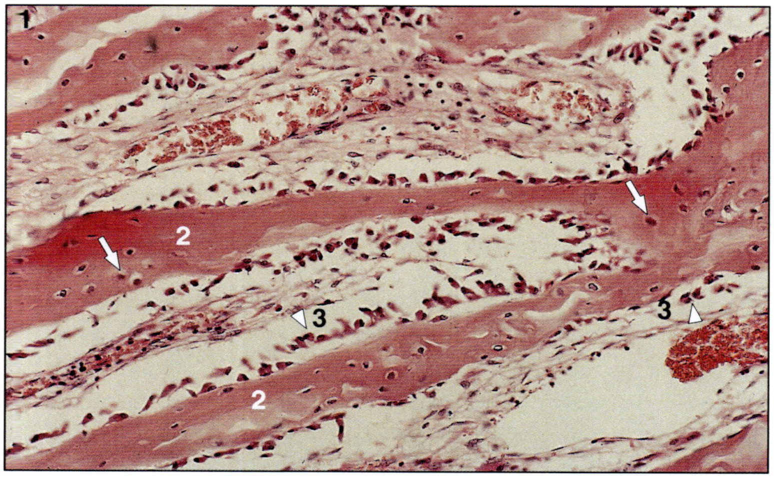

3.38 Spiculated bone (dog). (1) Periosteum. (2) Bone spicules with osteocytes in the lacunae (arrowed). (3) Bone marrow filled spaces lined by osteoblasts (arrowhead). H & E. ×100.

3.39

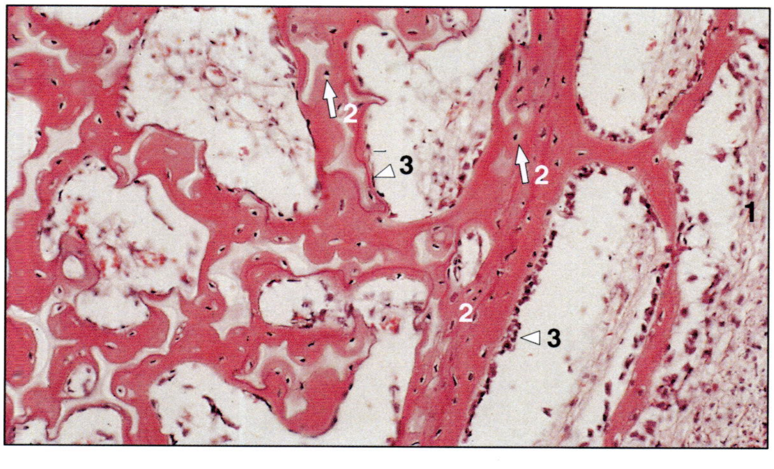

3.39 Spiculated bone (dog). (1) Periosteum. (2) Bone spicules with osteocytes (arrowed). (3) Osteoblasts (arrowhead) on the free surface of the bone. H & E. ×160.

.40

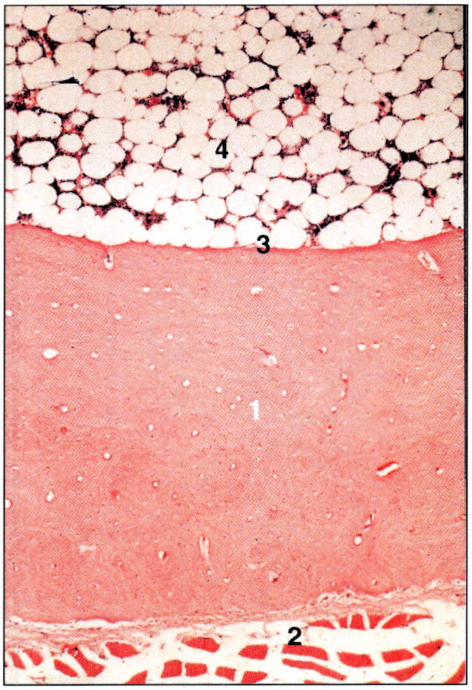

3.40 Compact bone (dog). (1) Compact bone of the diaphysis of the femur. (2) Periosteum. (3) Endosteum. (4) Marrow with a high proportion of fat cells. H & E. ×20.

3.41

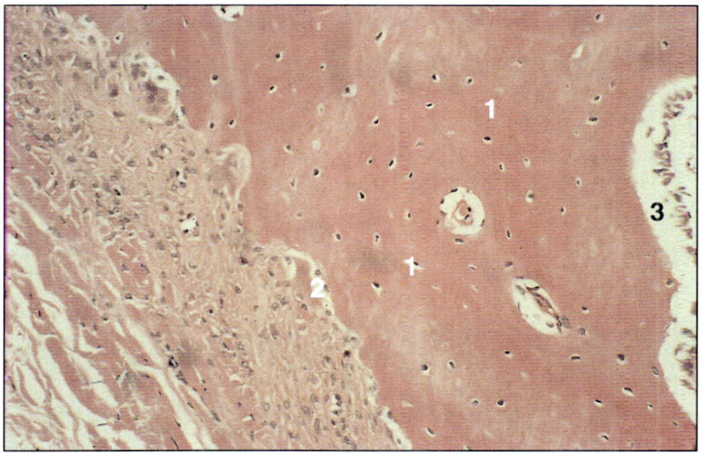

3.41 Compact bone (dog). (1) Compact bone with osteocytes in lacunae arranged in lamellae with a central canal carrying blood vessels and nerves. The canal is lined by endosteum. (2) Periosteum. (3) Endosteum of the marrow cavity. H & E. ×62.5.

.42

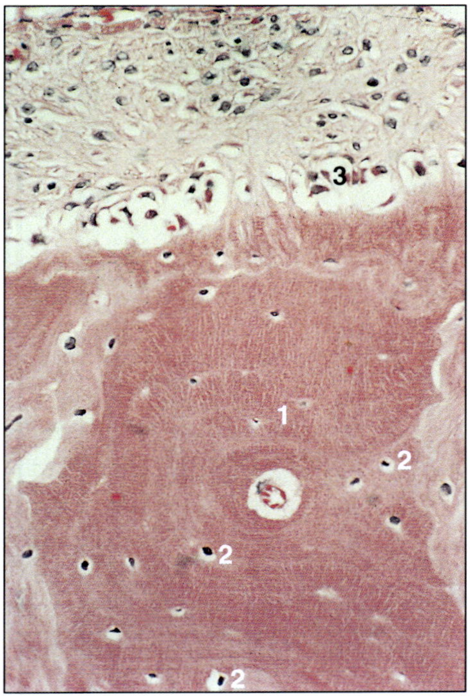

3.42 Compact bone (dog). (1) The osteon fills the field. The central canal is lined by endosteum and carries blood vessels and nerves. (2) Osteocytes in lacunae in the circumferential lamellae. (3) Periosteum. H & E. ×100.

3.43

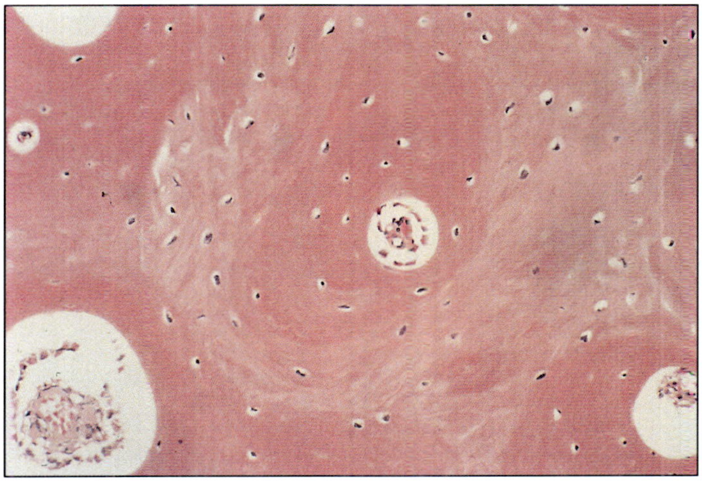

3.43 Compact bone (dog). This is a high power view of Fig. 3.42. H & E. ×250.

branches of the perpendicular canals (of Volkmann). These are part of the main blood supply to the bone and link the endosteal and periosteal surfaces. The lamellae may be regular circular rings as in the osteon, surround the shaft of the bone as circumferential lamellae, or fill in the angular spaces between lamellae as interstitial lamellae. They are often the result of bone remodelling. Bone contains a vast continuous network of canals that are essential for the nutrition of the bone cell in the lacuna, the osteocyte (**3.41–3.45**). The cell body lies in the lacuna and extends in long processes into the canaliculi to contact similar processes from adjacent osteocytes.

Bone is a living tissue and is constantly being remodelled; osteoclasts are multinucleate non-dividing cells that are found in resorption bays (Howship's lacunae) at the site of bone remodelling (**3.46**). Osteoclasts are derived from a progenitor cell in bone marrow. The cell migrates to the developing tissue. The ruffled (brush) border is the undulating mobile cell membrane.

Osteoblasts are present on the inner surface of the periosteum and endosteum, and cover the surface of bone spicules in an active osteogenic area (**3.38, 3.39** and **3.46**). The cell has a central or slightly eccentric nucleus with chromatin granules, and the cytoplasm stains deeply with haematoxylin because of the concentration of organelles. Long cytoplasmic processes extend out from the osteoblast and the matrix is deposited around them. This provides a fine canalicular network and allows nutrients to pass to the bone cells. Unlike cartilage there is no diffusion in bone. Once the bone has been deposited the trapped cells (osteocytes) function to maintain the bone and retain contact with the blood vessels through the canalicular system.

3.44

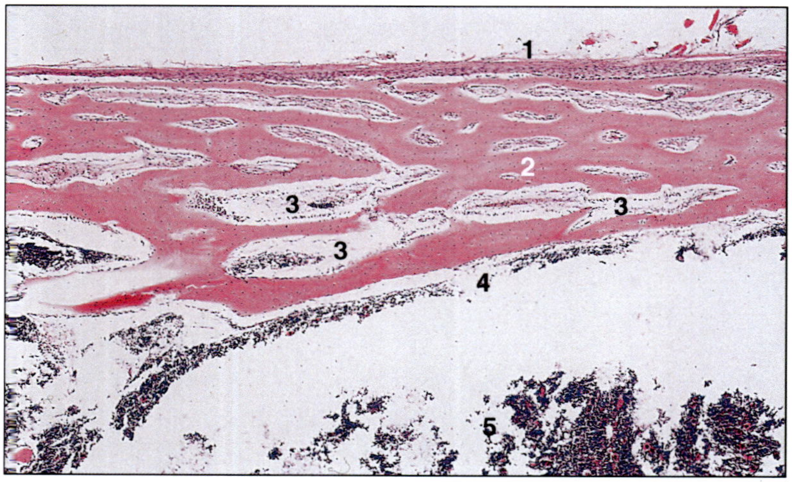

3.44 Developing periosteal bone (foal). (1) Periosteum. (2) Bone spicules. (3) Osteogenic tissue fills the spaces between the spicules. (4) Endosteum. (5) Marrow. H & E. ×62.5.

3.45

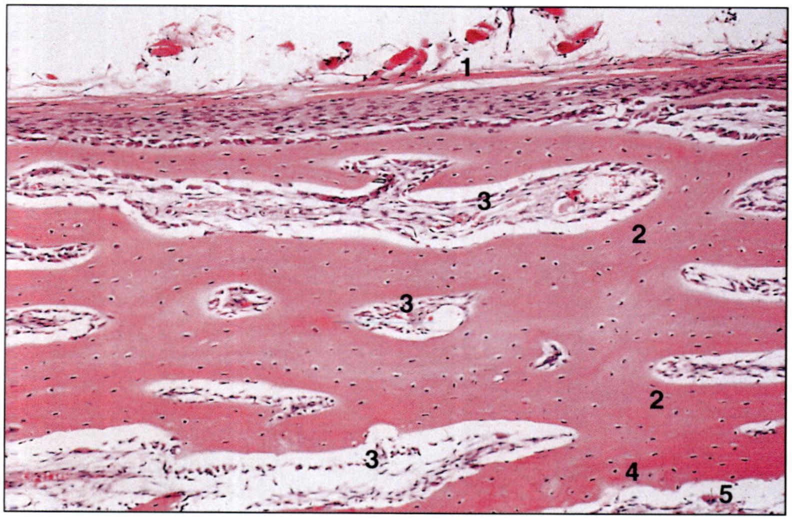

3.45 Developing periosteal bone (foal). (1) Periosteum. (2) Bone spicules. (3) Osteogenic tissue fills the spaces between the spicules. (4) Endosteum. (5) Marrow. H & E. ×125.

Endochondral ossification

In the embryo, mesenchymal cells at predetermined sites differentiate into chondroblasts and lay down cartilage models of the long bones (3.47). Later in gestation, the mesenchyme surrounding the cartilage model becomes very vascular and the cartilage matrix is calcified. Nutrients are unable to diffuse through this calcified cartilage and the cells die. Cell death is followed by breakdown of the matrix. Vascular mesenchymal tissue moves in, differentiates into osteogenic tissue and deposits bone on the remains of the calcified cartilage (3.48 and 3.49).

3.46

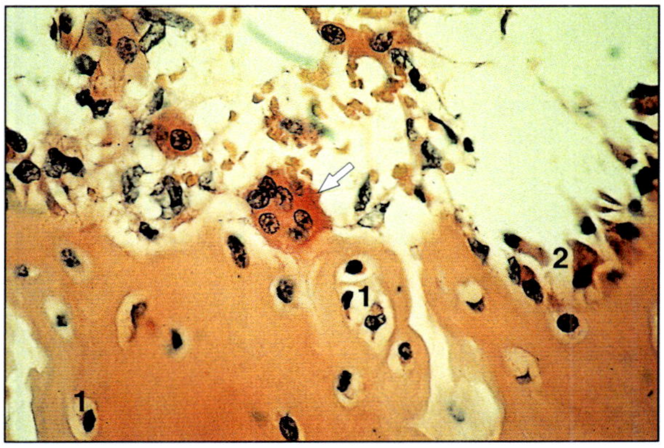

3.46 Compact bone (cat). Osteoclast (arrowed). (1) Osteocytes in lacunae. (2) Osteoblasts on the free surface of the bone. H & E. ×250.

3.47

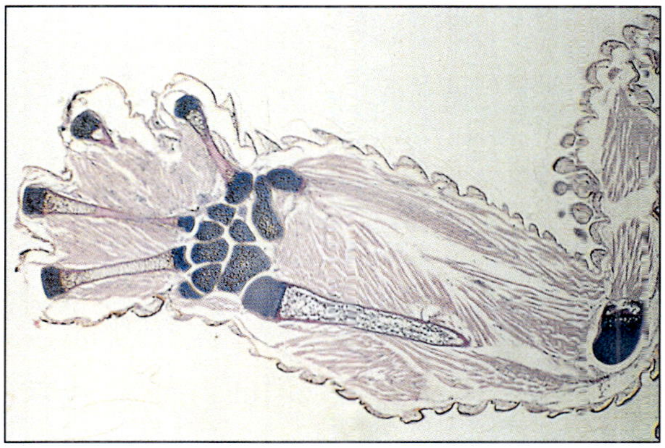

3.47 Whole mount section of the left forelimb of a small viviparous yucca night lizard (*Xantusia vigilis*). Note the transition between the blue staining cartilaginous ends and the mineralized diaphyseal compact bone. H & E. ×5.

3.48

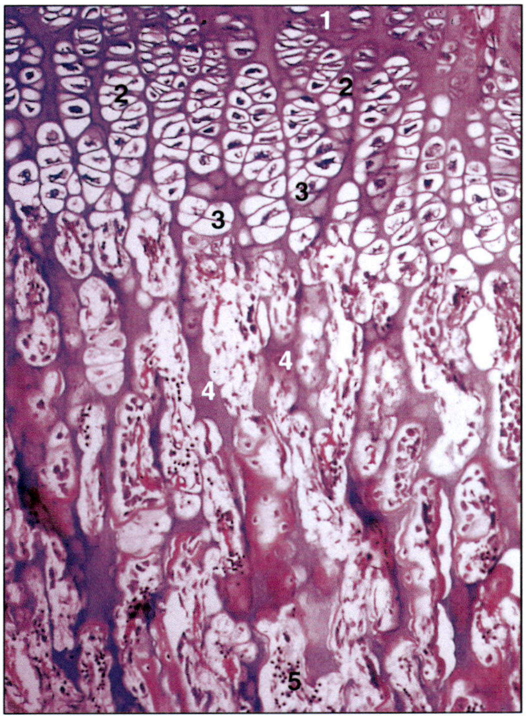

3.48 Endochondral ossification (cat). (1) Zone of resting cartilage. (2) Zone of proliferating cartilage. (3) Zone of hypertrophied chondrocytes. (4) Basophilic calcified cartilage with freshly deposited eosinophilic bone. (5) Osteogenic tissue. H & E. ×62.5.

3.49

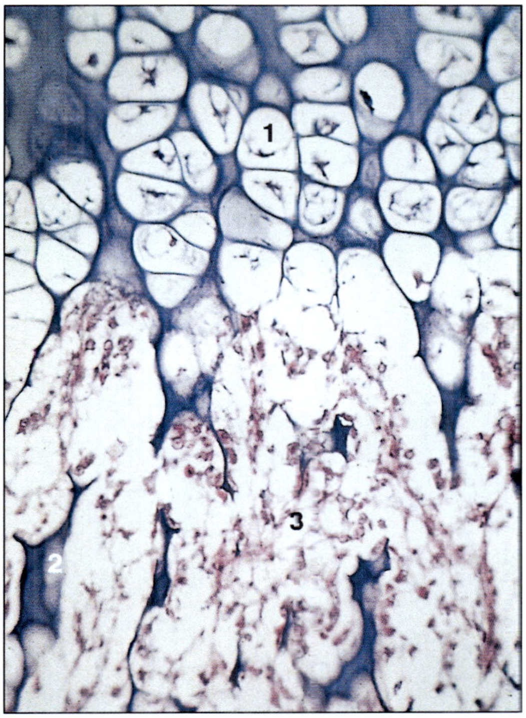

3.49 Endochondral ossification (cat). (1) Zone of hypertrophied chondrocytes. (2) Calcified cartilage with bone deposits. (3) Osteogenic tissue. H & E. ×160.

This is an ossification centre. The cartilage is replaced by bone beginning at the centre of the diaphysis and extending to the epiphysis. The epiphysis has a separate centre of ossification and a plate of cartilage persists, the epiphyseal plate; this separates the epiphysis from the diaphysis (**3.50**). The perichondrium becomes the periosteum.

Multinucleated osteoclasts remove mineralized osseous matrix (**3.52**). In metabolic bone disease (fibrous osteodystrophy, secondary nutritional hyperparathyroidism, 'rubber jaw', 'renal rickets'), which may be caused by an improper dietary calcium : phosphorus ratio, or in some cases of severe chronic renal disease the osteopenic bone is replaced by fibrous connective tissue (**3.51**).

Growth of a long bone

Bones are able to grow in width and length and do so until the adult size is reached. Thereafter, bone continues to remodel as circumstances demand. Growth in width is appositional from the osteogenic inner layer of the periosteum and new bone is formed locally, the periosteal collar (**3.44**). This ability to deposit bone is utilized in bone grafts. Growth in length is accomplished at the diaphyseal/epiphyseal junction at the persistent layer of the epiphysis. Cartilage grows interstitially on the epiphyseal side and dies on the diaphyseal side of the plate. Osteogenic tissue invades and deposits bone, the epiphyses are pushed apart and the bone grows in length (**3.50**).

3.50

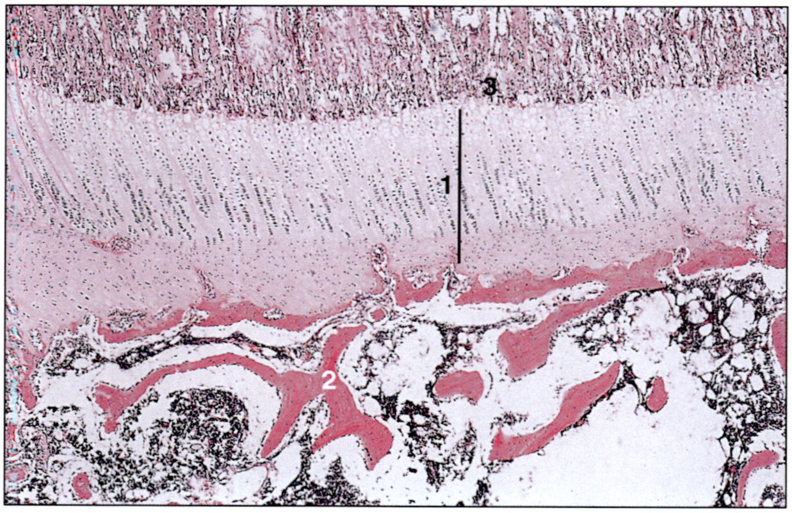

3.50 Epiphyseal plate (cat). (1) Epiphysis. (2) Spiculated bone. (3) Growth area of endochondral ossification. H & E. ×25.

3.51

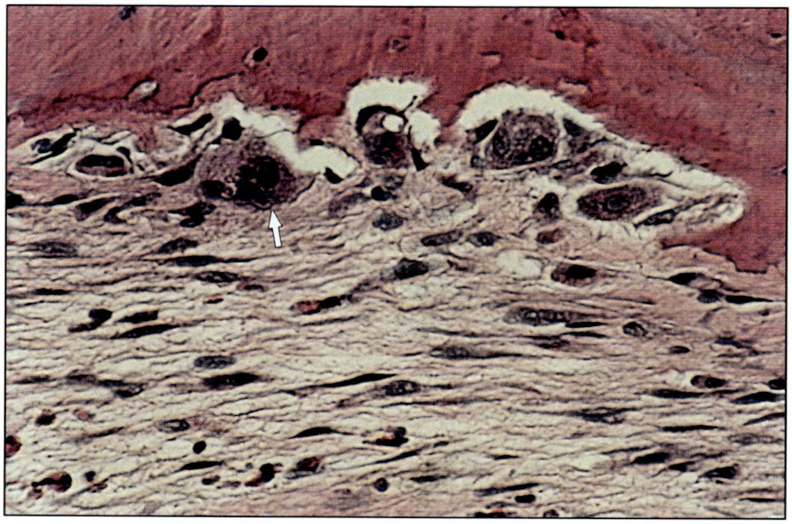

3.51 Section of femur from a green iguana (*Iguana iguana*) with metabolic bone disease. Note the multinucleated osteoclasts (arrowed) that have been removing ossified tissue and fibrous connective tissue that has replaced the cancellous bone. H & E. ×250.

Intramembranous ossification

Small bones and flat bones develop directly from mesenchymal cells; these differentiate into osteoblasts. Bone is laid down as a network of bony spicules that are gradually enlarged by the deposition of new bone lamellae. The spaces are filled in and compact bone is formed in the outer plates which are continuous with the more central cancellous bone. The surrounding mesenchyme condenses to become the periosteum; the inner layer is osteogenic (*see* 3.44). The osteoblasts on the inner surface lining the spicules of cancellous bone also retain their osteogenic ability.

Clinical correlates

Although a variety of benign and malignant tumours of various origins arise in the skeleton, osteosarcomas, a malignant mesenchymal tumour in which the neoplastic cells produce tumour osteoid or bone, account for approximately 80% of canine and 50% of feline skeletal neoplasms. Osteosarcomas can be subdivided according to their location within bone or histological appearance. An osteogenic, or bone producing, osteosarcoma that has multifocal formation of well mineralized new bone is shown in 3.52. This was taken from an 8-year-old St Bernard dog. An example of a giant cell osteosarcoma (3.53) from a German Shepherd dog shows numerous multinucleate syncytia formed by fusion of the neoplastic cells.

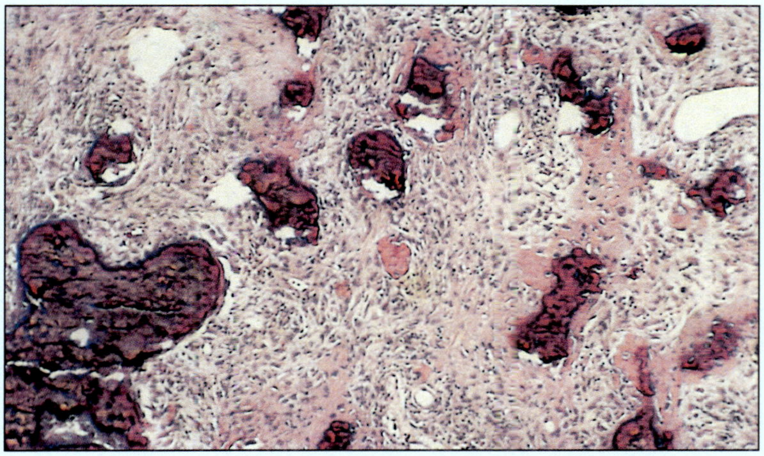

3.52

3.52 Osteogenic osteosarcoma (dog) showing tumour bone formation. H & E. ×20.

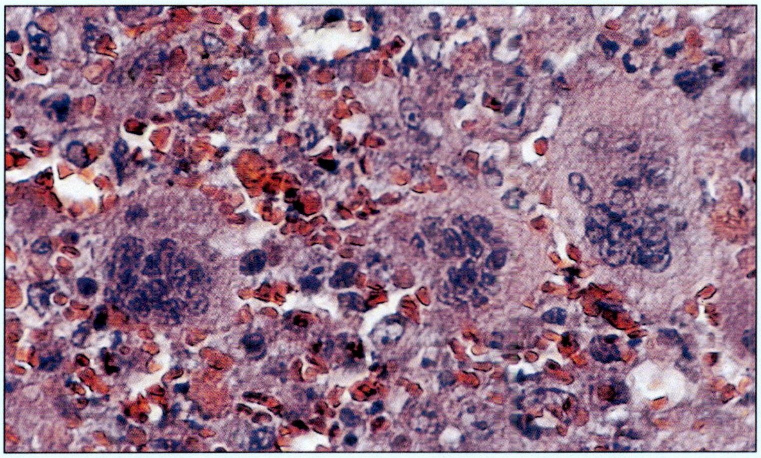

3.53

3.53 Giant cell osteosarcoma (dog). Note the numerous multinucleate cells. H & E. ×250.

Arthritis is a general term for inflammatory disease of the joints. There are many causes and many types of arthritis but often a similar pattern of reaction and joint damage may be observed. A synovial biopsy from an adult German Shepherd dog in which the thickened synovial membrane is invaded by large numbers of plasma cells is shown in **3.54**. The predominance of this cell type suggests an immunological basis for the disease in this case.

3.54

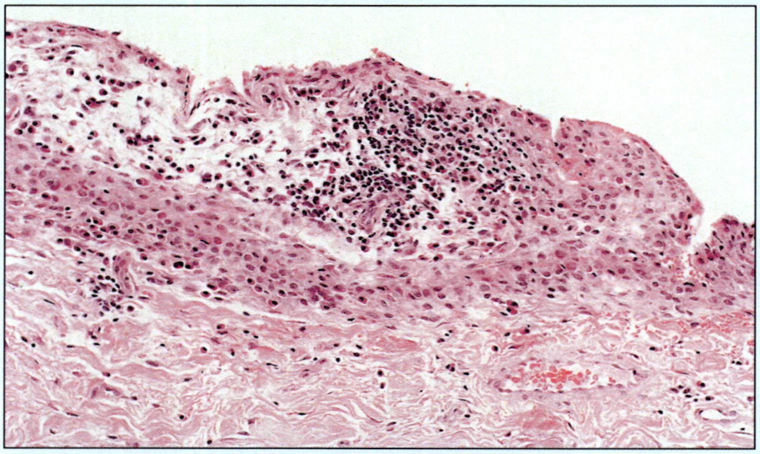

3.54 Plasmacytic arthritis in the dog. The synovial membrane is infiltrated by plasma cells. H & E. ×125.

4. BLOOD

Blood is a special type of connective tissue: the intercellular matrix, the plasma, is a fluid, and the cells are red and white blood corpuscles. Small fragments of cells, the platelets, and large proteins such as fibrinogen, albumin and globulin are non-cellular elements carried in the plasma. Both red and white blood cells are derived from the same primitive cell, the haemocytoblast. The red blood cells, or erythrocytes, are contained within the blood vessels and carry oxygen and carbon dioxide. The white blood cells, or leucocytes, are part of the body's defence mechanism and use the circulation as a means of transport to particular sites where they leave the blood vessel and enter the tissues. The cellular elements account for 40% of whole blood and the plasma for 60%.

The preparation of blood for histological examination is remarkably simple. A drop of blood is spread on a glass slide, fixed immediately in air and by immersion in absolute methanol, and stained with one of the Romanowsky dyes, mixtures of methylene blue and the derivatives azure blue and eosin. Cell nuclei stain purple; the haemoglobin-containing erythrocytic cytoplasm stains pink or tan; and the cytoplasm of leucocytes assumes a blue to blue–grey hue. Cytoplasmic granules react either with eosin and are eosinophilic, or with the blue stains and are basophilic. They often display some degree of refractility. Erythrocytic and leucocytic haemoparasites stain variably, depending upon their type. Some granules do not stain with either and are regarded as neutral. This method allows for identification of all the cell types in a blood smear, and differential cell counts are used to assess the blood picture (see Appendix Table 2 for species variation).

Blood cells and platelets

Erythrocytes

The mature mammalian erythrocyte is a highly differentiated cell lacking a nucleus, ribosomes and mitochondria. It is a biconcave disc with the cell membrane enclosing the cytoplasm, and is filled with haemoglobin, the protein carrier of oxygen and carbon dioxide (**4.1, 4.2**; *see* also Chapter 1, **1.21**). The diameter varies in size according to species. Mammalian erythrocytes are round and they measure from 4.1 µm in the goat to 7 µm in the dog. The erythrocytes of birds, fish, amphibians and reptiles are elongated and they can measure nearly 20 × 100 µm in some amphibians and reptiles. Erythrocytes from one animal are the same size, except in the cow and sheep where variation in size (anisocytosis) is not unusual. The erythrocyte is flexible enough to pass through the smallest capillary. The average life span is 3 months in mammals, but in some reptiles it is as long as 3 years. Immature erythrocytes may appear in the

4.1

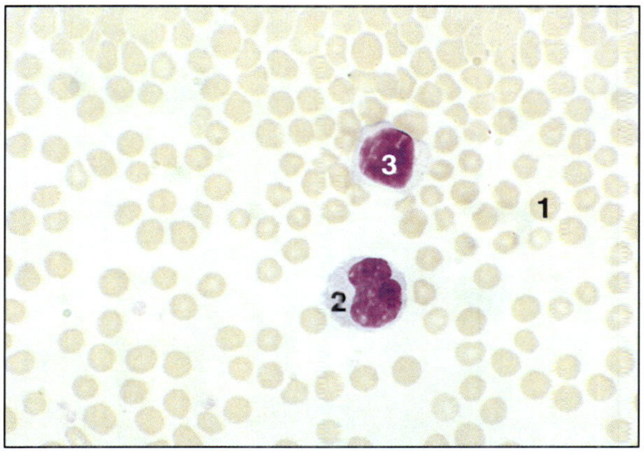

4.1 Blood (ox). (1) Erythrocytes. (2) Large lymphocyte. (3) Small lymphocyte. Leishman. ×200.

Clinical correlate

4.2

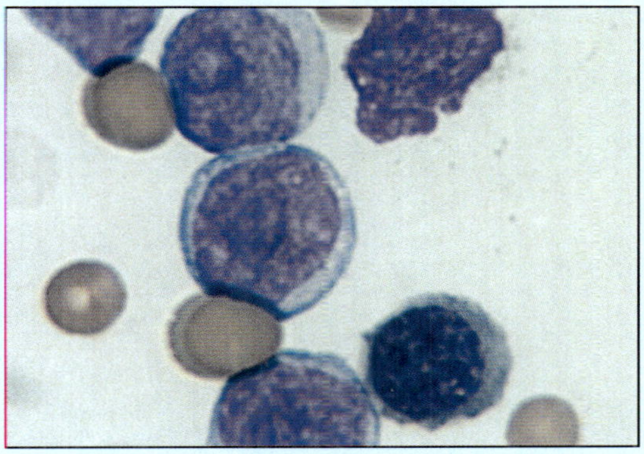

4.2 Feline prolymphocytic leukaemia. The nuclei are large, and the nucleoli are retained. Wright's. ×625.

circulation in response to urgent need; the commonest of these is the reticulocyte (**4.3** and **4.4**). Proerythroblasts, basophilic erythroblasts and the metarubricyte are also seen occasionally (**4.5**). The nuclei of avian, amphibian and reptilian erythrocytes are elongated and retained into maturity. Nucleus-free, but otherwise intact, erythrocytes (erythroplastids) are occasionally found in reptilian blood. Similarly, nuclei with a tiny amount of haemoglobin-containing cytoplasm may be seen. These cell-like objects, called haematogones, appear to be intact erythrocytic nuclei or nuclear remnants that have been extruded from other red blood cells. Because they are nucleated, the cells of birds, fish, amphibians and reptiles are capable of mitosis and amitotic division even after they have matured. Although the erythrocytes of the lower vertebrates retain their nuclei, the presence of their immature phase, the reticulocyte, is easily demonstrated by staining unfixed blood films with the supravital dye new methylene blue.

During metamorphosis in amphibians, the erythrocytes change from the larger larval cells to the smaller adult cells. The nucleus is retained in both, but the amount of endoplasmic reticulum is greater in the adult cells. The haemoglobin also changes during the development of larval amphibians into adults. Larval haemoglobin possesses a greater affinity for oxygen; this is consonant with the aquatic habitat. Larval erythrocytes are more able to incorporate the amino acids uridine and thymidine than are the adult cells. The site of haemopoiesis shifts during larval and metamorphic development. As an embryo, the erythrocytes are formed in the ventral blood islands. Later, the pronephric and nephric kidneys are major sites for red blood cell production. In late metamorphosis and into adulthood, the liver and then the spleen and bone marrow predominate as the sites where erythropoiesis occurs.

4.3

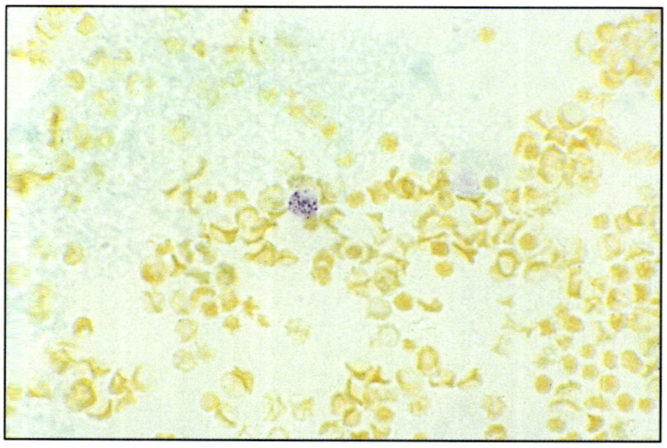

4.3 Reticulocytes (cat). Early stage erythrocytes; the nucleus has just been extruded and a fine network of residual nuclear material is still present. Leishman. ×160.

4.4

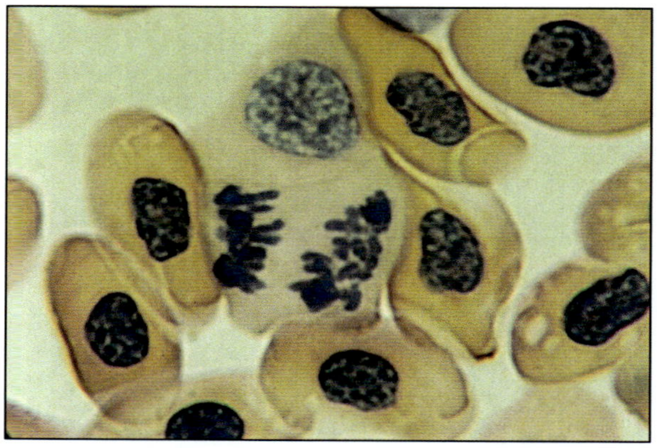

4.4 Mitotic division in a previously mature, haemoglobin-containing erythrocyte of a western diamondback rattlesnake (*Crotalus atrox*) demonstrates the ability of these cells, under certain conditions of anaemia, to revert to a blastic phase and undergo mitosis. Benzidine peroxidase. ×625.

4.5

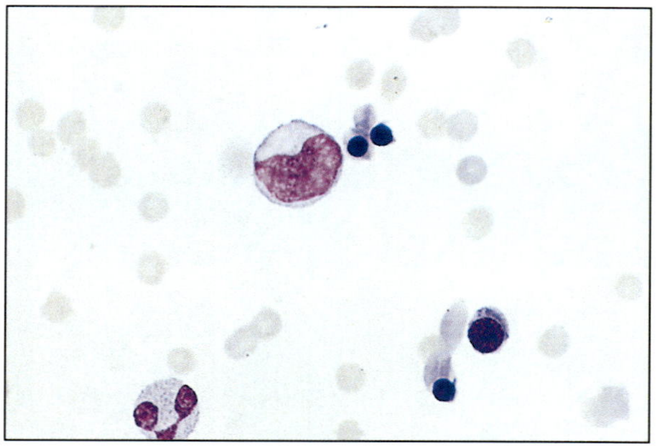

4.5 Blood (dog). Metarubricyte (or normoblast) is a nucleated early stage erythrocyte seen on rare occasions in circulating blood. Leishman. ×200.

Leucocytes

There are two main types of leucocytes, granulocytes and agranulocytes, both of which can leave and enter the circulating blood by crossing the capillary wall between the endothelial cells. They are part of the body's defence system and involved in the immune response. The most numerous of the white cells in domestic animals, with the exception of oxen and sheep, are the polymorphonuclear leucocytes (PMLs), large granulocytes (10–12 μm in diameter) with lobed nuclei, usually five lobes joined by thin strands of chromatin. They are described as PMLs (**4.6**). Staining of the granules is very variable and the individual granules are small and difficult to identify. The eosinophilic leucocytes (eosinophils, acidophils) have large red granules in the cytoplasm (particularly large in the horse), bilobed nuclei and form about 5% of the white cell population (**4.7**). They are associated with response to parasitic infections and allergic reactions.

The heterophil is another granulocyte that is present in the lower vertebrates. It is the functional and numerical equivalent of the PML in mammals. Heterophils display the greatest diversity in size and granule shape from species to species of any of the leucocytes. In most amphibians, lizards, snakes and crocodilians, the heterophil granules are small, round and orange. In chelonians (turtles, tortoises and terrapins) they are elongated, needle-shaped and often a muddy brown colour. Like their mammalian PML counterpart, the heterophils are lysosomally active, recruited to sites of bacterial infection and can act as phagocytes. Because of their reddish-orange coloured granules, heterophils are often mistaken for eosinophils.

The basophilic leucocytes (basophils) are the rarest of the granulocytes in mammals, forming only 0.5% of the white cell population. However, as one descends the phylogenetic scale, the number of basophils enumerated in a differential blood cell count increases markedly to as many as 10% in some species. Characteristically large basophilic granules, containing histamine and heparin, obscure the bilobed, multilobed, or unlobed nuclei, and the cells are essentially similar to mast cells (**4.8**).

4.6 Blood (dog). Polymorphonuclear leucocytes are arrowed. Leishman. ×160.

4.6

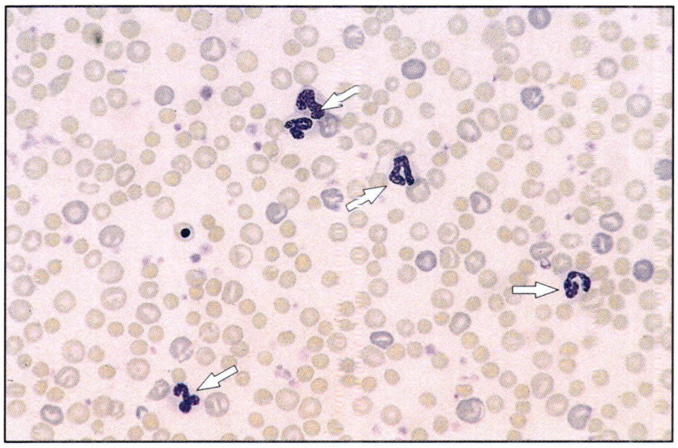

4.7

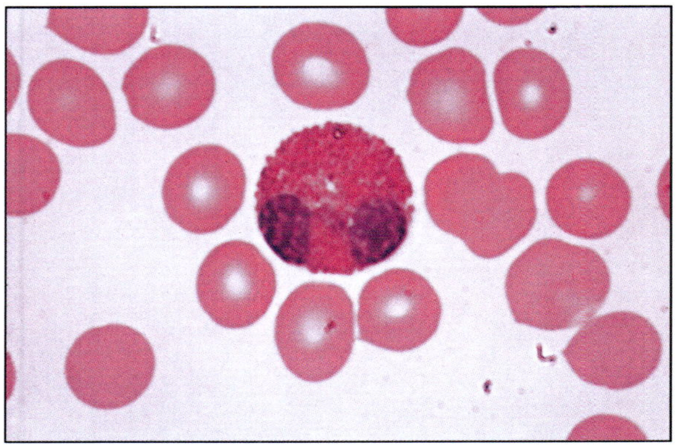

4.7 Eosinophil. Blood (dog). Large rod-shaped granules are present in the cytoplasm. Leishman. ×625.

4.8

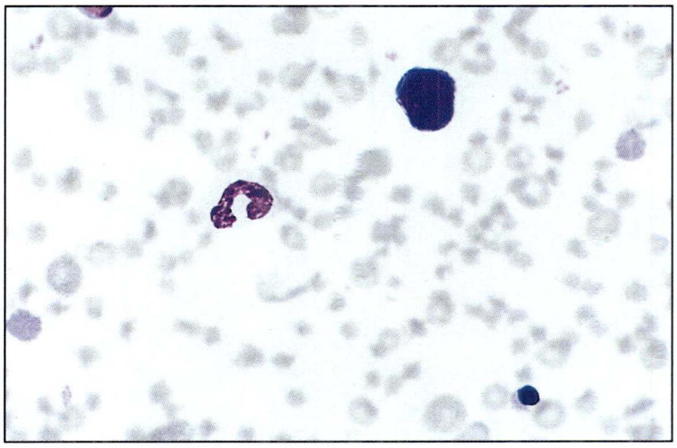

4.8 Basophil. Blood (dog). The dense basophilic granules obscure the cell. Leishman. ×200.

4.9

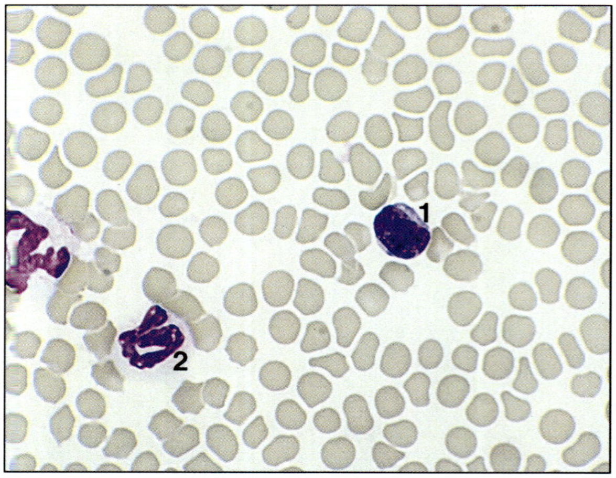

4.9 Blood (dog). (1) Small lymphocyte. (2) Polymorphonuclear leucocytes. Leishman. ×200.

The most common of the agranulocytes is the small lymphocyte, which constitutes 30% of the white cell population, except in oxen and sheep where it makes up 70% of the total. It is 7–8 µm in diameter, with a dark blue nucleus and a thin rim of cytoplasm (**4.1, 4.9** and **4.10**). Medium and large lymphocytes are up to 10 µm in diameter with a dark blue nucleus and pale blue cytoplasm (**4.11** and **4.12**). The largest cell of the agranulocytic series is the monocyte, which is 12–20 µm in diameter, with a horseshoe-shaped nucleus lying in abundant cytoplasm (**4.13**). It leaves the blood and transforms into a variety of macrophages at various sites in the body as part of the mononuclear phagocyte system.

4.10

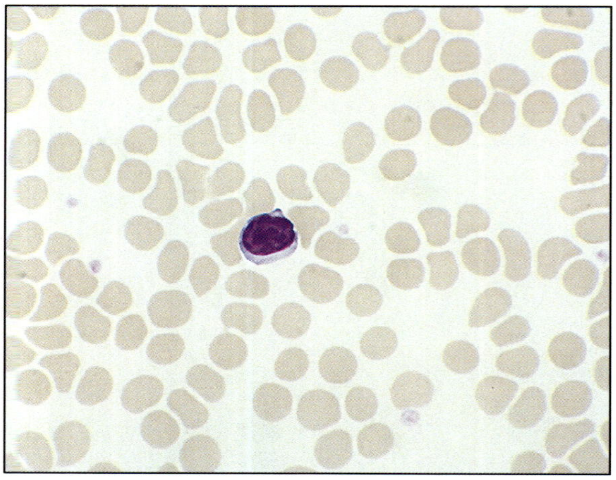

4.10 Lymphocyte. Blood (dog). A small lymphocyte lies in the middle of the field. Leishman. ×200.

4.11

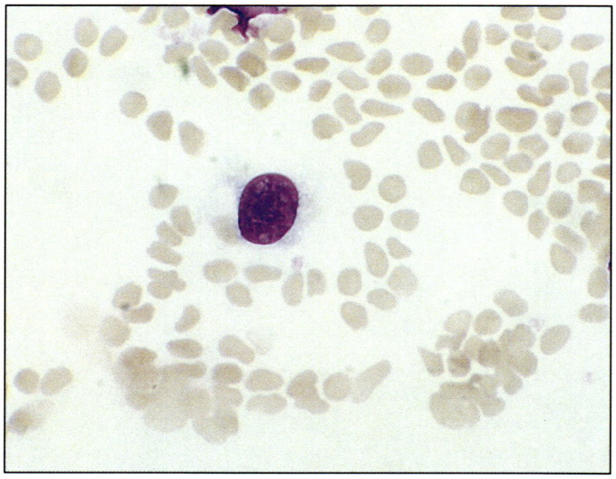

4.11 Lymphocyte. Blood (ox). A large lymphocyte lies near the middle of the field. Leishman. ×200.

4.12

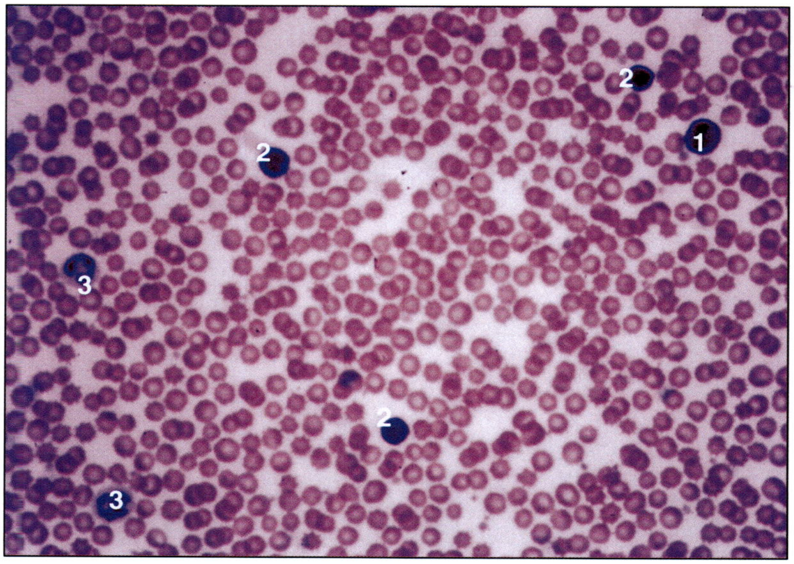

4.12 Blood (ox). (1) Large lymphocyte. (2) Small lymphocytes. (3) Polymorphonuclear leucocytes. Leishman. ×160.

4.13 Monocyte. Blood (dog). A monocyte is the largest cell present. Leishman. ×200.

4.13

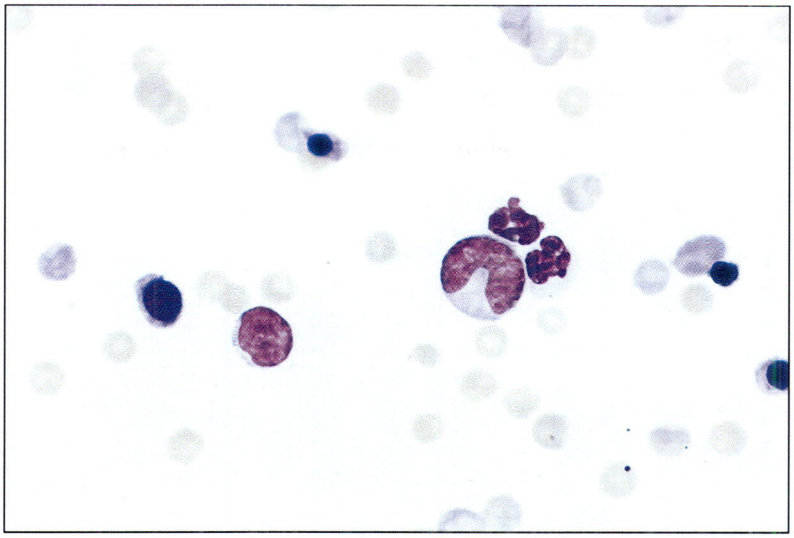

Platelets

Platelets are cytoplasmic fragments, about 3 μm in diameter, derived from large multinucleated cells in the bone marrow called megakaryocytes. These cells function with fibrinogen to repair damaged blood vessels by forming a thrombus or clot (**4.14**). In birds, fish, amphibians and reptiles, thrombocytes are responsible for blood clotting; this cell is not present in mammalian blood. The thrombocyte is nucleated, elongated and usually somewhat smaller than an erythrocyte. It possesses a pale blue, agranular cytoplasm, and is capable of active phagocytosis, amitotic division and, amazingly, pluripotentiality inasmuch as it has the ability under conditions of severe acute and chronic blood loss to be transformed into a haemoglobin-rich, respirationally functional erythrocyte. Whether the thrombocyte, like its mammalian stem cell cousin, can transform into other cell types is unknown. In reptiles, thrombocytes bud off from large multinucleated cells with distinctly granular cytoplasm that are present in the bone marrow. Under conditions of severe anaemia, they can also be found in extramedullary sites such as the liver and spleen. Because of their delicacy, the megakaryocyte-like giant cells are best seen in bone marrow *touch* preparations (**4.15**).

.14

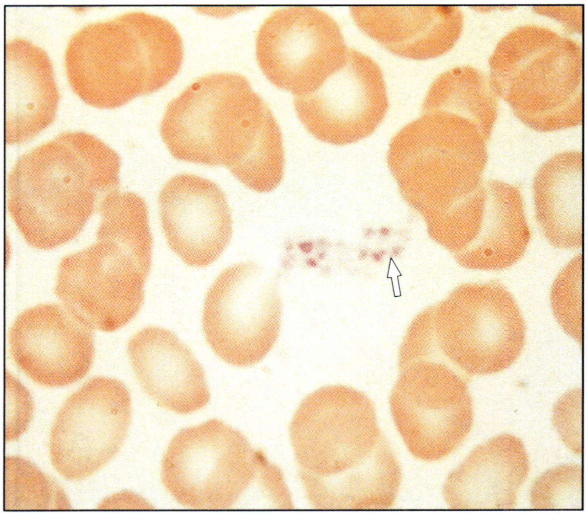

4.14 Platelets. Blood (dog). A group of platelets are arrowed. Leishman. ×625.

4.15

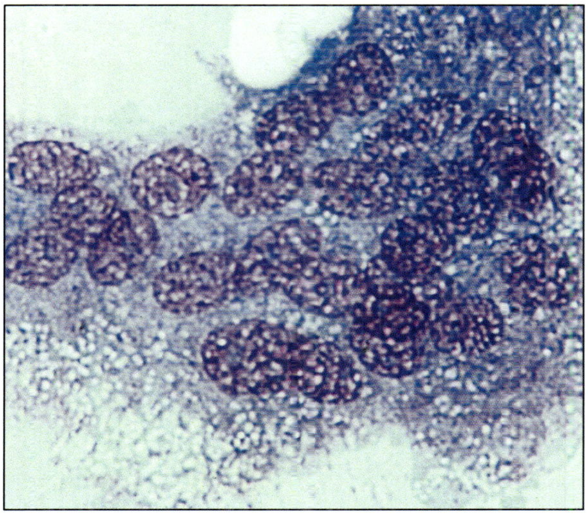

4.15 Megakaryocytic-like multinucleated cell from which reptilian thrombocytes originate. Jenner–Giemsa. ×200.

Avian blood cells

The various corpuscles of mammalian blood are present in birds, but exhibit distinctive features. These include retention of the nucleus by the mature erythrocyte and the presence of a true thrombocyte, in contradistinction to the mammalian blood platelet. The erythrocyte is a nucleated oval cell with an eosinophilic cytoplasm, measuring approximately 9–12 μm in diameter (**4.16**). The thrombocyte is analogous to the mammalian platelet, is oval or round in shape and is smaller than the erythrocyte. The nucleus stains deeply basophilic, as does the cytoplasm. Prominent red granules are commonly present in vacuoles adjacent to the nucleus (**4.17**).

Granular leucocytes account for approximately 24% of the white cells and are classified as heterophils, eosinophils and basophils. The heterophils are 8–10 μm in diameter and are so-called because of the variable staining of the cytoplasmic rods; the nucleus is bilobed or trilobed (**4.18**). The eosinophils are about 7 μm in diameter and rounded granules are present in the cytoplasm. They are less regularly rounded than are the heterophils and most have a bilobed nucleus. The specific granules are round or oval and smaller than the granules of the heterophils. The cytoplasm is basophilic (**4.20**). The basophil is more numerous than in the mammal; the granules are deep blue staining. Agranular leucocytes are identical to the lymphocytes and monocytes of the mammal and form 72% of the white cell population (**4.18, 4.21** and **4.22**). The bone marrow haemopoietic tissue is basically similar to the mammalian, with the notable absence of megakaryocytes.

4.16

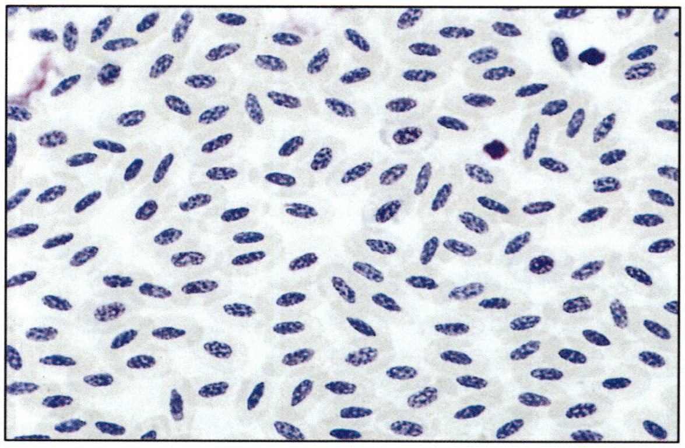

4.16 Blood (bird). The avian erythrocytes are nucleated. Leishman. ×200.

4.17

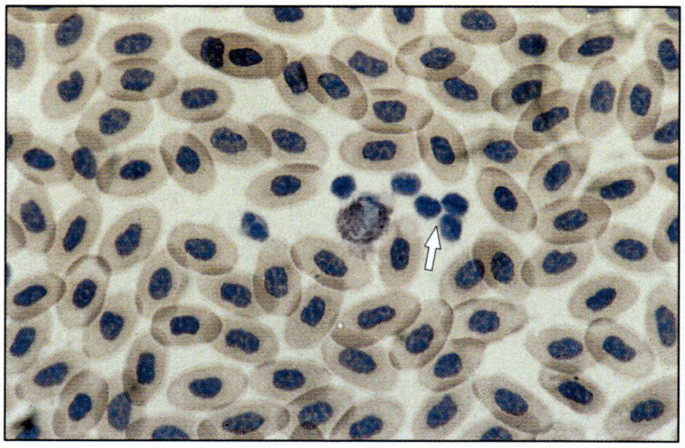

4.17 Blood (bird). A group of thrombocytes are arrowed. Leishman. ×250.

4.18

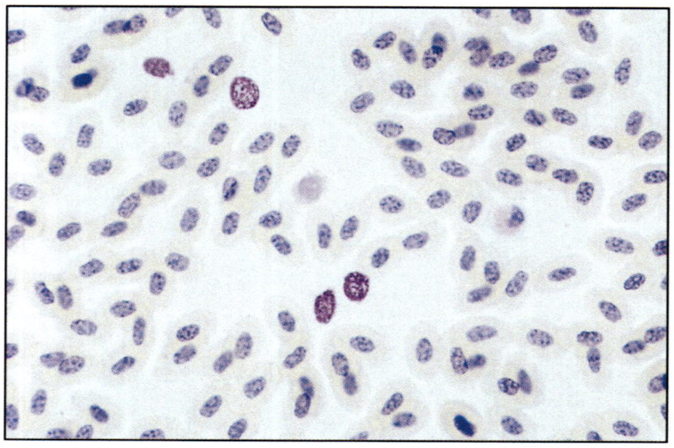

4.18 Blood (bird). The cytoplasm of the avian heterophil is filled with eosinophilic granules. Leishman. ×480.

4.19

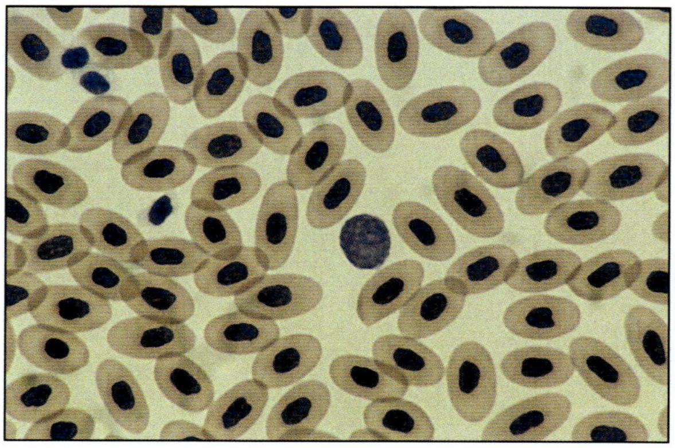

4.19 Blood (bird). A small lymphocyte. Leishman. ×480.

.20

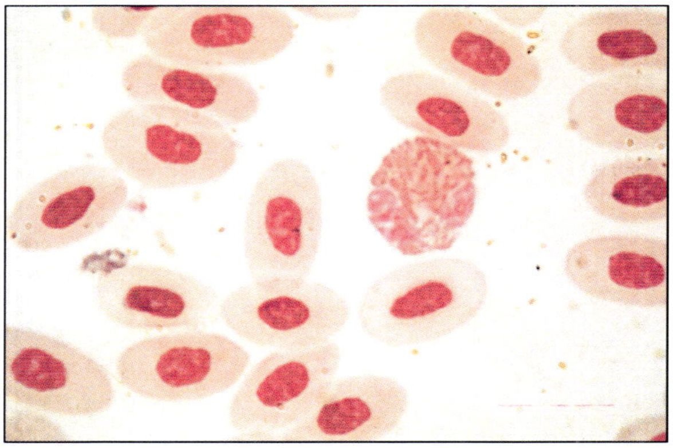

4.20 Blood (bird). Eosinophil. Leishman. ×480.

4.21

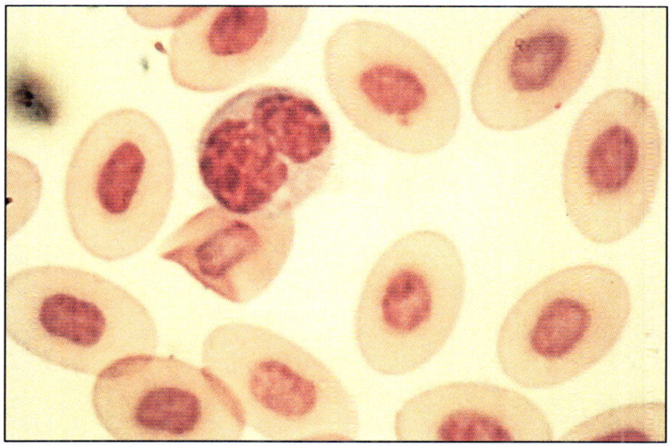

4.21 Blood (bird). Monocyte. Leishman. ×480.

.22

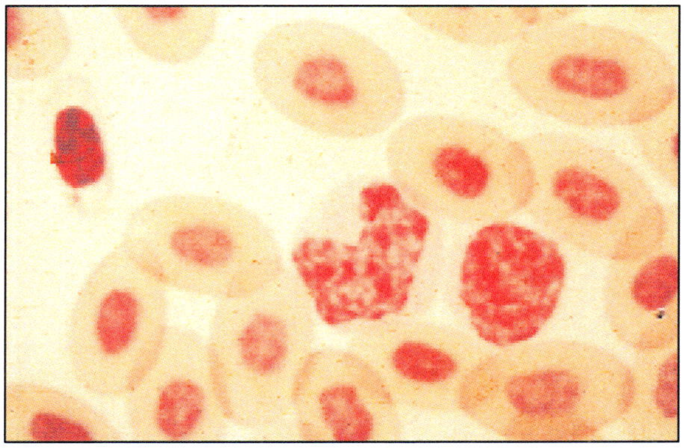

4.22 Blood (bird). Monocyte. Leishman. ×480.

Reptilian, amphibian and fish blood cells

The formed cellular components of amphibian and reptilian blood are similar to those present in avian blood. Erythrocytes are elongated and vary widely between species. The largest erythrocytes are found in the tuatara, *Sphenodon punctatus* (a quadruped reptile that superficially resembles a large lizard), and in some aquatic salamanders, particularly *Amphiuma* spp. In some instances the erythrocytes of animals are approximately 100 μm long and 20 μm wide. Generally, lizards and snakes possess smaller erythrocytes and leucocytes than do chelonians and crocodilians. However, there are individual variations between species.

Although all of the blood cells of fish, amphibians and reptiles retain their nuclei throughout their lifespans, true reticulocytes can be demonstrated by supravital staining (see 4.4). Because the blood cells retain their nuclei, it is not unusual to find both mitotic and amitotic division in stained films of peripheral blood from amphibians and reptiles. These cells in division usually reflect a response to blood loss and, thus, do not necessarily suggest neoplastic proliferation.

The leucocytes of amphibians and reptiles are also similar to those present in birds. The granulocytes include acidophils (amphiphils) comprising heterophils and eosinophils, the intracytoplasmic granules of which stain reddish-orange or muddy brown with Romanowsky dyes, are ovoid to distinctly spindle-shaped and possess pale blue lobed or unlobed nuclei that tend to be eccentrically placed. The heterophil is one of the major leucocytes that functions enzymatically in opsinization and chemotaxis in amphibians and reptiles. It is also capable of phagocytosing particulate matter, such as bacteria and cellular detritus. The percentage of heterophils in the differential leucocyte counts of reptiles and amphibians normally ranges widely from 2 to 65%, depending on the species, season of the year and sex of the animal from which they were obtained. Clinically, they usually range from 20 to 55%. The granules of eosinophils are spherical and stain deeply red with the identical dyes used to stain blood films of mammals and birds. In some instances, one or more giant red granules are found rather than dozens of smaller ones. The nuclei of eosinophils tend to be more centrally located and may be lobed, unlobed or concentric. Eosinophils may account for 0–10% (or more) of the differential leucocyte count of most reptiles. They increase during parasitism and other antigenic challenges. The basophil granulocytes are probably the most readily identified because of their uniformly dense and dark blue or purple staining. Their nuclei may be lobed or unlobed, and centrally or eccentrically located against the inner surface of the cell membrane. Basophils account for 0–10% of the leucocytes of most normal amphibians and reptiles.

Another granulocyte observed in amphibians and reptiles is the azurophil. This cell is characterized by its large, usually unlobed, nucleus composed of densely clumped chromatin and finely granular cytoplasm, which usually contains tiny azurophilic granules. Amphibian and reptilian azurophils are often called PMLs. In instances of bacteraemia, azurophils may engulf particulate matter. Azurophils account for approximately 2–10% of the differential cell count.

The mononuclear leucocytes of amphibians and reptiles include small and large lymphocytes, plasma cells and monocytes. Each of these cell types resembles its counterpart in mammals and birds.

Unlike mammals, for which the cellular component of the blood clotting mechanism involves nucleus-free platelets, fish, amphibians and reptiles possess nucleated thrombocytes. These elongated cells characteristically contain a pale blue, usually nongranular, cytoplasm and a single elongated central nucleus. Superficially, they resemble erythrocytes but they lack haemoglobin. Under certain conditions involving acute and chronic blood loss, thrombocytes display pluripotentiality: they can be transformed into erythrocytes. In doing so, they acquire increasing amounts of haemoglobin and may undergo mitotic or amitotic division. Like their leucocytic counterparts, the amphibian and reptilian thrombocytes can also serve as phagocytes and engulf bacteria and cellular detritus, including senescent erythrocytes.

Because they are nucleated, all of the cellular elements of amphibian and reptilian blood can be involved in haemopoietic neoplastic disorders (4.23), in addition to the many lymphoreticular and myelopoietic disorders that occur in mammals and birds.

4.23

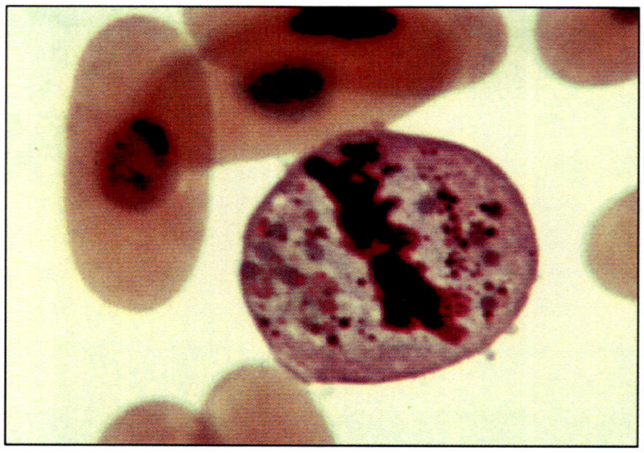

4.23 Baso-eosinophilic myelogenous leukaemia in a boa constrictor (*Boa C. constrictor*). Note the dual population of eosinophilic and basophilic granules that characterize a clonal population of neoplastic granulocytic leucocytes. Wright's. ×625.

4.24

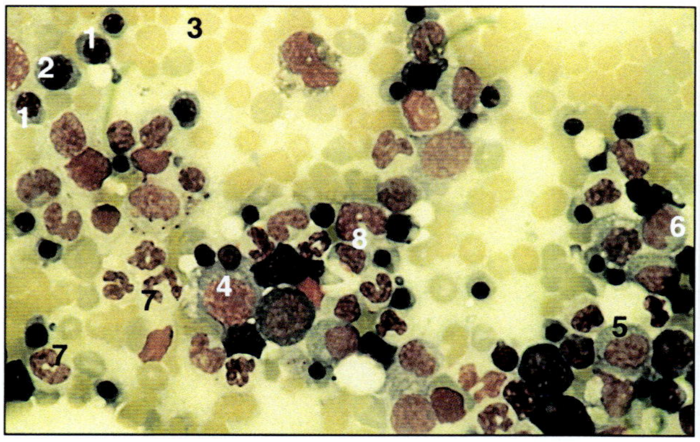

4.24 Bone marrow (dog). (1) Basophilic erythroblast, prorubricyte. (2) Polychromatophil erythroblast, rubricyte. (3) Erythrocytes. (4) Myeloblast. (5) Promyelocyte. (6) Myelocyte. (7) Polymorphonuclear leucocytes. (8) Monocyte. Giemsa. ×250.

4.25

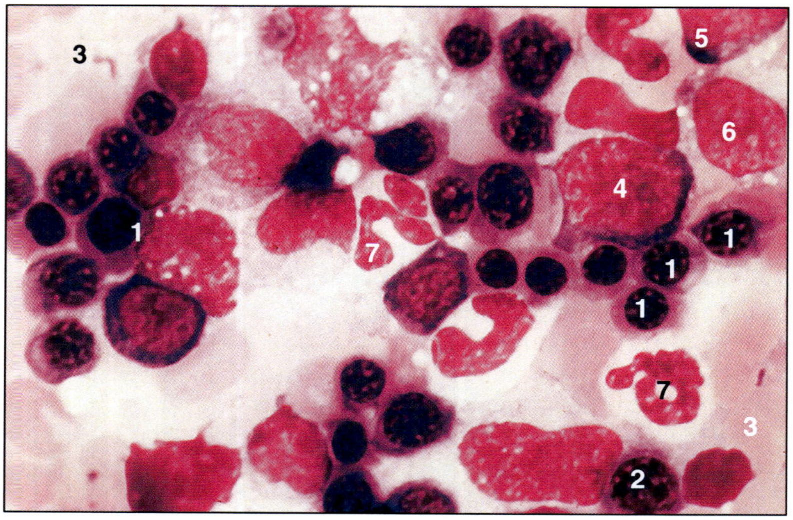

4.25 Bone marrow (dog). (1) Basophilic erythroblast, prorubricyte. (2) Polychromatophil erythroblast, rubricyte. (3) Erythrocytes. (4) Myeloblast. (5) Promyelocyte. (6) Myelocyte. (7) Polymorphonuclear leucocytes. Giemsa. ×500.

Bone marrow: production of blood cells

Haemopoietic tissue located in the adult bone marrow is responsible for the production of red cells, granular and agranular white cells, and platelets. The precursors of these cells are present in bone marrow (all of which derive originally from the multipotential stem cell, the haemocytoblast), but as they develop the individual characteristics of each cell type predominate and the various stages may be identified (4.24–4.29).

4.26

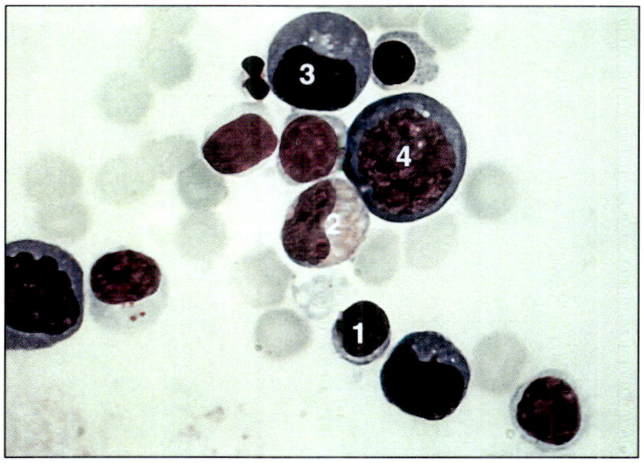

4.26 Bone marrow (dog). (1) Basophilic erythroblast, prorubricyte. (2) Polychromatophil erythroblast, rubricyte. (3) Promyelocyte. (4) Myelocyte. Giemsa. ×480.

.27

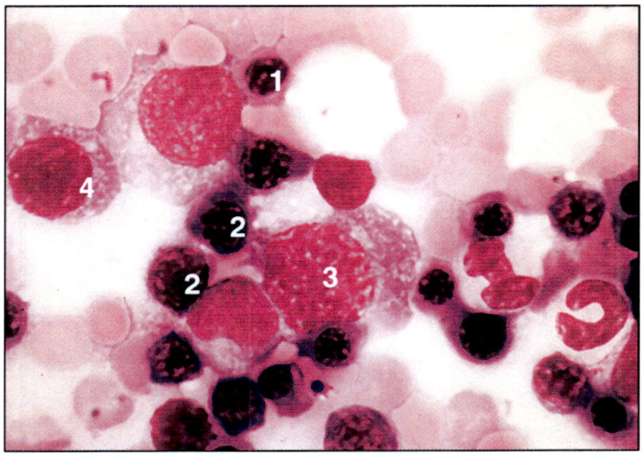

4.27 Bone marrow (dog). (1) Basophilic erythroblast, prorubricyte. (2) Polychromatophil erythroblast, rubricyte. (3) Promyelocyte. (4) Myelocyte. Giemsa. ×480.

4.28

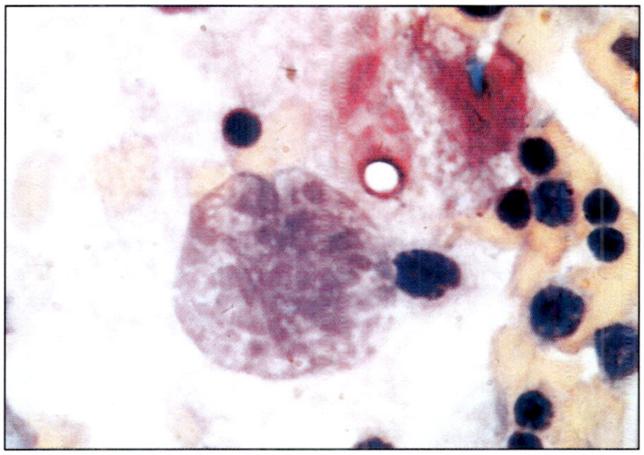

4.28 Megakaryocyte. Bone marrow (dog). Giemsa. ×480.

4.29 Red bone marrow (dog). (1) Megakaryocytes are separated by haemopoietic tissue. (2) Blood vessel. Giemsa. ×250.

4.29

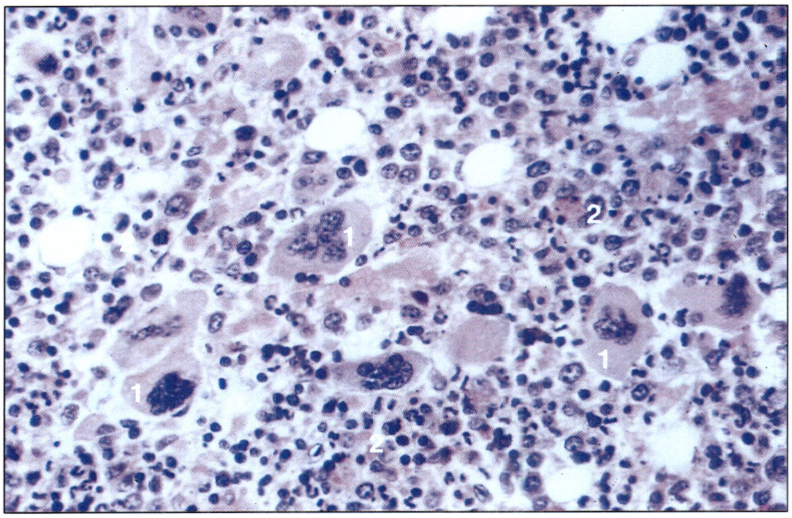

The erythrocyte series begins with the rubriblast (proerythroblast), a large cell with a large clear nucleus with two nucleoli in a basophilic cytoplasm. The prorubricyte (basophilic erythroblast) is smaller, with a dense nucleus and diffuse basophilic cytoplasm. The rubricyte (polychromatophilic erythroblast) has a dense nucleus in grey-pink cytoplasm, which is caused by the synthesis of haemoglobin. There are no further cell divisions; the nucleus condenses, the haemoglobin content of the cytoplasm increases and the cell is called a metarubricyte (normoblast). The nucleus then becomes extruded and the cell becomes a reticulocyte (an immature form of erythrocyte), small numbers of which are present in circulating blood.

A similar series forms the granulocytes, beginning with the myeloblast, a large cell with a clear nucleus and a pale rim of agranular cytoplasm. This divides and forms the promyelocyte, a very large cell with a large clear nucleus and some granules in the basophilic cytoplasm. The myelocyte is a markedly smaller cell. The deeply indented nucleus is eccentrically disposed in the cytoplasm, and specific granules indicate the type of leucocyte. Late metamyelocytes have a band nucleus; again, these are found in the circulating blood. The mature leucocyte has a lobed nucleus.

Where haemopoietic tissue predominates, with small amounts of adipose tissue, the active marrow is red in appearance (**4.24**, **4.25** and **4.29**). Where adipose tissue predominates the inactive marrow is yellow (**4.30**). Blood sinusoids lined by reticuloendothelial cells are present in marrow (**4.30**).

Lymphopoiesis is complicated by the fact that although lymphocytes arise from stem cells in the bone marrow, they become two separate and functionally different cell populations: T lymphocytes and B lymphocytes. T lymphocytes from the thymus are segregated from the blood by the thymic barrier and are responsible for cell-mediated immunity. When they leave the thymus T lymphocytes are found in diffuse sites in secondary lymphatic tissue, such as the paracortex of a lymph node. The B lymphocytes are present in bone marrow. As a result of antigen stimulus (the humeral response), they become plasma cells and produce immunoglobulin.

4.30

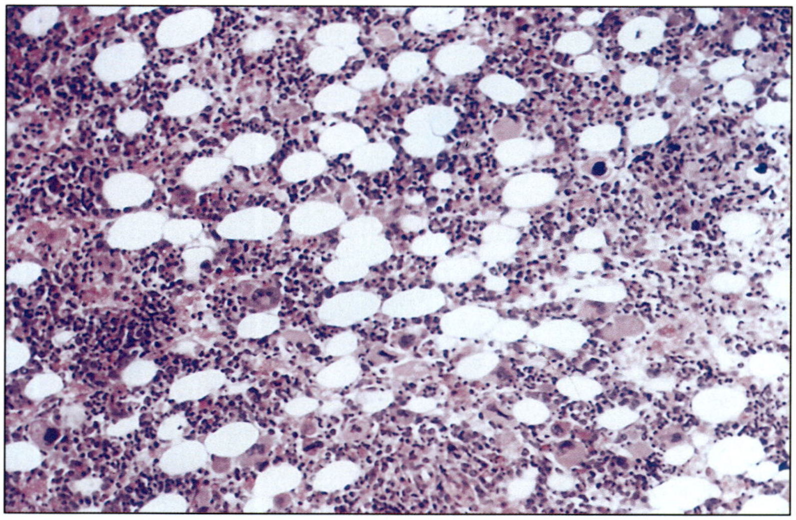

4.30 Yellow bone marrow (dog). The empty spaces indicate the site of the fat cells. Giemsa. ×250.

Clinical correlates

Disorders of the blood can be attributed to abnormalities in production of blood cells from the bone marrow or other central blood-forming organs or to abnormal loss or consumption of these cells. Anaemia, the deficiency of oxygen-carrying erythrocytes, can be regenerative (i.e. the bone marrow is able to respond by releasing new cells, including immature cells into the circulation) or non-regenerative (in which this response does not occur). A blood film that illustrates haemolytic anaemia in a dog is shown in **4.31**. In this regenerative anaemia there is variation in cell size (anisocytosis) with red cell precursors, such as the large, stippled reticulocyte (1) and nucleated normoblast (2), visible. Some of the red cells have small, dense dots (Howell–Jolly bodies), which represent remnants of nuclear chromatin and are characteristic of regenerative anaemias. Spherocytes, red cells that have lost their biconcave shape and become globular due to immunological attack, are present (3). There is an increased neutrophil count with some immature neutrophils (reactive neutrophilia with a left shift), which typically accompanies haemolysis. These findings are diagnostic of autoimmune haemolytic anaemia, the most common type of anaemia in the dog.

In immune-mediated anaemia, erythrocyte destruction follows the attachment of antibody to the cell membrane. In most cases the aetiology is unknown.

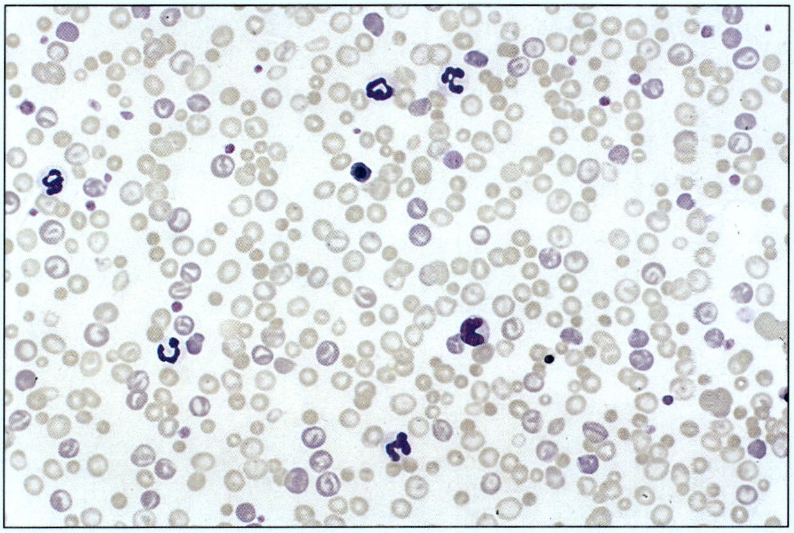

4.31

4.31 Haemolytic (regenerative) anaemia in a dog. Note the variation in appearance of the red cells. Reticulocytes, nucleated normoblasts and spherocytes are present. Giemsa. ×200.

The blood film in 4.32 was prepared from a dog with acute lymphoblastic leukaemia. Very high numbers of malignant lymphoblasts, which are larger than normal lymphocytes and have bluer cytoplasm, are seen. In some cases of leukaemia, although the bone marrow is invaded by neoplastic haemopoietic cells, no abnormal cells are released into the peripheral blood. Such cases may be termed aleukaemic leukaemias. Non-regenerative anaemia is a common finding with many leukaemias.

The liver of a cat in which the sinusoids (vascular channels) are heavily infiltrated by large neoplastic megakaryocytes with multilobed nuclei is shown in 4.33. This is megakaryocytic myelosis, a rare, chronic disease of dogs and cats characterized clinically by bleeding and thrombosis of the ear and tail tips.

4.32

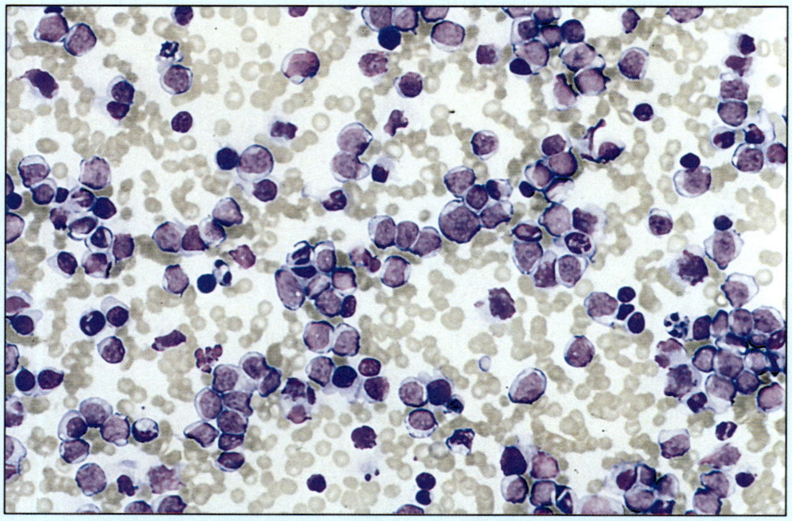

4.32 Acute lymphoblastic leukaemia (dog) showing large numbers of malignant lymphoblasts. Giemsa. ×255.

4.33

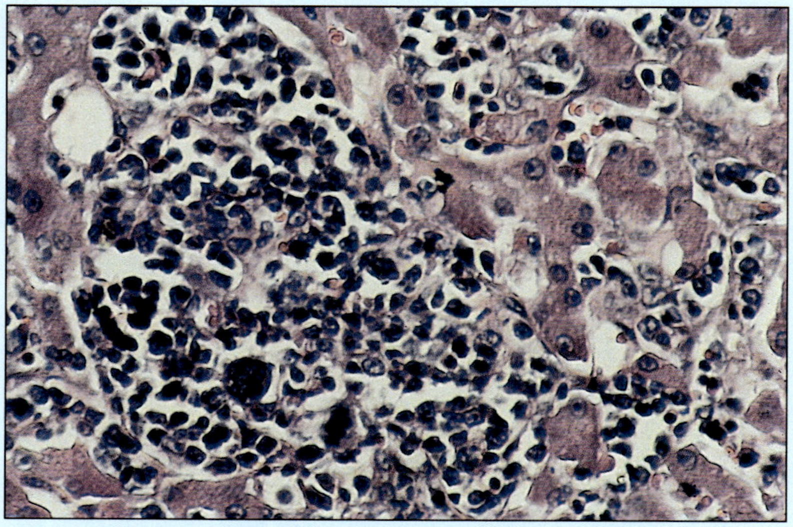

4.33 Megakaryocytic myelosis in the liver of a cat. Note the megakaryocyte with the multilobed nuclei in the cellular infiltrate. H & E. ×255.

Avian bone

A unique feature of avian bone in egg-producing birds is the accumulation of spiculated bone in the medullary cavity, under the combined influence of oestrogens and androgens. This medullary bone is particularly labile and the stored calcium is utilized in the formation of the calcareous egg shell. The medullary bone is basophilic and decreases during shell deposition and increases at other times. The basophilia is caused by a change in the density of the matrix and in the glycosaminoglycans that are present. During resorption, osteoclasts are active; during deposition, osteoblasts are prominent on the surface of the bone spicules (4.34 and 4.35).

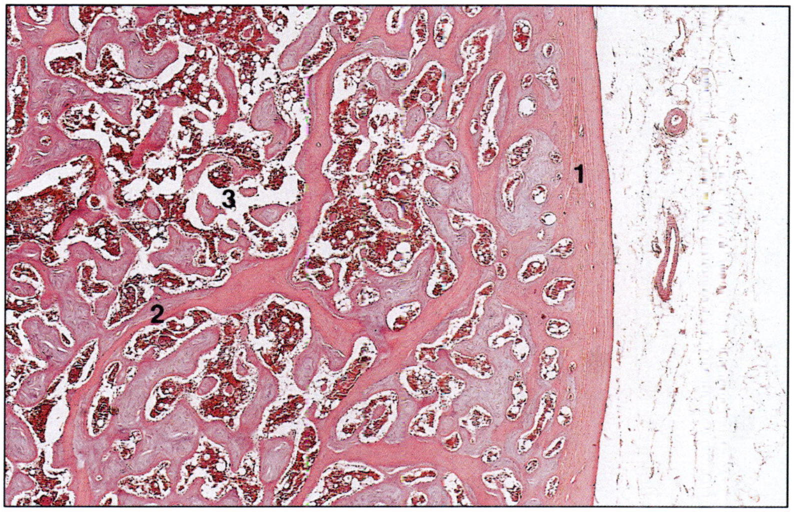

4.34 Head of the humerus (domestic hen). (1) Outer layer of eosinophilic cortical bone. (2) The spiculated medullary bone is basophilic. (3) The marrow cavity is lined by osteoblasts. H & E. ×62.5.

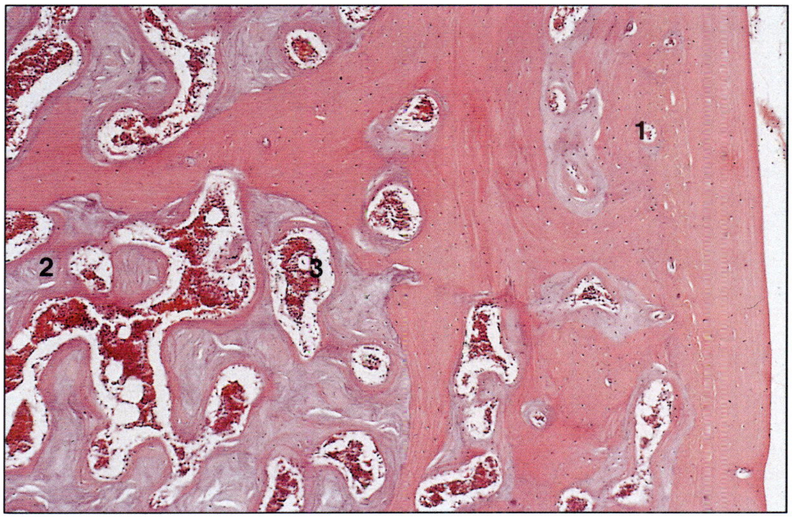

4.35 Head of the humerus (domestic hen). (1) The osteocytes in the eosinophilic cortical bone form an osteon. (2) Osteocytes in the open lacunae of the basophilic medullary bone. (3) Marrow cavity lined by osteoblasts H & E. ×125.

Reptilian, amphibian and fish bone and bone marrow

Reptiles do not possess pneumatized bone such as that found in birds capable of flight. The box-like carapace and plastron of chelonians are composed of specialized bone that must be both strong and relatively lightweight in order for this bone to protect efficiently the delicate internal structures. Compressional stresses applied to the dorsal and ventral surfaces are distributed widely and are then borne upon buttress-like vertical supporting pillars of bone that are at each end of the 'bridge' that joins the carapace to the plastron on each side. The strength of their shells is further enhanced by the curved shape and by additional internal struts that distribute compressive forces so that they are not concentrated onto a single focus. The shell is composed of parallel layers of inner and outer tables of compact bone with an intervening layer of spongy cancellous bone characterized by spaces filled with bone marrow. In form and function the bony shell resembles the calvaria that covers the brain case of a mammalian skull.

The bone of amphibians and reptiles contains numerous sites of haemopoiesis; long bones (*see* 3.29), ribs, skull and mandibles are locations in which active blood cell formation normally occurs. During severe blood loss and a few other conditions, sites other than bone marrow are recruited for extramedullary haemopoiesis; liver, spleen and kidney are then most often involved.

In fish, the major organ of haemopoietic activity is the cranial pole of each kidney (*see* Chapter 9), with lesser amounts occurring in other extramedullary sites during times of severe anaemia, infection or stress.

The presence of numerous megakaryocytes in the splenic red pulp is a common finding in the healthy house mouse, *Mus musculus*, whereas extramedullary haemopoiesis is usually considered an abnormal finding in most other animals (**4.36**).

4.36

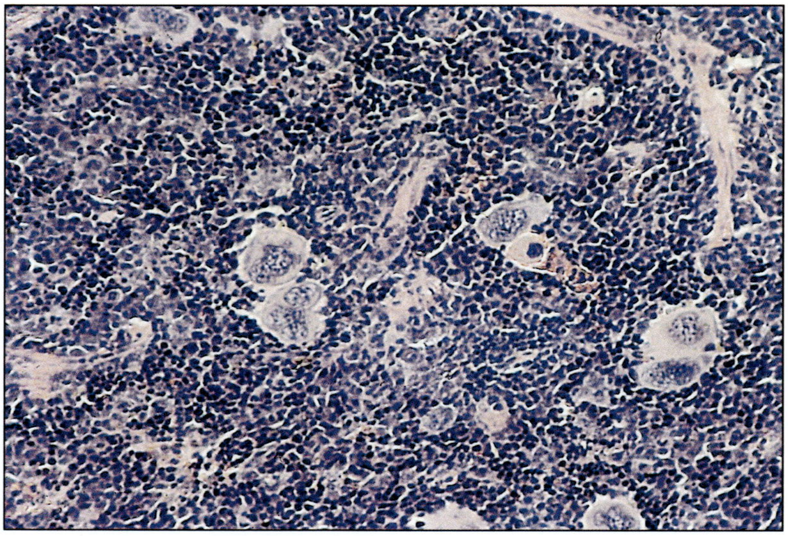

4.36 Extramedullary haemopoiesis in the spleen of a domestic mouse (*Mus musculus*). Note the multinucleated megakaryocytes which are normal in murine splenic tissue. H & E. ×125.

5. MUSCLE

Contractility, a fundamental property of cytoplasm, is developed to a highly specialized degree in muscle tissue. The elongated muscle cell is commonly referred to as a muscle fibre, the plasma membrane as the sarcolemma and the cytoplasm as the sarcoplasm. There are basically two types of muscle: smooth, visceral or involuntary muscle; and striated muscle, which is further subdivided into skeletal voluntary muscle and cardiac involuntary muscle.

Muscle contraction depends upon the proteins actin and myosin in the sarcoplasm. In skeletal and cardiac muscle the longitudinal arrangement of these proteins is aligned in register to give cross-striations, which are absent from smooth muscle.

Muscle types

Smooth muscle

Smooth muscle cells are elongated fusiform fibres (2–50 μm long) with a single, centrally located nucleus with several nucleoli. These fibres may occur singly, as in the lamina propria of intestinal villi, but are more commonly arranged in sheets or layers in the walls of a wide range of tubes of the alimentary, urogenital, respiratory and cardiovascular systems. The fibres are packed in a staggered fashion with the thickest nucleated portion of one fibre juxtaposed to the thin tapered end of an adjoining one. Individual smooth muscle fibres are supported by reticular fibres, with collagen and elastic fibres forming a supporting framework of connective tissue carrying blood vessels and nerves. Smooth muscle is under involuntary control; it is innervated by the autonomic nervous system (5.1–5.3).

5.1

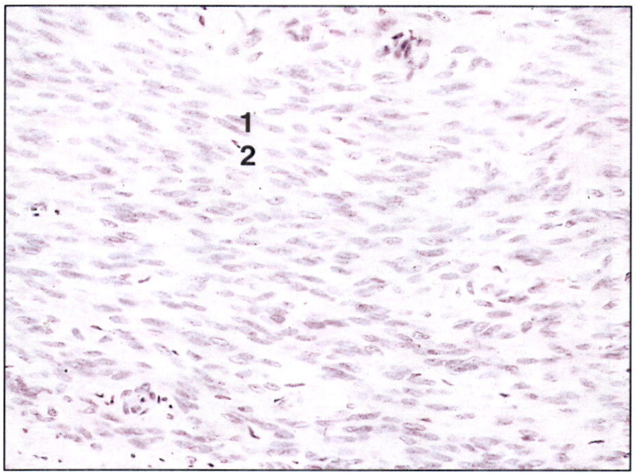

5.1 Smooth muscle. Uterus (cat). (1) Nucleus. (2) Sarcoplasm. H & E. ×100.

5.2

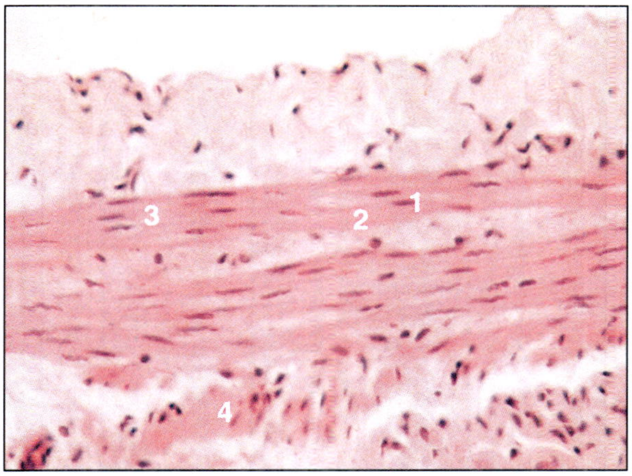

5.2 Smooth muscle. Uterus (cat). (1) Nucleus. (2) Sarcoplasm. (3) Longitudinal fibres. (4) Transverse fibres. H & E. ×200.

5.3

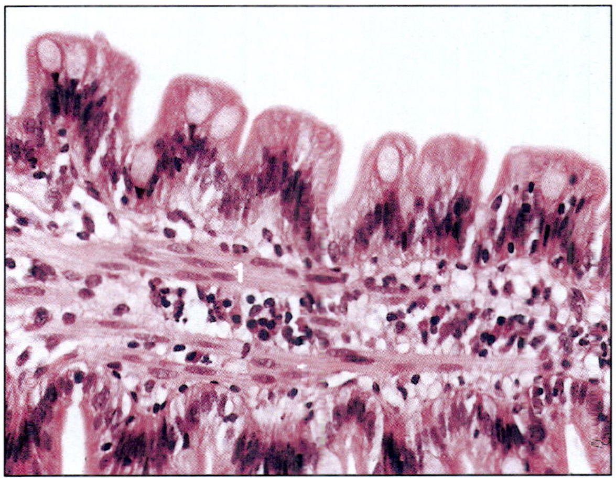

5.3 Smooth muscle. Duodenum (dog). (1) Fusiform smooth muscle fibre. H & E. ×200.

Striated (skeletal) muscle

Skeletal muscle fibres are multinucleated giant cells that range in length from a few millimetres to several centimetres. The nuclei lie immediately beneath the sarcolemma, and the myofibrils give both a longitudinal and a cross-striation arrangement. The contractile myofilaments are arranged in alternating isotropic I bands and anisotropic A bands. This imparts the cross-striated effect.

Skeletal muscle fibres are bound into large bundles by an outer connective tissue investment, the epimysium. This dips into the muscle and invests bundles of muscle fibres (fascicles) in connective

5.4 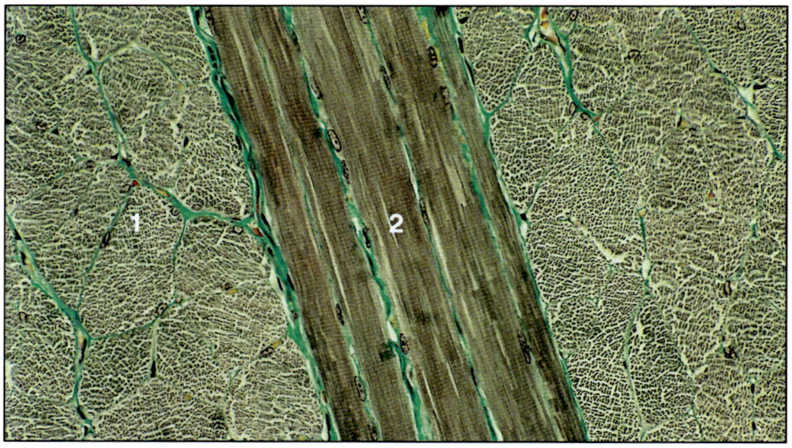

5.4 Striated muscle. Tongue (ox). (1) Transverse section (TS) muscle fibres. (2) Longitudinal section (LS) muscle fibres. Masson's trichrome. ×125.

5.5 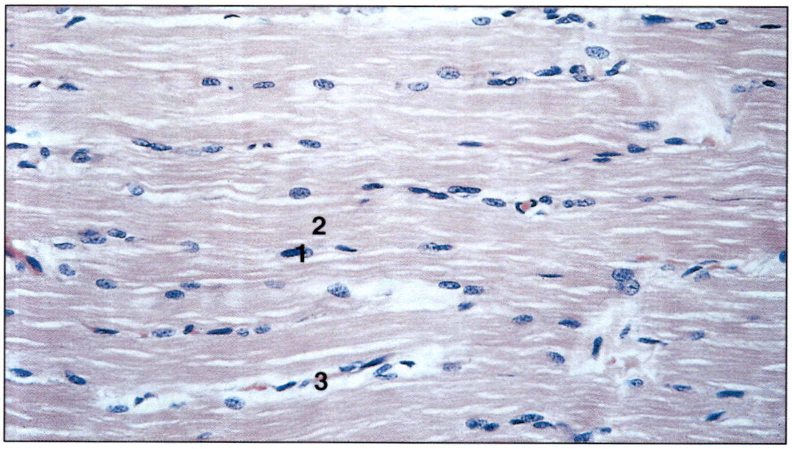

5.5 Striated muscle. Tongue (cat). (1) Nucleus. (2) Sarcoplasm. (3) Endomysium. H & E. ×200.

5.6 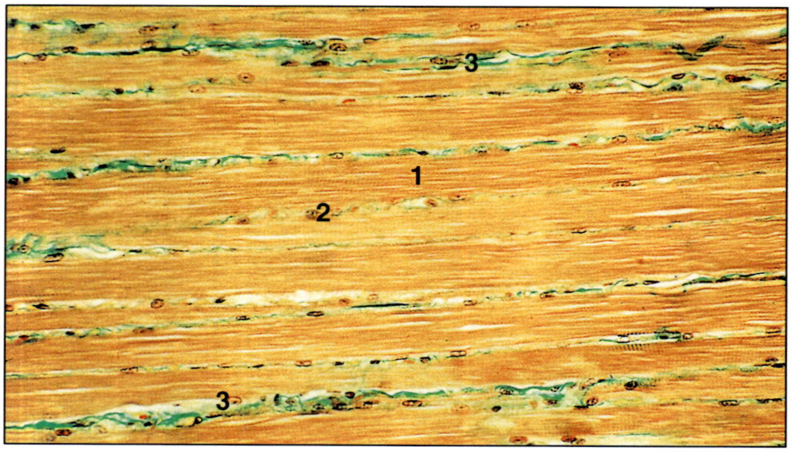

5.6 LS striated muscle. Tongue (cat). (1) Longitudinal striated muscle. (2) Nuclei. (3) Endomysium stained green. Masson's trichrome. ×200.

tissue, the perimysium. This in turn invests each muscle fibre in a vascular loose connective tissue, the endomysium. A fine network of reticular fibres lies against the sarcolemma. The collagen fibres of the tendon extend into the epimysium and allow muscular contraction to effect movement (5.4–5.9).

Every skeletal muscle fibre receives an axon terminal from a motor neuron at the myoneural junction, the motor endplate (see 13.27). Muscle spindles, which are attenuated skeletal muscle fibres, act as stretch receptors that are innervated both by motor and by sensory nerve terminals.

5.7

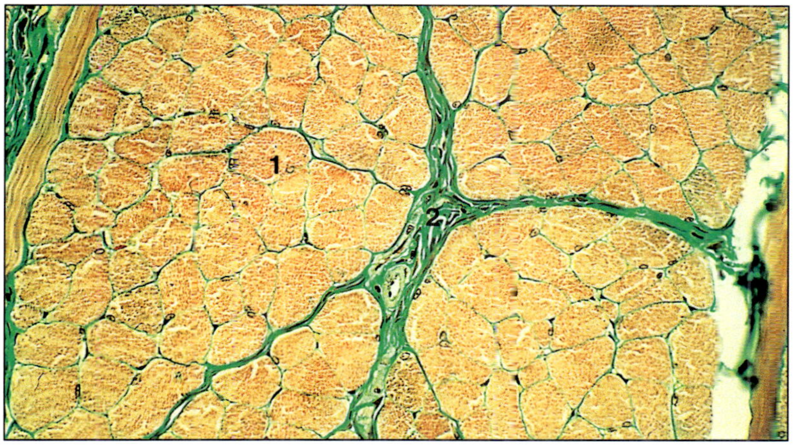

5.7 TS striated muscle. Tongue (cat). (1) Transverse section of muscle fibres. (2) Connective tissue perimysium. Masson's trichrome. ×62.5.

5.8

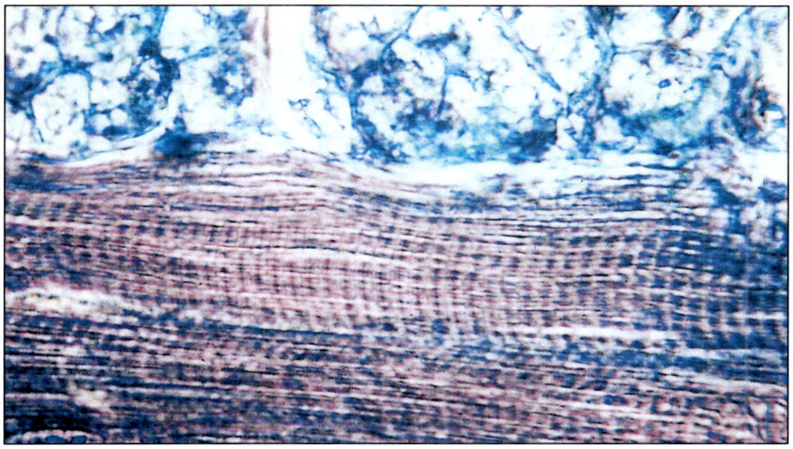

5.8 Striated muscle. Tongue (ox). Muscle fibres showing cross-striations. Masson's trichrome. ×625.

5.9

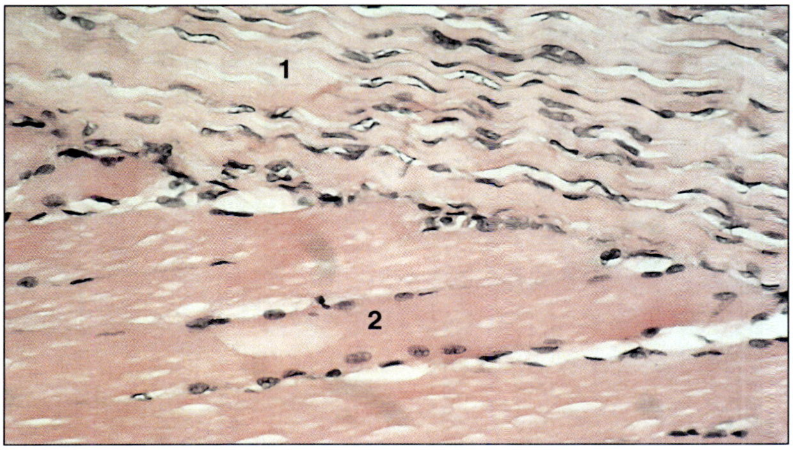

5.9 Tendon/muscle junction (dog). (1) Collagen fibres of the tendon. (2) Striated muscle fibres. H & E. ×200.

Cardiac muscle (myocardium)

Cardiac muscle is exclusive to the myocardium, the muscular wall of the heart. The fibres are smaller than skeletal muscle fibres and branch repeatedly (**5.10**). The nucleus lies in the centre of the fibre (occasionally two nuclei are present) and the fibres have strong areas of attachment at the intercalated disc. These are visible as a dark cross-striation at the end of one fibre and the beginning of the next, and confer structural integrity on the heart muscle to allow contraction to spread throughout the myocardium (**5.11** and **5.12**). These are represented at the ultrastructural level by tight junctions and gap junctions. The cardiac conducting system is composed of several specialized muscle fibres in the sinoatrial and atrioventricular nodes. In the sinoatrial node (**5.13**, **5.14**), small cardiac muscle fibres, which are low in myofilaments, have an intrinsic ability to contract at a species-specific rate and act as the pacemaker for cardiac muscle contraction. The atrial wave of depolarization converges on the second node, the atrioventricular node, from where specialized large muscle fibres spread throughout the ventricular muscle and initiate contraction. These specialized conducting fibres are binucleate and the nucleus lies in a clear area of sarcoplasm (**5.15**).

The various types of muscle tissue can be discerned, even in invertebrates low on the phylogenetic scale. For example, the striated muscle fibres of a spider are structurally similar to those found in mammals and the multiple heart-like pumping chambers that circulate the haemolymph and

5.10

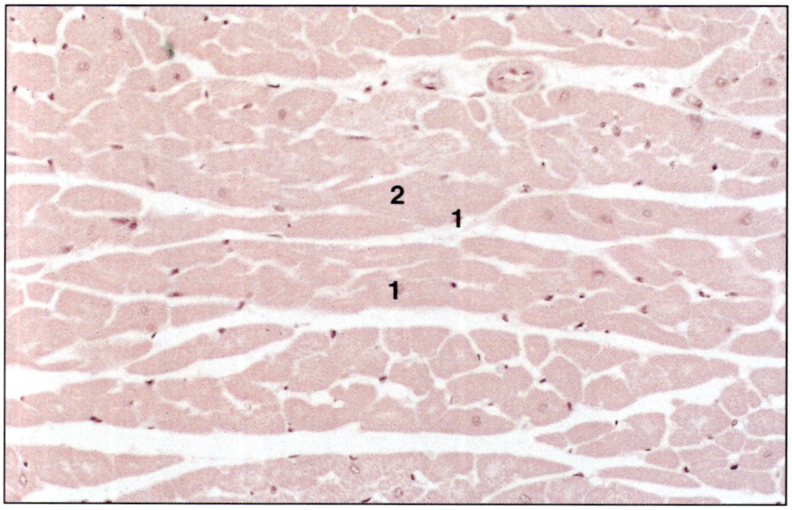

5.10 Cardiac muscle (horse). (1) Nucleus of the muscle fibre. (2) Sarcoplasm. H &.E. ×125.

5.11

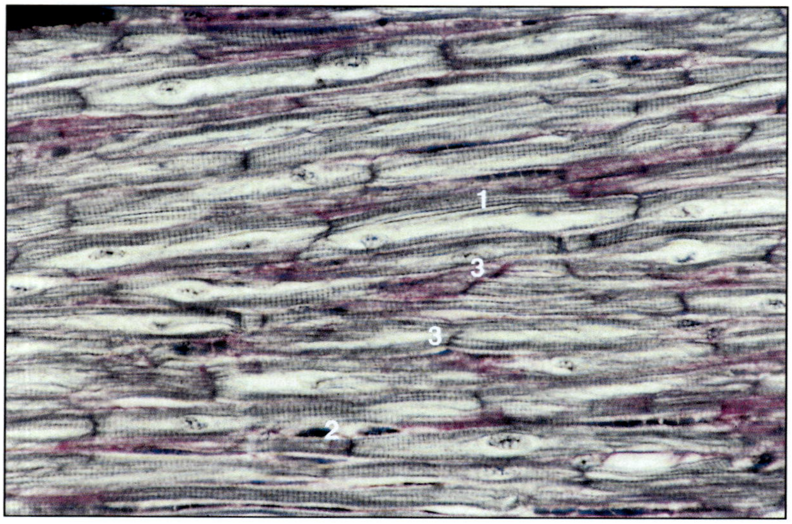

5.11 Cardiac muscle (horse). (1) Cardiac muscle fibre. (2) Vascular connective tissue of the endomysium. (3) Intercalated disc. Heidenhain's iron haematoxylin. ×625.

haemolymphocytes through the coelom of earthworms are formed from myocardium.

As all fish and amphibians and most reptiles (all except the crocodilians) possess a three-chambered heart with paired atria and a single ventricle, there are some structural differences between the hearts of these animals. For example, a ridge of myocardium helps direct the flow of blood through the ventricle so as to reduce the mixing of oxygenated and deoxygenated blood in non-crocodilian reptiles. Blood flow through twin aortic arches and atrioventricular valves is controlled by typical heart valve leaflets composed of myxoid connective tissue that are covered by a thin endothelial lining in all vertebrates.

5.12

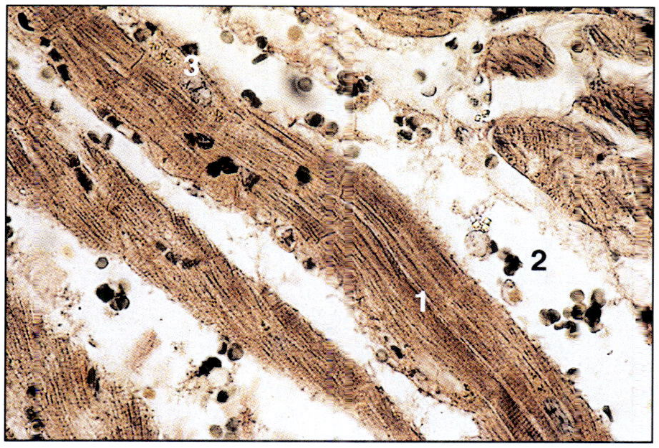

5.12 Cardiac muscle (horse). (1) Cardiac muscle fibre. (2) Vascular connective tissue of the endomysium. (3) Intercalated disc. Heidenhain's iron haematoxylin. ×200.

5.13

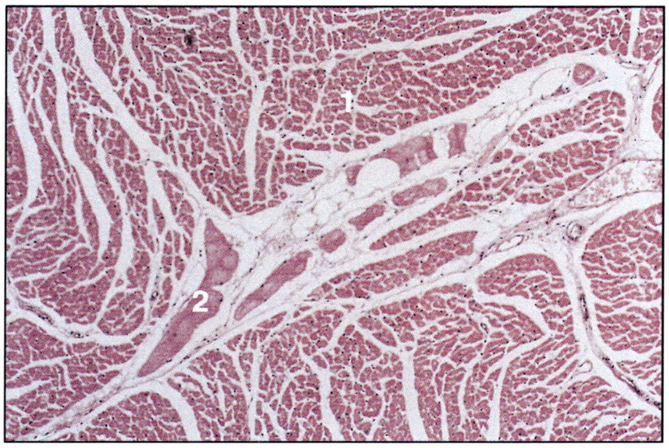

5.13 Cardiac muscle (horse). (1) Cardiac muscle. (2) Purkinje's fibres. H & E. ×62.5.

5.14

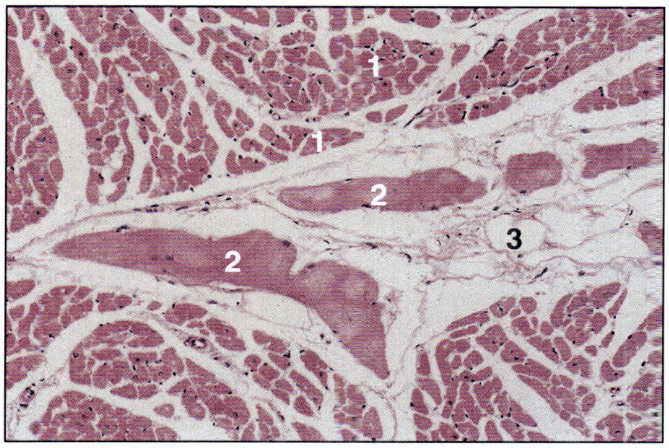

5.14. Cardiac muscle (horse). (1) Cardiac muscle. (2) Purkinje's fibres. (3) Loose vascular connective tissue. H & E. ×125.

5.15

5.15 Cardiac muscle (horse). (1) Endocardium. (2) Impulse-conducting fibres (Purkinje's fibres). (3) Muscle fibre. H & E. ×125.

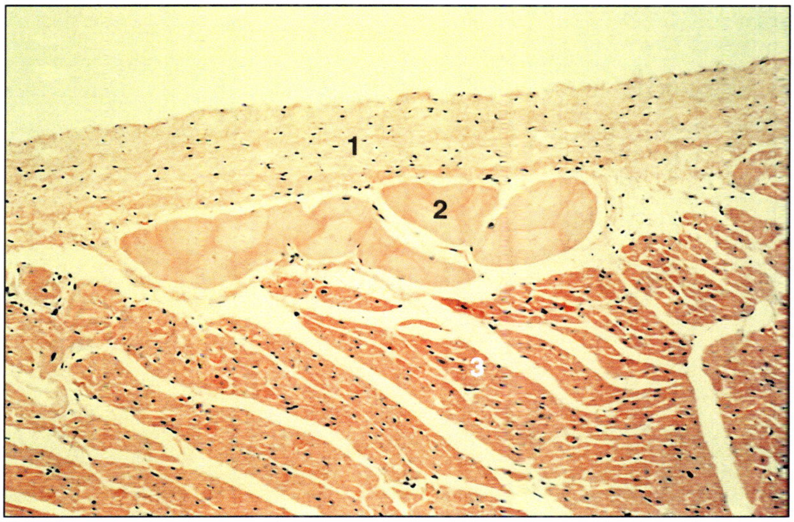

Clinical correlates

Myopathies, primary disorders of muscle structure, may be congenital, metabolic or inflammatory. Viral, bacterial, fungal, parasitic, protozoal and metazoal agents can be implicated in infective myopathies.

Where there is frank inflammation the disease would be termed a myositis. In eosinophilic myositis, a condition that affects the masticatory muscles of dogs, in particular in the German Shepherd breed (**5.16**), the affected muscle is diffusely infiltrated by numerous eosinophils accompanied by lesser numbers of lymphocytes and other inflammatory cells. There is muscle degeneration and atrophy. Production of abnormal antibodies which attack these muscles is believed to initiate the process, which then becomes dominated by a cellular response. Progressive destruction of these muscles leads to fixation of the jaws.

Other non-neoplastic conditions that affect the muscle may be loosely divided into neuropathies which result from disturbance of innervation and myasthenic conditions of the motor end plate. Muscle atrophy (reduction in cross-sectional area of the muscle fibres) will tend to occur.

Under certain circumstances, all types of muscle can be vulnerable to pathological deposition of mineral salts. This may be induced by conditions characterized by persistent hypercalcaemia (see **6.28**) or at sites of previous injury.

Primary neoplasms of muscle are quite rare with malignant tumours (rhabdomyosarcoma, **5.17**) outnumbering benign ones (rhabdomyoma). Muscle can also be affected by neoplasms of associated connective tissue origin.

5.16

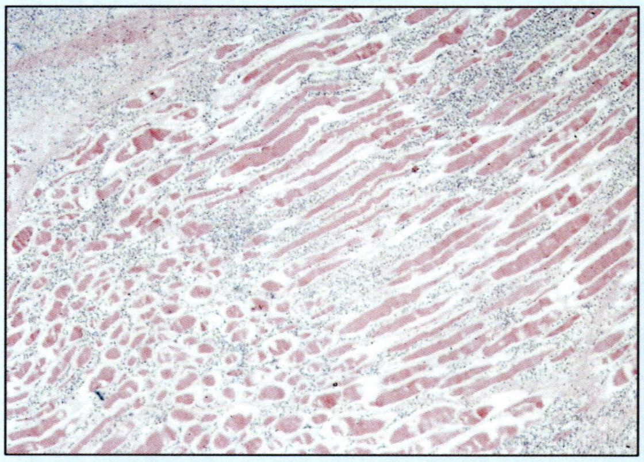

5.16 Eosinophilic myositis. Masticatory muscles from a dog. Phosphotungstic acid haematoxylin. ×125.

5.17

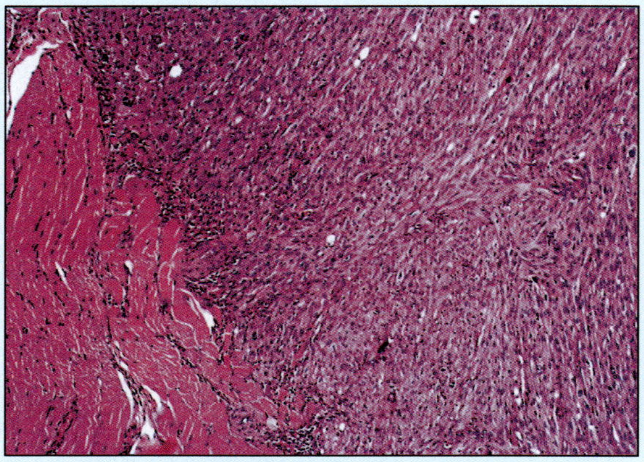

5.17 Rhabdomyosarcoma in a 10-year-old male cat. Large, rather pleomorphic, elongate to strap-like cells invade and replace skeletal muscle. These tumours, although uncommon, are highly malignant. H & E. ×100.

6. CARDIOVASCULAR SYSTEM

The mammalian circulatory system is a closed system of tubes with an endothelial lining from the heart through the arteries into the capillaries and back through the veins.

Arteries

Arteries are the conducting channels conveying blood from the heart to the capillary bed. There are three types of artery: elastic, muscular (distributing) and arteriole. The arterial wall has a common structure: tunica intima (inner lining layer), tunica media (middle layer) and tunica adventitia (outer layer; 6.1 and 6.2). The tunica intima consists of elongated flattened endothelial cells resting on loose areolar connective tissue.

The tunica media of the elastic arteries has a high proportion of concentric lamellae of fenestrated elastic fibres interspersed with smooth

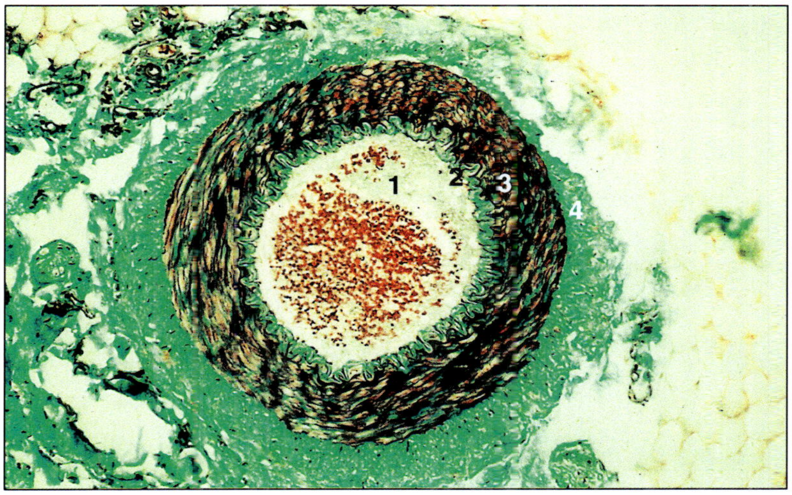

6.1

6.1 Artery (dog). (1) Lumen. (2) Tunica intima. (3) Tunica media. (4) Tunica adventitia. Masson's trichrome. ×62.5.

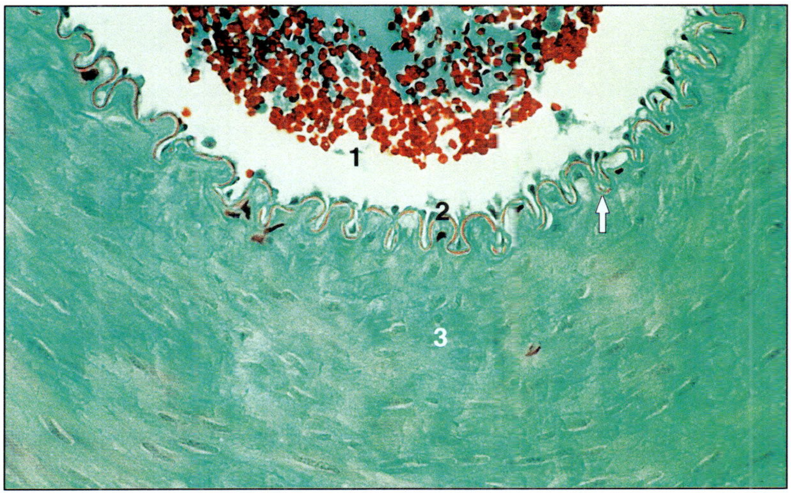

6.2

6.2 Artery (dog). (1) Lumen. (2) Tunica intima with the internal elastic lamina (arrowed). (3) Tunica media. Masson's trichrome. ×125.

6.3

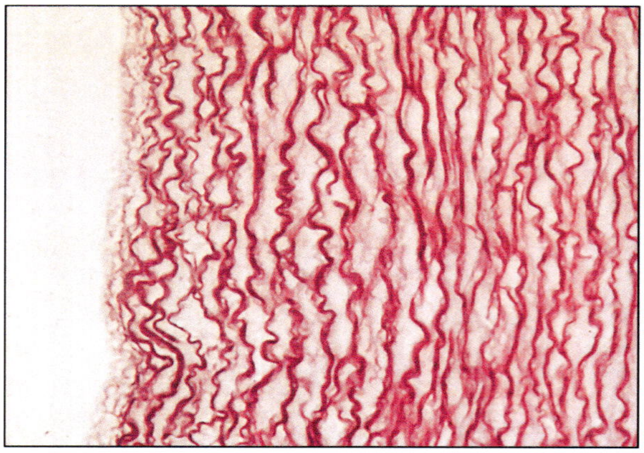

6.3 Aorta (horse). Elastic artery stained to illustrate the wavy elastic fibres. Weigert's elastin. ×100.

muscle fibres (**6.3**). These allow the vessels to dilate. The recoil sends the blood onwards, creating the pulse in the major elastic artery, the aorta.

In muscular (distributing) arteries, the elastic content is reduced and the smooth muscle increased. Internal and external elastic lamina are present (**6.2** and **6.4–6.6**).

The arterioles (**6.7**) reduce the pressure of the blood and supply the capillary bed. The tunica media may consist of only one layer of smooth muscle cells, and the luminal diameter is less than the thickness of the wall (**6.8**). The tunica adventitia is composed of collagen and elastic fibres, and contains the vasa vasorum, the small nutrient arteries and veins in the walls of the larger blood vessels.

6.4

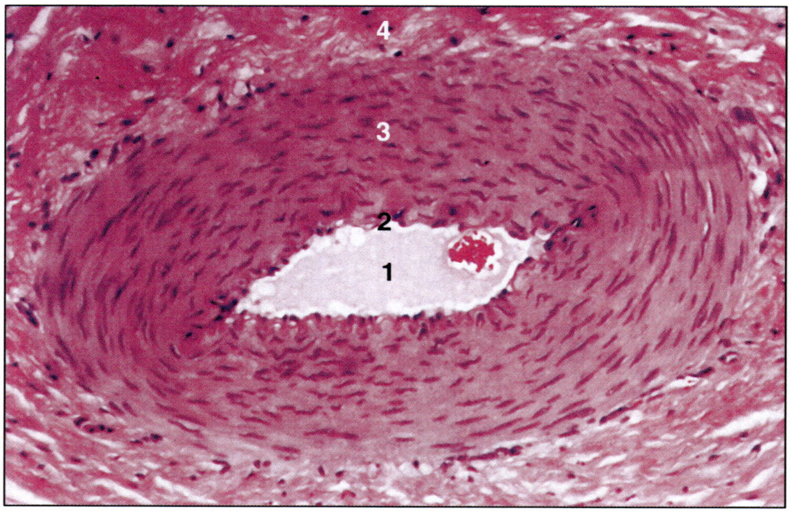

6.4 Muscular artery (sheep). (1) Lumen. (2) Tunica intima with the internal elastic lamina. (3) Tunica media. (4) Tunica adventitia. H & E. ×125.

6.5

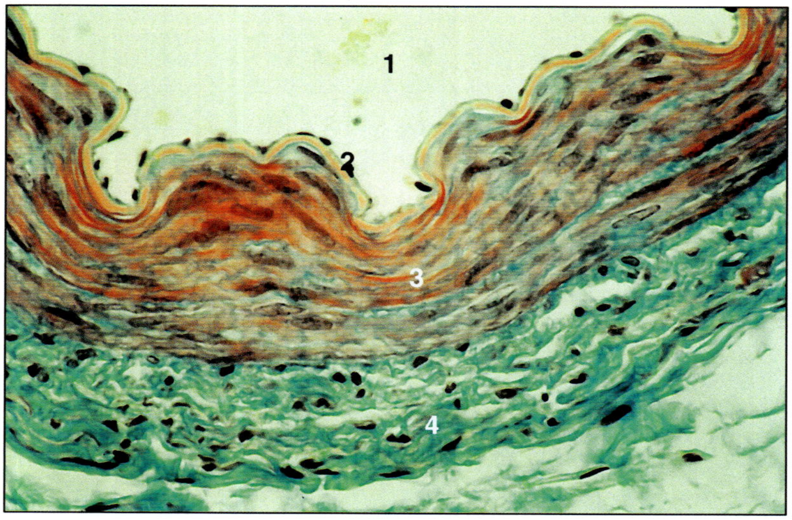

6.5 Muscular artery (sheep). (1) Lumen. (2) Tunica intima. (3) Tunica media. (4) Tunica adventitia. Masson's trichrome. ×250.

6.6 Artery and vein. Stomach (dog). (1) Small artery. (2) Small vein. (3) Lymphatic vessel. H & E. ×62.5.

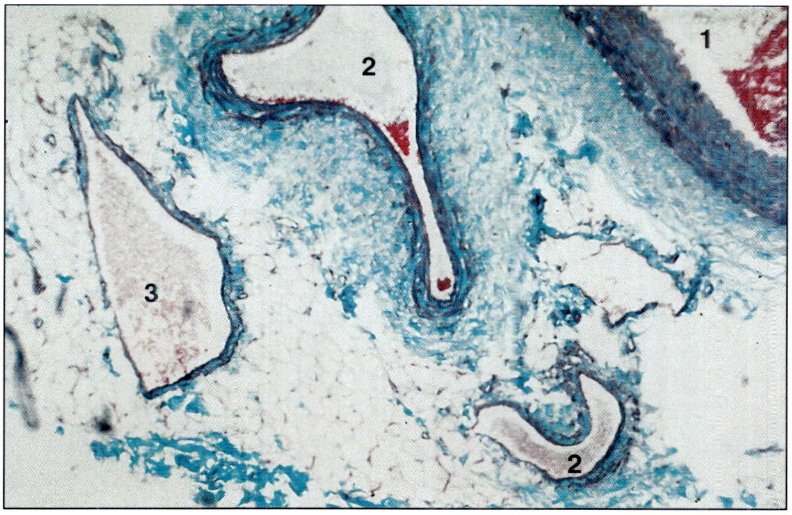

6.6

6.7 Arteriole, vein and a lymphatic vessel in connective tissue. Tongue (ox). (1) Arteriole. (2) Vein. (3) Lymphatic vessel. H & E. ×62.5.

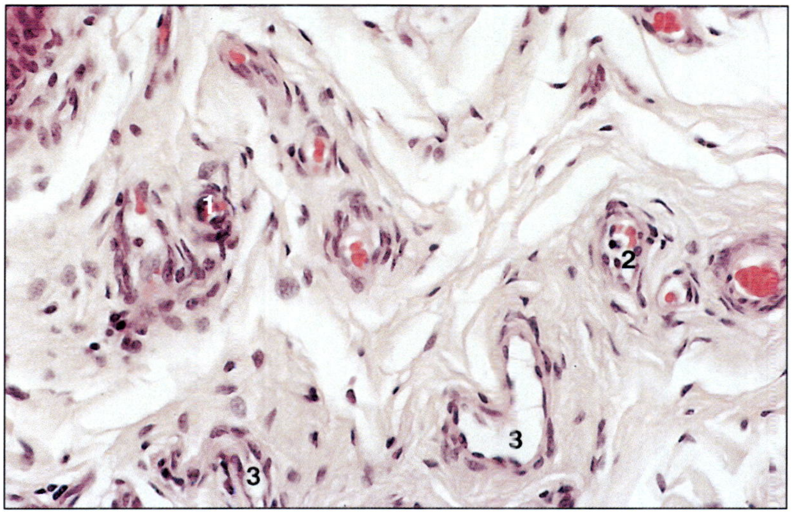

6.7

6.8 Arterioles in the wall of a small artery (horse). (1) Arteriole. (2) Veins. (3) Artery. H & E. ×160.

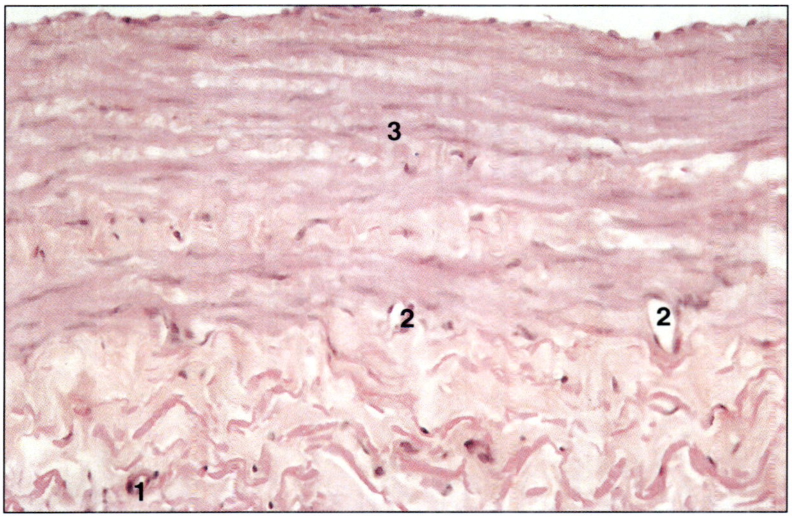

6.8

Capillaries and venules

The capillary is the smallest unit of the vascular system. The diameter of the lumen is no larger than an erythrocyte and permits these cells to pass in single file only (**6.9**). The capillary wall is two-layered: a tunica intima of one or two squamous endothelial cells resting on a basal lamina, and a fine tunica adventitia of collagen and elastic fibres. The endothelial cells usually form a continuous layer, but fenestrated capillaries occur in the renal glomerulus, the endocrine glands, intestinal villi and the choroid plexus where gaps are present between adjoining cells closed by a membrane diaphragm. The wall also contains pericytes: undifferentiated cells believed capable of becoming fibroblasts or muscle cells. Venules collect the blood from the capillaries. Their lumina are wider than those of the arterioles. The tunica intima (there is no tunica media and adventitia) in each venule consists of a continuous layer of endothelial cells and areolar connective tissue. Pericytes are also present.

6.9

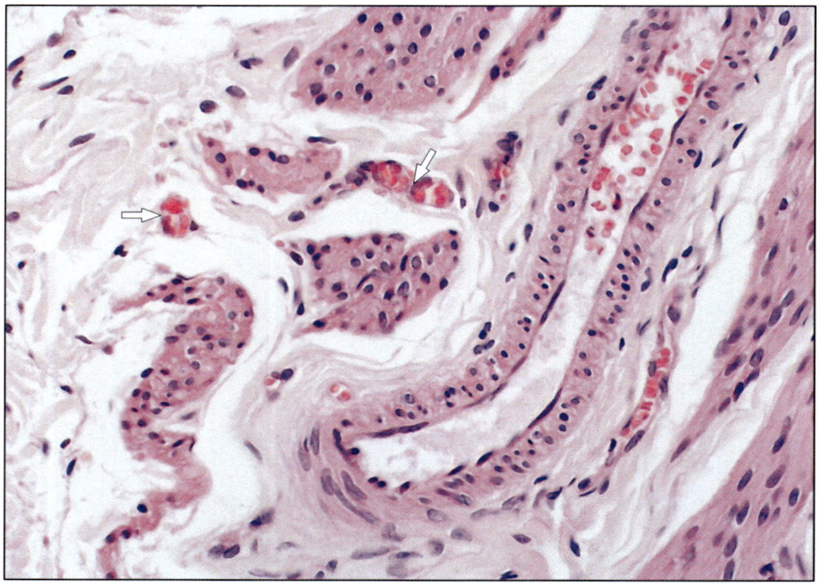

6.9 Capillaries (sheep) in the connective tissue of the cervix (arrowed). Masson's trichrome. ×125.

Sinusoids

Sinusoids are found in the liver, spleen, bone marrow and adenohypophysis. Their wide lumina are lined by endothelial cells interspersed with fixed macrophages of the mononuclear phagocyte scavenging and defence system of the body (**6.10–6.12**). Similar thin-walled venous sinuses are found in endocrine glands.

6.10

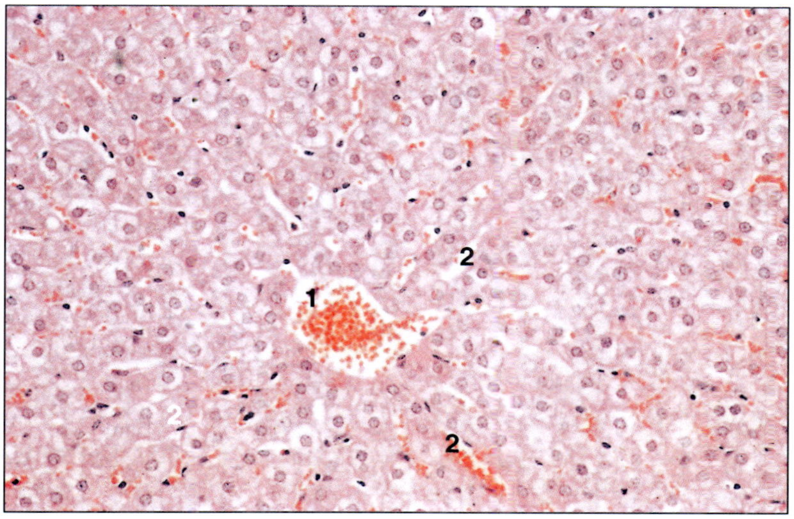

6.10 Liver (sheep). (1) Central vein. (2) Liver sinusoids. H & E. ×62.5.

6.11

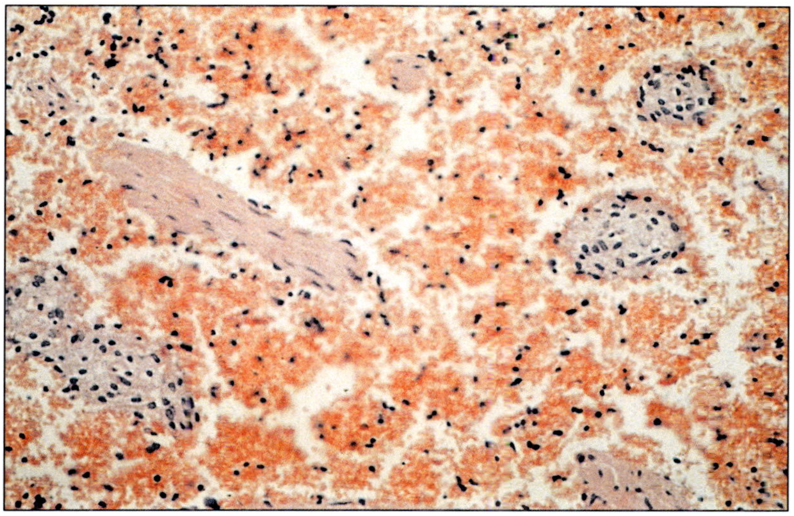

6.11 Spleen (horse). Sinusoids filled with erythrocytes. H & E. ×125.

6.12

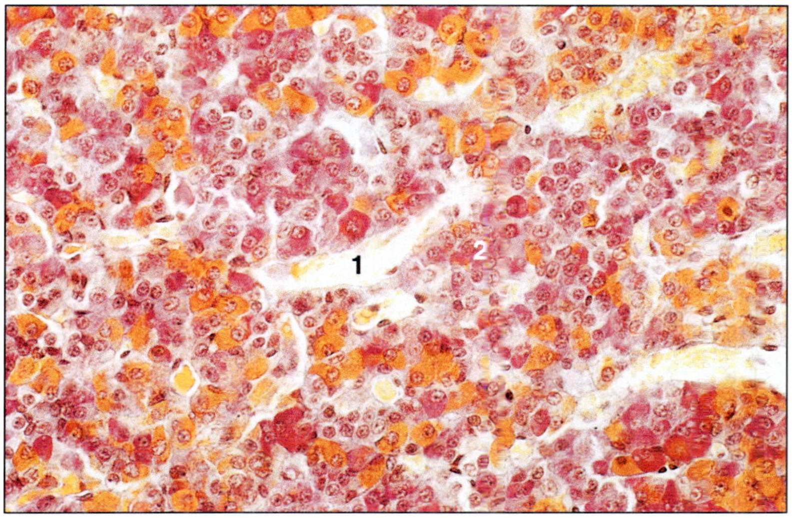

6.12 Pars distalis of the adenohypophysis (cat). (1) Sinusoids. (2) Cords of hypophyseal cells. Orange G. ×250.

6.13

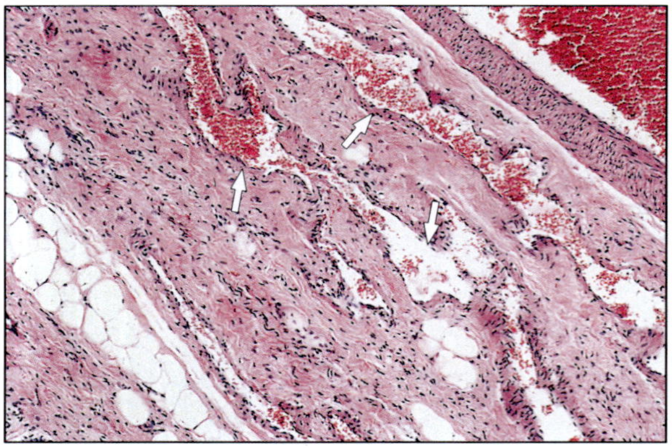

6.13 Spermatic cord (horse). Venous plexus (arrowed). H & E. ×62.5.

Veins

Veins are lined by a continuous layer of endothelial cells and areolar connective tissue. The tunica media, which is always narrow, contains a few circular smooth muscle fibres, some elastic fibres, but no elastic lamina. The tunica adventitia consists of longitudinal collagen fibres and, in the large veins, some smooth muscle (**6.13–6.16**). The lumen contains valves that are projections of the tunica intima; these allow only unidirectional blood flow (**6.17** and **6.18**).

6.14

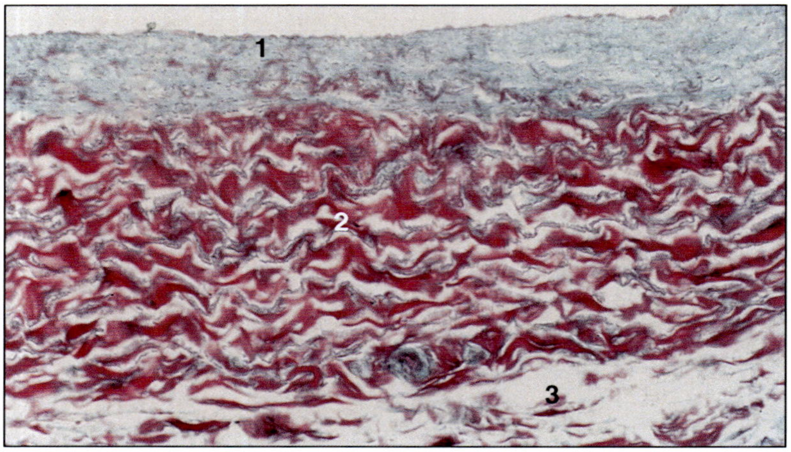

6.14 Caudal vena cava (dog). (1) Tunica intima. (2) Tunica media. (3) Tunica adventitia with vasa vasorum (arrowed). Gomori's trichrome. ×125.

6.15

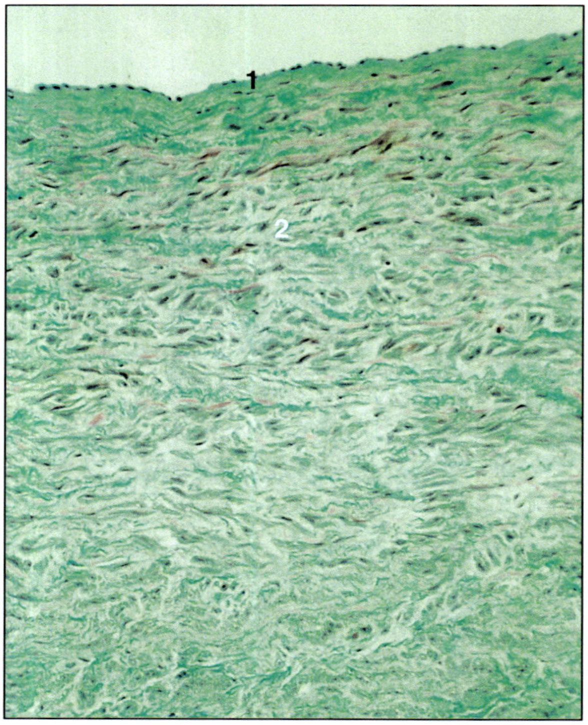

6.15 Caudal vena cava (horse). (1) Tunica intima. (2) Tunica media. Masson's trichrome. ×125.

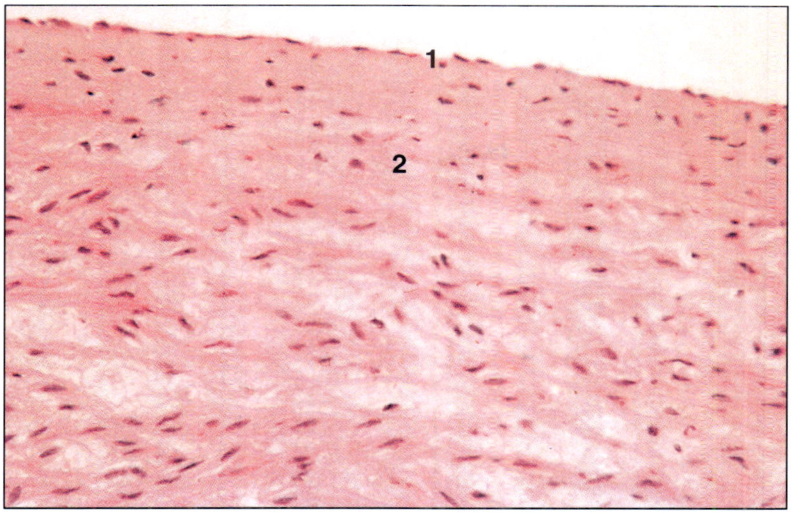

6.16

6.16 Cranial vena cava (horse). (1) Tunica intima. (2) Tunica media. H & E. ×125.

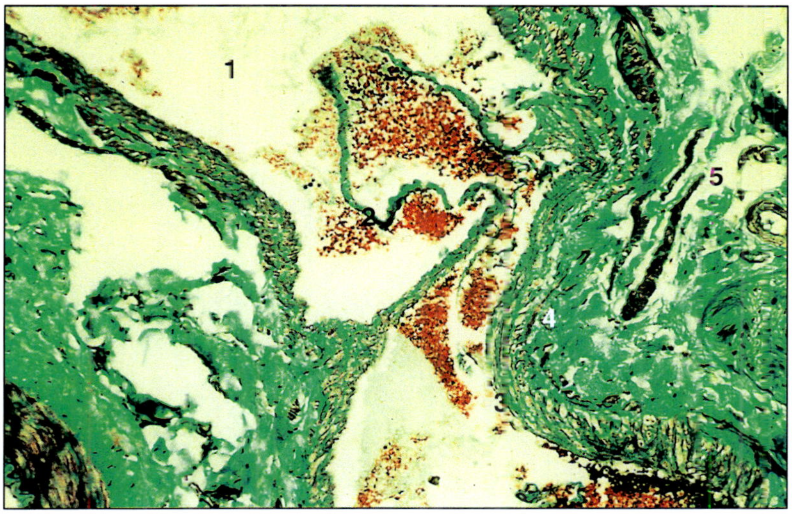

6.17

6.17 Femoral vein with valves (cat). (1) Lumen. (2) Valve. (3) Tunica intima. (4) Tunica media. (5) Tunica adventitia. Masson's trichrome. ×25.

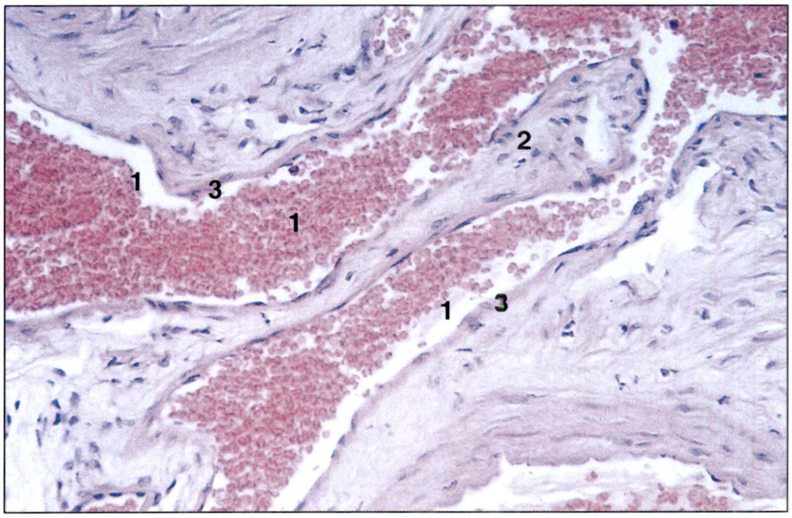

6.18

6.18 Valve in the brachial vein (cat). (1) Lumen filled with erythrocytes. (2) Valve. (3) Tunica intima. H & E. ×125.

Arteriovenous anastomoses

Arteriovenous anastomoses are special areas of the skin of the nose, lips and pads where the arteriole opens directly into a venule without going through the capillary bed (6.19). This provides an alternative channel of blood supply and regulation of heat loss.

6.19

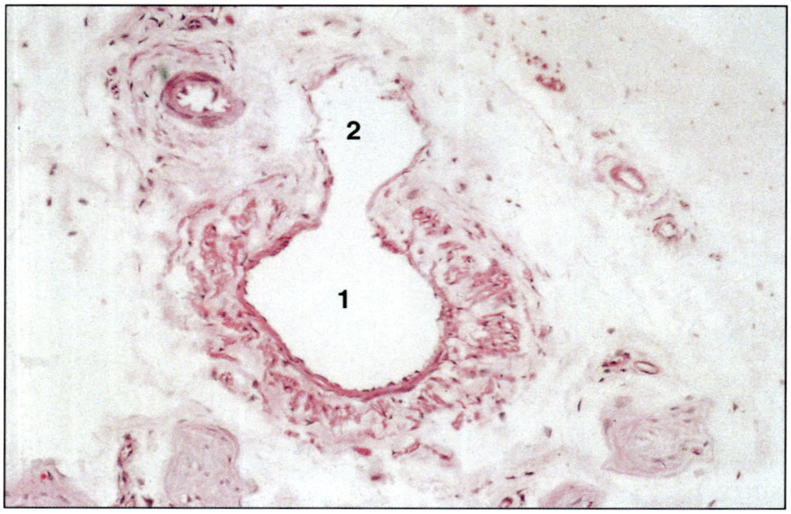

6.19 Arteriovenous anastomosis in loose connective tissue (cat). (1) Artery. (2) Vein. H & E. ×62.5.

Heart

The cardiac wall consists of three layers: endocardium (inner), myocardium (middle) and epicardium (outer).

The endocardium contains continuous squamous endothelial cells, vascular areolar connective tissue and conducting fibres. The myocardium is composed of cardiac muscle and also contains vascular areolar connective tissue. The epicardium is thicker than the endocardium, and fat deposits in the rather dense connective tissue and coronary blood vessels are often found (6.20 and 6.21). Fibrous rings support the heart valves (6.22). They provide a means of insertion for the cardiac muscle and may be referred to as the fibrous or cardiac skeleton (6.23). In older horses the aortic rings may become calcified to form the ossa cordis. Two bones form in the aortic rings of cattle, the ossa cordis.

6.20

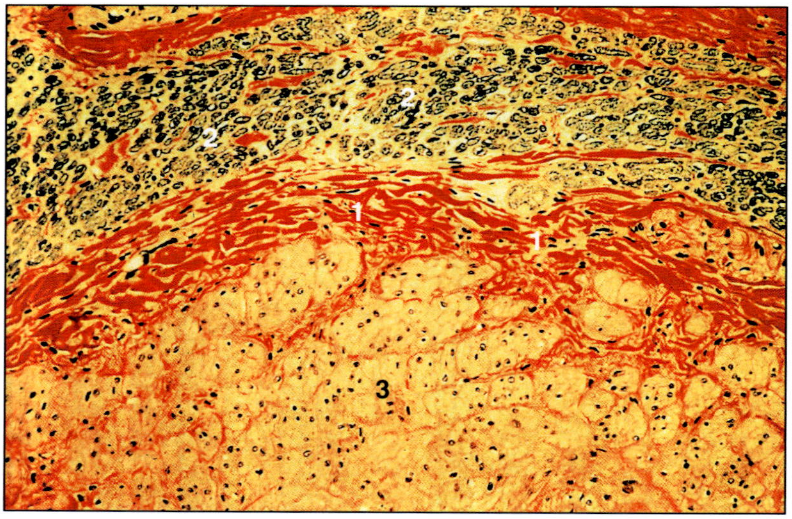

6.20 Cardiac muscle (ox). (1) Cardiac muscle. (2) Connective tissue of the fibrous skeleton. (3) Atrioventricular node. Masson's trichrome. ×125.

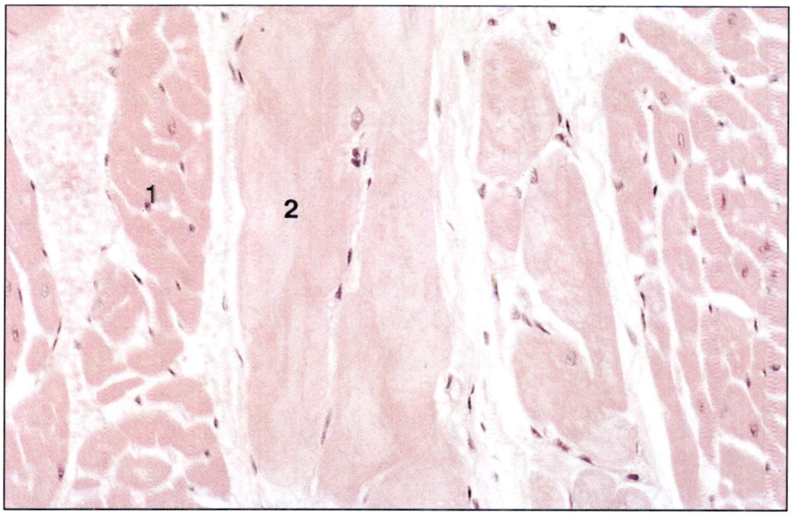

6.21

6.21 Cardiac muscle (horse).
(1) Cardiac muscle fibres.
(2) Conducting (Purkinje) fibres.
H & E. ×125.

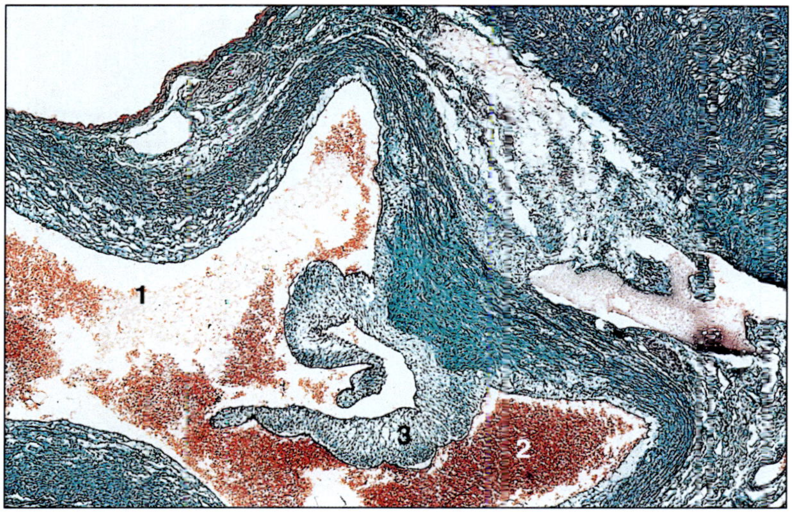

6.22

6.22 Heart (dog). (1) Lumen of the atrium. (2) Lumen of the pulmonary artery. (3) Valve cusps. Masson's trichrome. ×62.5.

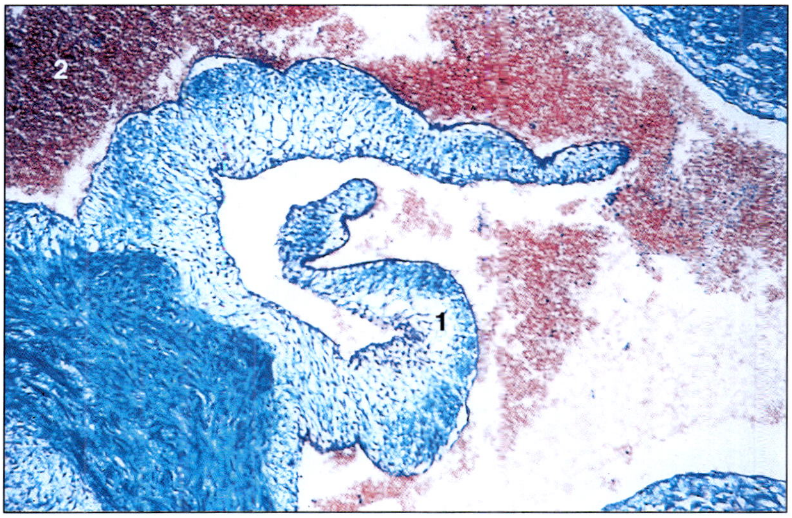

6.23

6.23 Heart (dog). (1) Valve cusps. (2) Dense connective tissue part of the fibrous skeleton of the heart. Masson's trichrome. ×62.5.

Lymphatic vessels

Lymphatic vessels drain excess fluid from the tissues and are made up of a thin layer of connective tissue with an endothelial lining. Larger lymphatic vessels, such as the thoracic duct, may have a few smooth muscle fibres in the wall.

Amphibians and reptiles have perilymphatic and endolymphatic systems that are particularly well developed in some species. These lymph-filled structures serve several functions. Perilymphatic pathways encircle the auditory apparatus and may participate in the transmission of sounds. The endolymphatic system consists of receptor organs of the inner ear as well as either bilateral separate or fused thin-walled sacs. These communicate with the skull via narrow ducts and serve as reservoirs for the storage of calcium carbonate microcrystals. In some amphibians, endolymphatic sacs form a ring-like extension of the vertebral canal around the brain.

Clinical correlates

A range of cardiovascular diseases are important in veterinary medicine. The heart itself can be affected by congenital, degenerative, inflammatory and neoplastic conditions with a variety of underlying causes. Disease caused by congenital malformations is naturally recognized most often in the young animal. Mitral valve dysplasia in an 11-week-old Bearded Collie is shown in **6.24**. The heart is opened to show the left atrioventricular (mitral) valve. The valve leaflets are thickened and malformed and the chordae tendinae are short, thick and partially fused. This congenital defect leads to mitral valve incompetence and produces a holosystolic murmur centred around the fifth intercostal space near the left sternal border.

In adult animals primary cardiac disease is most often encountered in the form of cardiomyopathy or degenerative change in the muscle of the heart. In **6.25** and **6.26** special stains have been used to highlight features of interest. Both are from the same case, a 12-year-old dog with myocardial degeneration. In **6.25** a Sirius Red stain, which colours collagen red, demonstrates the large amount of fibrosis replacing muscle bundles, which are stained yellow. In **6.26** a Masson's trichrome stain highlights muscle fibres undergoing degeneration. Myocardial degeneration and fibrosis may be found in cases of dilated cardiomyopathy or as a non-specific response of the cardiac muscle to injury or insult.

One of the most important diseases to affect the blood vessels is haemangiosarcoma, a malignant tumour of the endothelial cells that line blood vessels. In dogs the spleen, right atrium and skin are common primary sites and metastasis can be very widespread. Other species are also affected. A haemangiosarcoma in a 6-year-old thoroughbred gelding is shown in **6.27**.

The smooth muscle in the tunica media of blood vessels can be affected by the deposition of calcium salts. This change is frequently induced by oversupplementation of the diet of herbivorous reptiles or amphibians with vitamin D_3 either directly or by inclusion of commercial dog, cat or primate food. Similarly hypervitaminosis D_3 may be induced when supplemented goldfish are fed to fish-eating reptiles and amphibians. Early arteriosclerotic mineralization of the tunica media in a large pulmonary artery in an iguana is shown in **6.28**.

6.24

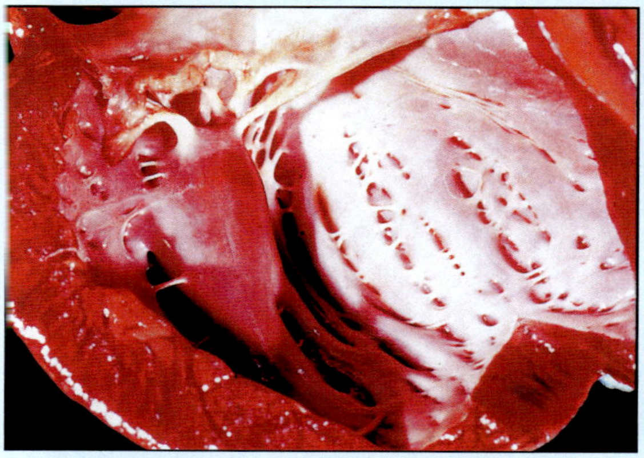

6.24 Mitral valve dysplasia in an 11-week-old Bearded Collie. Note the thickened, distorted chordae tendinae.

6.25

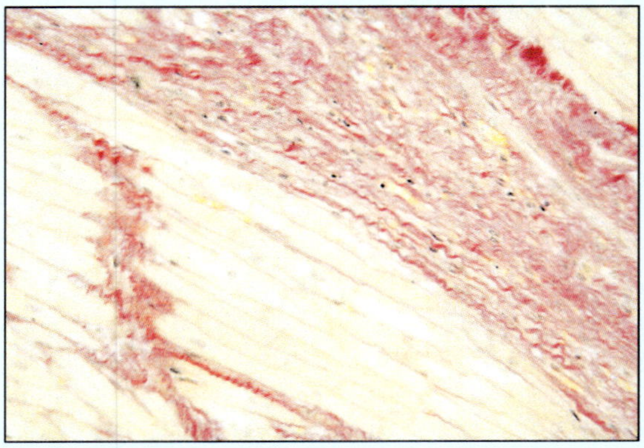

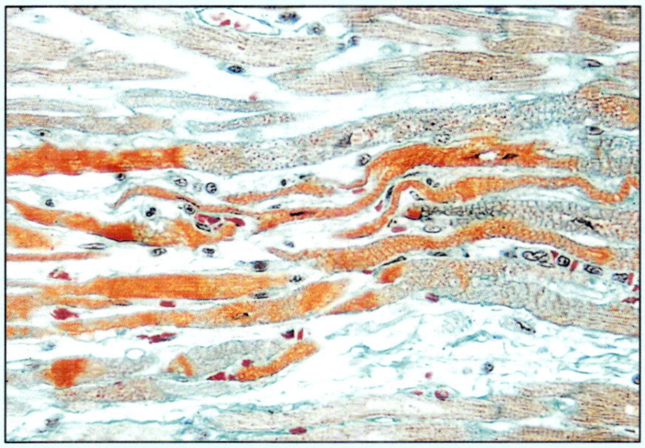

6.26

6.25, 6.26 Myocardial degeneration and fibrosis in a 12-year-old dog with cardiomyopathy. In **6.25**, the collagenous tissue which replaces muscle bundle is stained red. Sirius Red. ×45. In **6.26**, degenerative muscle fibres are seen stained strongly orange in the centre. The striations of the muscle fibres are also demonstrated with this stain. Masson's trichrome. ×180.

6.27 Haemangiosarcoma in a horse. The tumour cells are spindle-shaped with large, often hyperchromatic, nuclei and are arranged into loosely interlacing bundles that form irregular, blood-filled channels and spaces. H & E. ×125.

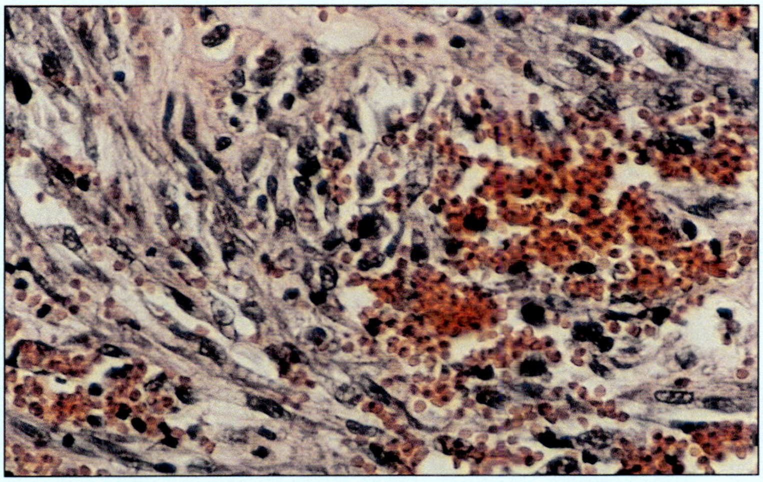

6.27

6.28 Early arteriosclerotic mineralization in a large pulmonary artery (iguana). The mineral deposition is highlighted in red. Alcian blue/PAS. ×125.

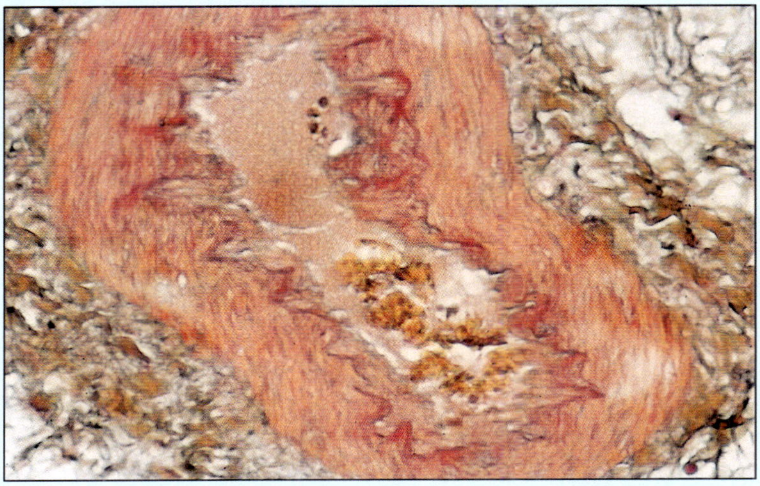

6.28

7. RESPIRATORY SYSTEM

The respiratory system has two functions: conduction and respiration. Conduction is carried out via a continuous system of tubes carrying air from the nostrils into the nasal cavity through the nasopharynx and larynx to the trachea and bronchi. The air is warmed, moistened and filtered in these passages before reaching the organs responsible for respiration: the lung parenchyma, the respiratory bronchioles, alveolar sacs and alveoli. It is between the alveoli and the capillaries that gas exchange takes place.

The paranormal sinuses are cavities found in skull bones. The mucoendosteum lining these cavities is continuous with the mucous membrane of the nasal cavity.

Conduction of air

The skin around the nostrils has long tactile hairs and numerous sebaceous and sweat glands (7.1). Respiratory epithelium lines all but the finer divisions of the respiratory tract and consists of pseudostratified columnar ciliated cells and mucus-secreting goblet cells. The lamina propria is continuous with the perichondrium or periosteum where appropriate, is very vascular, contains both collagen and elastic fibres, and warms the inspired air. Seromucous glands secrete into the lumen through the epithelium (7.2–7.4).

7.1

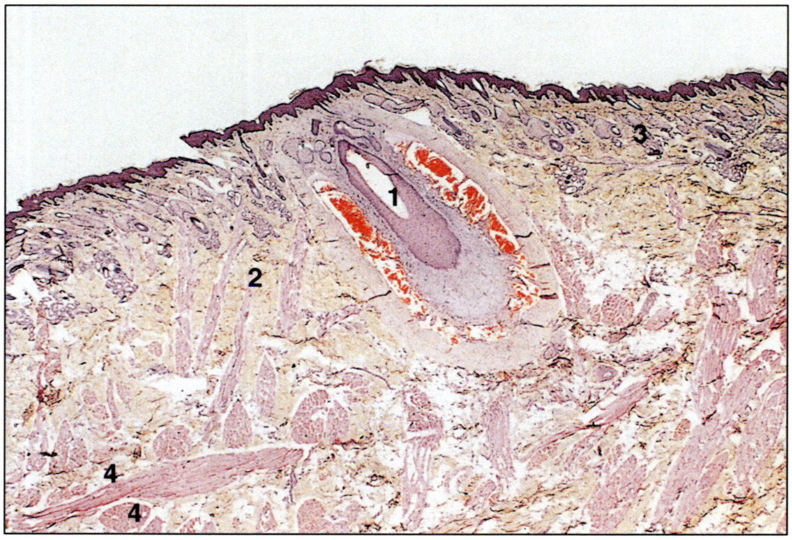

7.1 Skin. Nostril (horse). (1) Sinus hair. (2) Lamina propria. (3) Sebaceous glands. (4) Sweat glands. H & E. ×20.

7.2

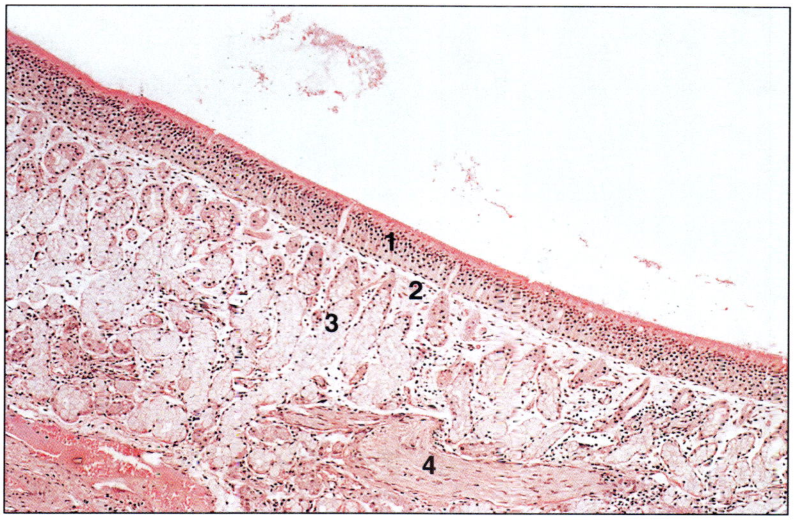

7.2 Respiratory epithelium (horse). (1) Pseudostratified columnar ciliated epithelium with goblet cells. (2) Lamina propria. (3) Seromucous glands. (4) Smooth muscle. H & E. ×62.5.

7.3

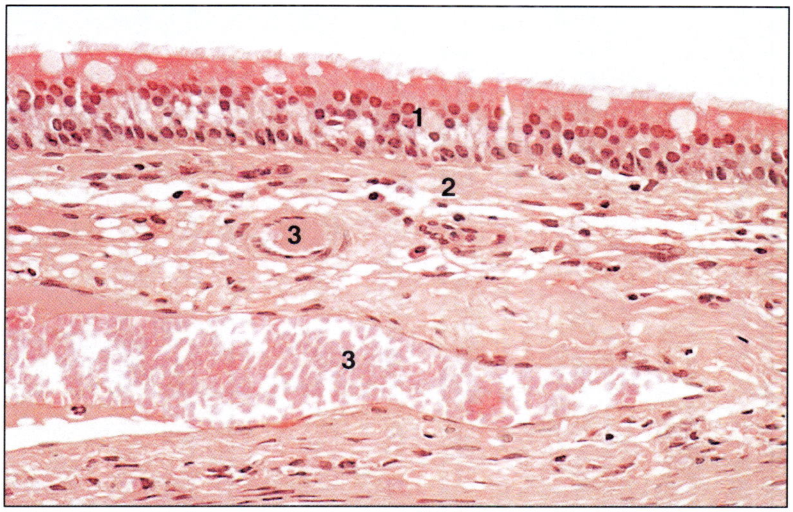

7.3 Respiratory epithelium (horse). (1) Pseudostratified columnar ciliated epithelium with goblet cells. (2) Lamina propria. (3) Blood vessels. H & E. ×160.

7.4

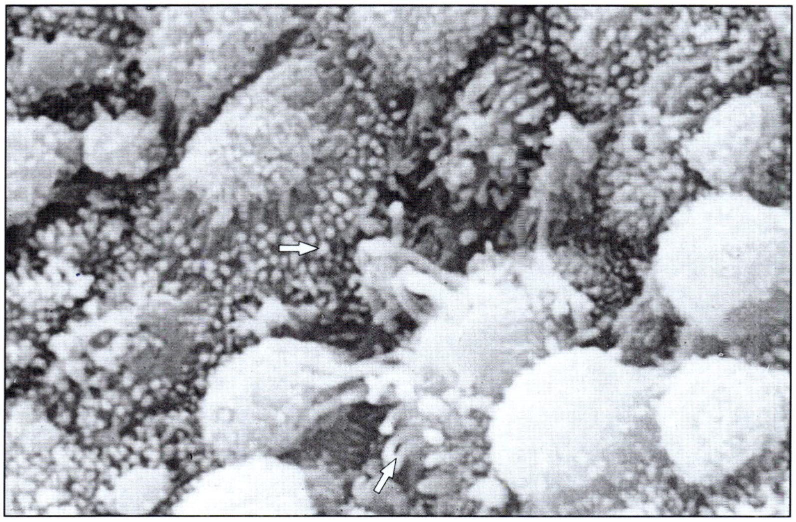

7.4 Respiratory epithelium (horse). The cilia project from the surface of the epithelial cell as fine strands; active mucus-secreting cells lie between the ciliated cells (arrowed). Scanning electron micrograph. ×1500.

Cilia beat towards the pharynx, an area common both to the digestive and to the respiratory system. The auditory tube connects the pharynx to the middle ear and is common to the digestive, respiratory and auditory systems (7.5). The guttural pouch of equids is a diverticulum of the auditory tube. The digestive surface is covered by a stratified squamous epithelium that is continuous with the oral cavity, and the respiratory surface by respiratory epithelium continuous with the nasal cavities (7.6 and 7.7). The epiglottis is a flap-like structure projecting into the pharynx. A plate of elastic cartilage provides internal support. The upper digestive surface mucous membrane is covered by a non-keratinizing stratified squamous epithelium (7.8) and the lower respiratory surface by respiratory epithelium (7.9). Taste buds may be present on the laryngeal aspect.

7.5

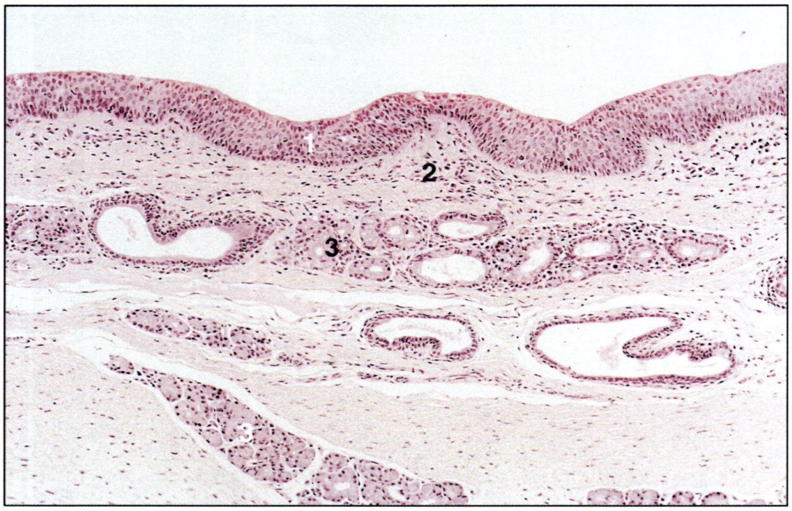

7.5 Auditory tube (horse). (1) Respiratory epithelium. (2) Lamina propria. (3) Seromucous glands. H & E. ×100.

7.6

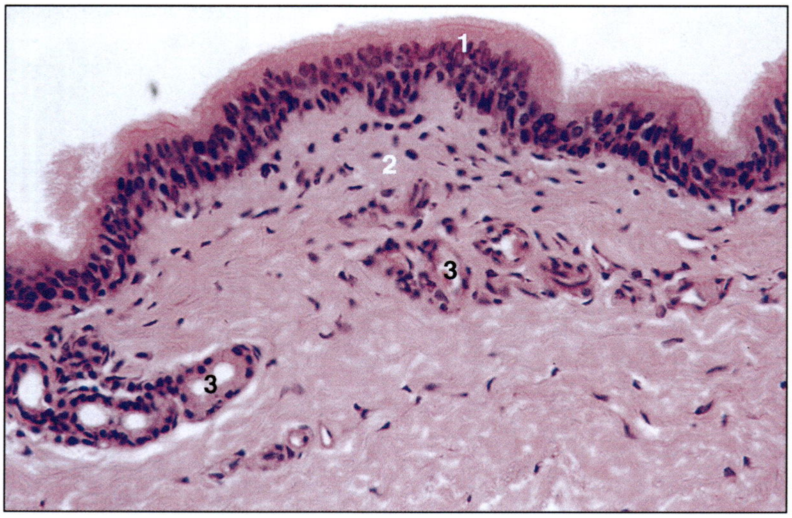

7.6 Guttural pouch (horse). (1) Respiratory epithelium. (2) Lamina propria. (3) Seromucous glands. H & E. ×250.

7.7 Guttural pouch (horse). (1) Respiratory epithelium; the goblet cells are individually stained blue. (2) Lamina propria. (3) Seromucous glands. Alcian blue/PAS. ×200.

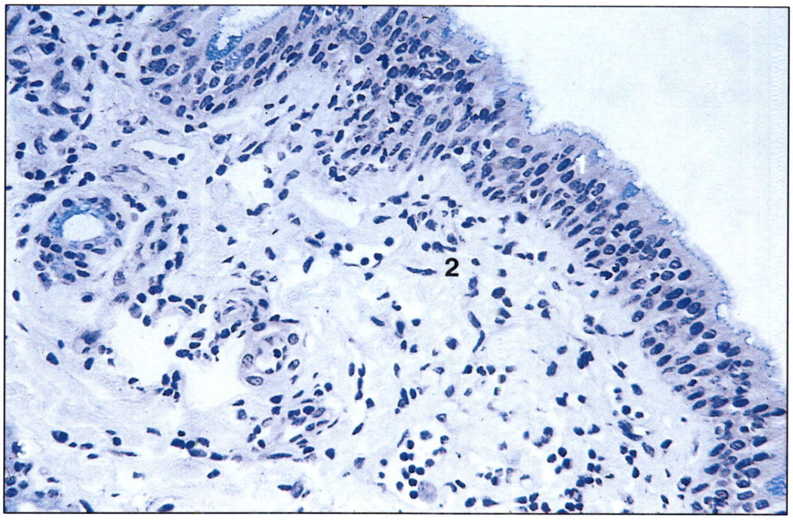

7.7

7.8 Epiglottis (horse). (1) Stratified squamous epithelium. (2) Lamina propria. (3) Seromucous glands. H & E. ×200.

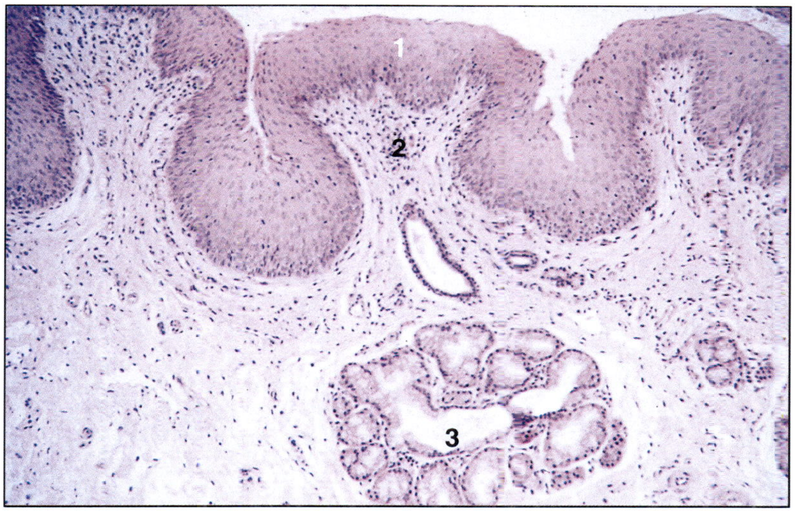

7.8

7.9 Epiglottis (horse). (1) Stratified columnar epithelium with mucus-secreting cells stained blue. (2) Lamina propria. (3) Seromucous glands. Alcian blue/PAS. ×125.

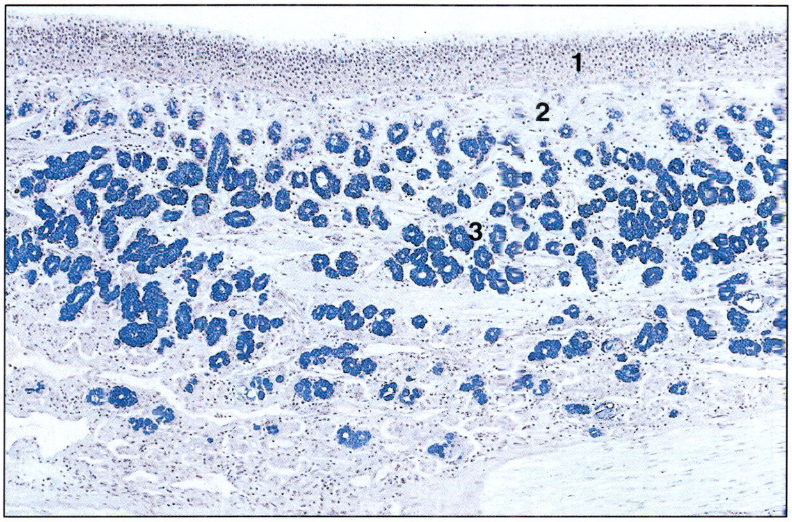

7.9

The larynx is lined by respiratory epithelium. The lamina propria is continuous with the perichondrium of the laryngeal cartilages. The vocal cords are covered by stratified squamous epithelium (**7.10** and **7.11**). The trachea extends from the larynx to the bifurcation of the extrapulmonary bronchi. These tubes have the same structure: a lining of respiratory epithelium rising on a lamina propria of loose connective tissue with elastic fibres and mixed seromucous glands opening into the lumen. Incomplete rings of hyaline cartilage keep the lumen patent and smooth muscle fibres bridge the gap at the dorsal aspect of the trachea (**7.12**). In the bronchus the hyaline cartilage has a plate-like arrangement. The smooth muscle forms a spiral and appears as discontinuous blocks in transverse sections (**7.13** and **7.14**). A fibrous adventitial coat covers the trachea and the extrapulmonary bronchi.

7.10

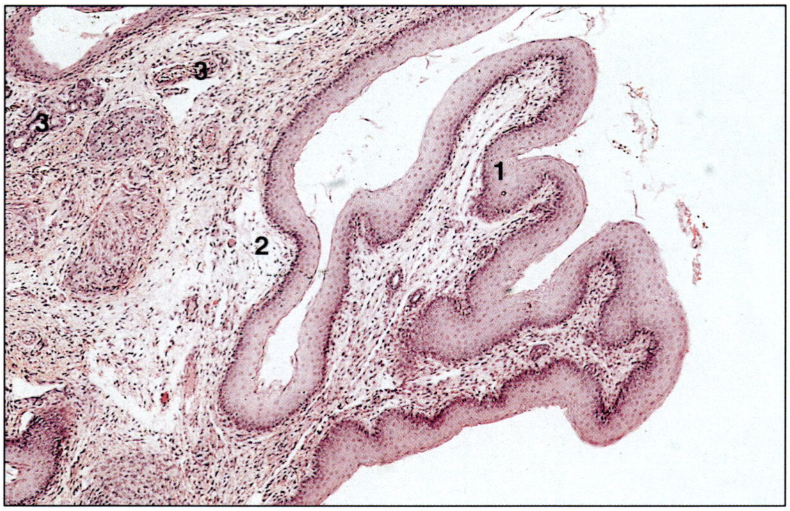

7.10 Larynx (vocal cord; dog). (1) Stratified squamous epithelium. (2) Lamina propria. (3) Simple tubular glands. H & E. ×62.5.

7.11

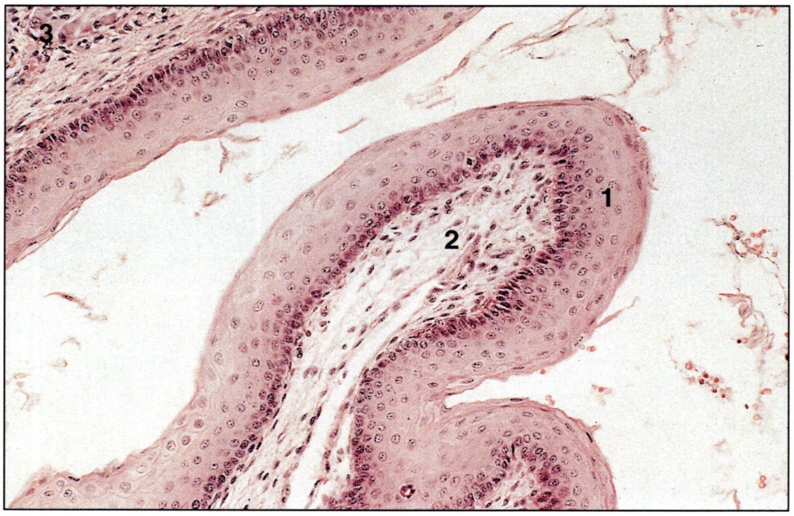

7.11 Larynx (vocal cord; dog). (1) Stratified squamous epithelium covering the vocal cord. (2) Connective tissue core of the lamina propria. (3) Parasympathetic ganglion. H & E. ×160.

7.12 Trachea (sheep). (1) Respiratory epithelium. (2) Lamina propria. (3) Seromucous glands. (4) Hyaline cartilage. Gomori's trichrome. ×25.

7.12

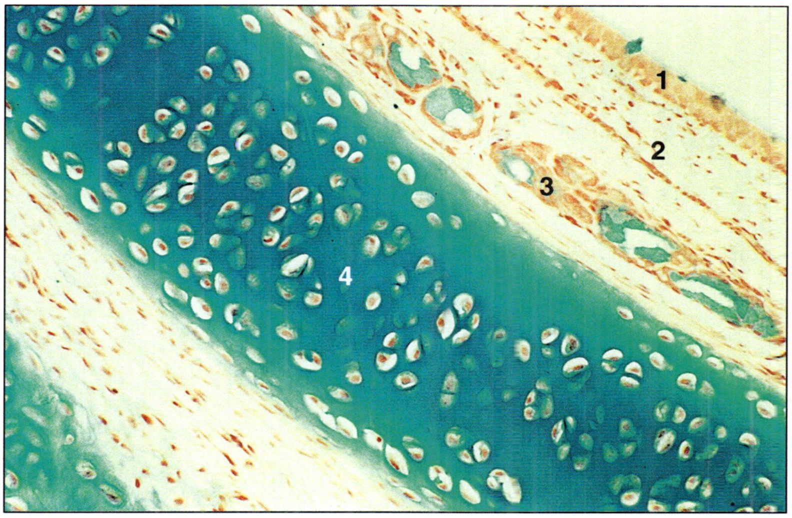

7.13 Bronchus (sheep). (1) Respiratory epithelium. (2) Lamina propria. (3) Smooth muscle. (4) Simple tubular glands open into the lumen through the epithelium. (5) Perichondrium. (6) Hyaline cartilage. H & E. ×25.

7.13

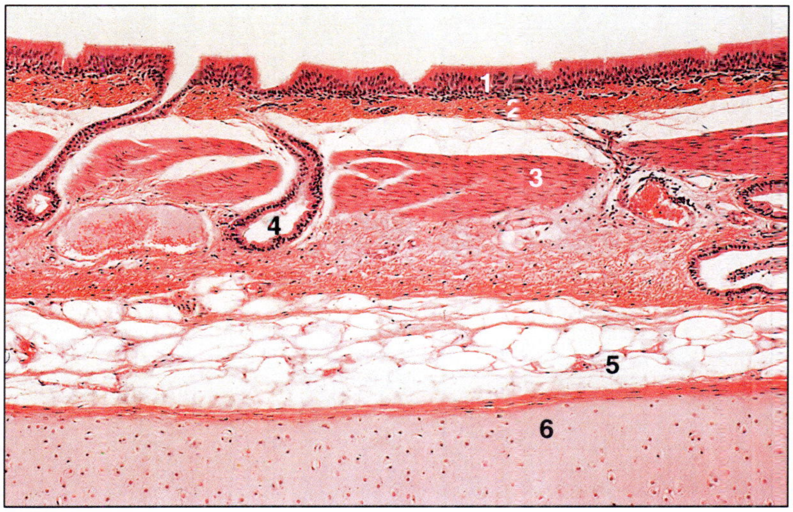

7.14 Bronchus (ox). (1) Respiratory epithelium; the goblet cells are stained specifically. (2) Lamina propria. (3) Smooth muscle. (4) Simple tubular glands. Gomori/aldehyde fuchsin. ×200.

7.14

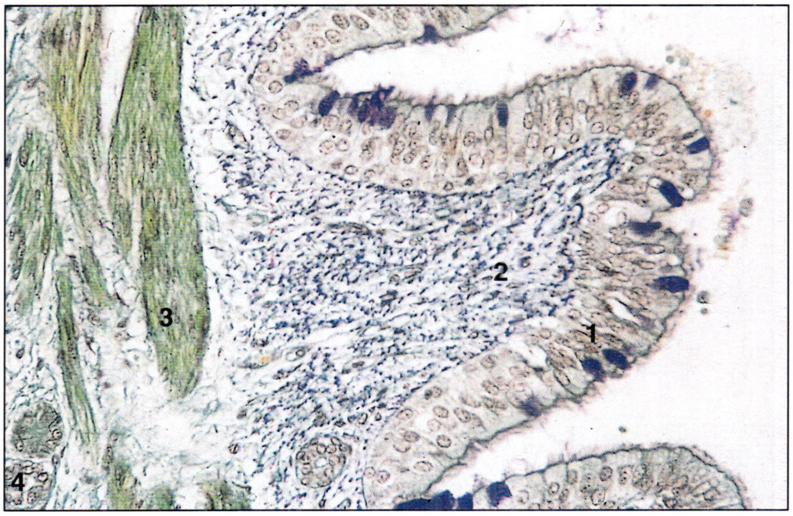

Respiration

The bronchi, both extrapulmonary and intrapulmonary, bring air to the lungs and branch out within the lungs into the bronchioles, which culminate in clusters of minute sacs: the alveoli. In the fetal lung the duct system is developed whereas the respiratory part develops slowly (7.15–7.17). Expansion begins with the first respiratory movements after birth. Thereafter, the lung expands in tandem with the growth of the animal.

Each lung is covered by elastic connective tissue with an outer layer of mesothelium, the visceral pleura (7.18). Connective tissue septa divide the lung into lobes and lobules and the intrapulmonary bronchi have the same structure as the extrapulmonary bronchi (7.19–7.23). The epithelium of

7.15

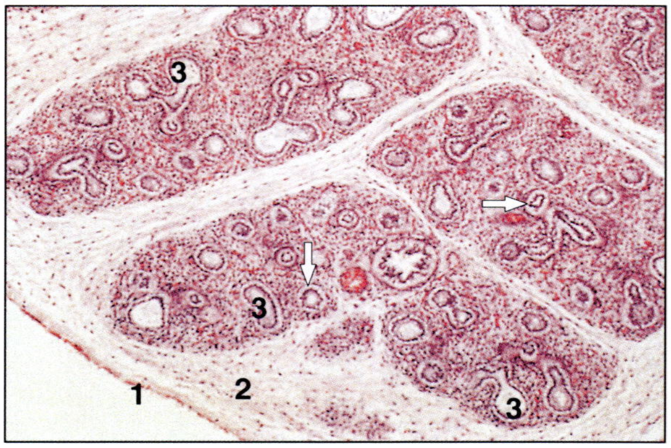

7.15 Bovine fetal (160-day) lung. Blood vessels (arrowed). (1) Pleural mesothelium. (2) Mesenchyme. (3) Duct system. H & E. ×5.

7.16

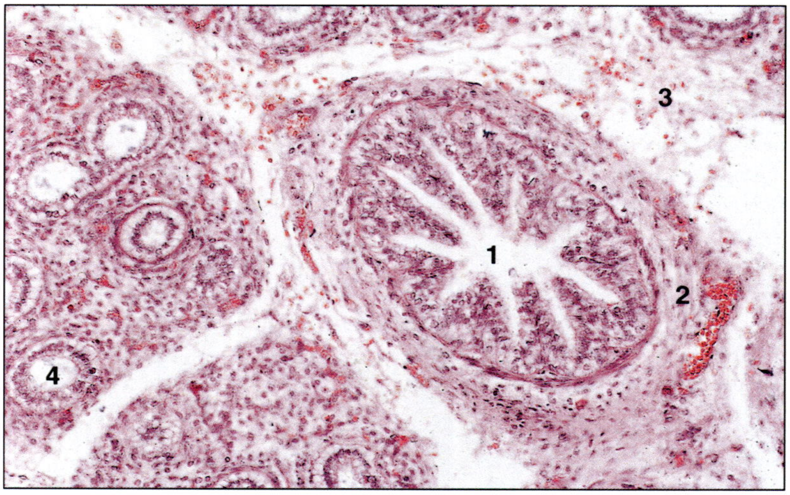

7.16 Bovine fetal (160-day) lung. (1) Large duct lined by a simple columnar epithelium. (2) Smooth muscle. (3) Vascular mesenchyme. (4) Small ducts. H & E. ×25.

7.17

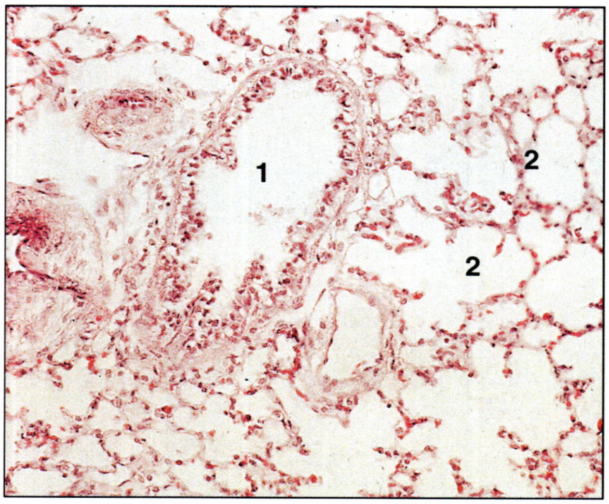

7.17 Fetal lung at term (cow). (1) Respiratory bronchiole lined by simple columnar epithelium. (2) Alveoli. H & E. ×62.5.

7.18

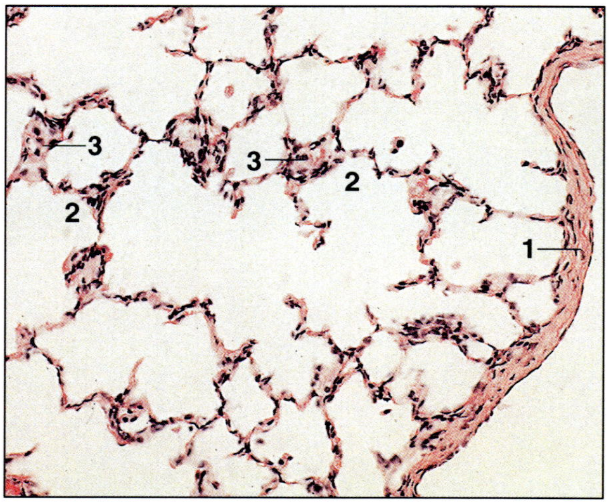

7.18 Adult lung (sheep). (1) Elastic connective tissue with an outer layer of mesothelium of the visceral pleura. (2) Alveoli. (3) Blood vessels. H & E. ×62.5.

7.19 Intrapulmonary bronchus. Lung (cow). (1) Lumen lined by respiratory epithelium. (2) Lamina propria. (3) Smooth muscle. (4) Hyaline cartilage. (5) Blood vessel. (6) Alveoli. Gomori/aldehyde fuchsin. ×52.

7.19

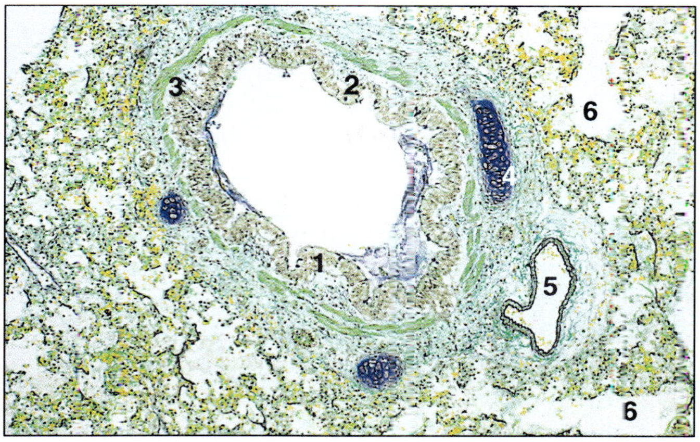

7.20 Intrapulmonary bronchus. Lung (sheep). (1) Lumen lined by respiratory epithelium. (2) Lamina propria. (3) Smooth muscle. (4) Hyaline cartilage. (5) Simple tubular glands. (6) Blood vessel. (7) Bronchiole. (8) Alveolar duct. (9) Alveoli. H & E. ×62.5.

.20

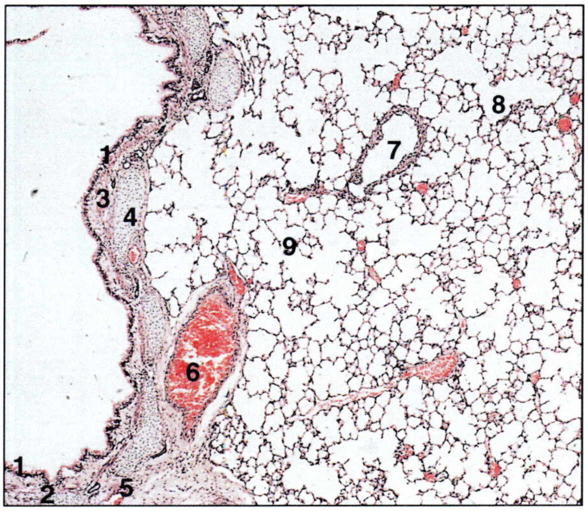

7.21

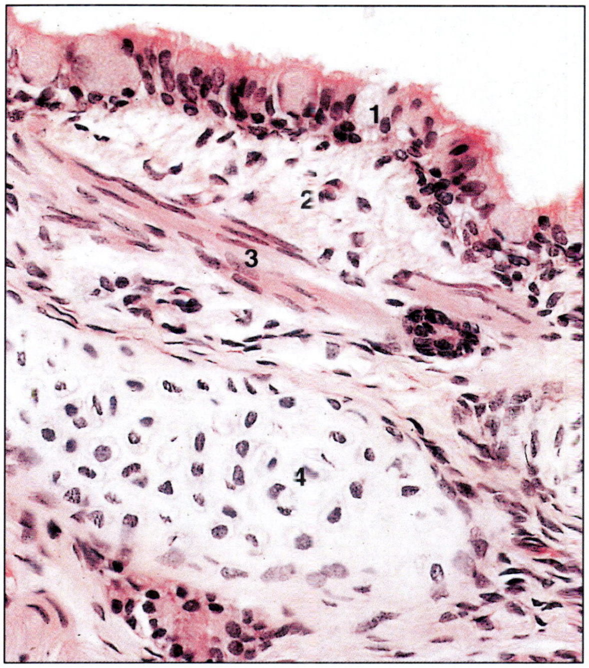

7.21 Intrapulmonary bronchus. Lung (sheep). (1) Respiratory epithelium. (2) Lamina propria. (3) Smooth muscle. (4) Hyaline cartilage. H & E. ×200.

.22

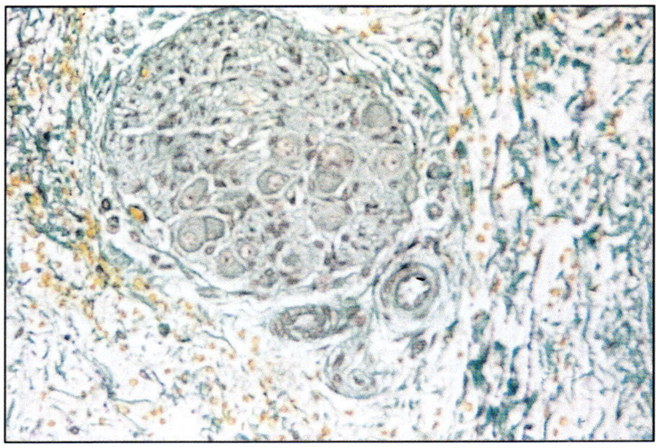

7.22 Intrapulmonary bronchus. Lung (cow). A parasympathetic ganglion is present surrounded by vascular connective tissue of the lamina propria.Gomori/aldehyde fuchsin. ×160.

7.23 Intrapulmonary bronchus (dog). (1) The intrapulmonary bronchus is lined by respiratory epithelium (arrowed). (2) Alveoli. Scanning electron micrograph. ×500.

7.23

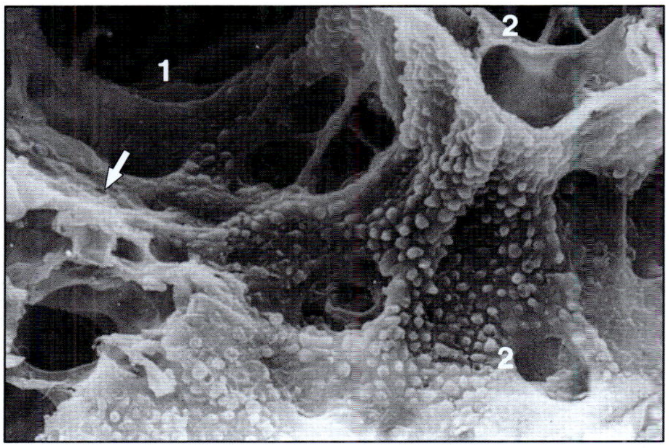

the bronchioles is columnar or even cuboidal and ciliated. In the smaller bronchioles the epithelium is thinner, the lamina propria is elastic, the smooth muscle forms a complete ring and there is no adventitia (7.24 and 7.25).

Non-ciliated bronchiolar cells (Clara cells) are tall, dome-shaped and protrude into the bronchiolar lumen. They replace the mucus-secreting goblet cells at this level. Both ciliated cells and Clara cells are present in the terminal and respiratory bronchioles (in the dog and cat they are lined by the latter exclusively). Clara cells divide to form other Clara or ciliated cells and have an important role in the repair of damaged epithelium. Their secretion also keeps the small airways patent.

Respiratory bronchioles are lined with a low columnar or cuboidal epithelium with ciliated and bronchiolar cells, an elastic lamina propria and a smooth muscle layer. This opens into the alveolar duct lined by squamous epithelium, interrupted by atria and alveoli along its length (7.26). Alveoli are the functional exchange part of the lung. The septa are very thin, with both elastic and collagen fibres, and contain one of the most extensive capillary networks in the body. Cells of the immune system, derived from blood monocytes, are also present and migrate through the alveolar epithelium into the air space, where they phagocytose particulate matter and micro-organisms to become dust cells (alveolar phagocytes). The respiratory membrane where gas exchange takes place consists of capillary endothelial cells, alveolar epithelial cells and a fused basement membrane (7.27). The squamous alveolar cell, the lining cell responsible for gas exchange, is a type I pneumocyte. The great alveolar cell secretes surfactant to reduce surface tension. It is a type II pneumocyte, is cuboidal and projects into the lumen.

7.24

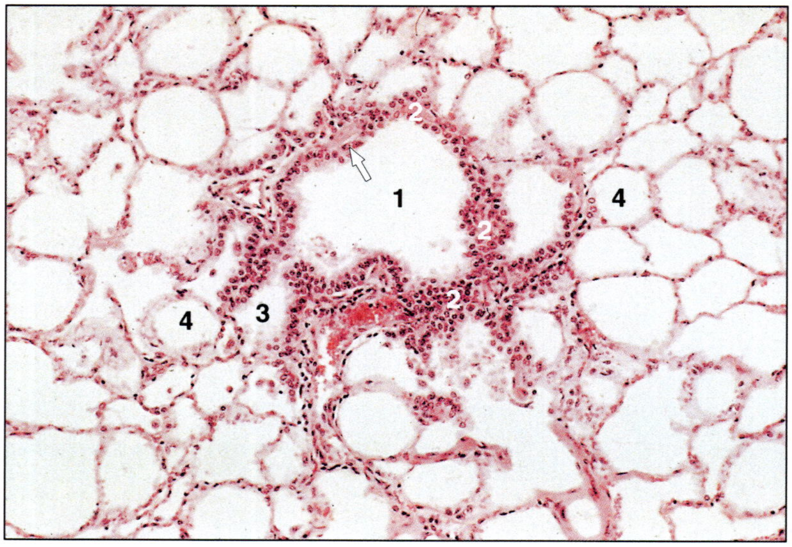

7.24 Bronchiole. Lung (sheep). (1) The bronchiole is lined by cuboidal/low columnar epithelium with ciliated and non-ciliated cells (arrowed). (2) Smooth muscle. (3) Alveolar duct. (4) Alveoli. The free cells in the lumen are macrophages. H & E. ×125.

7.25 Bronchiole. Lung (sheep). (1) The bronchiole is lined by cuboidal epithelium. (2) Respiratory bronchiole. (3) Alveolar duct. (4) Alveoli. The free cells are macrophages. H & E. ×62.5.

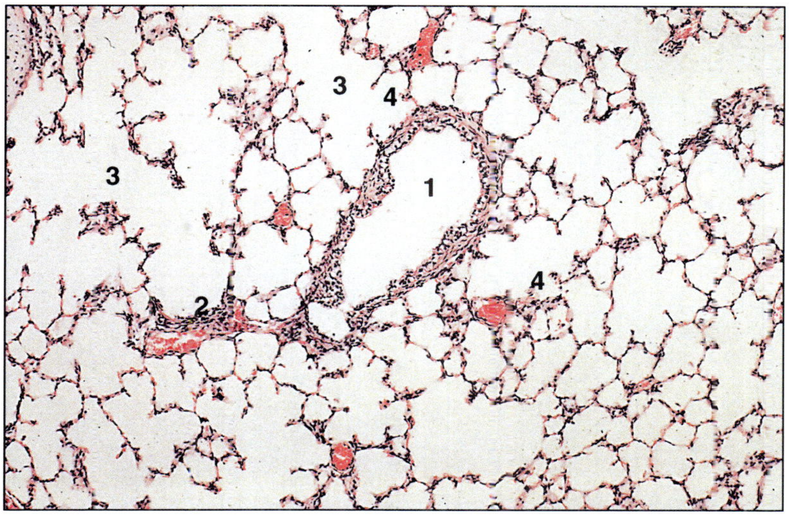

7.25

7.26 Bronchiole. Lung (sheep). (1) Respiratory bronchiole leading into (2) alveolar duct leading into (3) alveoli. H & E. ×80.

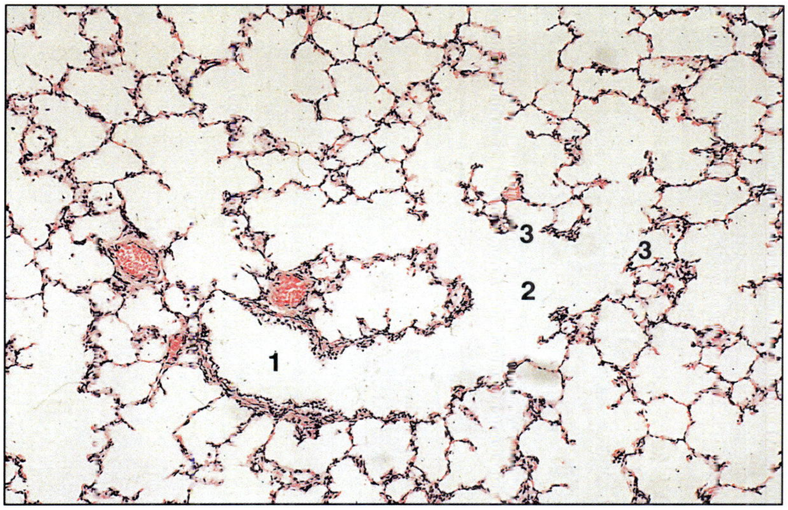

7.26

7.27 Lung (dog). The lung macrophages (dust cells) have phagocytosed the carbon particles. The alveolar lining cells are arrowed. Carbon-injected H & E. ×256.

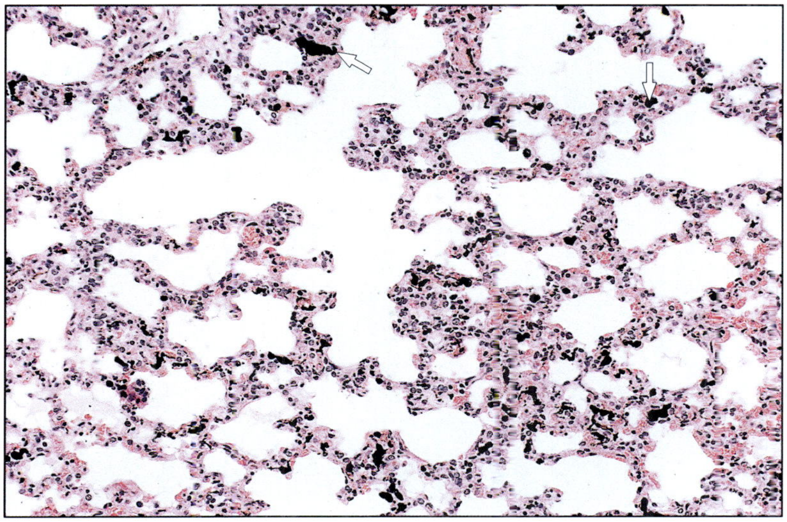

7.27

Clinical correlates

The patterns of disease seen in the respiratory system reflect its structure and function. The respiratory tract is constantly challenged by potentially injurious agents, by both the aerogenous (arrive in inspired air) and haematogenous (arrive in blood supply) routes.

These can include micro-organisms such as bacteria, fungi and viruses or toxic substances or particles (*see* 7.37) in the air. This is especially important where large numbers of animals are housed in the same airspace. A bronchiole surrounded by small cells with dark nuclei and scant cytoplasm is shown in 7.28. These cells, which are lymphocytes, also invade the bronchiolar wall. Often termed 'cuffing' pneumonia because of the arrangement of the lymphoid cells around the bronchioles, this is an example of a chronic, non-suppurative pneumonia, commonly seen in calves. Infection with *Mycoplasma* species is the most common cause.

The very rich blood supply to the lungs (which have the largest capillary bed in the body) also makes them a common target for haematogenous metastasis from tumours at other sites in the body. Primary lung tumours, both benign and malignant, are recognized in older animals. A bronchiolar–alveolar carcinoma, a malignant primary tumour of the lung is shown in 7.29.

7.28

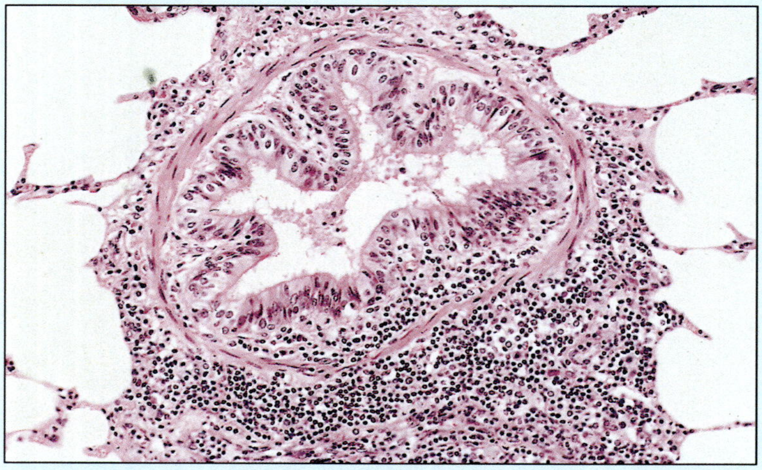

7.28 Cuffing pneumonia (calf). Lymphocytes cluster around a bronchiole. H & E. ×125.

7.29

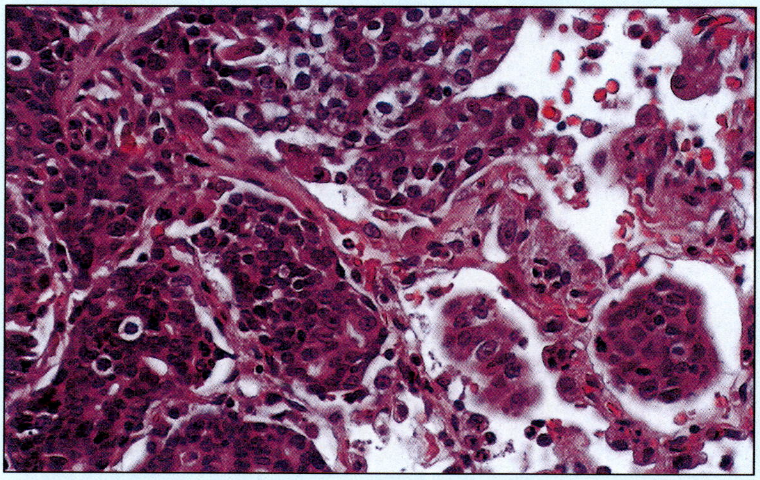

7.29 Bronchiolar–alveolar carcinoma in an 11-year-old entire bitch. Nodules of tumour, composed of convoluted layers of cuboidal epithelium, infiltrate interstitial tissue and fill alveolar spaces. Several mitoses are seen. H & E. ×250.

Avian respiratory system

Vestibule and conducting passages

In birds the vestibule is lined with a distinctive keratinized stratified squamous epithelium, and the conducting passages with pseudostratified columnar ciliated epithelium with simple alveolar mucous glands (7.30 and 7.31).

Trachea

The trachea and intraepithelial tracheal glands are lined with respiratory epithelium and rest on a connective tissue lamina propria. Overlapping rings of ossified hyaline cartilage form the wall. The trachea is compressed just cranial to the bifurcation into the primary bronchi. Thin vertical bars of cartilage fuse to form the pessulus, a single cartilage rod in the angle of the bifurcation (7.32). This is

.30

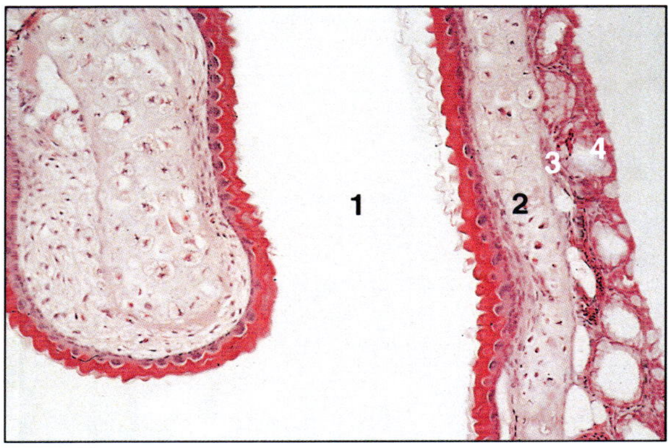

7.30 Avian vestibule. (1) The vestibule is lined by distinctive stratified squamous keratinized epithelium. (2) Hyaline cartilage. (3) Perichondrium. (4) Pseudostratified columnar ciliated epithelium with intraepithelial alveolar mucus-secreting glands, respiratory epithelium. H & E. ×5.

7.31

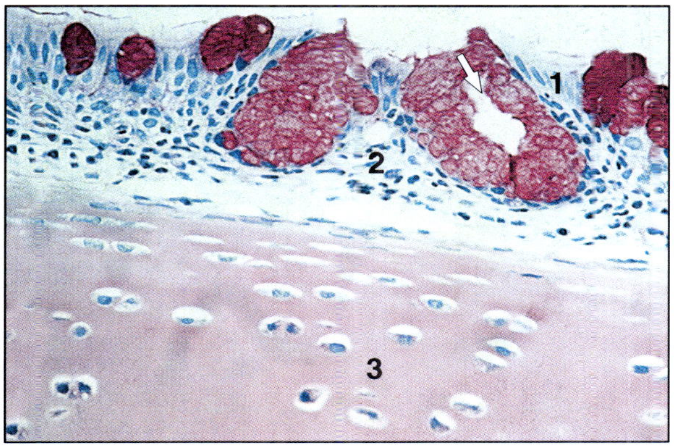

7.31 Respiratory epithelium (bird). (1) Pseudostratified columnar epithelium with intraepithelial mucus-secreting glands (arrowed). (2) Lamina propria and perichondrium. (3) Hyaline cartilage. Haematoxylin/PAS. ×160.

7.32

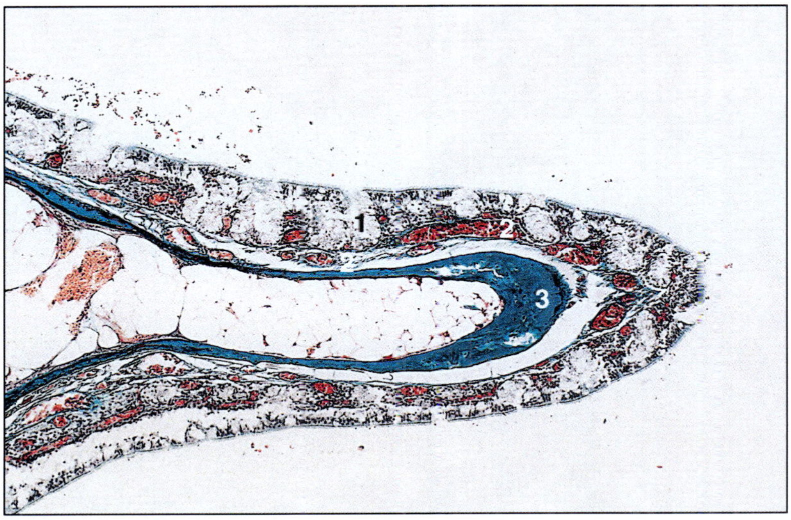

7.32 Avian syrinx, pessulus. (1) Respiratory epithelium. (2) Vascular lamina propria and perichondrium. (3) Hyaline cartilage. Gomori's trichrome. ×5.

the tracheobronchial syrinx, the avian sound box. The tympaniform membranes analogous to the mammalian vocal cords are covered with a stratified squamous epithelium (7.33).

Bronchi

The primary bronchi are lined with respiratory epithelium that rests on a connective tissue lamina propria with hemirings of cartilage embedded in fibrous connective tissue and smooth muscle. The primary bronchi pass into the lung, where they give off secondary bronchi. The epithelium of the secondary bronchi contains goblet cells rather than glands, and cartilage is absent. The secondary bronchi branch into anastomizing parabronchi. Each parabronchus forms the centre of a pulmonary lobule and is lined with simple squamous epithelium. Bundles of smooth muscle form spiral bands that are encased by a thin layer of connective tissue.

The parabronchial wall is perforated with openings leading to spaces lined with squamous or cuboidal epithelium: the atria. The air capillaries arise from the base of the atria via infundibula and radiate towards the periphery of each lobule. The air capillaries are lined with type I epithelial cells forming the respiratory surface and surrounded by a mass of blood capillaries to form the air exchange tissue (7.34).

7.33

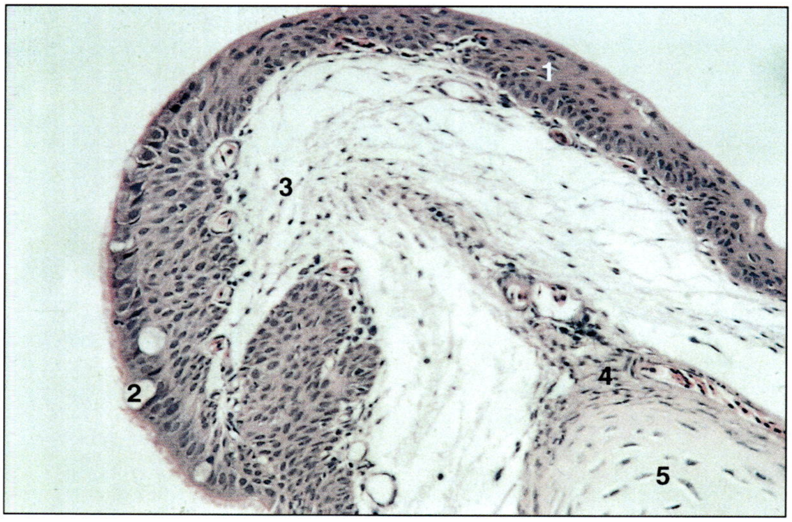

7.33 Avian bronchotracheal larynx. (1) The tympanic membrane is covered by a stratified squamous epithelium. (2) Respiratory epithelium. (3) Lamina propria. (4) Perichondrium. (5) Hyaline cartilage. H & E. ×200.

7.34

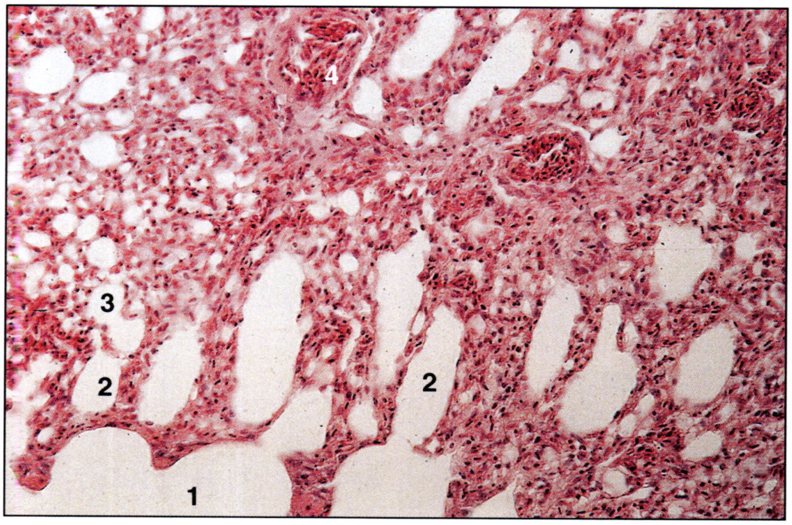

7.34 Lung (bird). (1) Lumen of the parabronchus (tertiary bronchus). (2) Conical ducts, atria. (3) Air capillaries. (4) Blood vessels filled with nucleated erythrocytes. H & E. ×62.5.

Air sacs

Air sacs are thin-walled structures lined by a squamous epithelium (they may be ciliated or columnar) resting on a thin layer of connective tissue. The blood supply is poor and, with the exception of the abdominal air sac (10 branches), they are connected to the secondary bronchi. The humerus and the sternum are some of the bones penetrated by extensions of the air sacs.

Reptilian, amphibian and fish respiratory systems

Most fish (except lungfish, the bowfin, some catfish and a few other teleosts) either lack lungs or possess only primitive elongated sac-like lungs. They must rely upon vascularized gills in order to extract oxygen from and excrete carbon dioxide into their aquatic environment. Gills are composed of parallel rows of gill filaments, the primary lamellae, which are supported by cartilaginous or bony rays forming semilunar folds: the secondary lamellae. The gill arches contain a fine vascular network of branchial arteries, arterioles and capillaries, across which respiratory gases are exchanged and osmoregulation (in conjunction with the kidneys) is maintained. In salmonids, eels and other fish that alternate between freshwater and marine aquatic environments during their life cycles, the electrolyte secreting cells of the gills play major cyclic roles in osmoregulation. Teleost fish also possess a pseudobranch, which is a moderately compressed gill-like structure that is derived during embryological development from the first gill arch (7.35). Its function is believed to be the regulation of blood oxygenation.

The gills of amphibians are similarly structured and function in a similar manner. Some amphibians possess both external gills and internal sac-like lungs, which serve not only as organs of respiratory gas exchange but also have a hydrostatic function. When the sac-like lungs are filled with air, the amphibian becomes more buoyant. When these lungs are empty, buoyancy is lost and the animal sinks to the bottom of the water, thereby requiring little or no effort to remain submerged. Adult plethodontid salamanders lack lungs entirely; their gas respiratory exchange is accomplished solely by diffusion across the well vascularized moist integument. In some amphibians, lungs are much reduced in size; in others, only a single lung is present. Many amphibians augment their pulmonary and integumentary respiration by buccal movements that help move gases across their oropharyngeal mucosae where some gas exchange occurs.

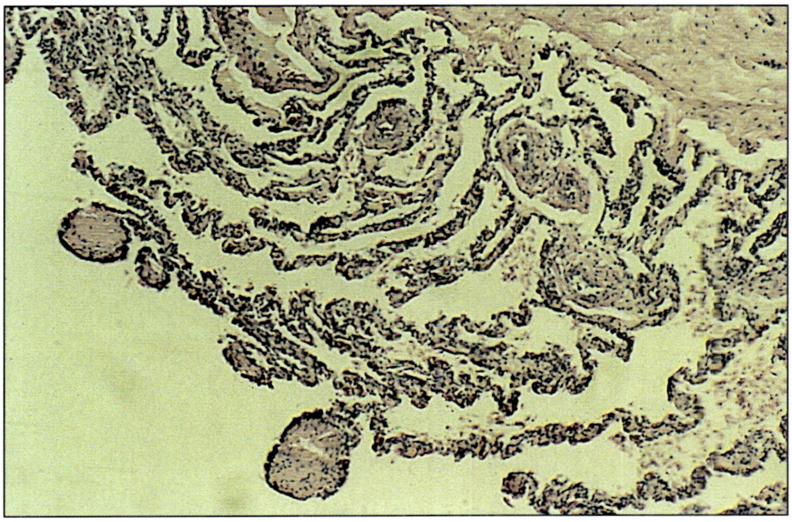

7.35

7.35 Pseudobranch gland of a zebra danio fish. This structure is unique to teleost fish and is derived embryologically from the first gill. It is composed of a cartilaginous 'skeleton' from which parallel lamellae that resemble compressed gill filaments intersect perpendicularly. This organ is thought to function in regulation of blood oxygenation. H & E. ×20.

Clinical correlates

The lungs of many diurnal amphibians and reptiles are heavily pigmented with melanin (*see also* Chapter 3). This pigment is believed to confer protection against the effects of solar radiation. A section of lung from a terrestrial frog (*Rana pipiens*) is shown in 7.36.

As described on page 92, lungs (and similarly gills) are vulnerable to pathogens present in both the external environment and the blood (7.37). In addition, the delicate capillary bed through which respiratory gases exchange is also predisposed to thromboembolism, because of the small cross-sectional area of these vessels.

7.36

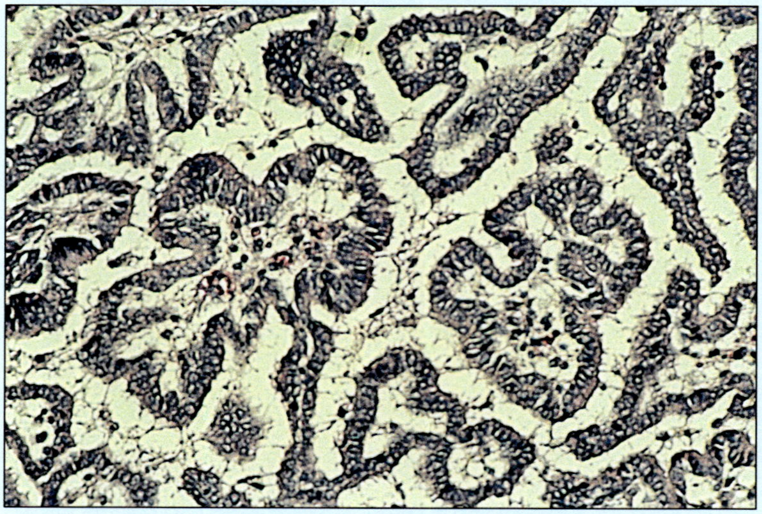

7.36 Lung of a terrestrial frog (*Rana pipiens*). H & E. ×200.

7.37

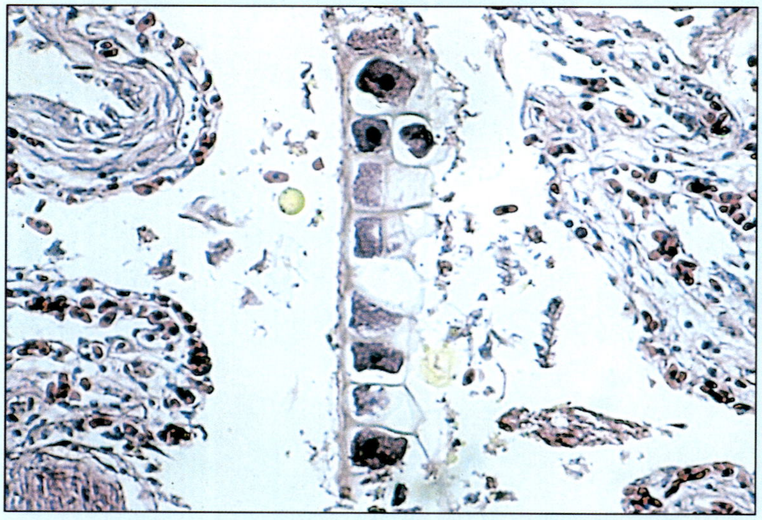

7.37 Aspiration pneumonia in a lizard. Note the plant fibre within the airspace. H & E. ×125.

8. DIGESTIVE SYSTEM

The digestive or alimentary tract begins at the entrance to the oral cavity and terminates at the anus. It is a muscular tube lined with a mucous membrane, divided for convenience into the oral cavity and the alimentary canal.

Oral cavity

Tongue

The bulk of the tongue is made up of interlacing bundles of skeletal muscle fibres and loose connective tissue. The mucous membrane on the undersurface consists of non-keratinized stratified squamous epithelium with a lamina propria (8.1). The dorsal surface of the anterior part of the tongue, where the epithelium is keratinized, is rough. The lamina propria is raised in small projections: the lingual papillae. The filiform, conical and lenticulate papillae are non-sensory and are heavily keratinized, and give the tongue a distinctive rough feel (8.2 and 8.3). The circumvallate, fungiform and foliate papillae are sensory and are associated with small salivary glands in the lamina propria; the taste buds can be found in the lateral

8.1

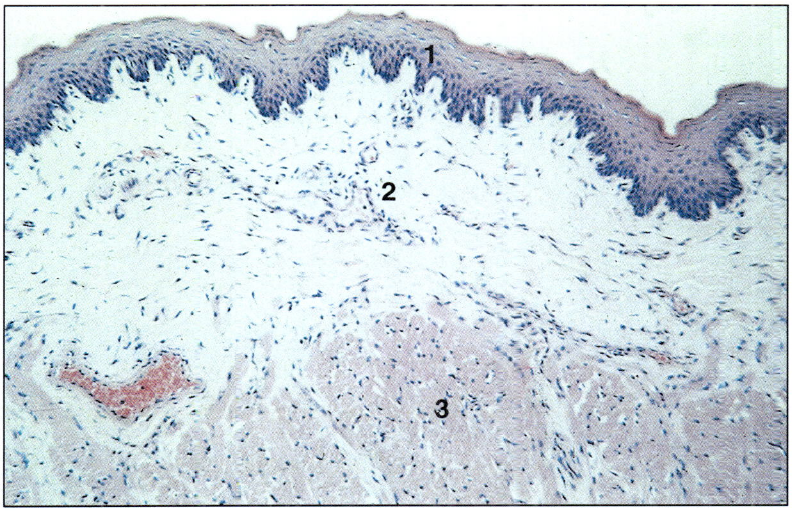

8.1 Tongue (cat). (1) Stratified squamous non-keratinized epithelium. (2) Vascular lamina propria with small projections. (3) Striated muscle fibres. H & E. ×25.

8.2

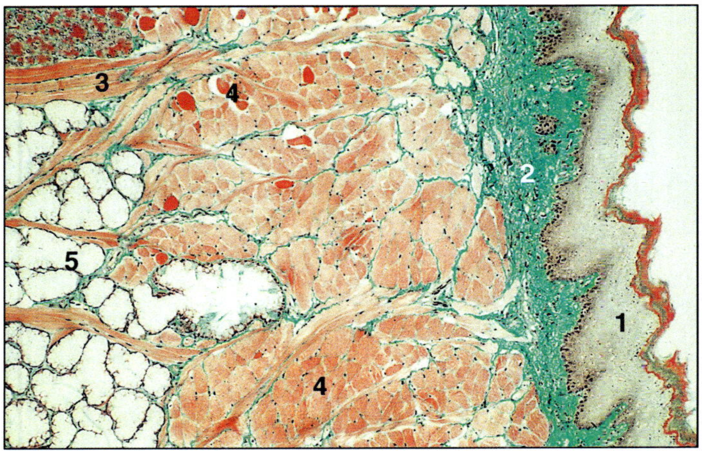

8.2 Tongue (dog). (1) Stratified squamous keratinized epithelium on the dorsum of the tongue. (2) Lamina propria. (3) Striated muscle fibres cut in longitudinal section and (4) in transverse section. (5) Mixed salivary gland. Masson's trichrome. ×25.

8.3

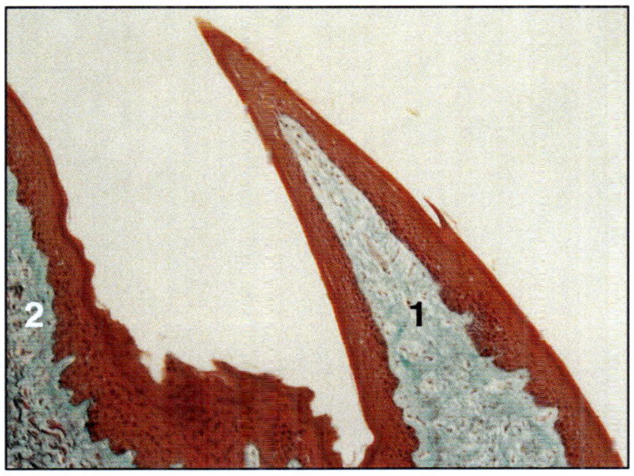

8.3 Tongue (cow). (1) Filiform papilla. (2) Lenticular papilla. Masson's trichrome. ×41.5.

walls. The circumvallate papilla is surrounded by a moat-like trough or vallum and is level with the surface of the tongue (8.4). The fungiform papilla is, as the term suggests, mushroom-shaped with a narrow base, is partly or non-keratinized, and projects above the surface of the tongue (8.5). The foliate papilla is large, non-keratinized and leaf-like, is crossed by transverse furrows and appears in section as a row of fungiform papillae (8.6).

8.4

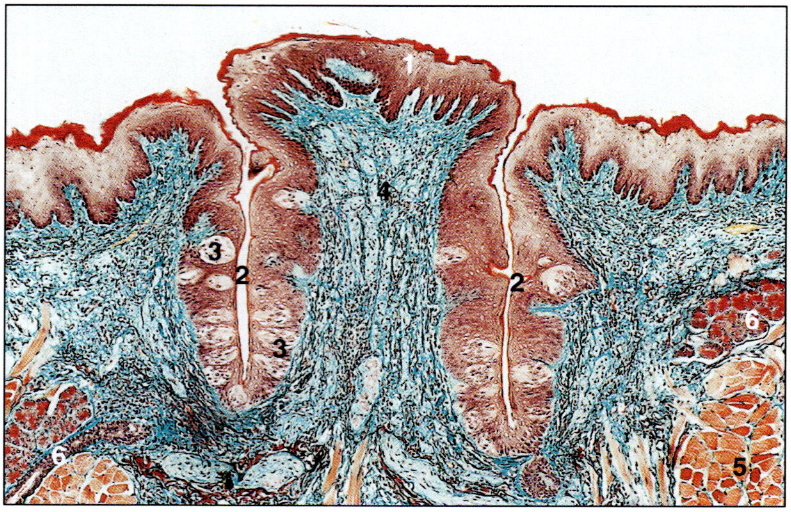

8.4 Circumvallate papilla. Tongue (cow). (1) Stratified squamous epithelium. (2) Vallum. (3) Taste buds. (4) Lamina propria. (5) Striated muscle. (6) Mixed salivary gland. Gomori's trichrome. ×100.

8.5

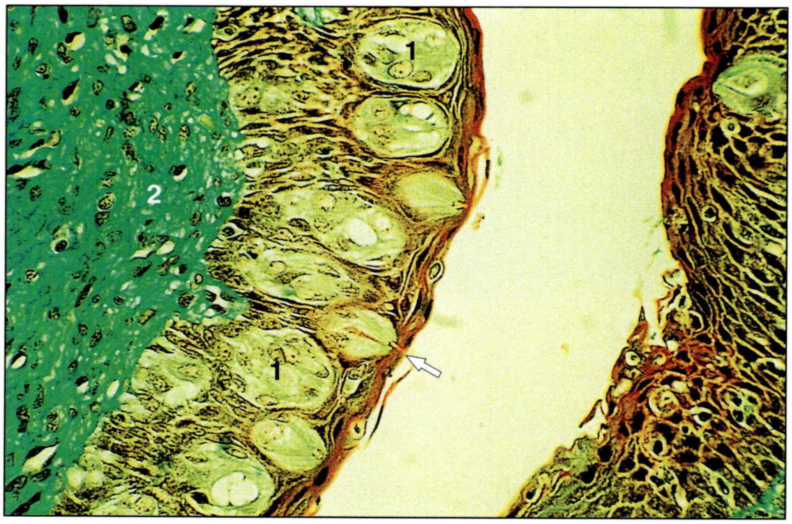

8.5 Tongue (cow). (1) Taste buds in the stratified squamous epithelium of the lateral wall of the papilla. The taste pore is arrowed. (2) Connective tissue lamina propria. Masson's trichrome. ×250.

Taste buds are epithelial structures associated with the terminal fibres of the facial and glossopharyngeal nerve. Within each bud is a taste pore, which opens onto the surface of the tongue, and a taste chamber lined with a taste receptor and sustentacular (supporting) cells. Food dissolved in the salivary gland secretion passes into the reservoir of the taste chamber (8.7).

The lingual tonsil is a localized mass of lymphoid tissue that is often present in the base of the tongue.

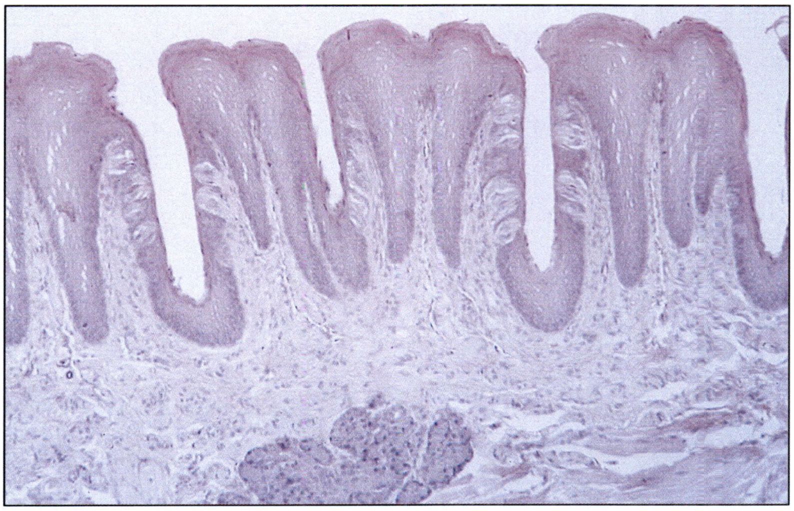

8.6

8.6 Foliate papilla. Tongue (rabbit). This papilla appears as a row of fungiform papillae. The taste buds are arranged along the lateral walls. H & E. ×62.5.

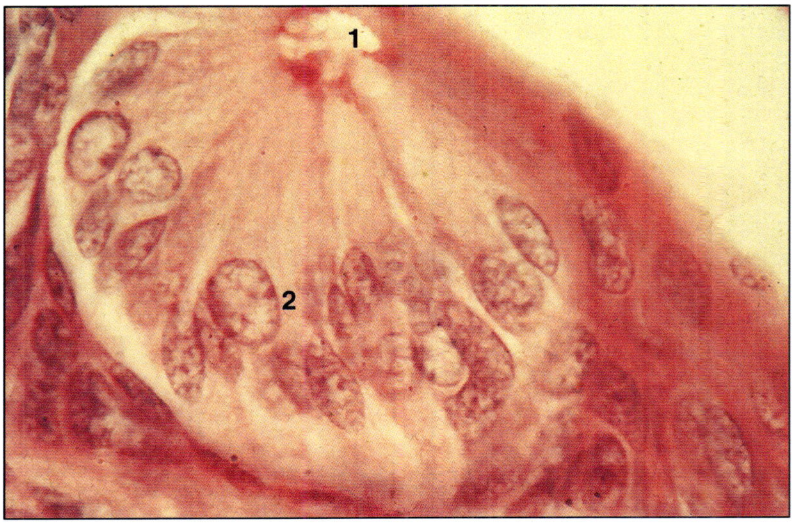

8.7

8.7 Taste bud. Tongue (cow). (1) Taste pore. (2) Taste receptor and sustentacular cells. H & E. ×62.5.

Salivary glands

Salivary glands are compound tubuloacinar exocrine glands. They secrete enzymes or, as seromucous or mixed salivary glands, a mixture of enzymes and mucus. The secretory component of each gland is the parenchyma and the supporting connective tissue is the stroma (**8.8–8.10**). In mixed salivary glands the serous and mucous units may be separate or the serous cells may form a distinctive cap on one side of a mucous unit: a serous demilune (**8.11**). The serous cell is columnar with a basal nucleus and basal basophilia caused by the presence of rough endoplasmic reticulum. The luminal eosinophilia is caused by the secretory granules accumulating before secretion. The mucous cell is triangular with a basal flattened nucleus and a pale staining vacuolated cytoplasm. Specialized epithelial cells, the myoepithelial or basket cells, are capable of contracting: these lie between the secretory cells and the basement membrane (*see* Chapter 2).

The dilute salivary secretion leaves the acinus and is concentrated in the first part of the duct system: the striated duct. The basal cell membrane is infolded and the cytoplasm is lined by mitochondria. This allows water to be removed, passed into the tissue fluid and back to the blood.

Palate

The hard palate is lined with stratified squamous epithelium with the lamina propria continuous with the underlying periosteum (**8.12**). The oral surface of the soft palate is also lined with stratified squamous epithelium, but the lamina propria has mucus-secreting glands and lymphatic nodules. The nasal surface is covered by respiratory epithelium (**8.13**).

8.8

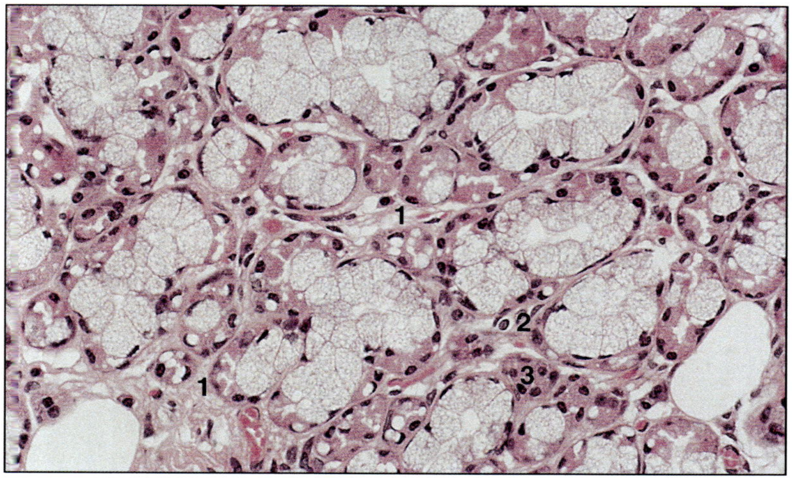

8.8 Mixed salivary gland (cow). The main mass of tissue is secretory units of seromucous acini. (1) Interlobular connective tissue with (2) blood vessels. (3) Interlobular ducts. H & E. ×125.

8.9

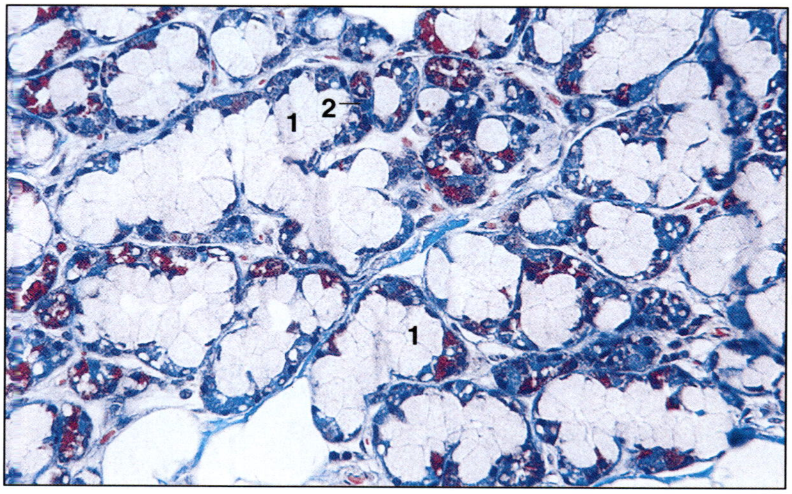

8.9 Mixed salivary gland (cow). Mixed seromucous acinus with (1) pale staining mucous cells and (2) darkly stained serous cells. Masson's trichrome. ×125.

8.10 Mixed salivary gland (dog). (1) Interlobular duct lined by a stratified columnar epithelium. (2) Connective tissue stroma. (3) Parasympathetic ganglion. (4) Seromucous acini. H & E. ×125.

8.10

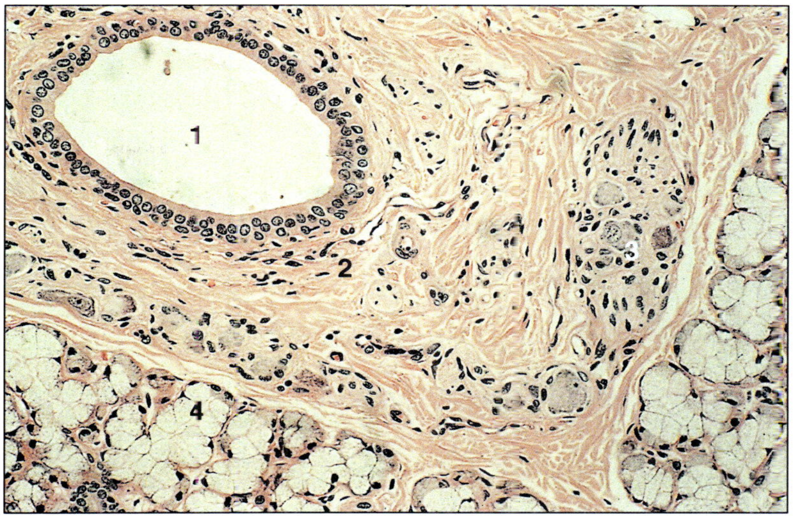

8.11 Mixed salivary gland (dog). (1) Pale staining triangular mucous cells with a basal nucleus. (2) Deeply staining serous cells with a round nucleus. Gomori's trichrome. ×125.

8.11

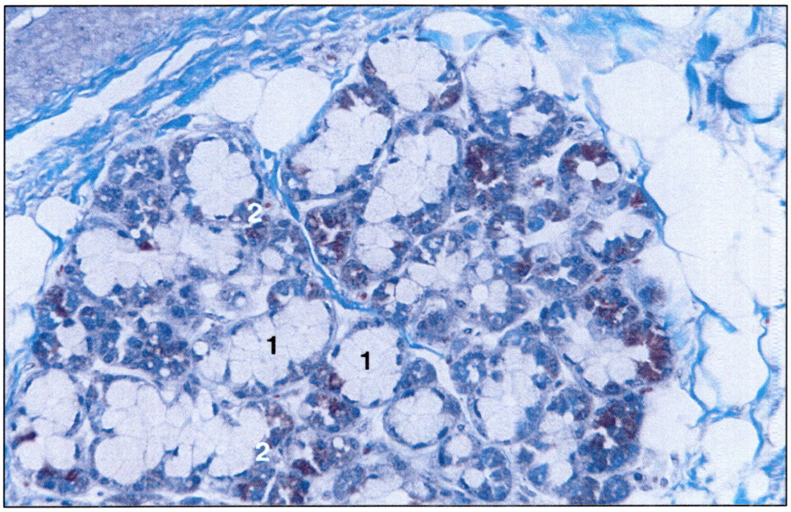

.12

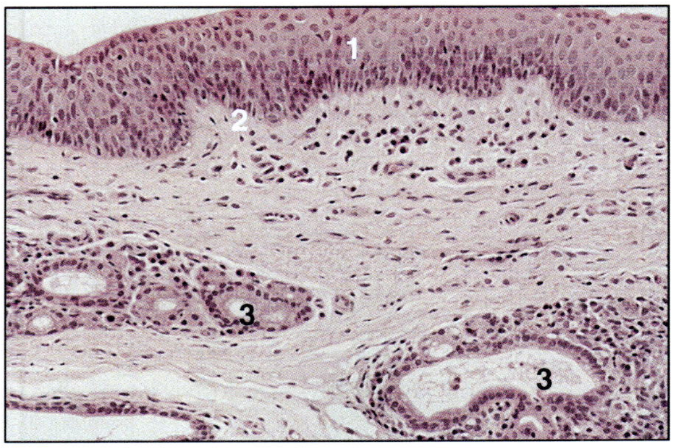

8.12 Hard palate (ox). (1) Stratified squamous epithelium. (2) Lamina propria. (3) Mucus-secreting glands in the lamina propria. H & E. ×125.

8.13

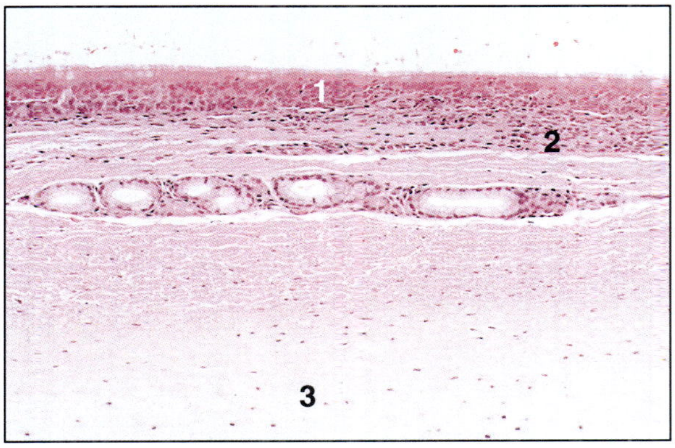

8.13 Soft palate (ox). (1) Respiratory epithelium. (2) Lymph nodule. (3) Bone. H & E. ×62.5.

Teeth

In the embryo teeth develop in the ectoderm as dental papillae within the enamel organs (**8.14**). The mesoderm invaginates each enamel organ into a bell shape, with an inner enamel epithelium of ameloblasts laying down enamel continuous with the outer enamel epithelium and enclosing the stellate reticulum (**8.15**). The mesenchymal cells of the papilla differentiate to become odontoblasts, the dentine-forming cells (**8.16**) and cementoblasts, and secrete cementum in a similar pattern to that of bone. Enamel and dentine are involved with the creation of the crown; dentine and cementum are involved in the root. The root is formed by an extension of the enamel organ at the junction of the inner and outer enamel epithelium: the root tubule (**8.17** and **8.18**). The tooth is held in the developing mandible and maxilla by the periodontal membrane of collagen fibres embedded in the cementum. Temporary teeth develop first. The permanent teeth are secondary offshoots on the lingual side of the

8.14

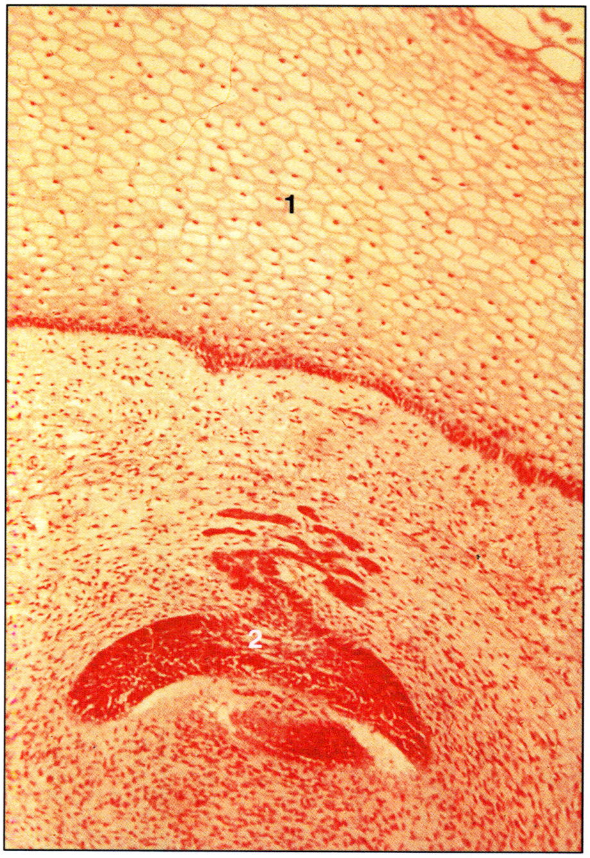

8.14 Developing tooth (cat embryo). (1) Oral epithelium. (2) Enamel organ surrounded by mesoderm. H & E. ×12.5.

8.15

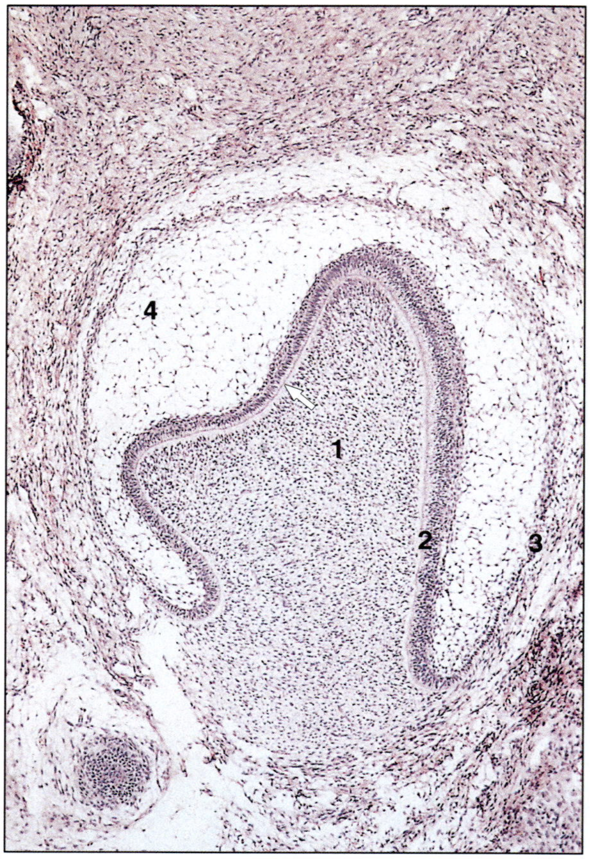

8.15 Developing tooth (cat embryo). (1) Mesenchymal papilla with a layer of odontoblasts (arrowed). (2) Inner enamel epithelium, continuous with (3) the outer enamel epithelium. (4) Stellate reticulum. H & E. ×62.5.

8.16

8.16 Developing tooth (cat embryo). (1) Mesenchymal dental papilla. (2) Ameloblasts in the inner enamel epithelium. (3) Outer enamel epithelium. (4) Stellate reticulum. H & E. ×62.5.

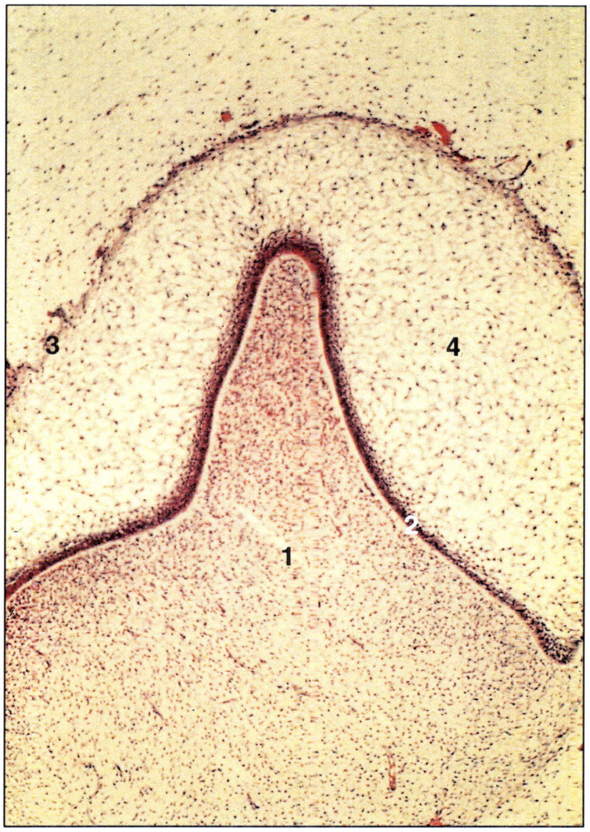

.17

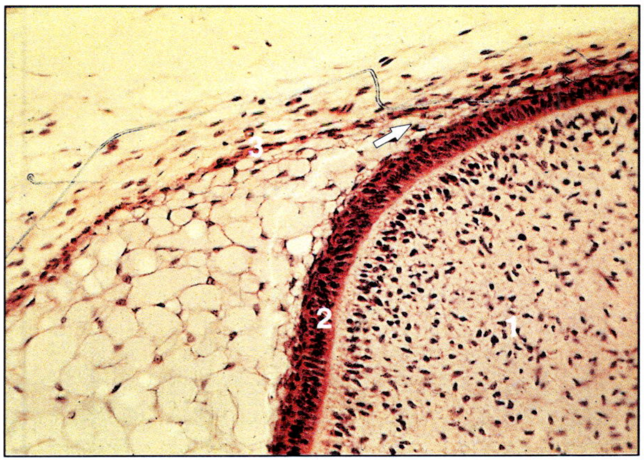

8.17 Developing tooth (cat embryo). (1) Mesenchymal dental papilla lined by odontoblasts. (2) Inner enamel epithelium, ameloblasts, turns to become (3) outer enamel epithelium at the point of root development (arrowed). H & E. ×125.

8.18

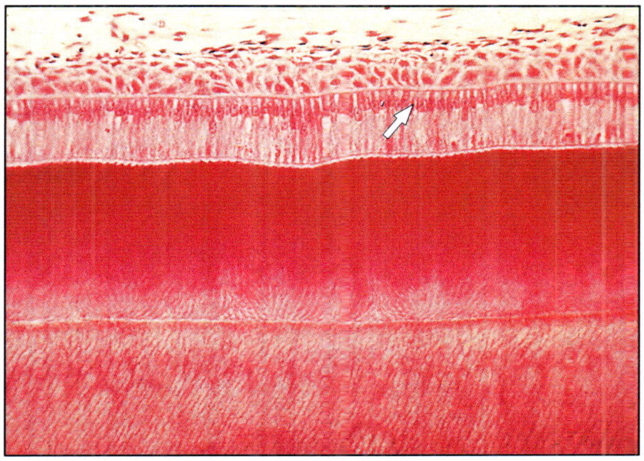

8.18 Developing tooth (cat). The ameloblasts are tall columnar cells with a basal nucleus (arrowed). H & E. ×125.

8.19

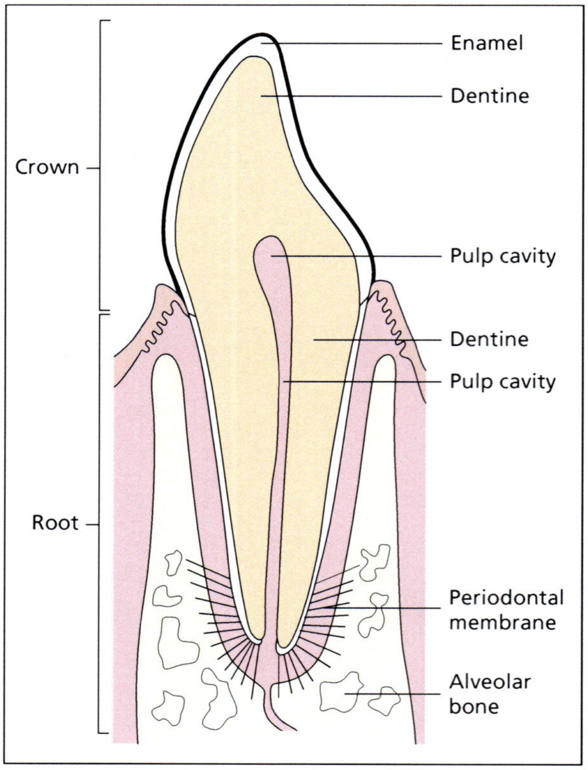

temporary teeth. The tooth is divided into a crown and a root (8.19). In the carnivore, teeth cease to grow after eruption and the ameloblast layer is lost: brachydont teeth. In the horse, ruminant and pig, teeth are much longer and continue to grow for all or part of adult life: hypsodont teeth. In these the dental sac covers the whole of the tooth before eruption and cementum covers the entire tooth, preventing loss of the ameloblasts and allowing continuing deposition of enamel and cementum and thus allowing for the wear and tear in these species (8.20), which include rodents and lagomorphs.

Oropharynx

This is a short junctional area between the oral cavity and the alimentary canal with some mucus-secreting glands (8.21).

8.19 Diagram of an incisor.

8.20

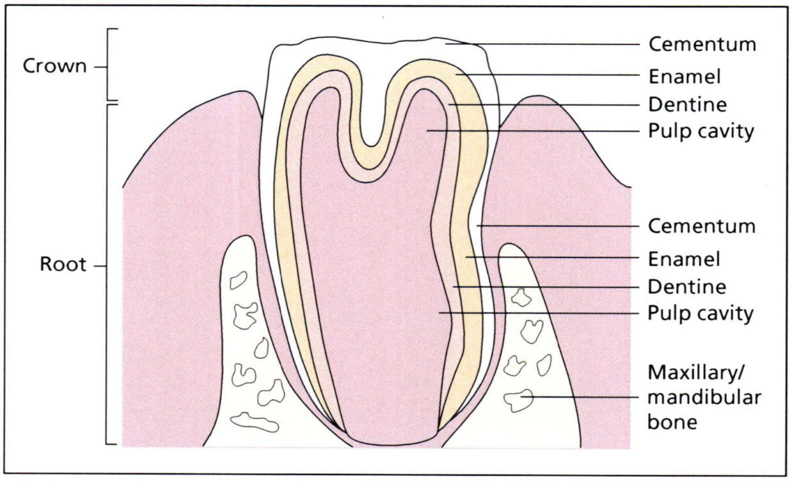

8.20 Diagram of a molar.

8.21

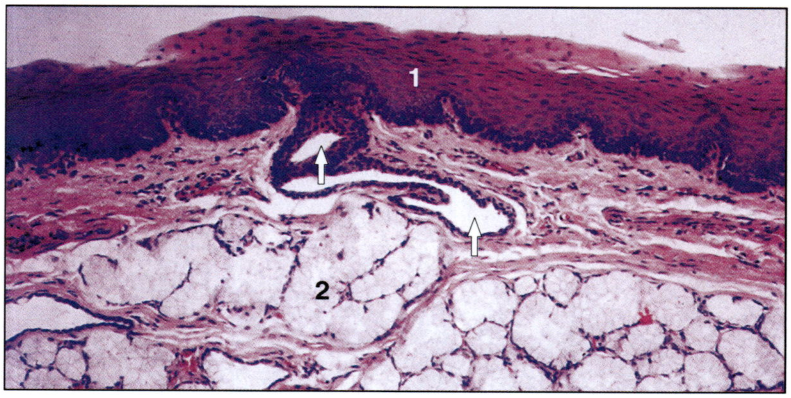

8.21 Oropharynx. (1) Stratified squamous epithelium. (2) Mucus-secreting glands open onto the surface (arrowed). H & E. ×62.5.

Clinical correlates

Any level of the intestinal tract can be affected by inflammation. Gingivitis, or inflammation of the gums, is common in dogs and cats, often in association with dental disease.

A gingival biopsy from a dog in which the gingival epithelium is irregularly hyperplastic is shown in 8.22. A dense inflammatory infiltrate occupies the superficial submucosa and extends into the mucosal epithelium. Plasma cells (mature immunoglobulin-secreting cells) predominate in the infiltrate. Their presence indicates a persistent antigenic stimulus. The initiating disease may be local or systemic.

8.22

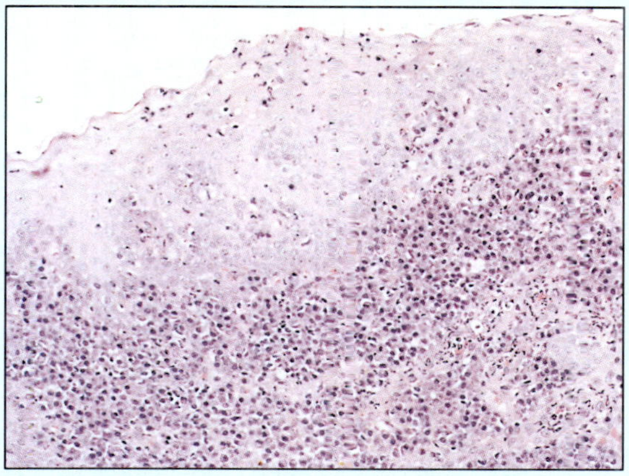

8.22 Plasmacytic gingivitis (dog). H & E. ×125.

Alimentary canal

The alimentary canal (digestive tract) is a muscular tube extending from the oropharynx to the anus, comprising the oesophagus, stomach, and small and large intestines. Two large glands, the liver and pancreas, are also derived from the embryonic alimentary canal. Each part of the canal has a specific function and the histology reflects this (8.23). The canal wall is derived from endoderm and splanchnic mesoderm and consists of four layers:

- Tuna mucosa (mucous membrane), with epithelial lining, supporting vascular lamina propria and lymphatic cells. Mucosal glands, which are derived from the epithelium, are variably present. The outer muscularis mucosae (absent from the mouth, pharynx, portions of the oesophagus and rumen) is smooth muscle.
- Tela submucosa: a connective tissue layer with lymphatic tissue and nerve plexi. Submucosal glands may be present.
- Tunica muscularis: smooth muscle (except in the oesophagus and the anus where the muscle is voluntary, striated muscle).
- Tunica adventitia/serosa (within the peritoneal cavity) or adventitia (retroperitoneal).

8.23 Diagram.TS. Alimentary canal.

8.23

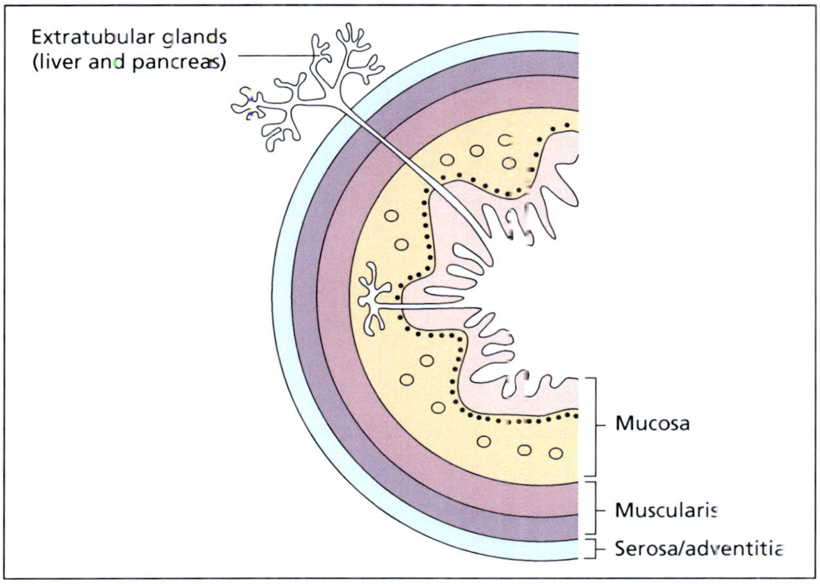

Oesophagus

The oesophagus is lined with stratified squamous epithelium, and both mucosal and submucosal mucus- or seromucus-secreting glands may be present. In ruminants the muscularis externa is skeletal muscle; in the pig and cat the distal part is smooth muscle (8.24–8.27).

8.24

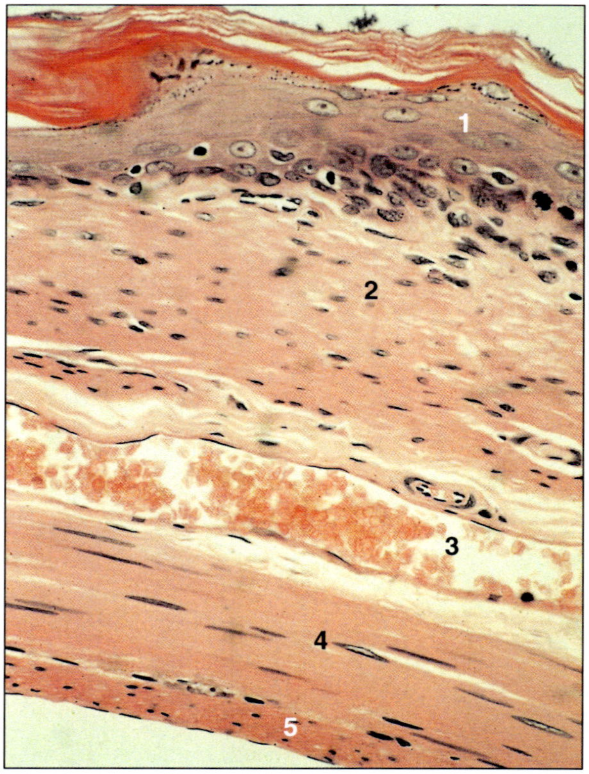

8.24 Oesophagus (cat). (1) Stratified squamous keratinized epithelium. (2) Lamina propria. (3) LS vein. (4) Inner layer of circular smooth muscle. (5) Outer layer of longitudinal smooth muscle. H & E. LP.

8.25

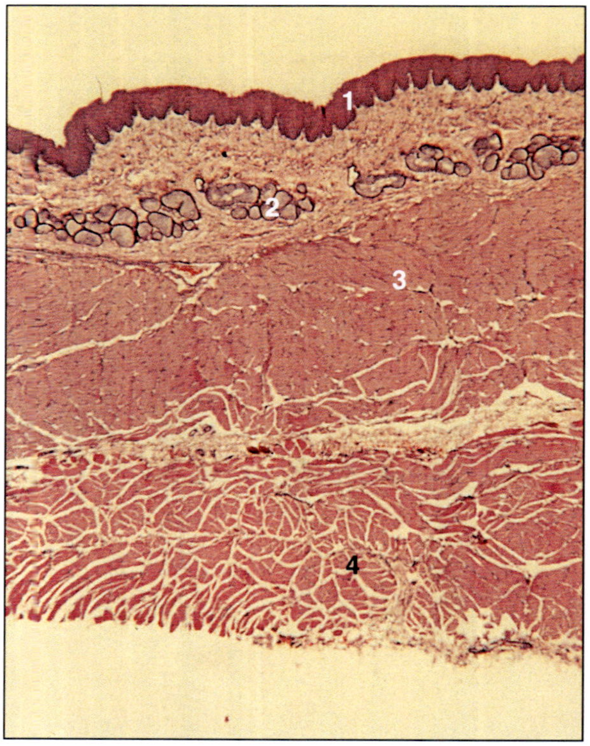

8.25 Oesophagus (dog). (1) Stratified squamous epithelium. (2) Mucus-secreting glands in the lamina propria. (3) Inner layer of circular skeletal muscle. (4) Outer layer of longitudinal skeletal muscle. H & E. ×12.5.

8.26

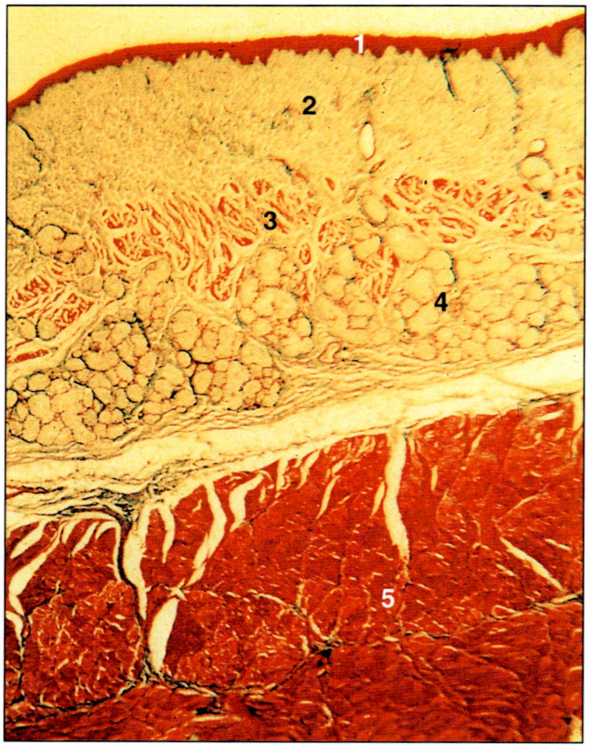

8.26 Oesophagus (cat). (1) Stratified squamous epithelium. (2) Lamina propria. (3) Muscularis mucosae. (4) Submucosal mucous glands. (5) Muscularis externa. Masson's trichrome. ×12.5.

8.27

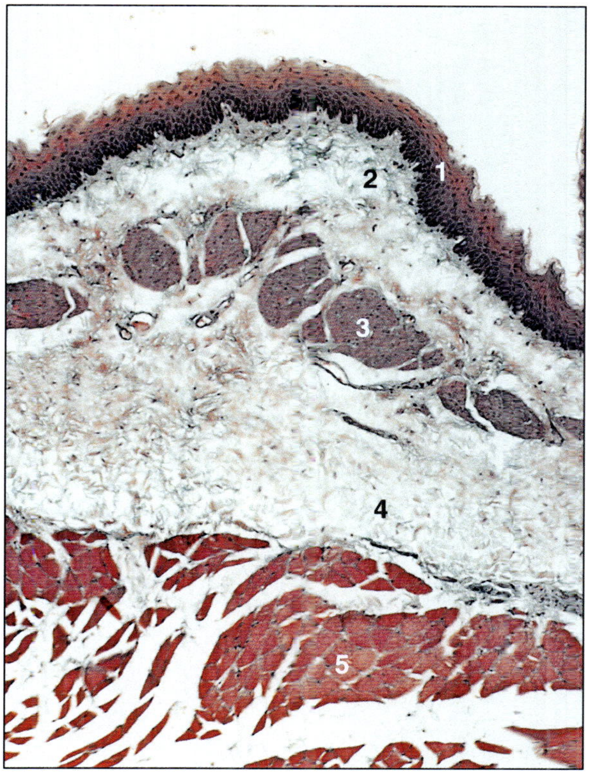

8.27 Oesophagus (dog). (1) Stratified squamous epithelium. (2) Lamina propria. (3) Muscularis mucosae. (4) Submucosal mucous glands. (5) Striated muscle of the muscularis externa. H & E. ×62.5.

Stomach

The stomach mucosa may be non-glandular or glandular in domestic animals. In the simple stomach of the dog and cat, the mucosa is glandular. In the pig and horse, there is a non-glandular (oesophageal) region and a glandular region (8.28 and 8.29). In the ruminant the non-glandular forestomach has three compartments: the rumen, the reticulum and the

8.28

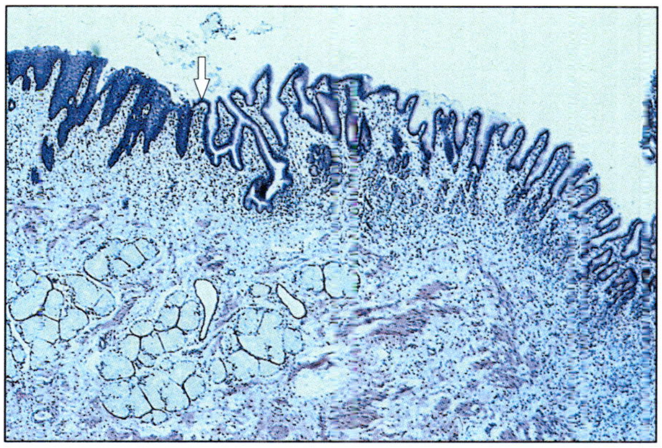

8.28 Oesophageal/stomach junction (horse). The epithelium changes abruptly from stratified squamous to simple columnar at the junction (arrowed). H & E. ×62.5.

8.29

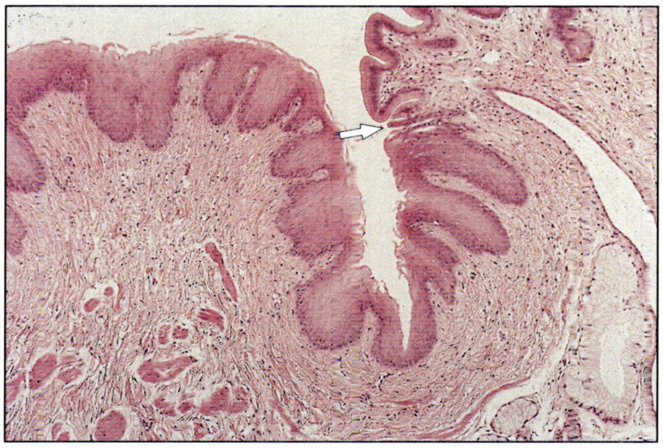

8.29 Oesophageal/stomach junction (horse). The epithelium changes abruptly from stratified squamous to simple columnar at the junction (arrowed). H & E. ×100.

8.30

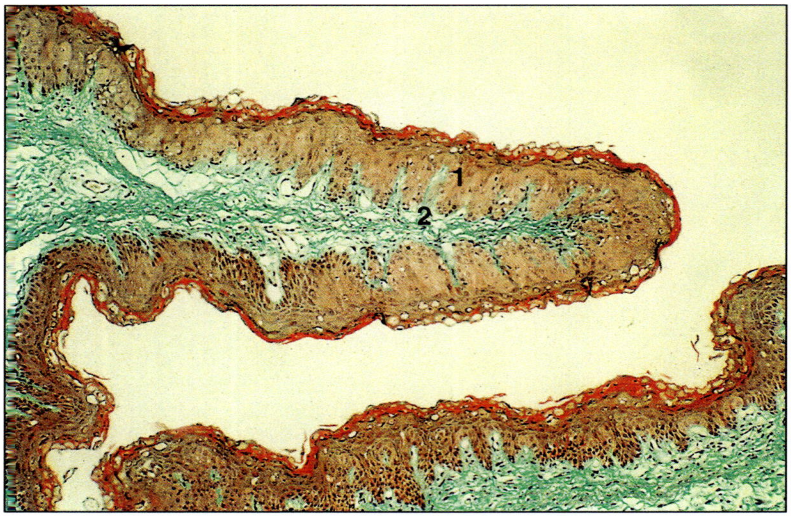

8.30 Rumen (sheep). (1) Stratified squamous epithelium lines the rumen. (2) Lamina propria. Masson's trichrome. ×12.5.

8.31

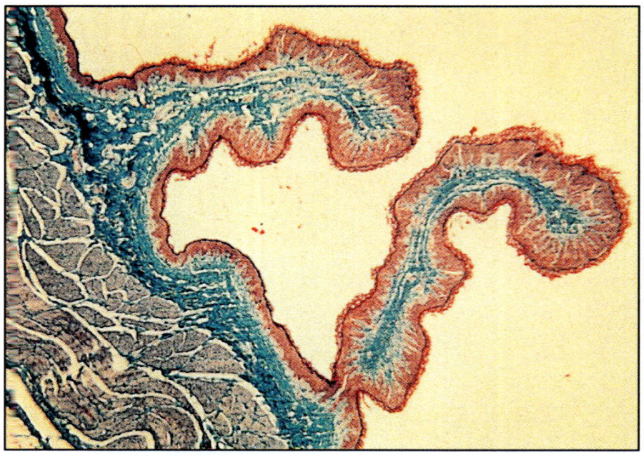

8.31 Rumen (goat). The lining epithelium is stratified squamous. The lamina propria is loose connective tissue, stained green. Gomori's trichrome. ×12.5.

8.32

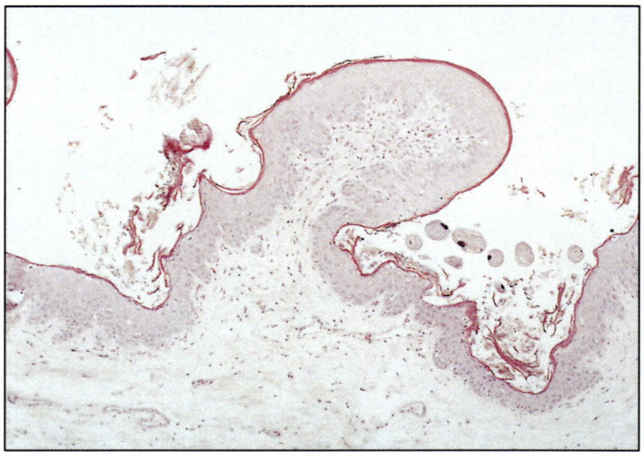

8.32 Reticular groove (goat). The mucosa is folded; this allows stretching. The lining epithelium is stratified squamous. H & E. ×12.5.

8.33

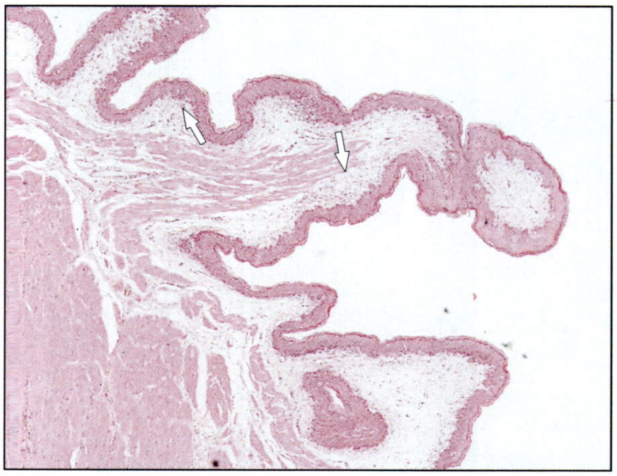

8.33 Omasum (sheep). The muscularis mucosae is present in the long omasal folds (arrowed). H & E. ×12.5.

omasum; the glandular stomach is a separate compartment: the abomasum (8.30–8.35).

The non-glandular stomach is lined with a stratified squamous epithelium with some keratinization. In the ruminant clear vacuolated cells in the epithelium give it a distinctive appearance and allow the transfer of water, electrolytes and short-chain fatty acids. Muscularis mucosae is present in the omasum and reticulum, but absent from the rumen.

The glandular mucosa of the stomach is folded and lined with a simple columnar mucus-secreting epithelium. The gastric pits, the foveoli, are surface depressions continuous with the simple tubular gastric glands (8.36). Three histological regions are

.34

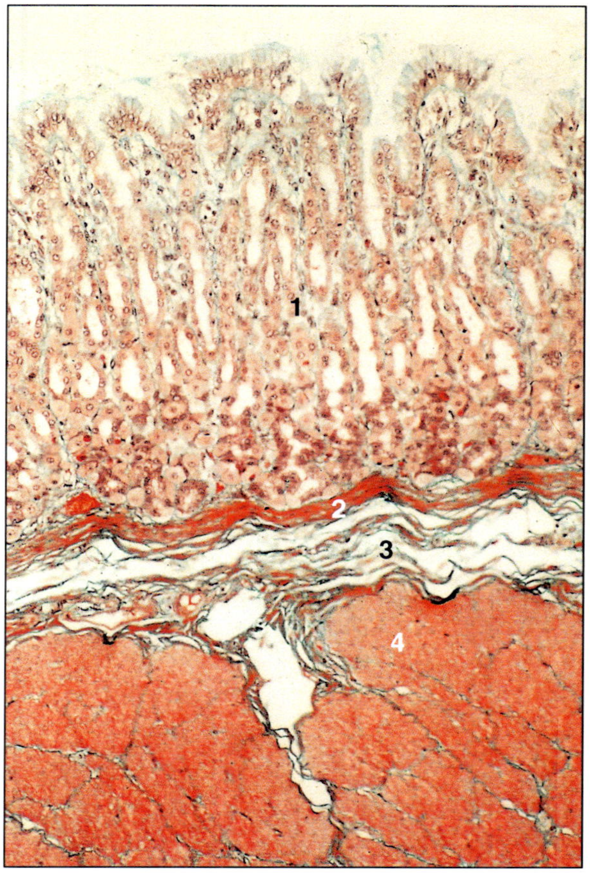

8.35

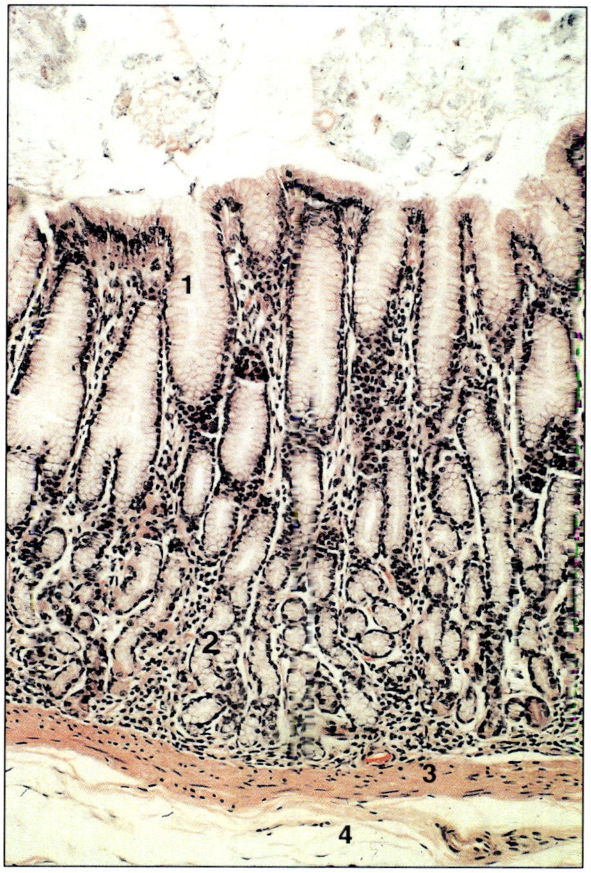

8.34 Abomasum. Fundic region (goat). (1) Mucosa. (2) Muscularis mucosae. (3) Submucosa. (4) Muscularis externa. Masson's trichrome. ×25.

8.35 Abomasum. Pyloric region (goat). (1) The lining epithelium is simple columnar and mucus secreting. (2) Simple tubular mucus-secreting glands. (3) Muscularis mucosae. (4) Submucosa. H & E. ×62.5.

8.36 Stomach (horse). (1) Simple columnar mucus-secreting epithelium. (2) Gastric pits. H & E. ×62.5.

8.36

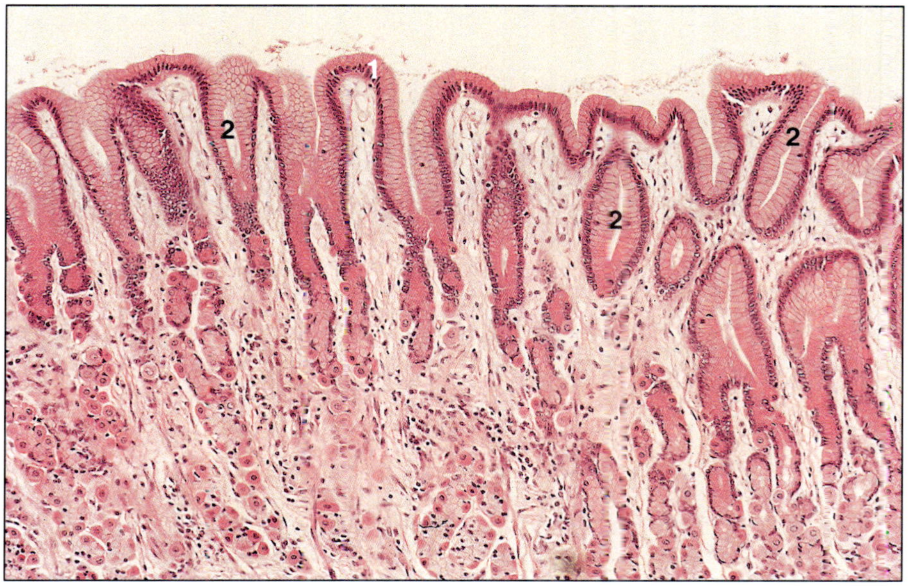

8.37

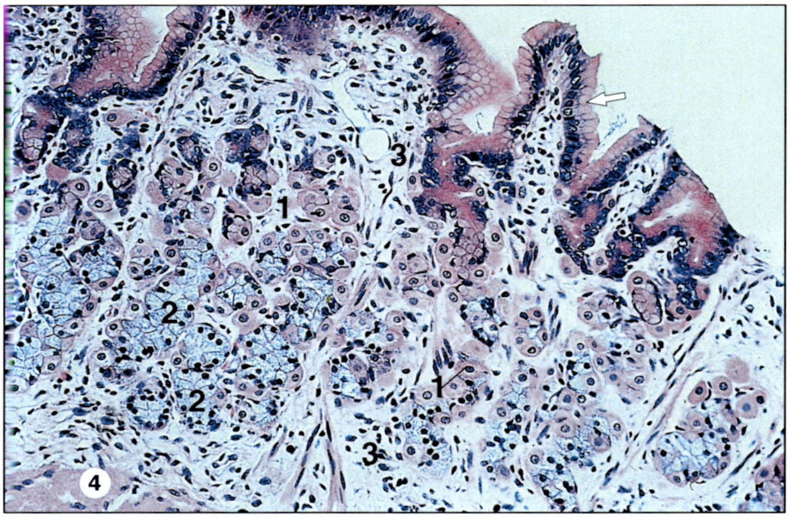

8.37 Cardiac glands. Stomach (horse). Simple columnar mucus-secreting epithelium lines the stomach (arrowed). (1) Parietal (oxyntic) cell, deep red staining. (2) Zymogen (chief) cell, basophilic staining. (3) Lamina propria. (4) Muscularis mucosae. H & E. ×125.

8.38

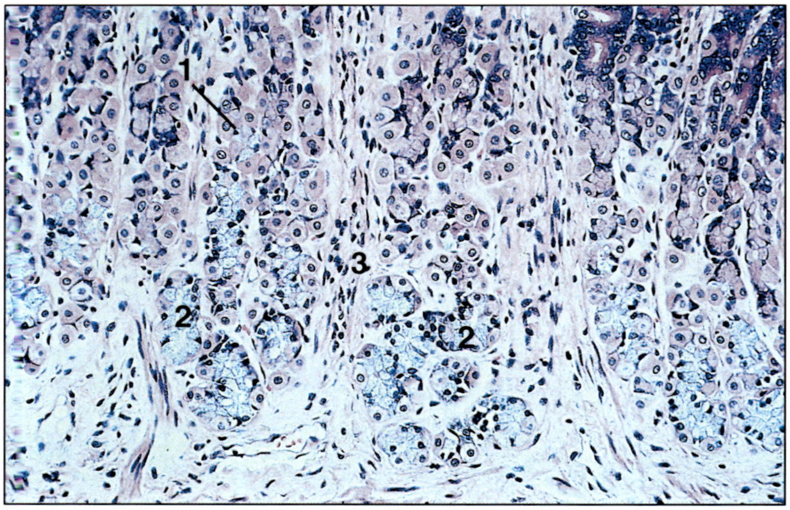

8.38 Cardiac glands. Stomach (horse). (1) Parietal cell. (2) Zymogen cell. (3) Lamina propria. H & E. ×125.

8.39

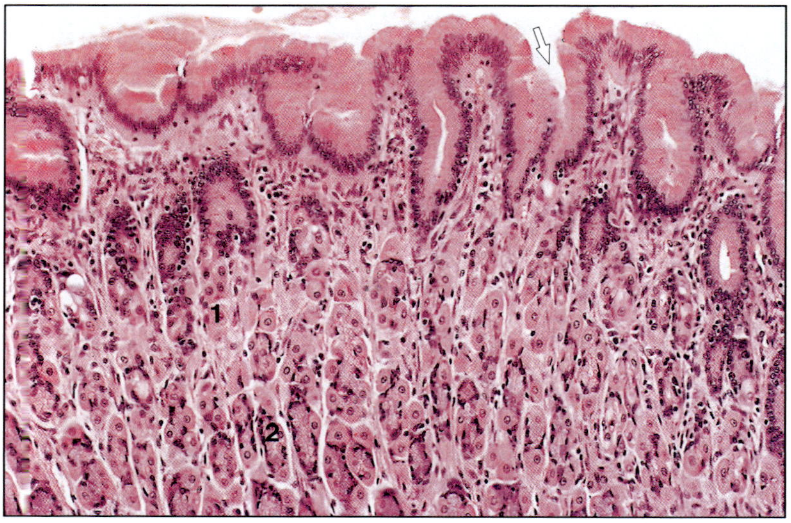

8.39 Fundic glands. Stomach (horse). Simple mucus-secreting epithelium extends into the gastric pits (arrowed). (1) Parietal cell. (2) Zymogen cell. H & E. ×250.

recognized: the cardia, the fundus and the pylorus. Glands are sparse with few cells in the cardia, but are abundant and cellular in the fundus (8.37–8.42).

8.40

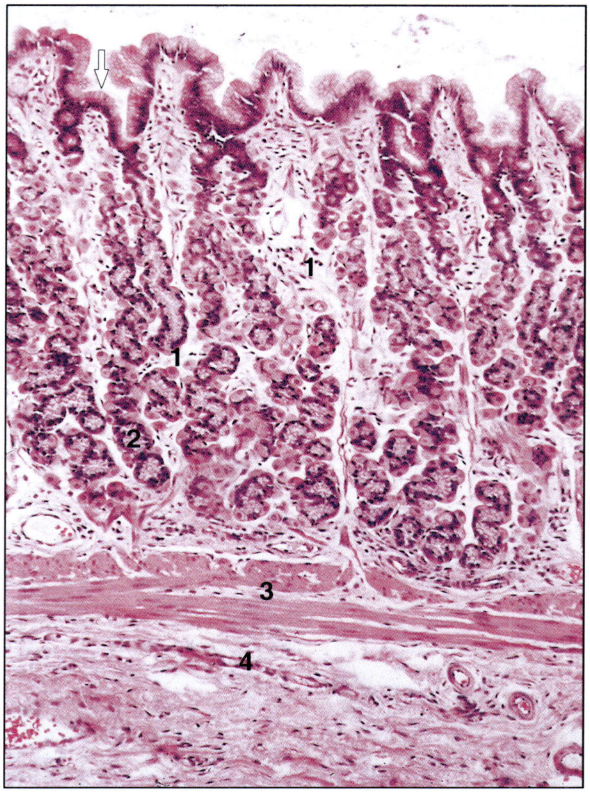

8.40 Fundic glands. Stomach (dog). Simple columnar mucus-secreting epithelium extends into the gastric pits (arrowed). (1) Parietal cell. (2) Zymogen cell. (3) Muscularis mucosae. (4) Submucosa. H & E. ×125.

8.41

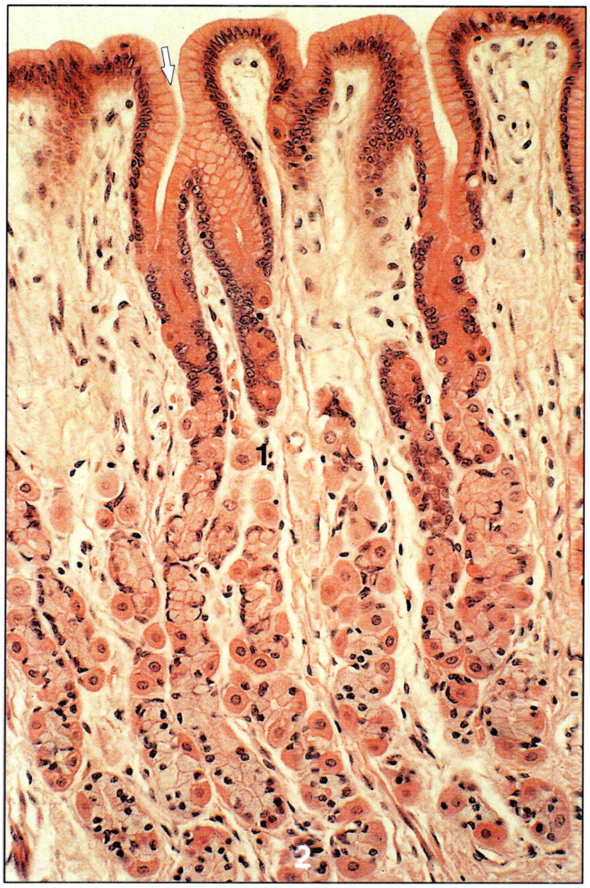

8.41 Fundic glands. Stomach (dog). Simple columnar mucus-secreting epithelium extends into the gastric pits (arrowed). (1) Parietal cell. (2) Zymogen cell. H & E. ×160.

8.42 Fundic gland. Stomach (cat). (1) Parietal cell. (2) Zymogen cell. H & E. ×250.

8.42

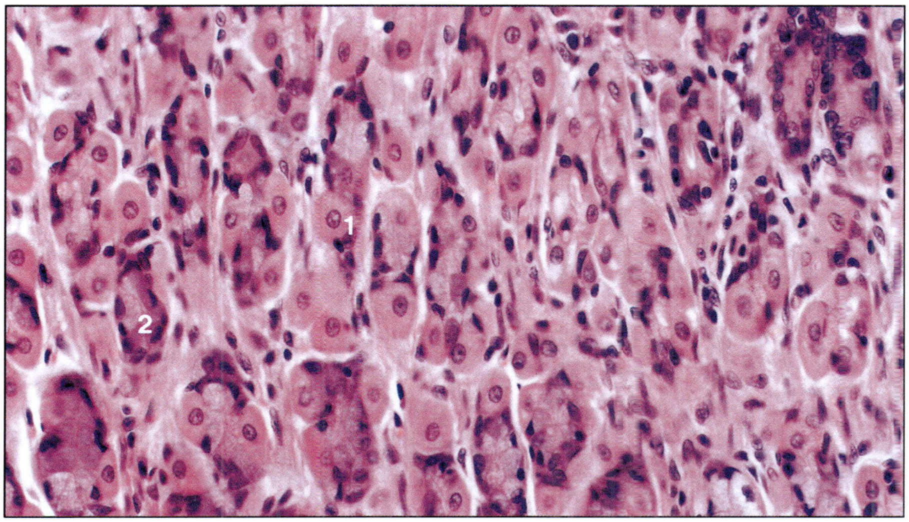

There are five cell types in the gastric glands:

- Stem cells at the neck of the gland divide and replace the surface epithelium.
- Mucous neck cells at the neck of the gland secrete mucus.
- Parietal (oxyntic) cells are large polyhedral cells with a central nucleus and eosinophilic cytoplasm. They secrete hydrochloric acid into canaliculi and elaborate invaginations of the plasma membrane.
- Chief (zymogenic, peptic) cells secrete the enzyme pepsinogen; this is converted into pepsin by the gastric acid. In common with all enzyme-secreting cells, the rounded basal nucleus is surrounded with basophilic cytoplasm (rough endoplasmic reticulum). The apical cytoplasm is eosinophilic (stored secretory granules).
- Enteroendocrine cells are a diffuse population that are identified with specialized silver stains and are also known as argentaffin and argyrophil cells. Chemical messengers (serotonin, gastrin, somatostatin and enteroglucagon) are secreted locally to control digestion. These cells are regarded as part of the 'amine–precursor–uptake–decarboxylation' (APUD) cell system, which is characterized by the ability to take up and process biogenic amines. However, not all of these cells process amines and the term 'diffuse neuroendocrine system' is more accurate.

The pyloric glands are mucus secreting (**8.43** and **8.44**).

The lamina propria is loose cellular connective tissue with lymphatic cells present as a local population and part of the gut-associated lymphoid tissue (GALT). The muscularis mucosae is composed of several layers of smooth muscle fibres. The submucosa is aglandular loose connective tissue with parasympathetic nerve plexi (**8.37–8.44**). The muscularis externa consists of three layers of smooth muscle: oblique, circular and longitudinal. The myenteric parasympathetic nerve plexus (Meissner's) lies between the muscle layers (**8.45**). The outer layer, the serosa, is vascular connective tissue covered with mesothelial cells continuous with the visceral peritoneum.

8.43

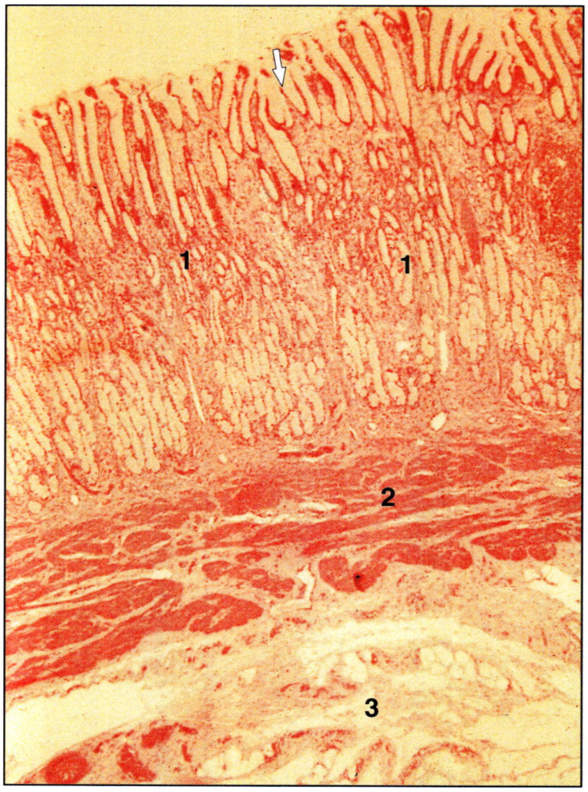

8.43 Pyloric glands. Stomach (pig). Simple columnar mucus-secreting epithelium extends into the gastric pits (arrowed). (1) Simple tubular mucus-secreting glands. (2) Muscularis mucosae. (3) Submucosa. H & E. ×25.

8.44

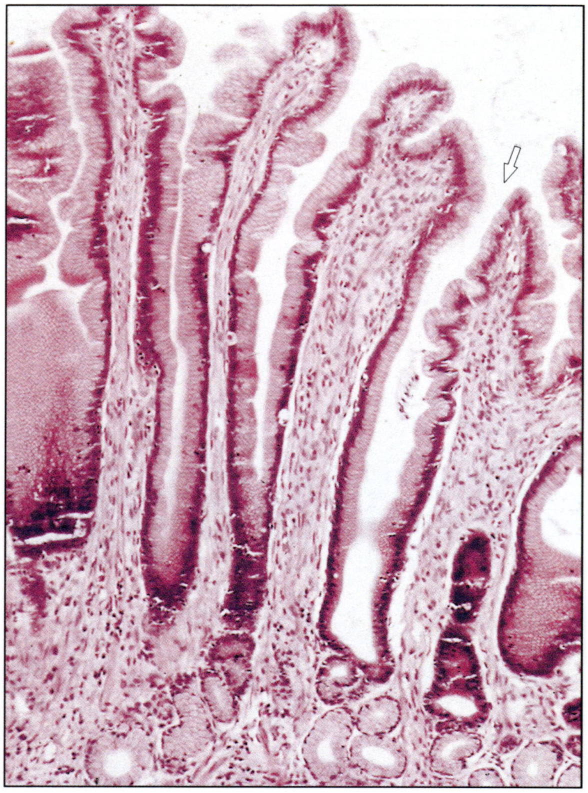

8.44 Pyloric glands. Stomach (dog). Simple columnar mucus-secreting epithelium extends into the gastric pits (arrowed). Simple columnar epithelium lines the gland tubule seen here cut in transverse section. H & E. ×100.

8.45

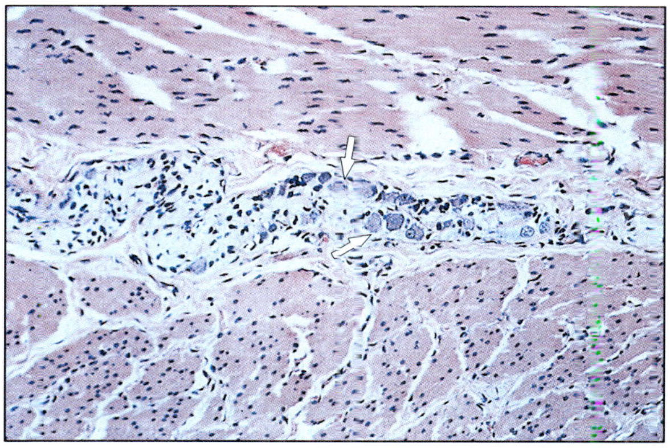

8.45 Myenteric nerve plexus. Stomach (horse). Parasympathetic neuron cell bodies (arrowed) lie in the connective tissue between the smooth muscle layers. H & E. ×125.

Clinical correlates

Gastric lesions may be associated with many conditions which have signs that also affect other body systems or other levels of the gastrointestinal tract. The aetiopathogenesis of peptic ulceration (8.46) is incompletely understood, but it results from an imbalance between the damaging effects of gastric acid and pepsin and the protective mechanisms of the gastric mucosa. Administration of non-steroidal anti-inflammatory drugs is known to predispose to gastric ulceration by inhibiting prostaglandin metabolism and damaging the gastric epithelium. Systemic disturbances, such as endotoxaemia or uraemia, may produce gastric lesions and complex factors associated with stress can also be implicated. Gastric ulceration can produce abdominal pain, vomition or haematemesis, melaena and anaemia.

8.46

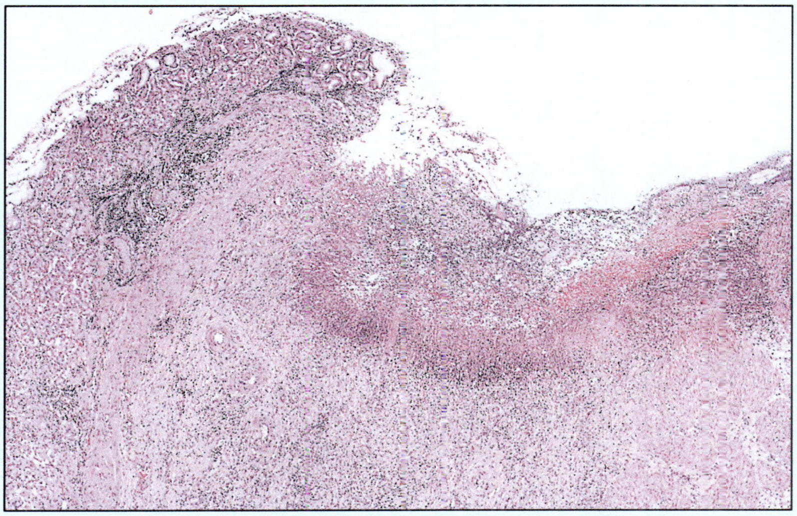

8.46 Peptic ulceration (dog). Loss of mucosal epithelium is seen, with eosinophilic necrotic debris within the defect. Granulation tissue is developing in the base of the ulcer. H & E. ×32.

8.47

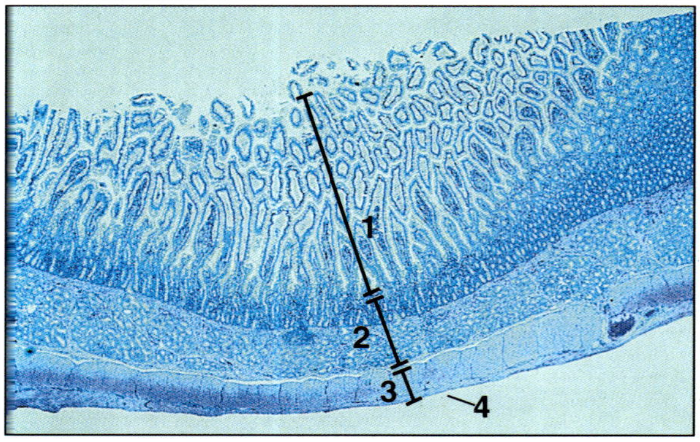

8.47 Duodenum (dog). (1) Mucosa. (2) Submucosa. (3) Muscularis externa. (4) Serosa. H & E. ×25.

Small intestine

The small intestine consists of the duodenum, jejunum and ileum (8.47–8.55). The function of the mucosa is absorption. Finger-like projections of the intestinal villi are long and thin in carnivores and short and thick in ruminants. They increase the surface area for absorption. The core of each villus is

8.48

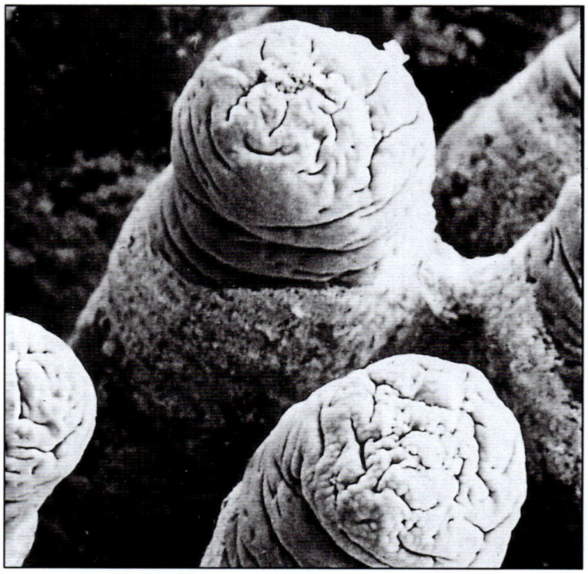

8.48 Duodenal villi (dog). The finger-like villi project into the lumen of the duodenum. Scanning electron micrograph. ×100.

8.49

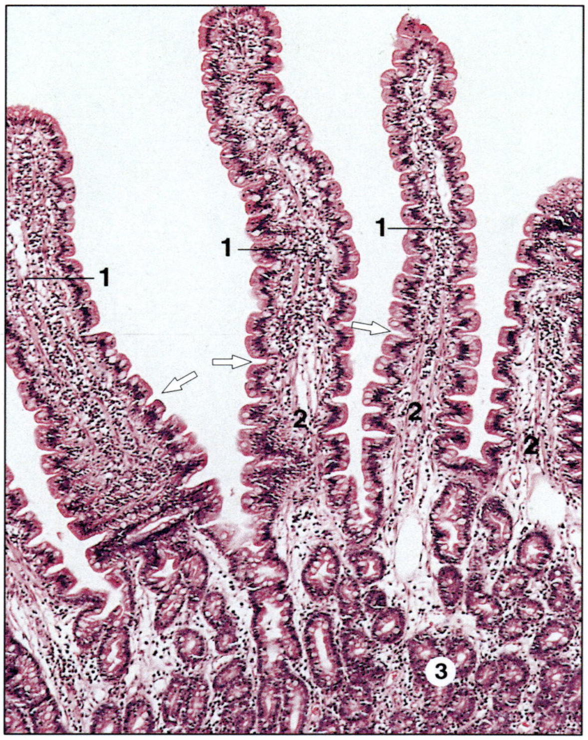

8.49 Duodenum (dog). (1) Villus covered by simple columnar epithelium. (2) Lamina propria forms the core of the villus; the contractile crypts are arrowed. (3) Mucosal glands. H & E. ×62.5.

8.50

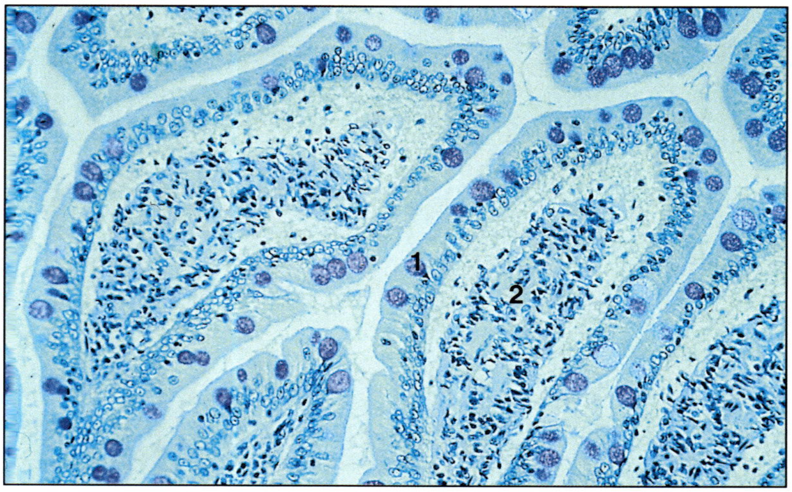

8.50 Duodenum (horse). (1) Goblet cells in the epithelium are stained deep pink. (2) Lamina propria. Haematoxylin/PAS. ×125.

formed by the lamina propria, which is vascular, cellular and reticular, with local aggregations of lymphoid cells. The tall columnar cells that line the intestine have a striated border containing mucus-secreting goblet cells; these increase in number with distance from the stomach. At the bases of the villi, the epithelium dips into the lamina propria to form mucosal intestinal glands (the crypts of Lieberkühn). The cells lining the crypts are columnar, secreting mucus, enzymes and local hormones, and are the stem cells that are active in the repair and replacement of the epithelium. Paneth cells,

8.51

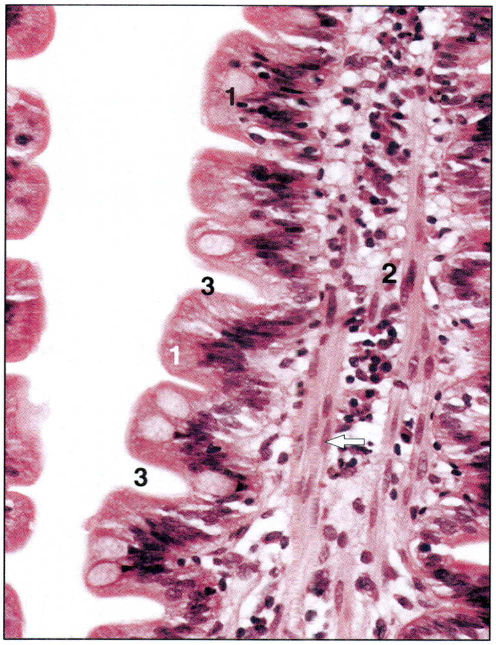

8.51 Duodenum (horse). (1) Simple columnar epithelium with goblet cells. (2) Lamina propria with smooth muscle fibres (arrowed). (3) Contractile crypts. H & E. ×250.

.52

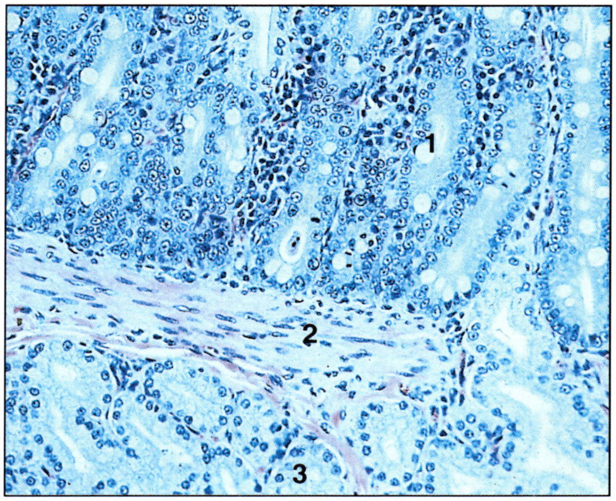

8.52 Duodenum (dog). (1) Mucosal glands. (2) Muscularis mucosae. (3) Submucosal glands. H & E. ×160.

8.53

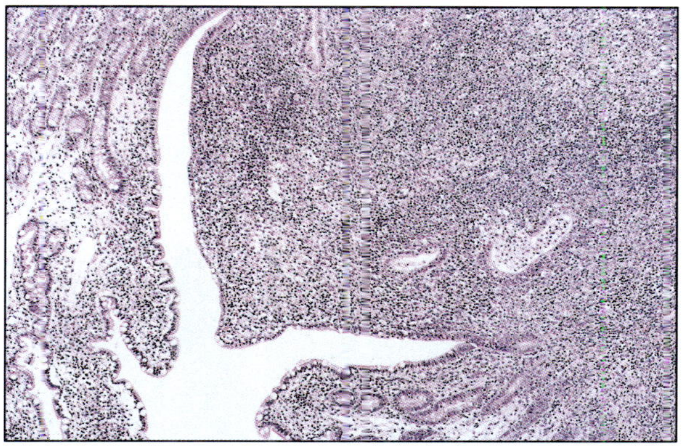

8.53 Duodenum (dog). The lamina propria is filled with lymphatic tissue and lymphocytes are seen migrating through the epithelium (a Peyer's patch). H.& E. ×12.5.

.54

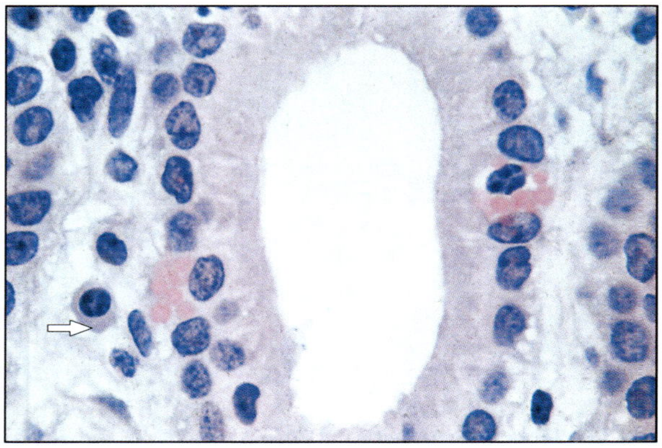

8.54 Globular leucocyte (horse). The globular leucocyte (function unknown) is in the epithelium of the intestinal gland. A plasma cell is present in the lamina propria (arrowed). H & E. ×500.

8.55

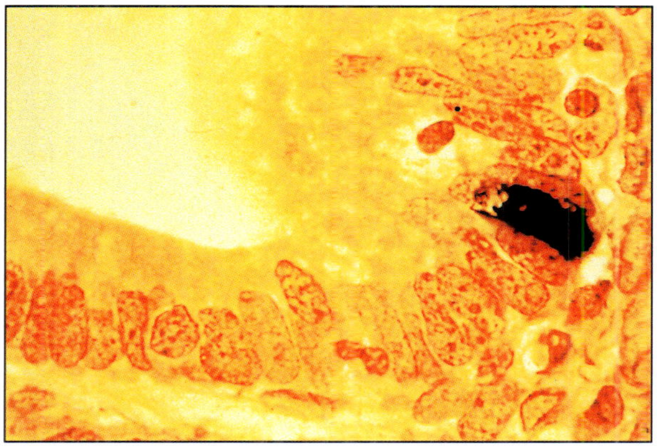

8.55 Enteroendocrine argentaffin cell (cat). Argentaffin cell stains black in the intestinal gland epithelium. Methanamine silver/safranin. ×500.

which contain secretory granules that contain pepsidase, may also be present in horses and ruminants.

The muscularis mucosae consists of two layers of smooth muscle, inner circular and outer longitudinal, and separates the crypts from the underlying mucosa. A strip of muscle extends into each villus from the muscularis mucosae; a lacteal (lymphatic that transports chyle) is also present. Indentations on the villi, called contractile crypts, are created by the contraction of the central strip of the muscle. Mucus- and seromucus-secreting submucosal glands are found in the horse in 6–7 m of the intestine, 3–5 m in the pig, 4 m in the cow and 60–70 cm in sheep.

The muscularis externa consists of two layers of smooth muscle dispersed in a gentle spiral, appearing as an inner circular and outer longitudinal layer. As in the stomach the myenteric parasympathetic nerve plexus (Meissner's) can be found between the layers.

The serosa consists of loose connective tissue, and the mesothelium is continuous with the visceral peritoneum.

Large intestine

There are no villi in the large intestine (caecum, colon, rectum and rectal canal). Goblet cells are abundant in the surface epithelium and in the mucosal glands, which are simple regular tubules. Lymphoid tissue is present in the lamina propria, as are eosinophil leucocytes associated with parasitic infestations. Lymphocytes are present in the epithelium when immunoglobulin, which bathes the epithelial cell surface as a defence against luminal antigen, is released. There are no submucosal glands.

A muscularis mucosae is present, and the muscularis externa consists of an inner circular and outer longitudinal layer of smooth muscle. The outer layer, or taenia coli, is arranged in bands and is characteristic of the colon of the horse and pig. In the horse, elastic fibres replace muscle fibres. The serosa is continuous with the peritoneum (**8.56** and **8.57**).

The rectum is lined with simple columnar epithelium. The mucosal glands decrease in number and may disappear entirely as the anus is approached, where there is an abrupt change to a stratified squamous epithelium. The muscularis externa is thicker here and becomes striated at the anal sphincter. Part of the rectum is covered by a serosa and the rest by adventitia. Tubuloacinar anal glands are present at the cutaneous–rectal junction where they secrete lipids in carnivores and mucus in the pig. In carnivores, circumanal, sebaceous-secreting glands are found in the anal canals. Anal sacs, opened by small tubular alveolar glands and lined with stratified squamous epithelium, open into the perianal region (**8.58**).

GALT is part of the immune system. Both T and B lymphocytes, as well as macrophages and eosinophils, are present. The tissue may be so profuse that the enterocytes are stretched over a bulging mass. Lymphocytes may migrate through the epithelium (*see* **8.53**).

8.56

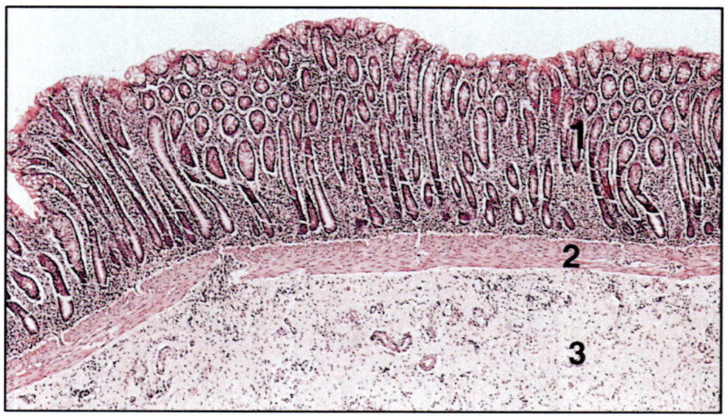

8.56 Colon (horse). (1) Mucosa. (2) Muscularis mucosae. (3) Submucosa. H & E. ×9.7.

8.57

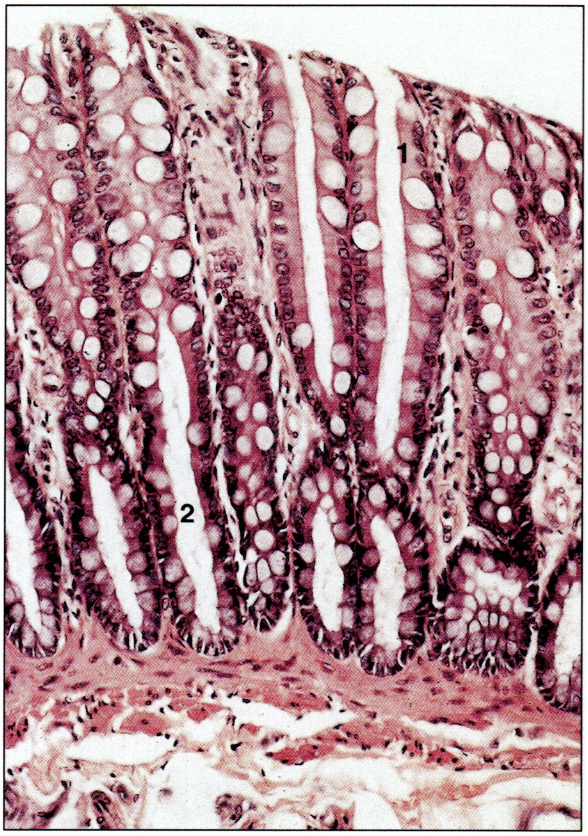

8.57 Colon (horse). (1) Simple columnar epithelium with goblet cells. (2) Intestinal mucosal glands. H & E. ×125.

8.58

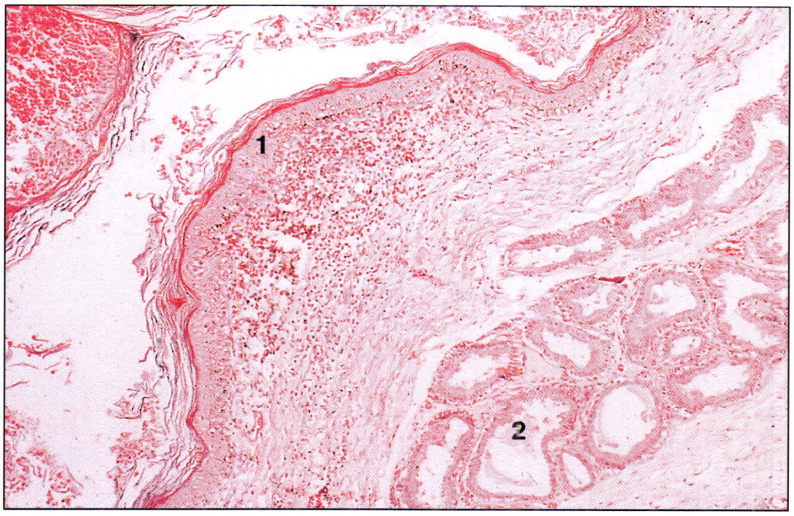

8.58 Anal sac (dog). (1) Stratified squamous keratinized epithelium lines the sac. (2) Tubuloalveolar glands in the lamina propria. H & E. ×12.5.

Alimentary system of reptiles and amphibians

When amphibians metamorphose from larvae to adults, significant changes take place in form and function. Many larval amphibians are facultative (or obligatory) herbivores, the alimentary tracts of which are elongated and often tightly coiled (particularly in frog and toad larvae). During the latter stages of metamorphosis, postlarval amphibians usually cease eating and, therefore, must subsist on their tails and other sources of readily catabolized tissue. As adults, most amphibians are carnivorous.

The lingual apparatus of many amphibians and reptiles is modified for the apprehension of prey: some contain glandular acini that secrete sticky mucus (8.59 and 8.60); others are characterized by numerous papillary projections at the lingual tip to which food particles stick and are then brought into the mouth. When not being used, the tongue of snakes retracts into a lingual sheath that is lined by

8.59

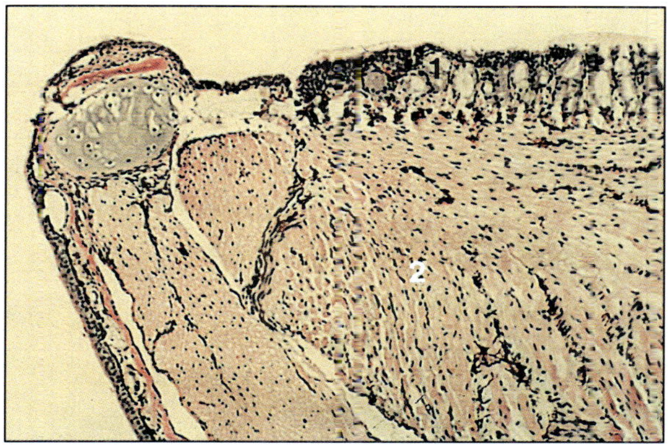

8.59 Tongue of a poison-arrow frog (*Dendrobates* spp.). The dorsal lingual surface (1) is covered by an unusual and complex epithelium composed of small, dark-staining cuboidal cells and acini of sticky mucin-secreting columnar cells that maintain a coating of adhesive mucus. The muscle fibres (2) are primarily arranged in a longitudinal direction and are attached at the front of the mandible. This facilitates the tongue being rapidly protruded and retracted in order to catch small invertebrates. H & E. ×12.5.

8.60

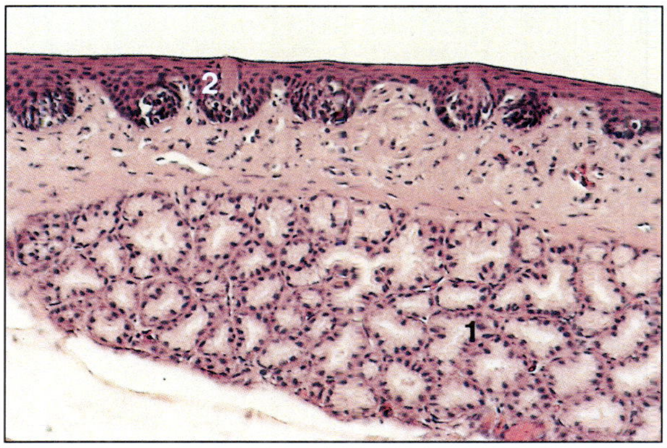

8.60 The tongue of some lizards overlies a sublingual salivary gland (1), as is illustrated by this longitudinal section of the tongue of a small skink (*Scincella lateralis*). The dorsal surface is covered by a non-keratinized stratified squamous epithelium (2) in which cup-shaped taste receptors are embedded. Some lizards (for example, many iguanines) possess tongues with a terminal tip composed of papillary projections that are kept moist and sticky with mucus secreted by goblet cells and several salivary glands. H & E. ×62.5.

mucus-secreting glands. It does not contain glands but is lubricated when it comes into contact with the luminal surface of the lingual sheath. The tongues of other reptiles contain taste receptors that are similar to taste buds found in the tongues of mammals.

The dental histology of amphibians and reptiles is similar to that in mammals, although the teeth of these animals are periodically and continually shed throughout life. Chelonians (turtles, tortoises and terrapins) lack teeth entirely. Their premaxillae, maxillae and mandibles are covered with hard and horny keratinous surfaces, called ramithecae, with which these animals cut their food items.

The salivary glands of amphibians and reptiles are similar to those found in mammals. They may be either entirely serous, entirely mucus-secreting or a mixture of the two.

In venomous snakes and helodermatid lizards (the Gila monster lizard, *Heloderma suspectum*, and the Mexican beaded lizard, *Heloderma horridum*) some salivary glands are greatly modified into structures (*see* Chapter 2) that secrete extremely toxic secretions that help these animals capture their prey and defend themselves. In venomous snakes the secretions from these glands are conducted to the hollow needle-like fangs through coiled venom ducts. The passage of venom through these ducts is aided by the contraction of the temporal and masseter skeletal muscles that surround the glands and myoepithelial cells that surround the ducts (*see* Chapter 2). The fangs are replaced periodically throughout a snake's life. They are formed with a separate hollow channel (**8.61**). Some nominally non-venomous snakes, especially many colubrids, possess modified salivary (Duvernoy's) glands (**8.62**), the secretions

8.61

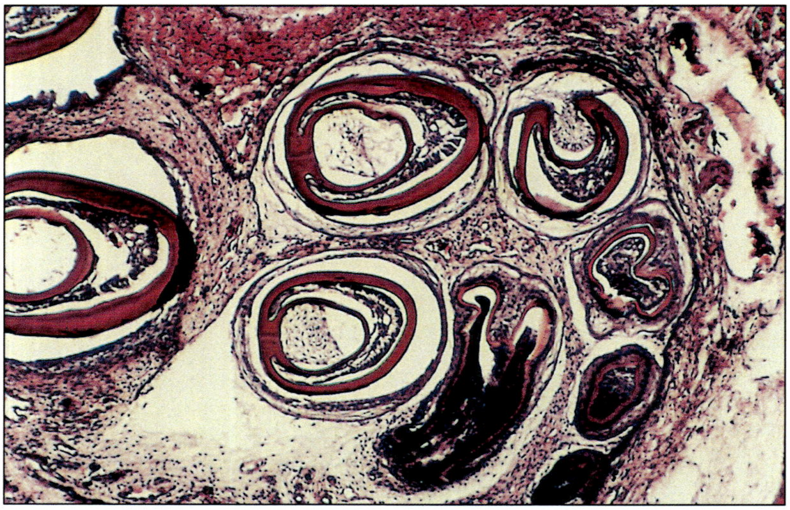

8.61 The fangs of venomous snakes are continually being renewed. Illustrated are several teeth primordia of a juvenile rattlesnake (*Crotalus* spp.), forming modified fangs with a central enamel-lined channel through which venom is conducted. H & E. ×12.5.

8.62

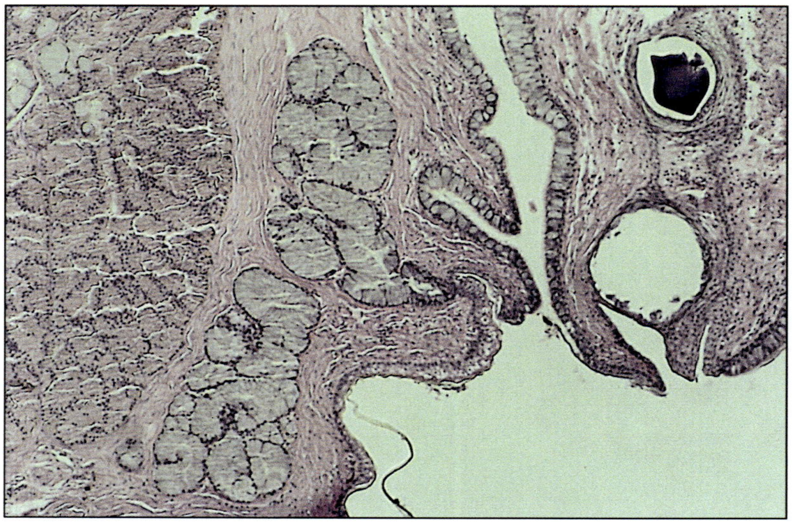

8.62 Some non-venomous snakes possess modified (Duvernoy's) maxillary and premaxillary salivary glands connected to short ducts that empty into the oral cavity. Current studies indicate that the secretions from some of these glands manifest venom-like bioactivity on the lower vertebrate prey of these snakes. Also, mild clinical envenomation of sensitive humans bitten by these snakes has been reported. Illustrated are two lobules of gland from a watersnake (*Natrix cyclopion*). H & E. ×62.5.

of which induce a toxic reaction when injected into particularly sensitive prey and humans.

Generally, the alimentary system of the lower vertebrates is similar to that found in mammals, but major variations exist in species that are highly adapted to a particular diet. Folivorous (leaf eating) reptilian herbivores utilize hindgut rather than foregut fermentation to accomplish the processing of cellulose and other complex carbohydrates. Modifications that aid in this process are an expanded sacculated colon, which is similar in function to the sacculus rotundus of lagamorphs (rabbits and hares) and some herbivorous rodents, and to the massive caecum and colon of equids. In all of these organs, the surface of the luminal lining is augmented by numerous mucosal villous projections, which greatly increase the area available for microbial digestion and nutrient absorption. Thus, the sacculated colon of reptilian folivores serves the same purpose as the large rumen complex of ruminants, even though it is part of the hindgut rather than the foregut.

The anterior alimentary tracts of various reptiles are modified. The oropharynx and oesophagus of some sea turtles have a heavily keratinized lining (8.63) that helps to protect the lumen from trauma when scabrous food items such as rocky and silica-rich coral are swallowed. The egg-eating snake (*Dasypeltis scabra*) ingests eggs with calcareous shells. As the egg enters the cranial oesophagus, the snake contracts its throat and thereby compresses the egg against multiple horny ridges that extend from the ventral region of the cervical vertebrae. After the eggshell is slit, the snake swallows the fluid and/or embryonic contents and regurgitates the shell fragments *en masse*. Most snakes and many lizards possess an oesophagus with walls formed into multiple longitudinal plaits that permit the swallowing of enormous meals (8.64), many times the diameter of their necks. Other reptiles, such as most

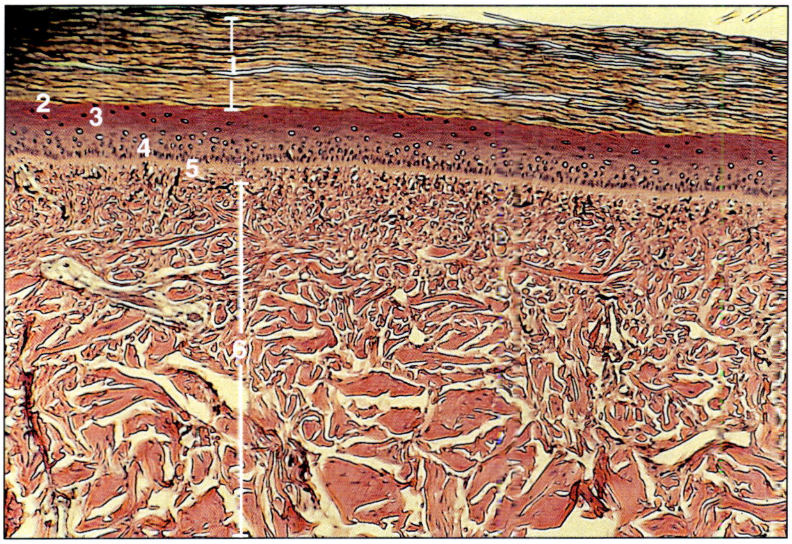

8.63

8.63 The oesophageal lumen of many chelonians, such as this green sea turtle (*Chelonia mydas*), is heavily keratinized and lacks mucus-secreting goblet cells. These characteristics reflect the scabrous diet of these marine animals. (1) Stratum corneum. (2) Stratum lucidum. (3) Stratum granulosum. (4) Stratum spinosum. (5) Stratum basale. (6) Muscularis externa. H & E. ×12.5.

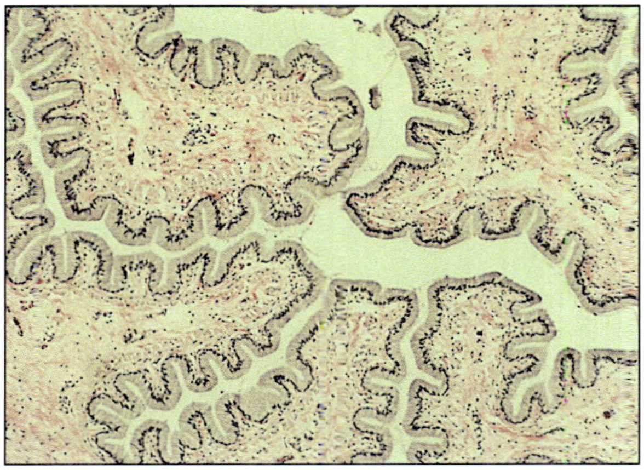

8.64

8.64 The oesophagus of most snakes and many lizards is characterized by its extensive plaiting which permits the oesophagus to stretch to accommodate enormous prey. Illustrated is a cross-section of the oesophagus of a kingsnake (*Lampropeltis triangulum*). Because of the necessity for abundant lubrication during the swallowing of furry, feathered or scaly prey, the oesophageal lumen is lined by a mucous epithelium composed of simple non-keratinized columnar cells bearing basal nuclei. H & E. ×62.5.

crocodilians, have thick-walled muscular stomachs in which their prey are macerated with the aid of ingested stones.

The gastric mucosa of reptiles is similar to that found in mammals, except that only chief and clear cells are present; parietal cells are lacking (8.65 and 8.66). The small intestine lacks Brünner's glands (*see* Chapter 3). The serosa covering most or all of the coelomic viscera of many diurnal lizards is heavily pigmented (8.67). Lymphoid patches or aggregates are scattered throughout the length of the alimentary tract. Discrete lymph nodes are not present.

Many lizards and some snakes possess salt-secreting glands through which hyperosmolar solutions containing sodium, potassium and chloride ions are secreted. In many lizards these glands are situated in the nasal cavity. Some sea snakes possess sublingual salt glands. In some crocodilians, particularly crocodiles that inhabit salt marshes and travel between oceanic islands, salt-secreting glands are located on the dorsal surface of the tongue. All of these aforementioned glands permit the non-renal secretion of electrolytes without the appreciable loss of water.

8.65

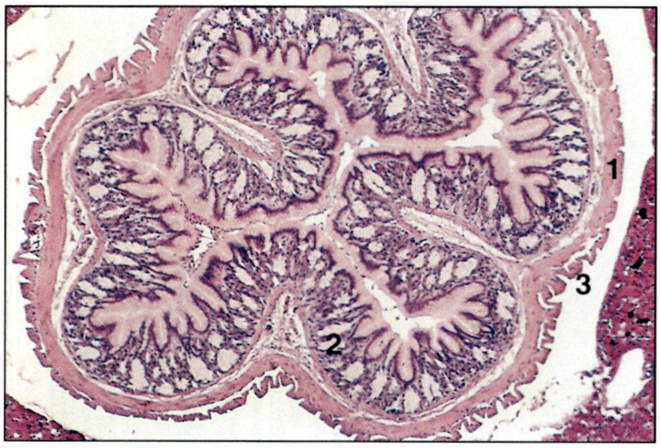

8.65 Whole mount cross-section of the fundic stomach of a small skink (*Scincella lateralis*). A very thin serosa covers the outermost visceral surface. The gastric wall is composed of an outer external longitudinal muscularis externa (1), a circular muscularis externa, the muscularis mucosa), and immediately beneath is the glandular mucosa (2) which is composed of pink staining granular chief cells and clear cells. The lumen is lined by tall mucus-secreting columnar cells. Parietal cells, present in mammalian gastric mucosae, are lacking in amphibians and reptiles. The outermost surface of the stomach is covered by a delicate serosa (3) formed of non-keratinized squamous cells. H & E. ×12.5.

8.66

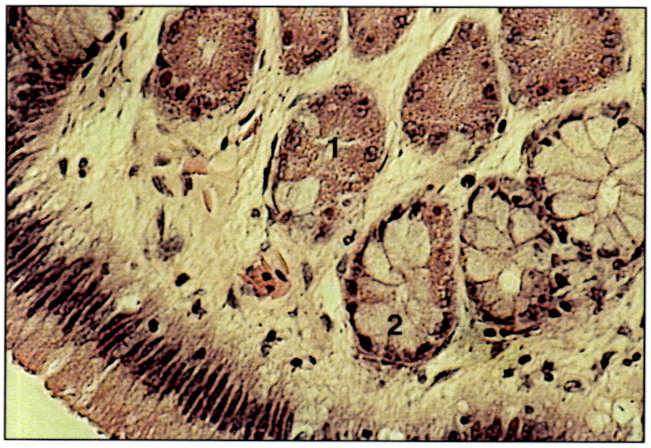

8.66 Gastric mucosa of a boa constrictor (*Boa constrictor*). The lumen is covered by tall columnar epithelium. The gastric glands consist of only granular, cuboidal, pink staining chief cells (1) with large vesicular nuclei, and pale staining clear cells (2) whose nuclei are dark and basal. Some gastric pits are lined by both cell types. H & E. ×250.

8.67

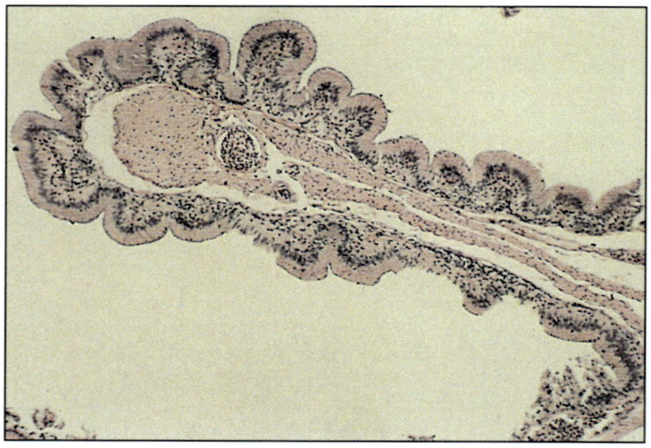

8.67 The colon of some lizards, particularly folivorous species, is a highly modified sacculated organ divided into multiple chambers that are functionally analogous to the hindgut of lagamorphs and some (herbivorous/folivorous) rodents, and the forestomachs of ruminants. Digestion is enhanced because the villous surface of the colon is covered by a highly absorptive columnar mucosa across which nutrients processed from cellulose-digesting micro-organisms are assimilated. The elongated villi that cover the surface are supported, and stiffened, by thin cores of smooth muscle. Illustrated is the sacculated colon of a green iguana (*Iguana iguana*). H & E. ×12.5.

Clinical correlates

Alimentary system of reptiles and amphibians

Squamous metaplasia of the nasal and pharyngeal mucosa (8.68 and 8.69) is a frequent clinical condition in reptiles fed diets deficient in vitamin A or β-carotene. Once this alteration occurs, the lubricative mucoid glandular secretion ceases and the affected animal becomes more susceptible to respiratory and oropharyngeal disorders.

Ulcerative stomatitis is one of the most common conditions found in the cranial alimentary tract of captive snakes. This infectious inflammatory disease is caused by a variety of pathogenic Gram-negative and some Gram-positive bacteria. Depending upon the aetiologic agent, the inflammatory response may be suppurative or non-suppurative. In suppurative lesions, heterophil granulocytes predominate; in non-suppurative inflammations, heterophils may be entirely absent.

Glossitis, pharyngitis, oesophagitis and gastritis also occur in captive amphibians and reptiles.

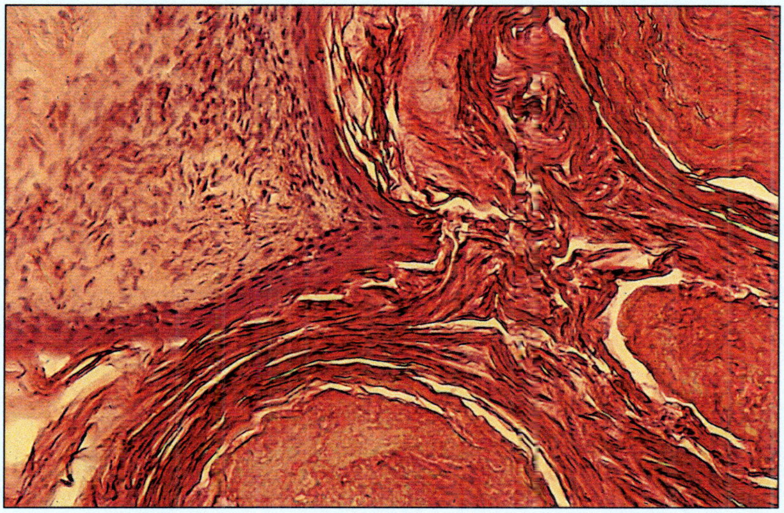

8.68

8.68 Massive pharyngeal hyperkeratosis in a desert tortoise (*Xerobates agassizi*). The pharyngeal glands are replaced by pearl-like masses of desquamated keratin. The luminal epithelial surface is thickened and covered by dense keratin debris. A similar alteration is seen in birds and mammals suffering from vitamin A deficiency. H & E. ×12.5.

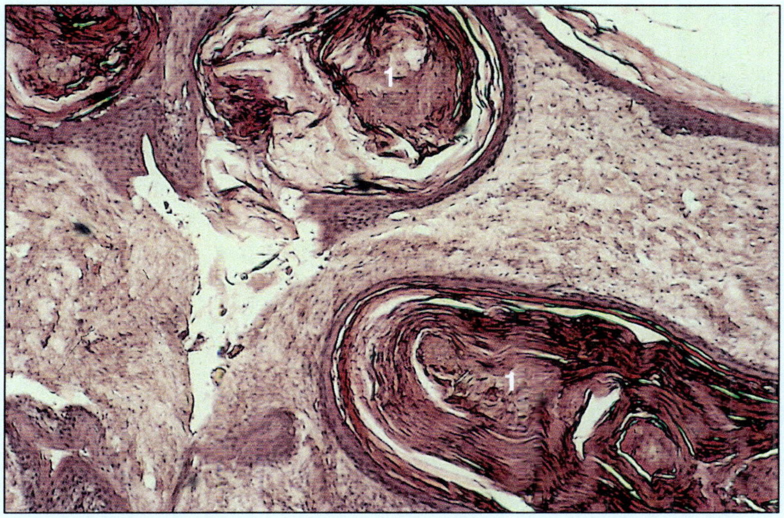

8.69

8.69 Cross-section of the pharynx of a red-eared slider turtle that was fed a diet seriously deficient in β-carotene or preformed vitamin A. The pharyngeal glands display squamous metaplasia and, as a result, have lost their mucus-secreting, goblet-cell-rich glands, which have been replaced by masses of desquamated keratin debris (1). The stratified squamous epithelium lining the pharyngeal lumen is thickened and hyperplastic. H & E. ×12.5.

These inflammatory conditions are often caused by items in the diet that injure the delicate mucous membranes that cover the tongue or line these cavities. In snakes, and to a lesser extent in lizards, gastric cryptosporidiosis is a serious clinical problem. Although typically termed 'hypertrophic' gastritis in the literature, the anatomical and histological features of gastric cryptosporidiosis in snakes are a marked hypertrophy of the muscular tunica comprising the wall of the stomach, together with an atrophy of the gastric mucosa. Gastric biopsy (or gastric lavage) specimens of infected snakes reveal myriad numbers of protozoan organisms attached to the brush border of the epithelial cells lining the gastric lumen and gastric pits (8.70).

Usually, enteritis is accompanied by an overproduction of protective mucus by the goblet cells. The inflammation may be suppurative, in which heterophils are easily identified, or nonsuppurative, in which the predominant leucocytes are mononuclear (8.71). The aetiologic agent may or may not be immediately apparent.

Intussusception (the telescoping of one segment of intestine into another, or into the stomach) occurs relatively frequently in some reptiles, particularly in iguanas and Old World chameleons (8.72 and 8.73). The reasons for this high incidence are unknown, but endoparasitism and dietary problems, especially hypocalcaemia, are suspected as predisposing factors.

Benign and malignant neoplasia of the stomach and small intestine are relatively common in captive reptiles, particularly snakes and lizards. This may be a consequence of living considerably longer while in captivity than under natural (wild) conditions. Adenomata, carcinomata, leiomyoma and leiomyosarcoma have been recorded in many snakes and in fewer lizards.

Preneoplastic leukoplakia and invasive squamous cell carcinoma have been described in chelonians. These proliferative lesions are similar to those observed in mammals.

Adult green iguanas (which are folivorous herbivores) have a simple stomach and a short small intestine that transports the partially processed leafy ingesta into the sacculated and much expanded colon. Villous projections (8.67), covered with pseudostratified, non-ciliated columnar epithelium overlying a thin lamina propria and a core of smooth muscle and blood vessels, extend into the colonic lumen and create a larger surface area for the processing of cellulose and absorption of nutrients.

8.70

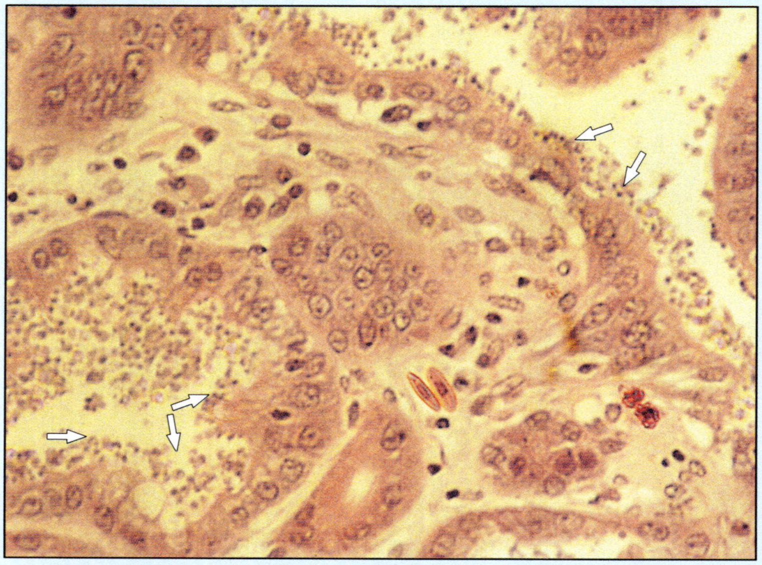

8.70 Gastric cryptosporidiosis in an Australian tiger snake (*Notechis scutatus*). A myriad number of round organisms (arrowed) are attached to the brush border of the mucosal cells lining the gastric lumen and gastric pits. H & E. ×250.

8.71 Non-suppurative enteritis in a desert tortoise. Most of the leucocytes are lymphoplasmacytic. H & E. ×62.5.

8.71

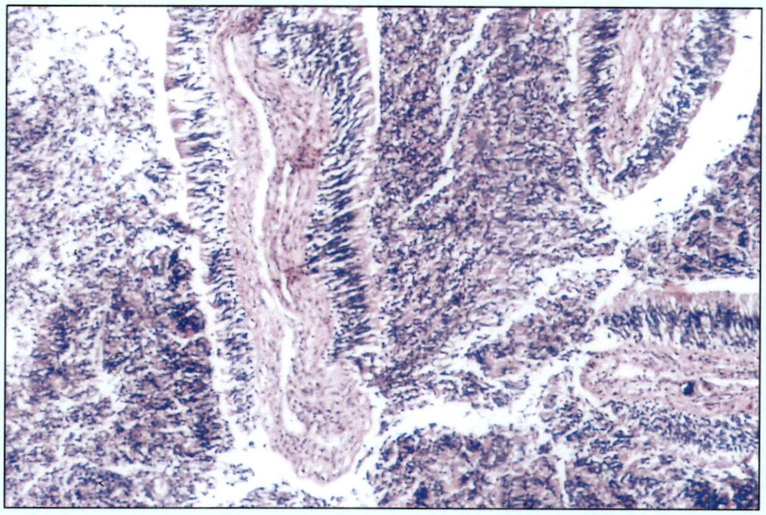

8.72, 8.73 Duodenal-jejunal intussusception in a Fisher's chameleon (*Chamaeleo fisheri*; **8.72**) and an iguana (**8.73**). A segment of duodenum has telescoped into the jejunum causing the two serosal layers to lie adjacent to each other. H & E. ×12.5.

8.72

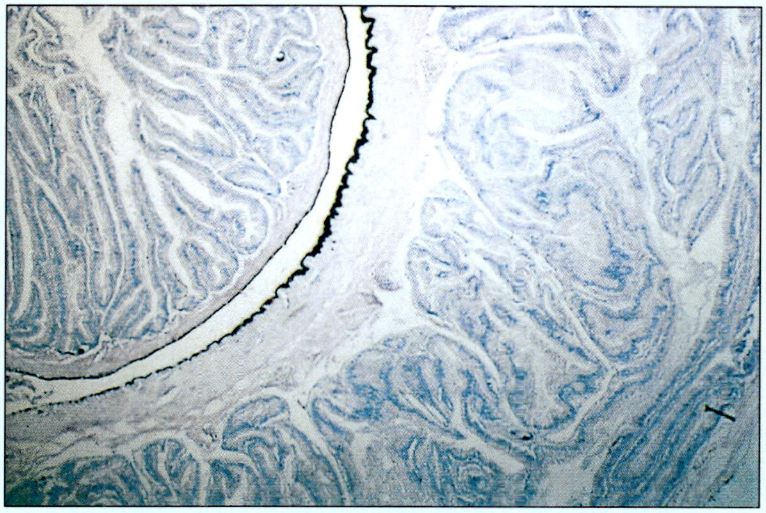

8.73

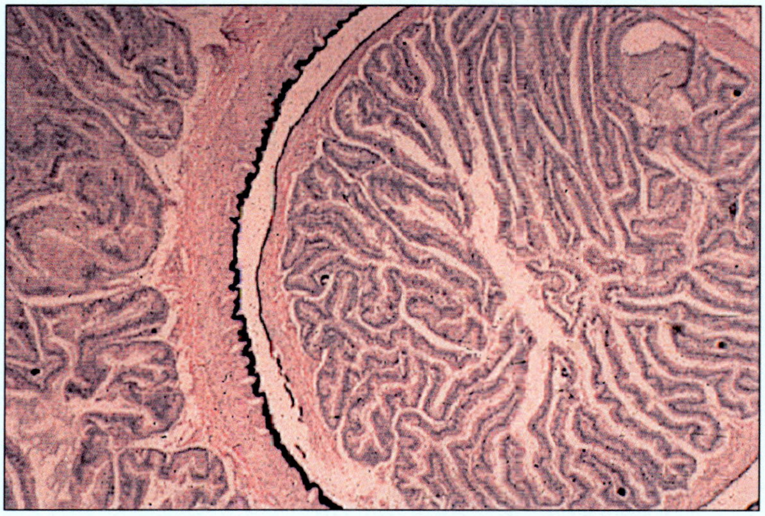

Liver

The liver is the largest gland in the body. Blood drains to it from the intestines in the hepatic portal vein, and the products of digestion are metabolized, harmful material detoxified, senescent erythrocytes removed from the circulation and bile secreted. The liver is surrounded by mesothelium. The connective tissue capsule extends into the gland and divides it into lobes and lobules. The structure of the classic lobule is most clearly visualized in the pig because of its plentiful array of connective tissue dividing the liver into discrete hexagonal lobules with a portal area at the corners of each hexagon. This is not the case in the other domestic animals, except under pathological conditions such as cirrhosis. The portal areas (triads) occur between three or more lobules and each contains one or more branches of a hepatic artery, a hepatic portal vein, a lymphatic vessel and a bile duct. The parenchyma consists of polyhedral epithelial cells of endodermal origin, the hepatocytes, arranged in anastomosing rows separated by sinusoids converging on the central vein. The sinusoids are lined with fenestrated endothelial cells and macrophages, part of the mononuclear phagocyte system. Blood flows through the sinusoids to the central vein. This in turn leaves the liver lobule to travel separately as branches of the hepatic vein.

Bile is secreted by each hepatocyte into the bile canaliculi, channels that are lined with the plasma membranes of the hepatocytes, between adjoining liver cells. It flows from there to a small bile duct in the portal area. Where the bile duct is the central functional axis of the lobule instead of the central vein, the term 'portal lobule' is used. The liver acinus is the smallest functional unit of the liver. It consists of parenchyma served by a terminal branch of the portal vein and the hepatic artery, and is drained by two central veins and terminal branches of the bile duct. It has functional and pathological significance. Bile ducts are lined with cuboidal epithelium in the portal areas; the larger interlobular ducts are lined with columnar epithelium (8.74–8.80).

Reptiles, amphibians and fish

The livers of fish, amphibians and reptiles are superficially similar to those of mammals. However, there are some differences. Many of the lower vertebrates have abundant melanin pigment scattered through-

8.74

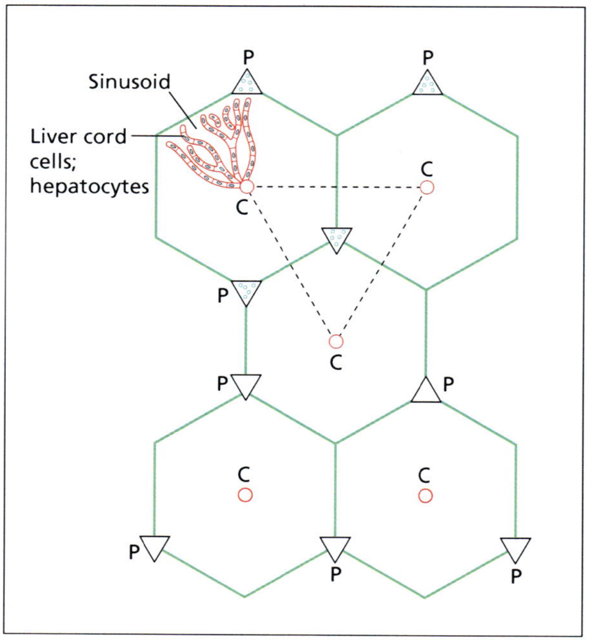

8.74 Hepatic lobule. The classic lobule is the hexagon, clearly seen in the figure by the outline (green) of connective tissue). Portal areas (P) occur between the lobules. A portal lobule is defined as the central functional axis of the lobule (the black dotted triangle).

8.75

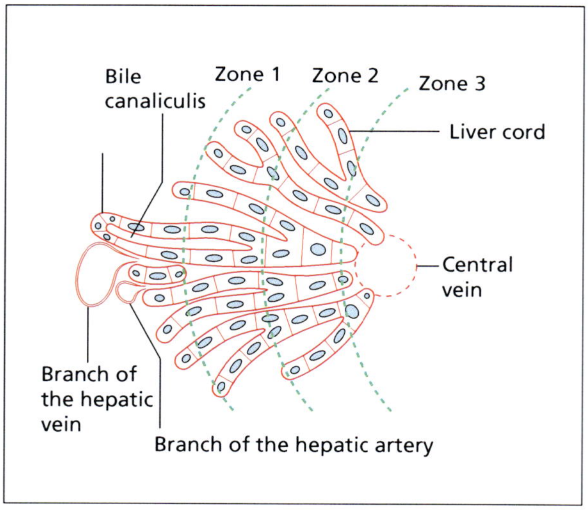

8.75 Liver acinus (functional unit). The liver parenchyma is served by the terminal branch of the portal vein and the hepatic artery. The acinus is divided into three zones, which indicate the relative position of the cells in realtion to the oxygen gradient. Hepatocytes in Zone 1 are closest to the fresh, oxygen-rich hepatic arterial blood, and those in Zone 3 are further away. Equally, cells in Zone 1 are first in line for toxins, etc., carried in the portal blood, with Zone 3 the cells the least affected by these.

out the hepatocellular parenchyma (*see* Chapter 3). Usually, this pigment is contained in melanophages that are aggregated together in packet-like groups of cells bearing fine dark-brown granules. In some species the liver is arranged in narrow cords radiating outward from a thin-walled central vein. It has one or more portal triads consisting of an arteriolar branch of the hepatic artery and one or more small bile ducts (as in mammals). In other species the central veins are scattered randomly throughout the liver and more than one portal triad or triads with multiple arterioles and bile canaliculi or ducts are present.

An admixture of hepatocellular and pancreatic tissues, thus forming a hepatopancreas, is present in many fish and in some amphibians and reptiles.

8.76

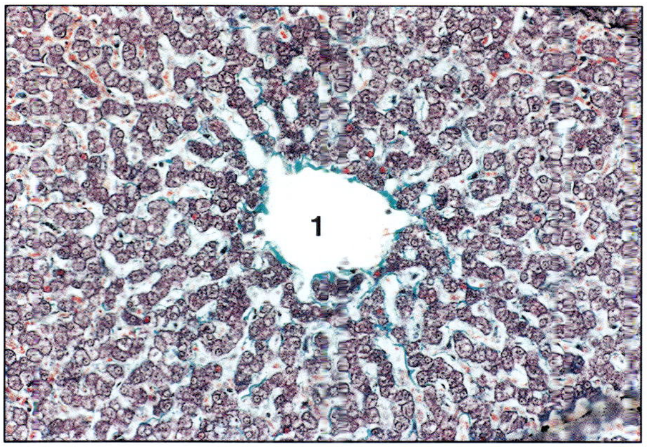

8.76 Liver (pig). The heaxagonal liver lobule is delineated by the green strands of the interlobular connective tissue. (1) Central vein. Masson's trichrome. ×125.

.77

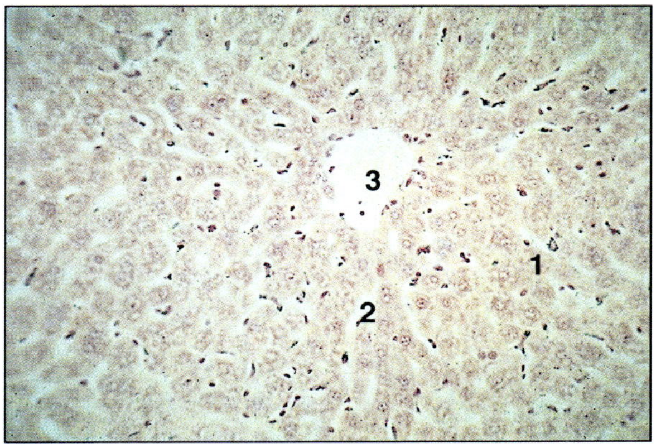

8.77 Liver (ox). (1) Hepatocytes arranged in cords. (2) Sinusoids lined by endothelial cells and macrophages open into (3) the central vein. Safranin/haematoxylin. ×125.

8.78

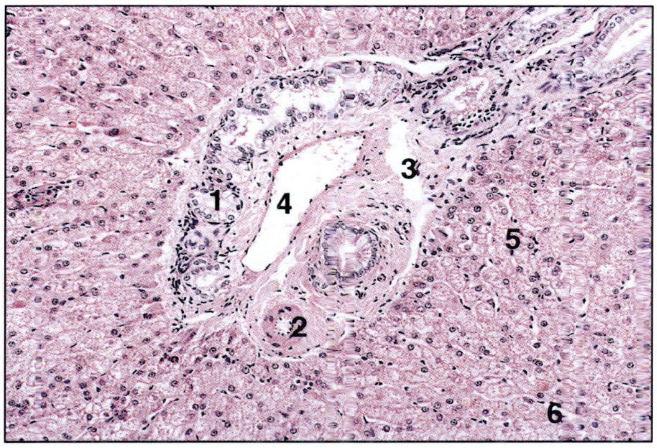

8.78 Portal canal (triad) (sheep). (1) Branch of the bile duct. (2) Hepatic artery. (3) Lymphatic vessel. (4) Hepatic portal vein. (5) Liver cords. (6) Sinusoids. H & E. ×125.

.79

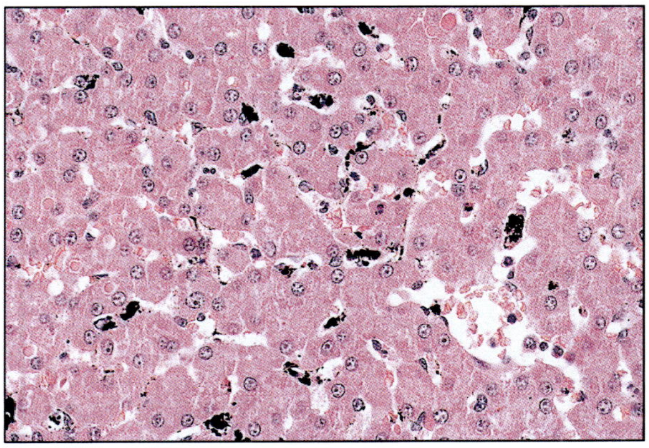

8.79 Liver (dog). The macrophages have taken up the injected carbon and appear as black areas between the cords of hepatocytes. Carbon-injected with H & E counterstain. ×125.

8.80

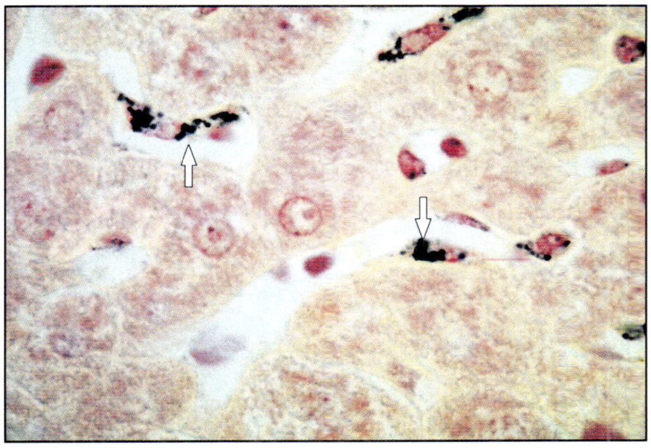

8.80 Liver (dog). The hepatocytes lie in anastomosing cords separated by sinusoids lined by macrophages (arrowed). Safranin/haematoxylin after carbon injection. ×250.

Clinical correlates

With its pivotal role in processing material carried from the intestine via the portal system, the liver is exposed to toxic factors and potentially harmful micro-organisms passing from the gut. Metabolic or nutritional disease (8.81), infectious disease (*see* 8.84) and neoplasia (8.82), both local and metastatic, can also affect the liver. Inflammation of the liver is termed hepatitis (8.83). Hepatic lipidosis, an excess fat storage in the liver, is seen as a clinical problem in obese animals under physiological stress: often pregnant pony mares, dairy cattle after parturition and ewes carrying twins in late pregnancy (pregnancy toxaemia). Mobilization of large amounts of triglycerides causes fatty acids to be presented to the liver in excess of its capacity to handle them. This problem may be quite rapidly fatal and cases of sudden death due to liver rupture are not uncommon.

The liver has a great capacity for regeneration of hepatocyte mass, but fibrosis is also a charac-

8.81

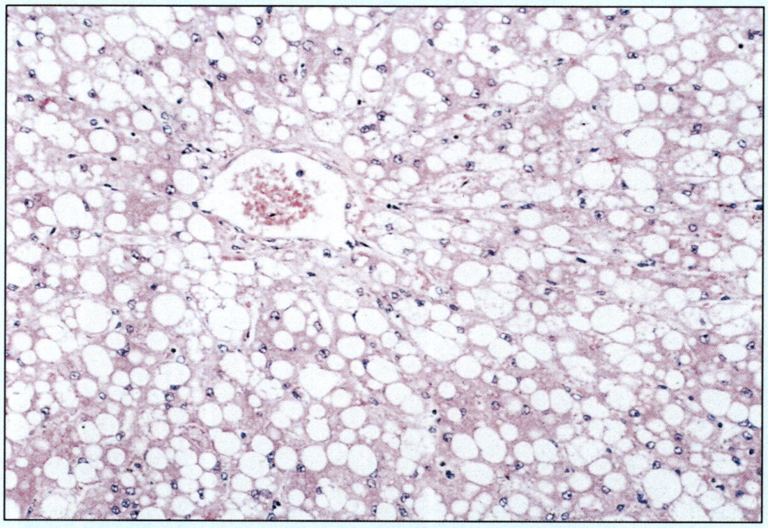

8.81 Hepatic lipidosis (horse).This micrograph of horse liver shows a central vein surrounded by radiating cords of hepatocytes that contain large, smoothly round vacuoles which occupy most of the cell and displace the nucleus to the periphery. These are fat vacuoles. The horse was hyperlipidaemic with hepatic lipidosis. H & E. ×250.

8.82

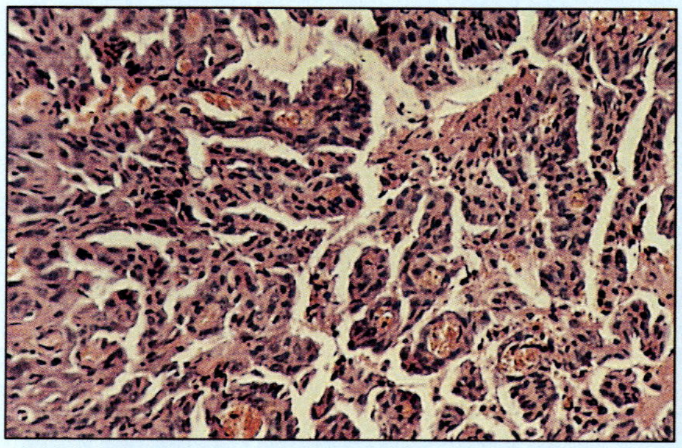

8.82 Cholangiocarcinoma in an Asiatic leopard (*Panthera pardus*). The cuboidal to columnar neoplastic cells form frond-like ducts and tubules with thin walls composed of two cell layers separated by a scant fibrovascular connective tissue stroma. H & E. ×125.

8.83

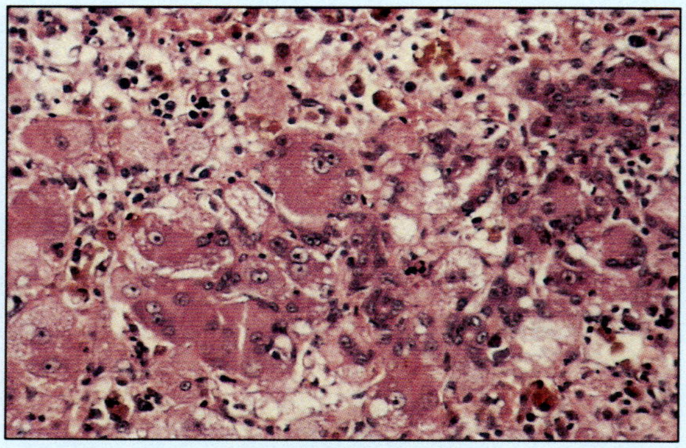

8.83 Giant cell hepatitis in a 5-year-old neutered female Siamese cat. Note that many of the hepatocytes are much larger than normal and frequently have multiple nuclei. A mixed mononuclear and polymorphonuclear leucocytic response is present. H & E. Haemosiderin is present. ×125.

teristic reaction of the liver to chronic injury. Any hepatic injury severe enough to result in hepatic necrosis results in some fibrogenesis, but progressive fibrosis can develop when the insult persists or when the initial damage is severe and provokes an extensive reaction. A canine liver with micronodular cirrhosis (8.84) shows progressive fibrosis in which the normal architecture of the liver is lost and cells are divided into small groups surrounded by fibrous tissue.

Amphibians and reptiles

As with domestic animals, numerous chemical and viral agents induce severe liver disease (8.85). The hepatic parenchyma is sensitive to changes in calcium and other minerals in the blood and, under conditions of hypervitaminosis D_3, may undergo severe mineralization and even ossification (8.86).

8.84

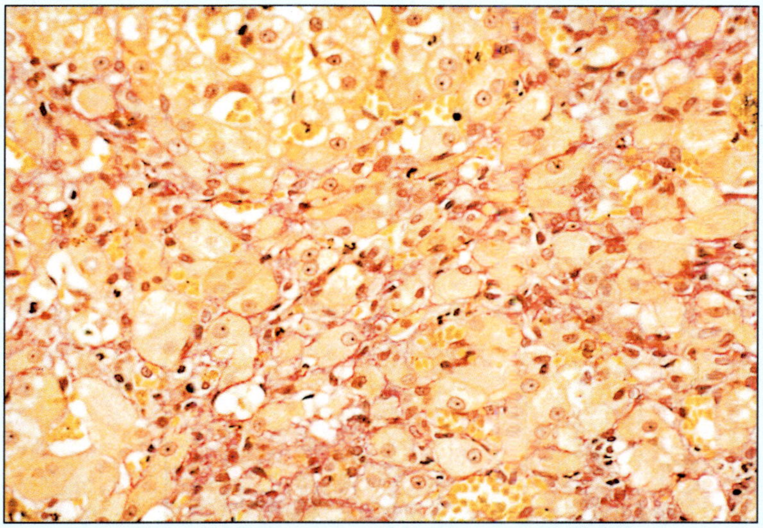

8.84 Micronodular cirrhosis in a 1-year-old Cocker Spaniel. The yellow-stained hepatocytes vary in size and shape and the developing fibrous tissue is stained red. With this technique, red blood cells stain yellow. Sirius Red. ×250.

8.85

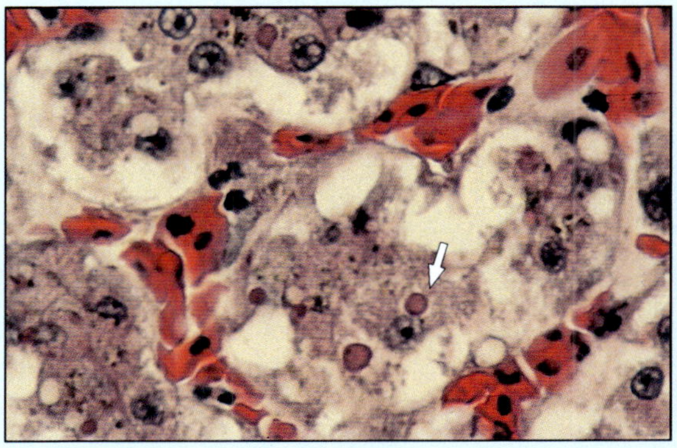

8.85 Viral hepatitis in a Colombian boa constrictor (*Boa C. constrictor*). Most of the hepatocytes contain eosinophilic, intracytoplasmic viral inclusion bodies (arrowed), most of which are surrounded by narrow clear 'haloes'. H & E. ×250.

8.86

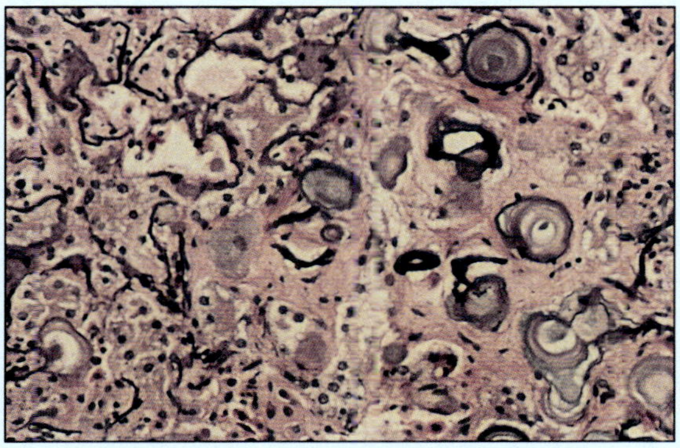

8.86 Nutrition related, massive hepatic mineralization secondary to hypervitaminosis D_3 in an African leopard tortoise (*Geochelone pardalis*). Most of the hepatocellular parenchyma has undergone gross alteration and is replaced by bone. As a consequence, few normal hepatocytes remain. Several osteocytes surrounded by concentric lamellae of compact bone are present. H & E. ×125.

Gall bladder

The gall bladder (absent in the horse, dolphins, rhinos and hippos) is a reservoir for bile and is attached to the visceral surface or between the lobes of the liver. The mucous membrane is folded in the flaccid state, and the epithelial lining consists of tall columnar cells with a striated border (8.87). Goblet cells and mucus- and serous-secreting glands may be present in ruminants. The muscularis externa is a circular layer of smooth muscle and the other serosa is continuous with the peritoneum.

The gall bladder of lizards and chelonians is embedded in or surrounded by the liver, as it is in mammals and birds (8.88). The gall bladder of snakes is located at a variable distance from the liver and is contiguous with the spleen and pancreas. A long bile duct transports bile from the intrahepatic bile duct(s) to the gall bladder for storage and eventual release into the duodenum.

Clinical correlates

The gall bladder can be a site of inflammation (cholangitis), calculi (choleliths), neoplasia and foreign bodies such as parasites (Fasciola hepatica).

8.87

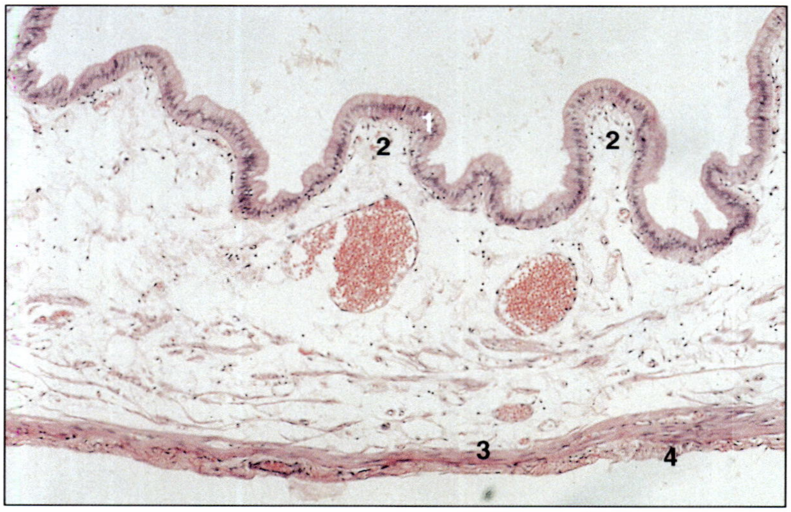

8.87 Gall bladder (cow). (1) Tall columnar epithelium lining the lumen. (2) Mucosal folds. (3) Muscularis. (4) Serosa. H & E. ×12.5.

8.88

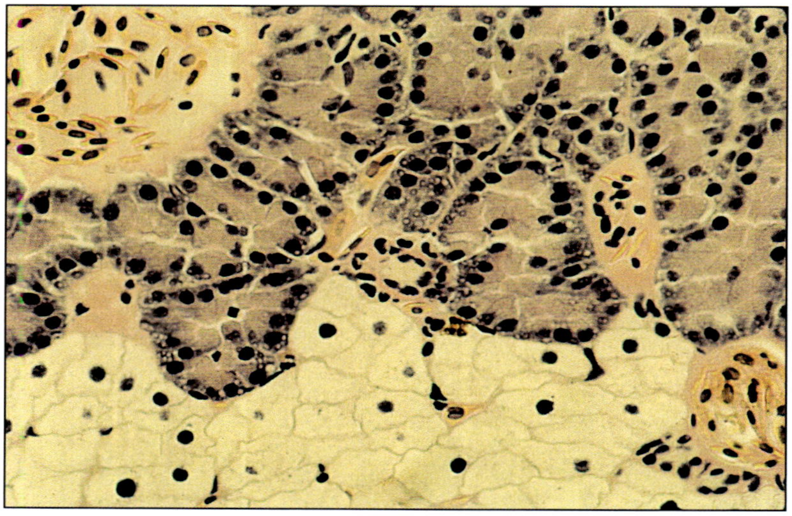

8.88 The liver and pancreas of some fish, amphibians and reptiles are fused or admixed with one another and form a hepatopancreas. Illustrated is a section of such a mixed organ in an axolotl, a neotenic form of the aquatic salamander (*Ambystoma maculatum*). The hepatocellular tissue is at the bottom of this section; the exocrine pancreatic portion is in the upper right; an islet is in the upper left. H & E. ×250.

Pancreas

A fine connective tissue capsule extends into the gland and divides it into lobules. The parenchyma is composed of exocrine and endocrine tissue; both are derived from the endoderm of the foregut. The exocrine portion of the pancreas is a compound tubuloacinar gland that secretes enzymes into the duodenum. The acinar cells are tall columnar with a basal nucleus in basophilic cytoplasm. Where the secretory granules are stored the luminal cytoplasm is eosinophilic. Projections of duct cells are commonly seen in the acinus; these are the centroacinar cells that are typical of the pancreas. Smaller ducts are lined with cuboidal epithelium and larger ducts with columnar epithelium (8.89–8.91).

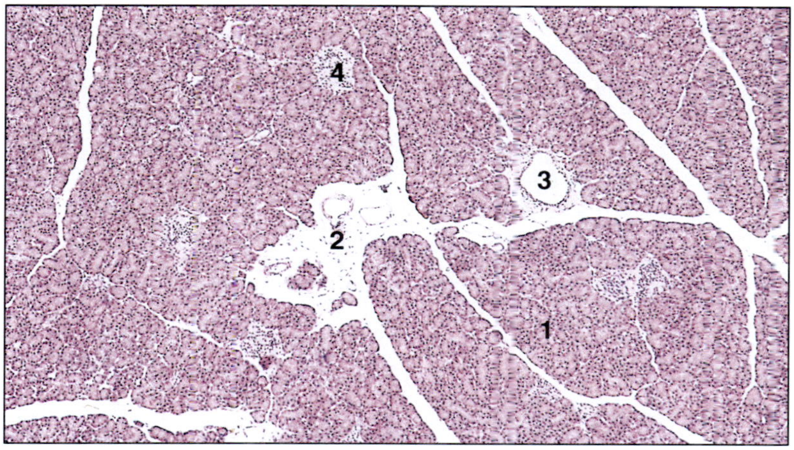

8.89

8.89 Pancreas (dog). (1) Serous acini of the exocrine pancreas. (2) Interlobular connective tissue. (3) Interlobular duct. (4) Pancreatic islet, the endocrine pancreas. H & E. ×12.5.

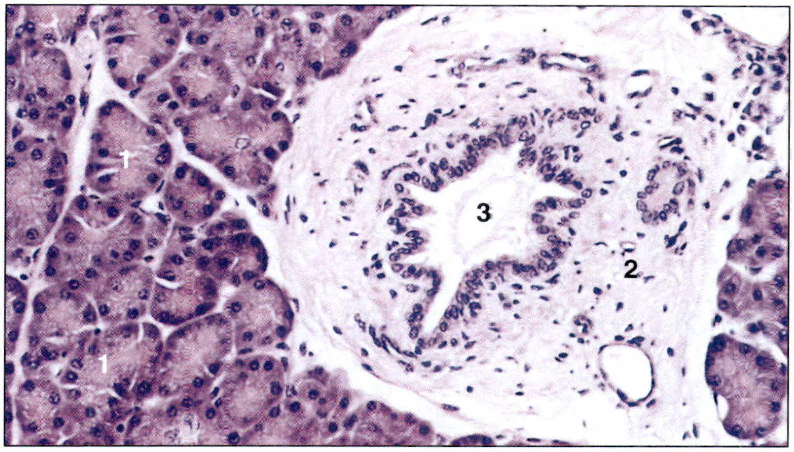

8.90

8.90 Pancreas (dog). (1) Serous acinus with a centroacinar cell (arrowed). (2) Interlobular connective tissue. (3) Interlobular duct. H & E. ×125.

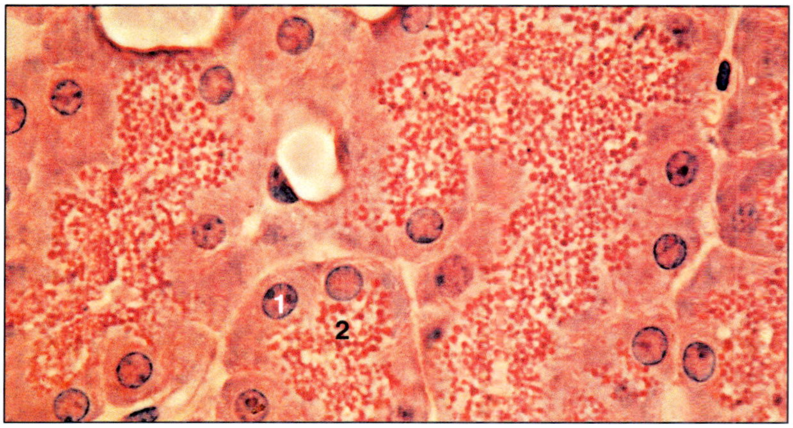

8.91

8.91 Pancreas (dog). (1) Nucleus lies in the basal basophilic cytoplasm of the serous cell. (2) Eosinophilic granules (the secretion) lie in the luminal cytoplasm. H & E. ×250.

The endocrine pancreas is responsible for the control of blood sugar concentrations, and isolated groups of pale staining islet cells (pancreatic cells or the islets of Langerhans) are found scattered among the secretory units (8.92). These have two main cell types: A, or alpha, cells secreting glucagon (a polypeptide hormone secreted in response to hypoglycaemia or to stimulation by growth hormone); and B, or beta, cells secreting insulin (a peptide hormone released into the blood in response to a rise in concentration of blood glucose or amino acids). Rare D, or delta, cells secrete somatostatin and F cells secrete pancreatic polypeptide. These cells belong to the APUD cell group (see enteroendocrine cells of the stomach).

8.92

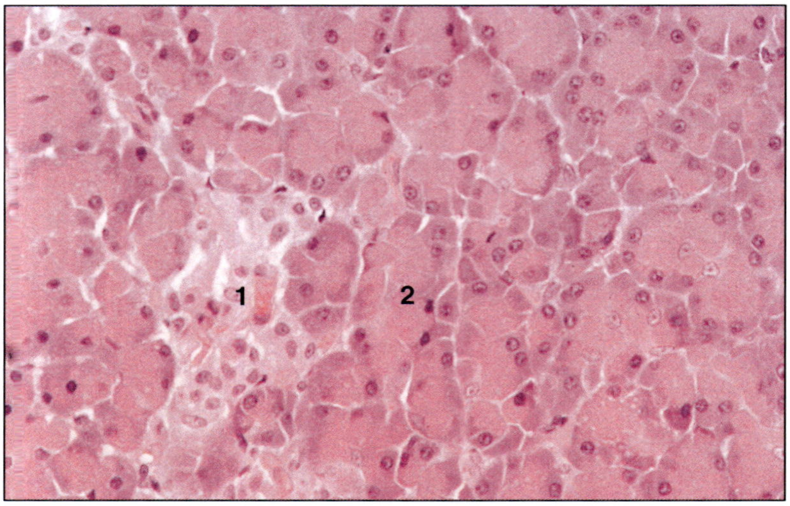

8.92 Pancreatic islet. Pancreas (cat). (1) Pale staining endocrine cells form cords associated with capillaries. (2) Exocrine acinus. H & E. ×125.

Clinical correlates

Essentially all of the various pancreatic disorders that occur in humans also occur in domestic mammals and in the so-called 'lower' vertebrates (8.93). Polycystic deformities, diabetes mellitus, pancreatic amyloidosis (8.94), acute and chronic pancreatitis, intraductal calculosis, and both benign and malignant neoplasms are recognized in diverse species.

8.93

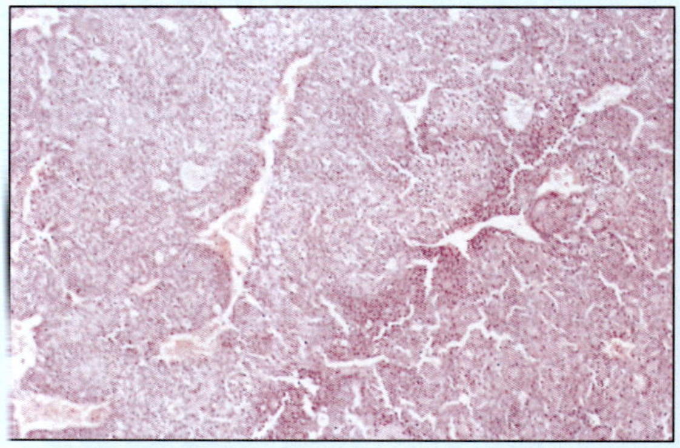

8.93 Pancreatic carcinoma in a 12-year-old dog. Part of a nodular mass with a mostly solid pattern of poorly differentiated or cuboidal-to-low columnar cells is shown. H & E. ×62.5.

8.94

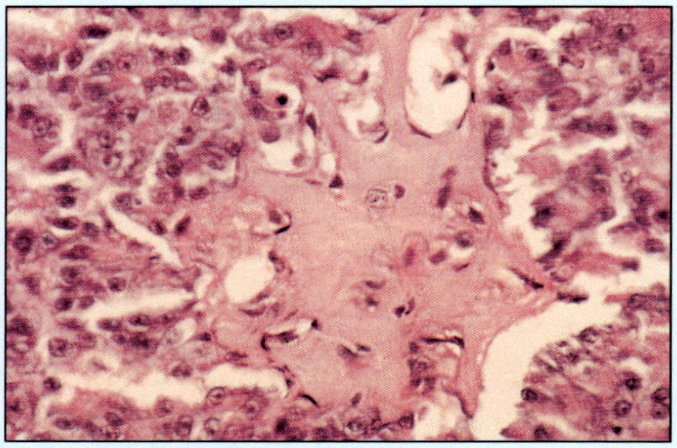

8.94 Pancreatic islet amyloidosis in a neutered female ocelot (*Felis padalis*). Essentially, this cat's islets are hyalinized and replaced with amorphous, eosinophilic amyloid. H & E. ×125.

Reptilian, amphibian and fish pancreas

Morphologically, the pancreas of teleost fish, amphibians and reptiles is similar to that found in mammals (8.95), but two major differences are observed in some species. Many fish, and some amphibians and reptiles, possess a pancreas that has an intimate association, and admixture of cells, with the spleen or liver (8.96). This combined organ is termed a 'splenopancreas' or 'hepatopancreas', respectively, and the cells and tissues of each organ receive blood from their respective splenic, pancreatic or hepatic branches of the splanchnic arteries and veins. Whereas the islet tissue in most reptiles tends to be conventionally arranged and evenly distributed, 'giant' islets of Langerhans are characteristic in the pancreatic tissues of some snakes, particularly members of the family Boidae (pythons and boas); rather than being scattered in a more or less random manner throughout the pancreatic exocrine tissue, these huge islets of endocrine cells tend to be localized in specific areas of pancreatic tissue (8.97).

.95

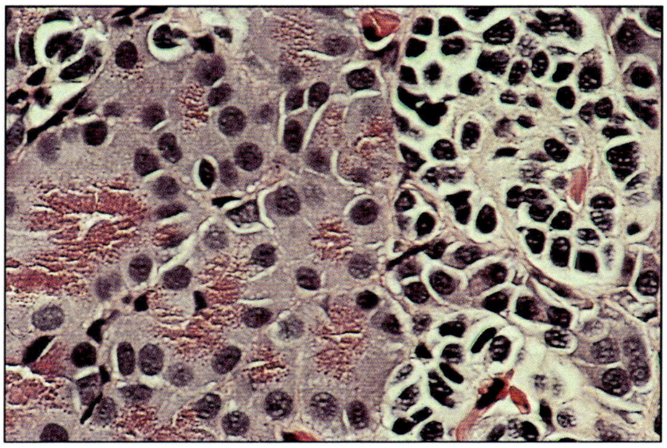

8.95 Pancreas of a salamander (*Amphiuma tridactyla*). Exocrine pancreatic cells characterized by their fine granular eosinophilic cytoplasm (on the left) extend a finger-like isthmus into the islet of paler staining endocrine cells bearing dense nuclei (on the right). The islet cells are arranged into nest-like lobules that are separated from each other and from the exocrine tissue by thin strands of connective tissue that support small blood vessels. H & E. ×250.

8.96

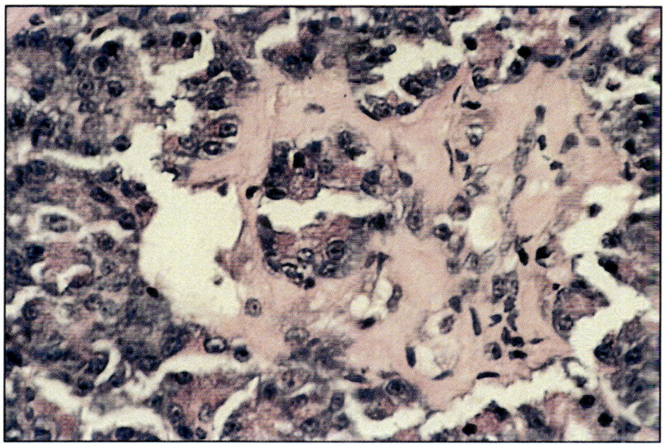

8.96 The splenopancreas of a milksnake (*Lampropeltis triangulum*). The spleen is on the right, a large aggregate of islet tissue is in the middle and a portion of the exocrine pancreatic tissue is on the left. The islet displays hyalinization. H & E. ×125.

8.97

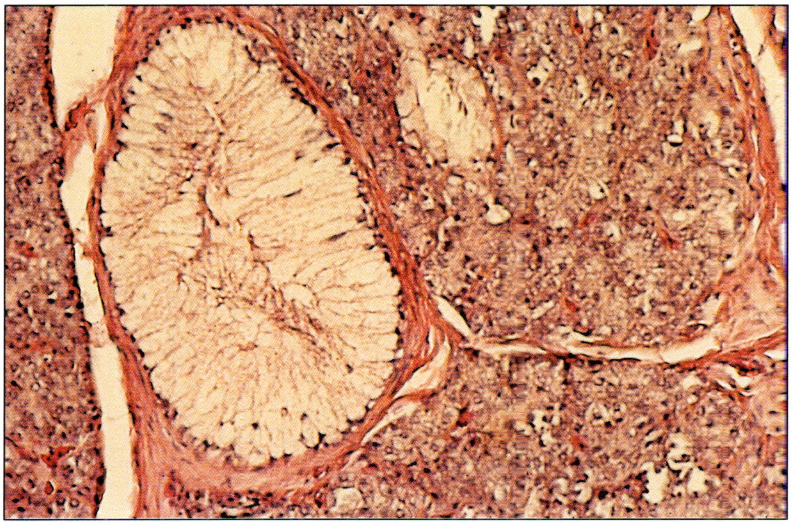

8.97 The pancreas of some snakes, particularly many pythons, is characterized by possessing endocrine cells formed into giant islets (often found at the edge of the lobule) rather than into many small nests of cells scattered randomly throughout the parenchyma. Illustrated is a section of the pancreas from a regal (ball) python (*Python regius*). H & E. ×125.

Clinical correlates

Reptilian pancreas

Certain species of reptiles appear to have a higher than expected incidence of some tumours. In captivity, some lizards, especially savanna monitors (*Varanus exanthematicus*), seem to show a high incidence of adult-onset diabetes mellitus and exocrine deficiency. No evidence suggests that diabetes mellitus or exocrine deficiency are as prevalent in wild savanna monitors. Therefore, these disorders seem to be artefacts of captive husbandry (caused particularly by overfeeding and lack of adequate exercise) resulting in spontaneous acute and chronic pancreatitis with subsequent autodigestion of the pancreatic parenchyma.

The migration of helminth larvae can also induce pancreatitis with secondary fibrosis and loss of secretory function both of exocrine and of endocrine components.

8.98

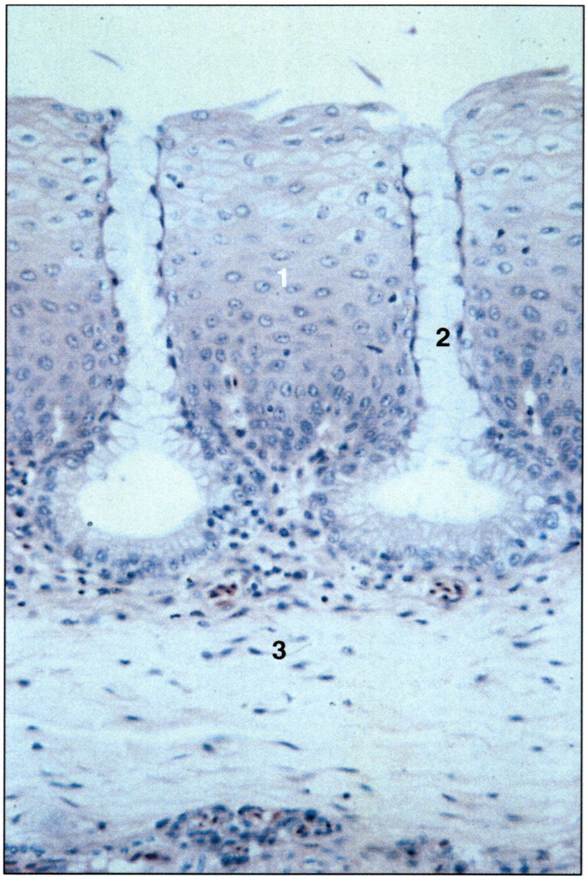

8.98 Oesophagus (bird). (1) Stratified squamous non-keratinizing epithelium. (2) Simple tubular mucosal glands. (3) Lamina propria. H & E. ×62.5.

Avian digestive system

The horny beak replaces functionally the lips and teeth of mammals.

Oral cavity and oesophagus

The oral cavity is lined with stratified squamous epithelium. The tongue is also lined with this type of epithelium, with some keratinized areas. The main mass of the tongue consists of striated muscle and a small bar of cartilage or bone: the entoglossal bone. There are no teeth. The glands in the lamina propria of the oral cavity, tongue and pharynx are simple-branched and mucus secreting.

The oesophagus is lined with stratified squamous non-keratinized epithelium, with simple mucous glands in the connective tissue lamina propria (8.98). The muscularis externa consists of a thick inner layer of circular and a thin outer layer of longitudinal smooth muscle. Lymphoid tissue accumulates in the caudal oesophagus as the oesophageal tonsil. The crop is an aglandular caudal diverticulum situated two-thirds of the way down the oesophagus (8.99). In the pigeon two lateral glomerular sacs secrete crop milk.

8.99

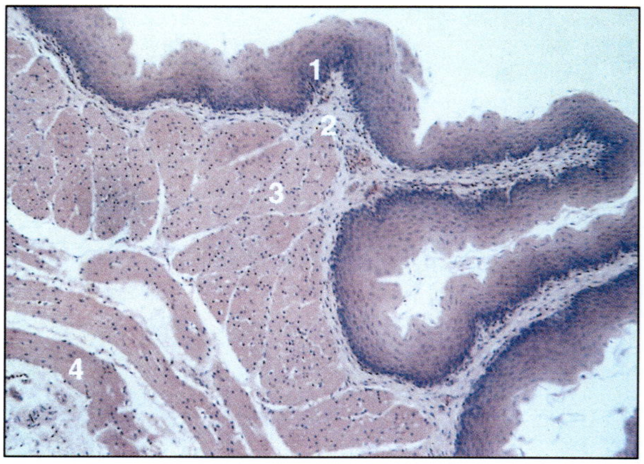

8.99 Crop (bird). (1) Stratified squamous non-keratinized epithelium. (2) Lamina propria. (3) Muscularis mucosae. (4) Muscularis externa. H & E. ×12.5.

Stomach

The stomach consists of the glandular proventriculus and a muscular ventriculus. The gastric epithelium of the proventriculus is simple columnar and mucus secreting. A thin lamina propria separates it from the lobules of the submucosal glands. These glands form an almost continuous mass of tissue, with adjacent lobules separated by fine strands of connective tissue. Each gland lobule contains a central cavity with straight secretory tubules radiating to the interlobular connective tissue. An excretory duct drains onto the gastric mucosal surface. The glands contain only one type of cell, which secretes acid and pepsinogen, thus combining the functions of both the chief and parietal cells of the mammal. The muscularis externa is arranged as inner circular and outer longitudinal layers of smooth muscle (8.100–8.102).

The ventriculus is the aglandular stomach or gizzard. The luminal surface is lined with secretory product of the mucosal glands, which solidifies at the surface to form a hard cuticle of koilin. The epithelium is low columnar and continues within the

8.100

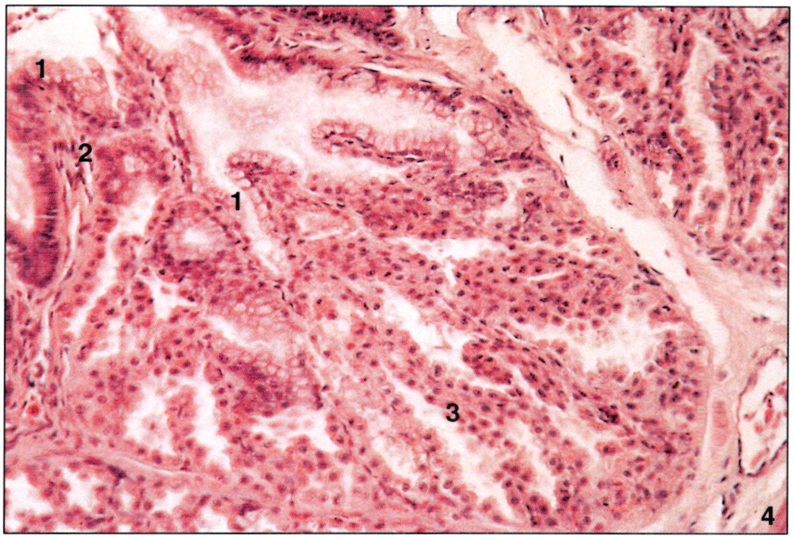

8.100 Proventriculus (bird). (1) Simple columnar mucus-secreting epithelium. (2) Lamina propria. (3) Submucosal glands. (4) Muscularis externa. H & E ×62.5.

8.101

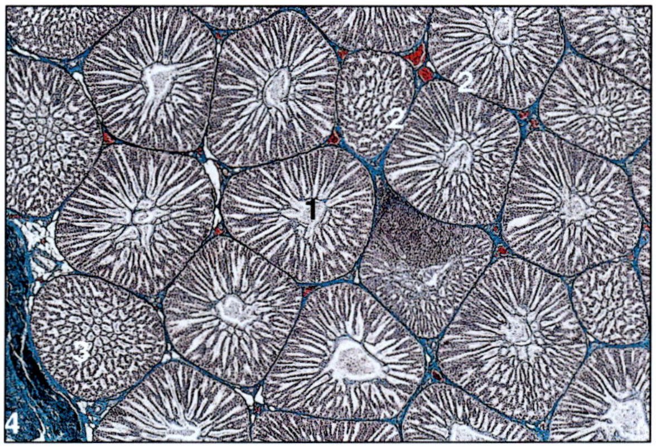

8.101 Proventriculus (bird). (1) Simple columnar mucus-secreting epithelium. (2) Lamina propria. (3) Submucosal glands. (4) Muscularis externa. Masson's trichrome. ×25.

8.102

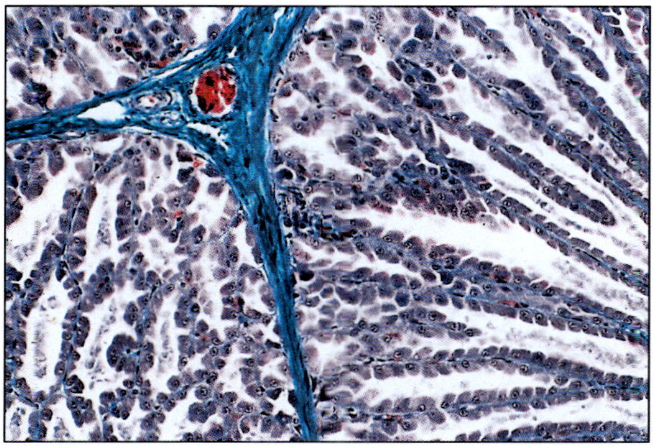

8.102 Proventriculus (bird). The submucosal gland lobules are separated by thin strands of connective tissue. Masson's trichrome. ×250.

8.103

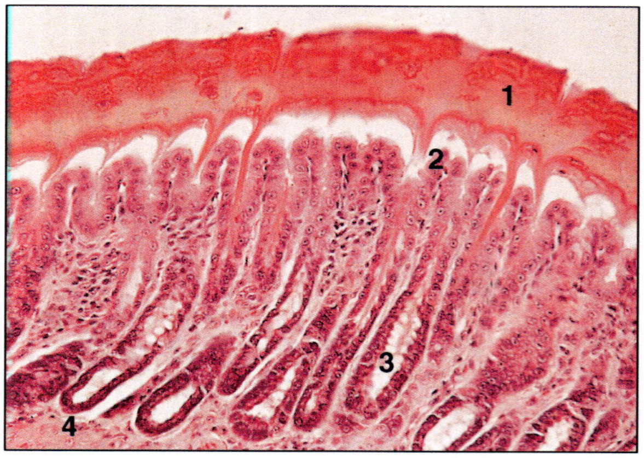

8.103 Ventriculus, gizzard (bird). (1) Cornified lining. (2) Epithelium lining the gizzard. (3) Mucosal glands. (4) Lamina propria. H & E. ×25.

simple straight tubular mucosal glands in the lamina propria. A submucosa is present, and the muscularis externa is a thick layer of smooth muscle (8.103 and 8.104). There is no muscularis mucosae.

Intestine

The small intestine is similar to that of mammals but is more uniform throughout its length. Diffuse lymphatic tissue is present in the lamina propria and the submucosa, and a third layer of circular smooth muscle may be present in the muscularis externa (8.105–8.107).

8.1

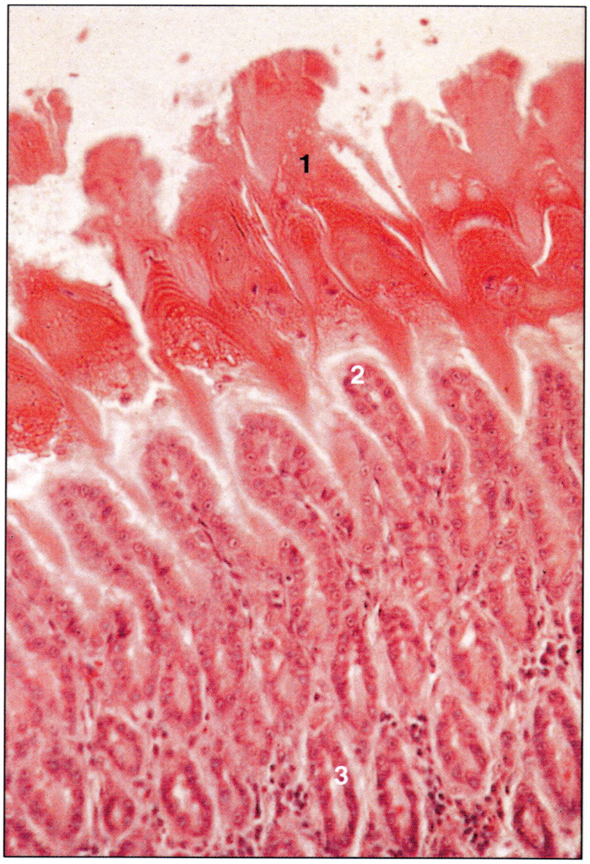

8.104 Ventriculus, gizzard (bird). (1) Cornified lining. (2) Lining epithelium. (3) Mucosal glands. H & E. ×125.

The caeca are two blind sacs at the junction of the small and large intestine and are of considerable size in domestic birds. The epithelium is simple columnar with mucous cells. Lymphatic tissue is particularly abundant, forming the caecal tonsil in the narrow proximal part of the caecum (8.108 and 8.109).

8.105

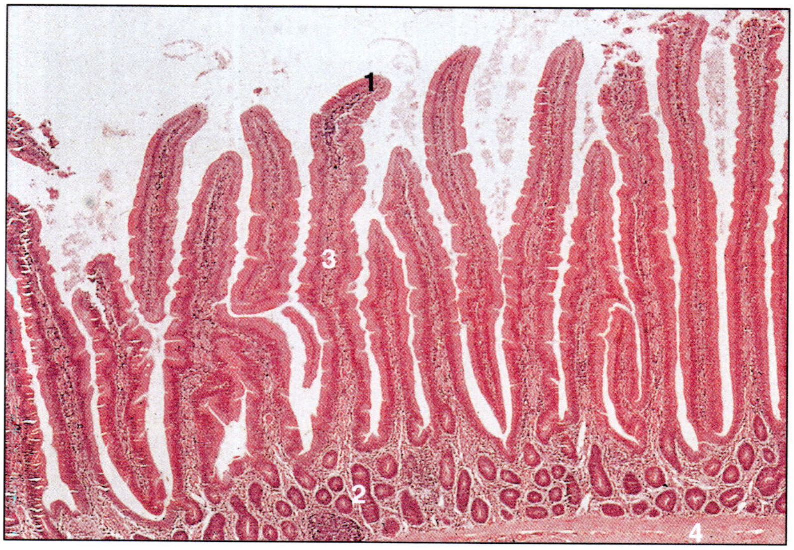

8.105 Duodenum (bird). (1) Simple columnar epithelium. (2) Intestinal mucosal glands. (3) Connective tissue core of the villus. (4) Muscularis mucosae. H & E. ×62.5.

106

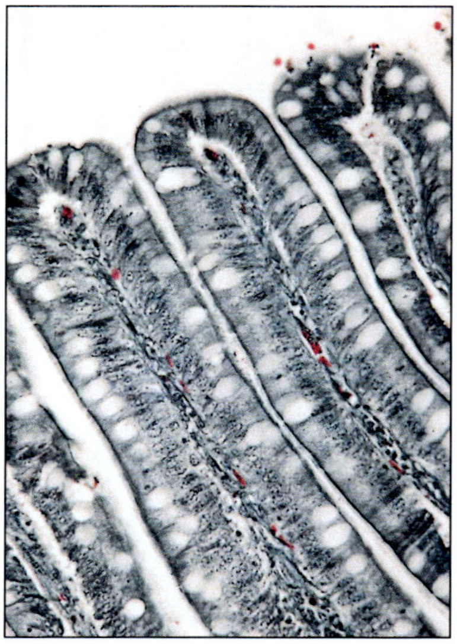

8.107

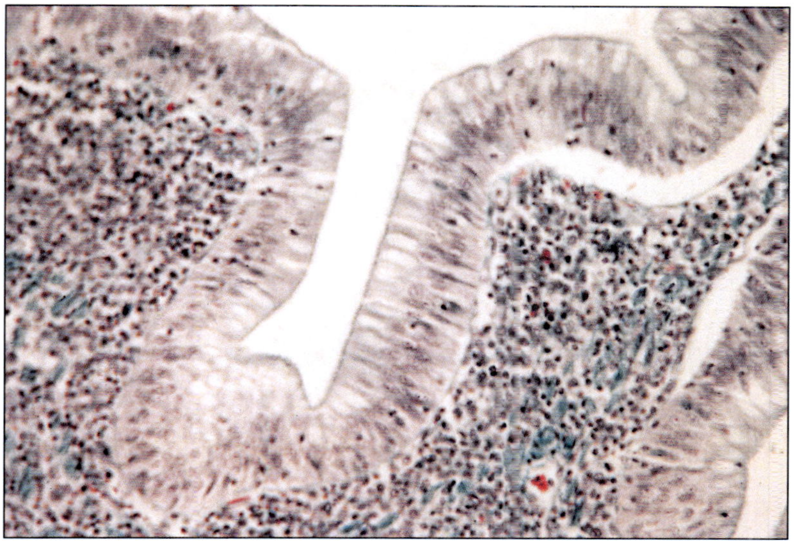

8.108

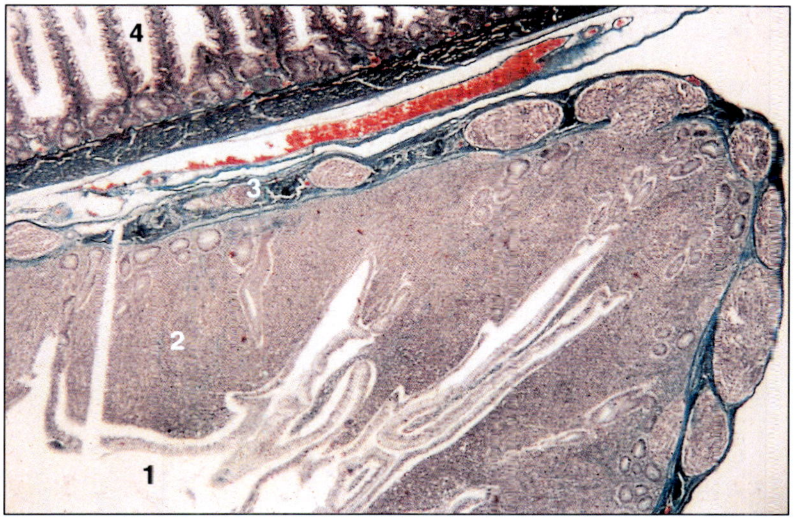

8.109

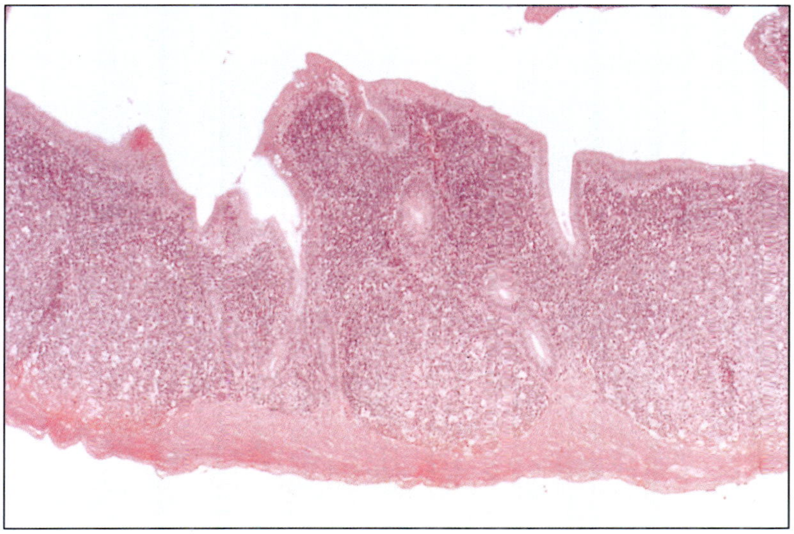

8.106 Duodenum (bird). The simple columnar epithelium lining the duodenum has a striated border to allow absorption and goblet cells. Masson's trichrome. ×125.

8.107 Duodenum (bird). The simple columnar epithelium rests on a lamina propria with numerous lymphatic cells. Masson's trichrome. ×250.

8.108 Caecum (bird). (1) Lumen of the caecum. (2) Mucosa consists of a columnar epithelium and a lamina propria with extensive deposits of lymphatic tissue. (3) Muscularis. (4) Lumen of the duodenum. Masson's trichrome. ×12.5.

8.109 Caecum (bird). Dense masses of lymphatic tissue fills the lamina propria. H & E. ×12.5.

The large intestine has the same histological appearance as the caeca (**8.110**). The cloaca is lined with tall columnar epithelium with a variable number of mucus-secreting cells. A vascular lamina propria separates it from the muscularis mucosae and externa (**8.111**). (See Chapter 15 for the cloacal bursa.)

The avian liver is very similar to the mammalian; the connective tissue capsule extends into the gland and divides it into lobes and lobules. The hepatocytes are arranged in rows, often two cells thick, separated by sinusoids.

The avian exocrine pancreas is similar to the mammallian, but has less interlobular connective tissue (**8.112**). The endocrine pancreatic islets are of three types: light (beta) islets, dark (alpha) islets and mixed.

8.110

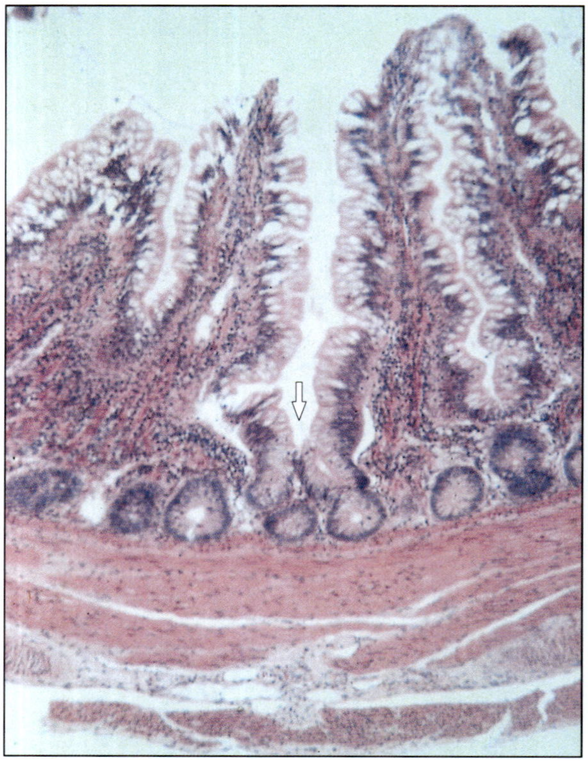

8.110 Rectum (bird). The lining epithelium is simple columnar with goblet cells extending into the simple tubular mucosal glands (arrowed). H & E. ×62.5.

8.111

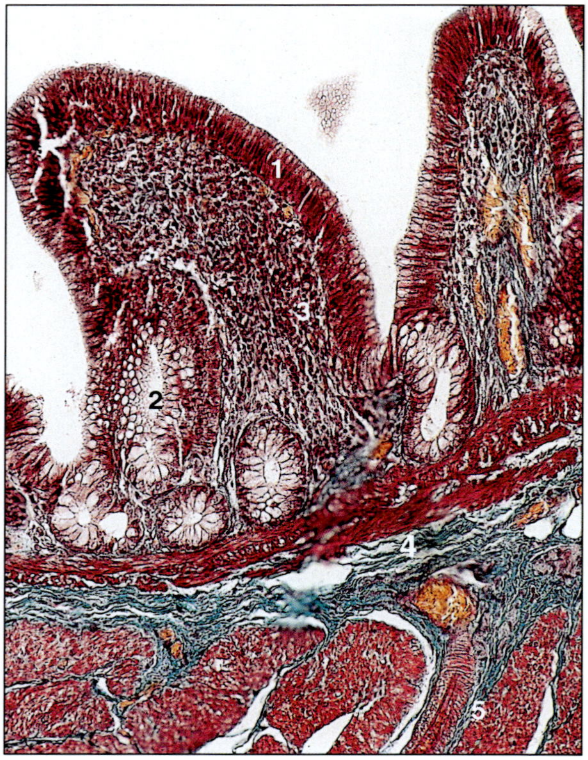

8.111 Cloaca (bird). (1) Simple columnar lining epithelium. (2) Simple tubular glands. (3) Lamina propria with lymphatic tissue. (4) Muscularis mucosae. (5) Muscularis externa. Alcian blue/PAS. ×62.5.

8.112

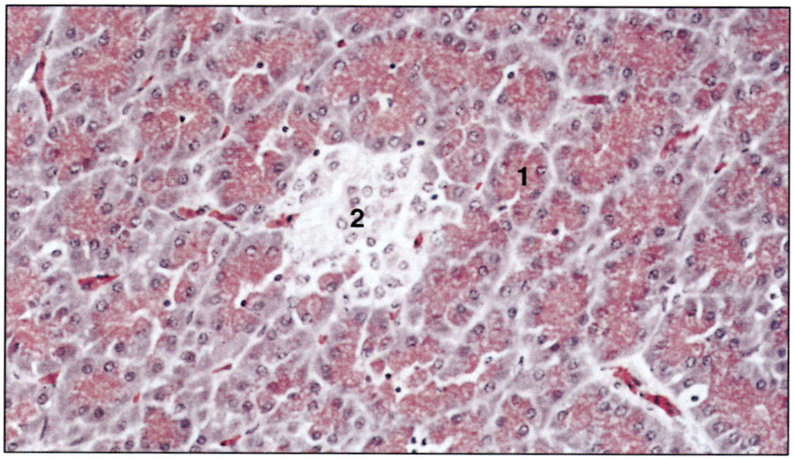

8.112 Pancreas (bird). (1) Serous units of the exocrine gland. (2) Pancreatic islet, the endocrine gland. H & E. ×125.

9. URINARY SYSTEM

The urinary system of mammals comprises the kidneys, renal pelvis, ureters, bladder and urethra.

Kidneys

The kidneys are highly vascularized organs that filter the blood and excrete waste materials, excess water and electrolytes via the ureters to the bladder as urine (see Appendix Figures **A1–A7**). The kidneys have an endocrine function: they secrete erythropoietin, which stimulates erythrocyte production in the bone marrow, and renin, which helps to regulate blood pressure. Each kidney is enclosed in a tough connective tissue capsule extending into the parenchyma and has two regions – the cortex and the medulla (**9.1–9.4**). Smooth muscle may be present in ruminants. The hilus is a deep fissure on the medial border of the kidney and contains the renal artery, the renal vein and the ureter.

9.1

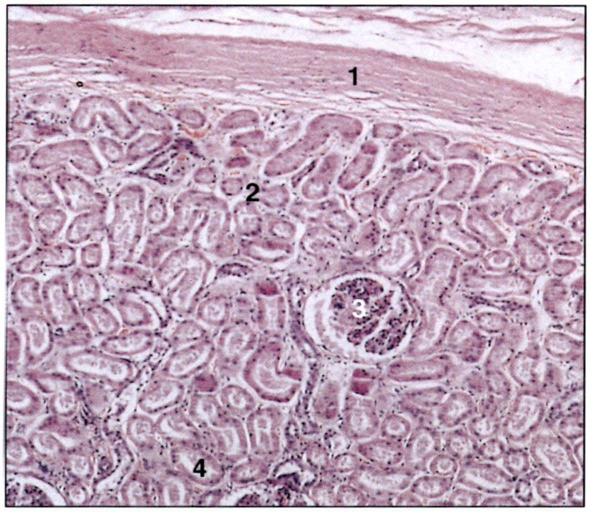

9.1 Kidney (horse). (1) Capsule. (2) Outer area of the cortex. (3) Renal corpuscle. (4) Uriniferous tubules. H & E. ×62.5.

9.2

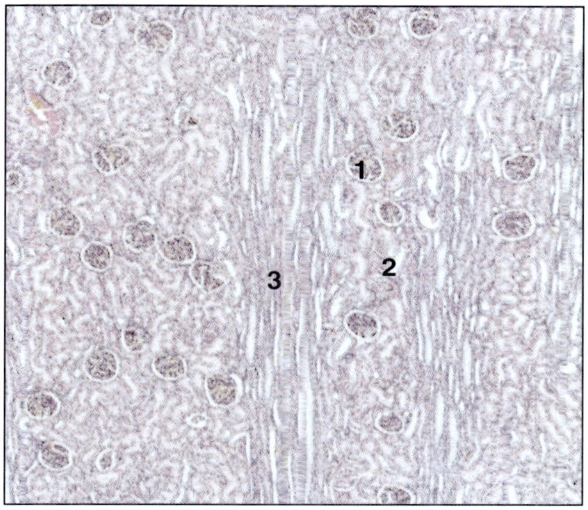

9.2 Kidney cortex (dog). (1) Renal corpuscle. (2) Uriniferous tubules. (3) Medullary ray. H & E. ×12.

9.3

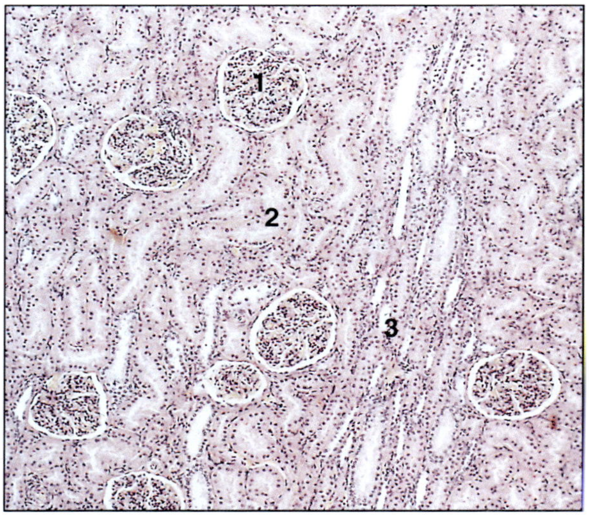

9.3 Kidney cortex (dog). (1) Renal corpuscle. (2) Uriniferous tubules. (3) Medullary ray. H & E. ×125.

9.4

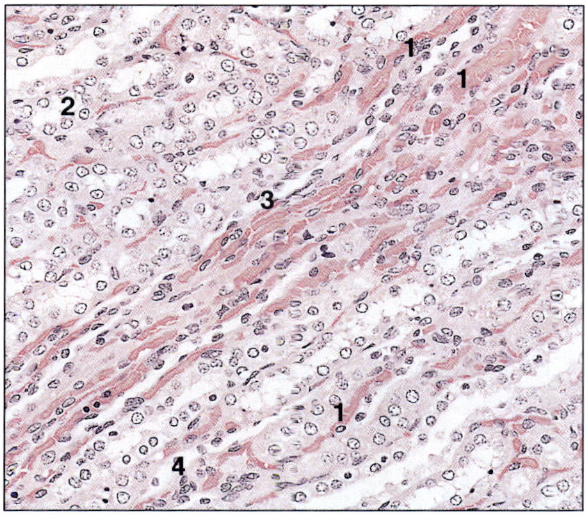

9.4 Kidney medulla (dog). (1) Blood vessels. (2) Collecting tubules. (3) Ascending thin limb. (4) Descending thin limb. H & E. ×125.

Nephron

The nephron is the functional unit of the kidney. The major subdivisions are the renal corpuscle and the uriniferous tubule.

Renal corpuscle

The blind end of the proximal tubule is indented with a network of capillaries and supporting cells to form a filtering system: the renal corpuscle. Each renal corpuscle consists of a glomerulus and a glomerular (Bowman's) capsule. The outer layer of the glomerular capsule is the capsular (parietal) wall, which is separated from the glomerular (visceral) layer by the capsular (urinary) space (9.5). The capillaries are lined with a fenestrated endothelium resting on a basal lamina. The visceral epithelial cells, or podocytes, closely invest the capillary endothelium of the glomerulus and develop primary processes wrapped around each capillary. These processes develop secondary foot processes called pedicles. The foot processes of adjacent podocytes interdigitate, resulting in the formation of small gaps called slit pores (9.6). The podocyte basal lamina is fused with the endothelial basal lamina and blood passing through the capillary is filtered through this common basal lamina into the capsular space (9.6 and 9.7). Mesangial perivascular cells are present between the endothelium and the basal lamina. The capillaries of the glomerulus are served by an afferent and an efferent arteriole, entering and leaving the renal corpuscle at the vascular pole (9.8). At the opposite pole is the capsular space, where the filtrate passes into the proximal tubule at the urinary pole of the renal corpuscle (9.8 and 9.9).

9.5

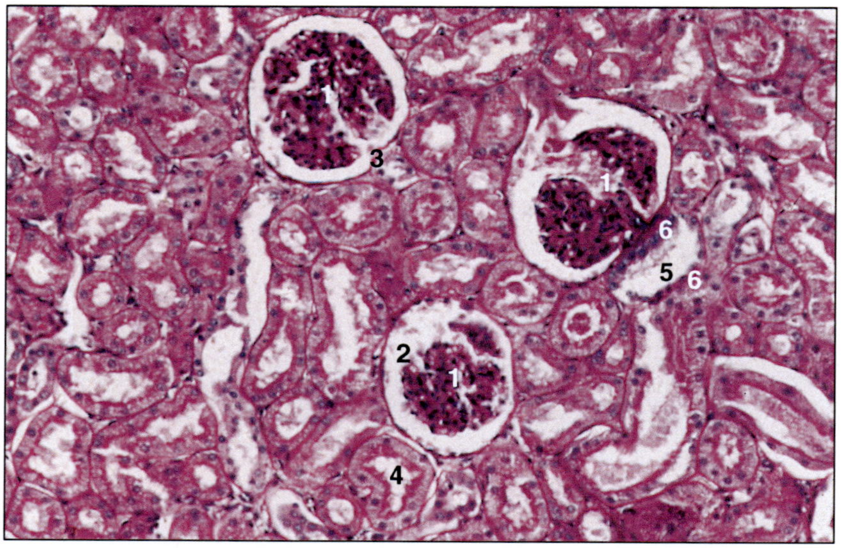

9.5 Kidney (horse). (1) Renal corpuscle with (2) capsular space (3) the urinary pole. (4) Proximal convoluted tubule. (5) Distal convoluted tubule with (6) the macula densa. H/PAS. ×250.

9.6

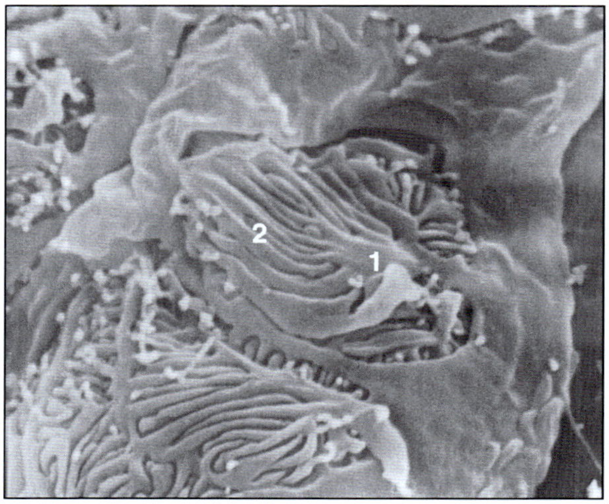

9.6 Kidney (dog). (1) Part of the podocyte. (2) Secondary foot processes, the pedicles – the filtration slit pores are the spaces between the solid pedicles. Scanning electron micrograph. ×1500.

9.7

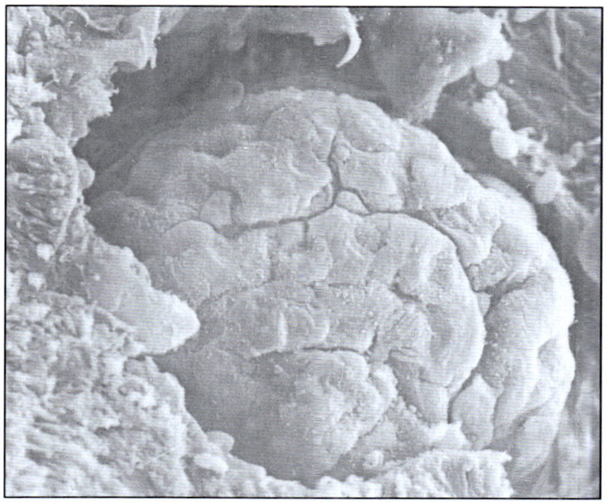

9.7 Kidney (dog). The renal corpuscle projects from the surrounding tissue. Scanning electron micrograph. ×500.

9.8

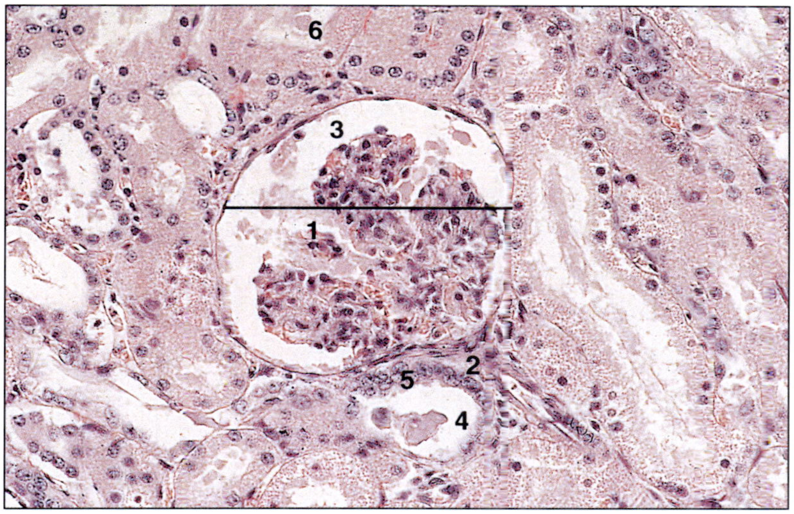

9.8 Kidney (horse). The width of the glomerular capsule is shown by the line. (1) Renal corpuscle with epithelial cells and mesangium. (2) Vascular pole. (3) Capsular space. (4) Distal convoluted tubule. (5) The macula densa. (6) Proximal convoluted tubule. H & E. ×250.

9.9

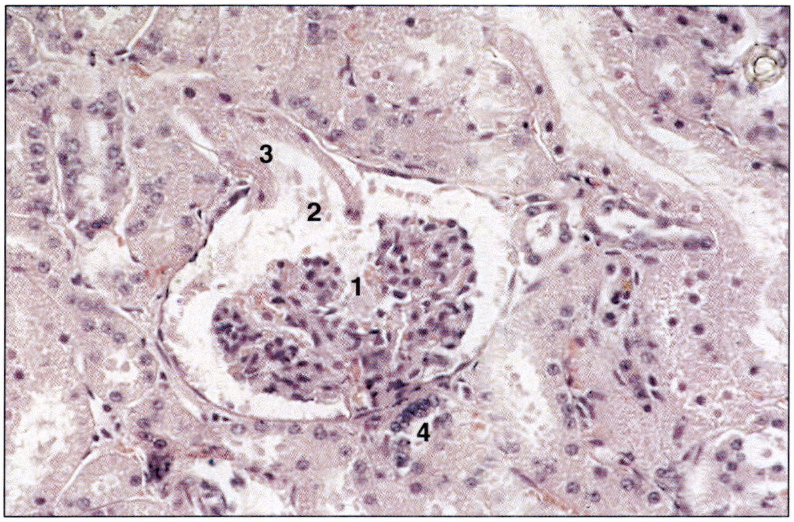

9.9 Kidney (horse). (1) Renal corpuscle with epithelial cells and mesangium. (2) Urinary pole opening into (3) the proximal convoluted tubule. (4) Distal convoluted tubule and macula densa. H & E. ×250.

Renal tubule

This nomenclature is based on the functional areas of the renal tubule. The proximal convoluted tubule (PCT) is long and lined with low columnar cells with a basal nucleus. The cytoplasm is deeply stained with eosin and the apical surface is a continuous brush border. The basal plasma membrane is folded, with mitochondria in the cytoplasm giving a striated effect, and functions to increase the surface for transport (cf. salivary glands striated duct). The PCT is continued with the proximal straight tubule. It is similar in appearance and extends towards the medulla where the epithelium changes abruptly to simple squamous. This part of the tubule descends into the medulla as the thin descending limb and bends sharply to return to the cortex as the thick ascending limb, which was previously known as the loop of Henle. In the cortex the epithelium becomes cuboidal or columnar and forms the distal straight tubule and coils near the glomerulus to become the distal convoluted tubule (DCT). The DCT is shorter than the PCT, the epithelium is cuboidal, the cytoplasm is paler and there is no brush border.

9.10

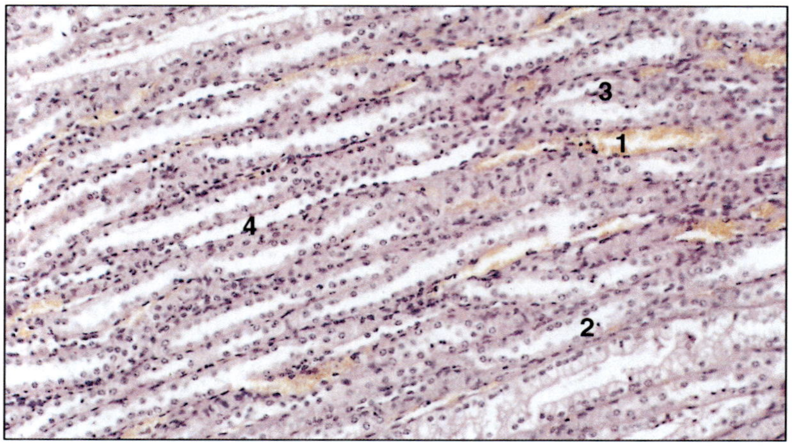

9.10 Kidney medulla (dog). (1) Capillaries lined by endothelium. (2) Collecting tubules lined by cuboidal cells. (3) Ascending limb lined by cuboidal epithelium. (4) Descending limb lined by squamous epithelium. H & E. ×125.

9.11

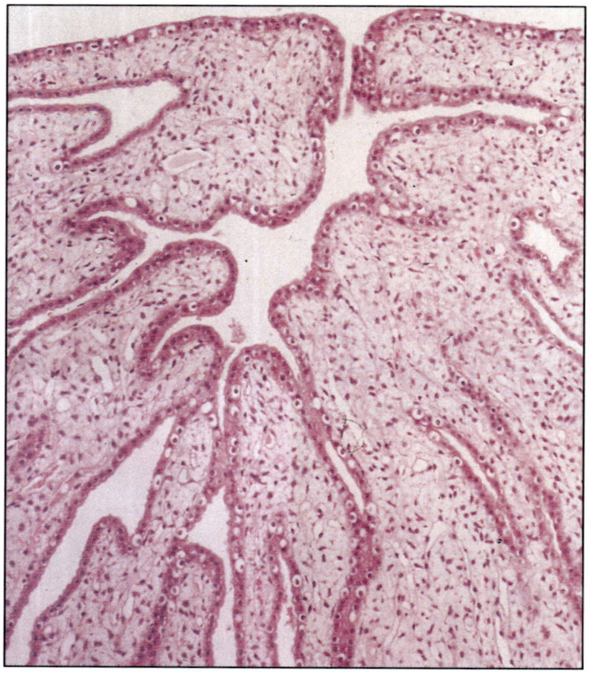

9.11 Kidney. Renal pelvis (sheep). The renal pelvis is lined by urethelium resting on a vascular lamina propria. H & E. ×62.5.

The DCT approaches the glomerulus at the vascular pole, where it thickens, and the cell nuclei of the tubule wall become crowded together to form the macula densa, part of the juxtaglomerular apparatus. Juxtaglomerular cells are modified smooth muscle cells in the walls of afferent arterioles close to the glomerulus. The cells are epithelioid, contain granules and produce renin (which plays a role in the regulation of blood pressure) and angiotensin (a vasoconstrictor and stimulus of aldosterone secretion) (**9.1–9.3** and **9.9**).

Collecting tubule

The collecting tubule or duct (lined with poorly staining cuboidal epithelium) is the terminal segment of the nephron, a continuation of the DCT within the medulla (**9.4** and **9.10**), joining with others to form straight ducts: the papillary ducts (of Bellini). Here the epithelium becomes columnar, and then becomes urethelium towards the opening into the renal pelvis (**9.11**).

Renal pelvis

This is the funnel-like dilatation at the cranial end of the ureter. It is usually within the renal sinus, but in certain conditions a large part may be extrarenal. It is lined with urethelium resting on a loose connective tissue lamina propria. In the horse there are numerous mucus-secreting glands (9.12 and 9.13). The muscularis is three ill-defined layers of smooth muscle. The tunica adventitia is loose connective tissue.

.12

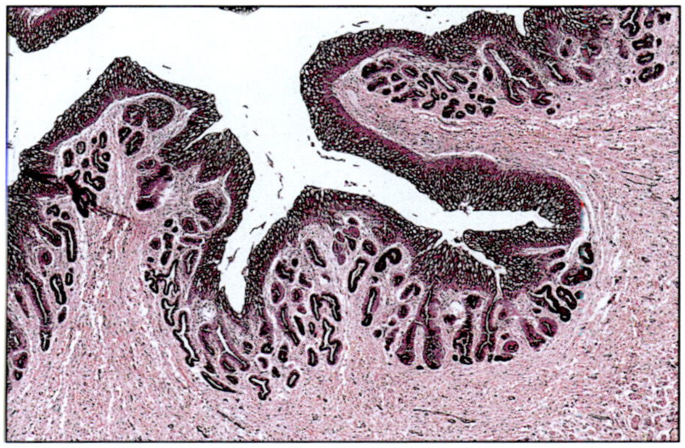

9.12 Kidney. Renal pelvis (horse). The renal pelvis is lined by urethelium; simple mucus-secreting glands are present in the lamina propria. H/PAS. ×62.5.

9.13

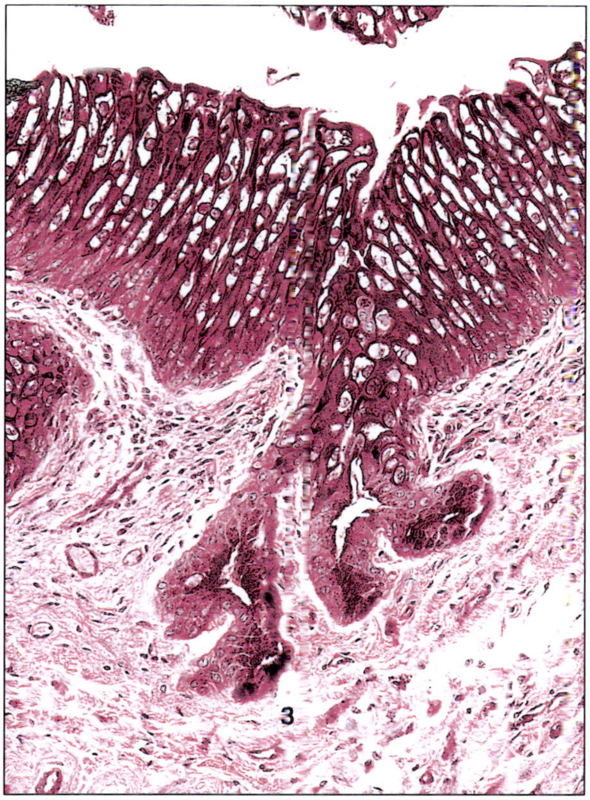

9.13 Ureter (horse). (1) Urethelium. (2) Simple mucus-secreting tubular glands. (3) Vascular lamina propria. H/PAS. ×250.

Ureter

The ureter leaves the kidney at the pelvis and runs to the bladder. The mucosa is formed into plait-like longitudinal folds, and elastic fibres allow stretching. The urethelium consists of at least five to six cell layers, and in the horse simple tubuloalveolar mucous glands are present in the lamina propria. There is no submucosa. The muscularis externa is ill-defined with connective tissue between the bundles of smooth muscle (9.14 and 9.15). The outer coat may be loose connective tissue adventitia or a serosa, depending on the part of the ureter that is examined.

.14

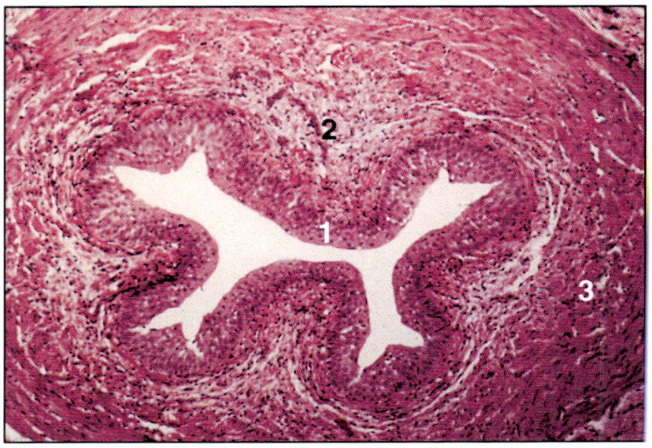

9.14 Ureter (dog). (1) Urethelium lines the lumen of the ureter. (2) Vascular lamina propria. (3) Muscularis externa. H & E. ×62.5.

9.15

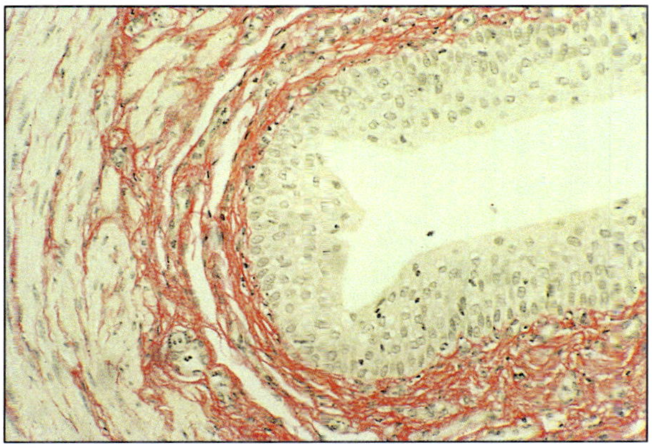

9.15 Ureter (dog). The elastic fibres are stained reddish-orange. Van Giesen. ×62.5.

Urinary bladder

The urinary bladder is lined by urethelium, the number of cell layers depending upon whether the bladder is stretched or unstretched. There are elastic fibres in the lamina propria. The muscularis is the same as in the ureter, and the outer layer may similarly be adventitia or serosa. Parasympathetic ganglia and nerve receptors are present (**9.16** and **9.17**).

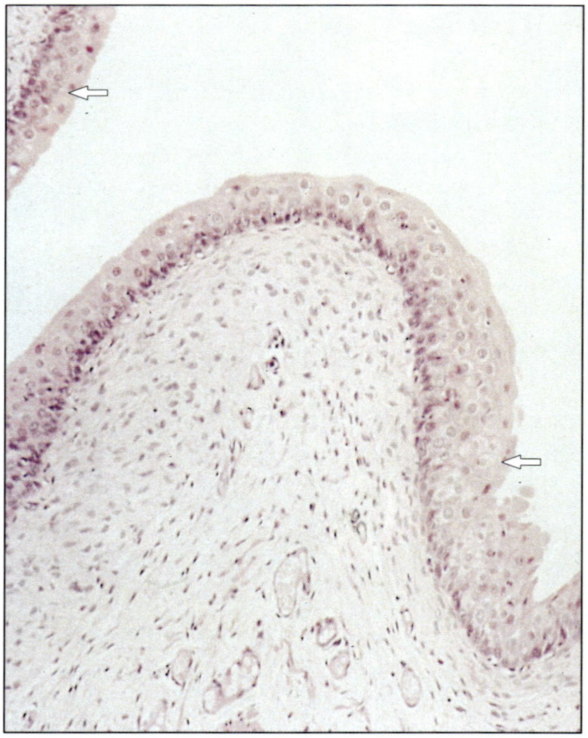

9.16

9.16 Urinary bladder (dog). The bladder is relaxed and the surface cells are rounded adjacent to the lumen (arrowed). H & E. ×125.

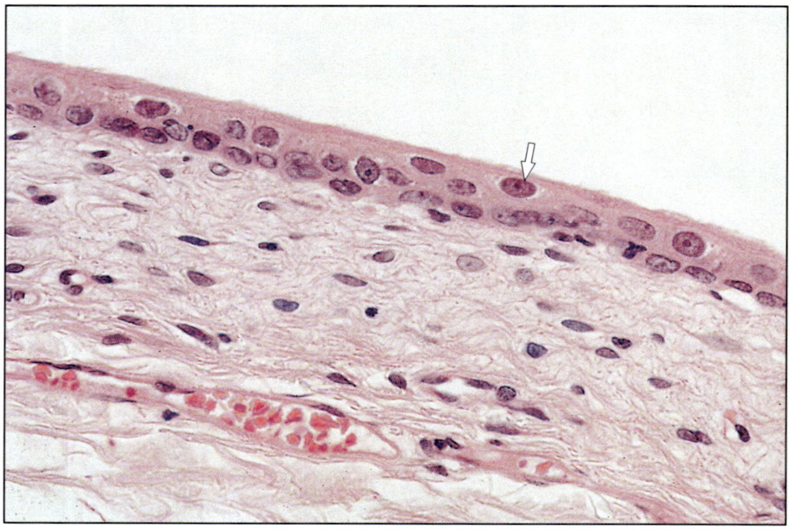

9.17

9.17 Urinary bladder (dog). The bladder is stretched and the surface cells are flattened (arrowed). H & E. ×250.

Urethra

The male urethra serves a genital function and is discussed in Chapter 11. The female urethra is short, running from the bladder to the external urethral orifice, and has a purely urinary function. The mucosa is folded longitudinally and the epithelium varies from urethelium at the bladder to stratified squamous at the urethral orifice. (See **11.14–11.17** and **12.26**.)

Avian urinary system

Each kidney consists of three pyramidal divisions: cranial, middle and caudal. These are not comparable to the lobes of the mammalian kidney. Each division receives a branch of the renal artery, a branch of the great renal vein, and in the renal portal vein this is a branch of the internal iliac. The avian renal division is composed of a number of indistinct lobes made up of lobules, the structural unit of the kidney. Lobules that drain into a single branch of the ureter constitute a lobe. Each lobule is pear-shaped; the wider part is cortical tissue and the tapering part is medullary tissue. In histological sections the appearance is of the larger cortical areas surrounding cone-shaped islands of medullary tissue, called medullary tracts. The interlobular veins are wedged between the lobules.

There is no renal pelvis or urinary bladder.

There are two types of uriniferous tubules: the mammalian (metanephric) tubule extends into the medullary tissue and the shorter 'reptilian' (mesonephric), or cortical, tubule lacks a loop (of Henle). Both types begin with a renal corpuscle. The reptilian renal corpuscle is smaller than the mammalian, but more numerous, and has a prominent central mass of mesangial cells. The PCT is about half of the tubule and is connected by a short intermediate segment to the DCT. In the medullary tubule the intermediate segment is the loop descending into the medullary tissue. A juxtaglomerular complex is present as in the mammal. The DCTs are joined by collecting tubules, lined with mucus-secreting cuboidal to low columnar epithelium, to the perilobular collecting ducts. These fuse with other ducts to form larger ducts and lead to a secondary branch of the ureter. Five or six secondary branches fuse to form a primary ureteral branch (9.18 and 9.19).

The ureters are lined with a mucus-secreting, pseudostratified epithelium supported by a cellular lamina propria with variable amounts of diffuse lymphoid tissue. The thick muscularis consists of an inner longitudinal and an outer circular layer of smooth muscle (9.20). The ureter drains into the middle compartment of the cloaca: the uroceum.

.18

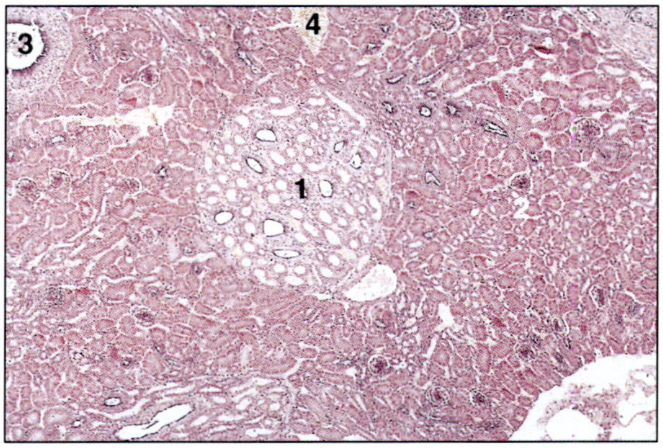

9.18 Kidney (bird). (1) The central, pale staining medullary area is surrounded by (2) the much denser staining cortical area. (3) Lobar duct. (4) Renal vein. H & E. ×25.

.19

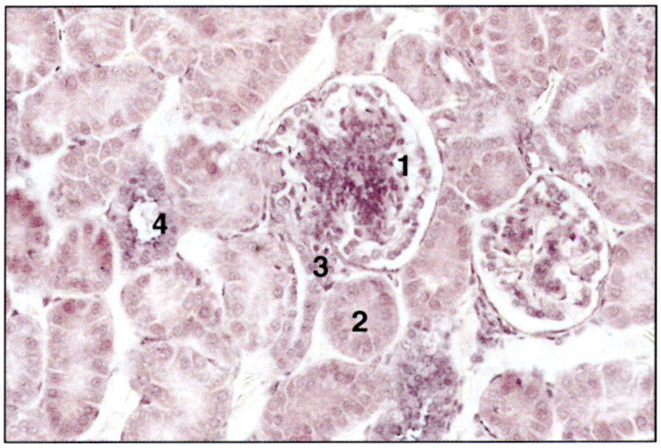

9.19 Kidney cortex (bird). (1) The renal corpuscle has a central mass of epithelial cells and mesangial cells. (2) Proximal convoluted tubule. (3) Distal convoluted tubule. (4) Small collecting tubule with low columnar mucus-secreting epithelium. H & E. ×125.

9.20

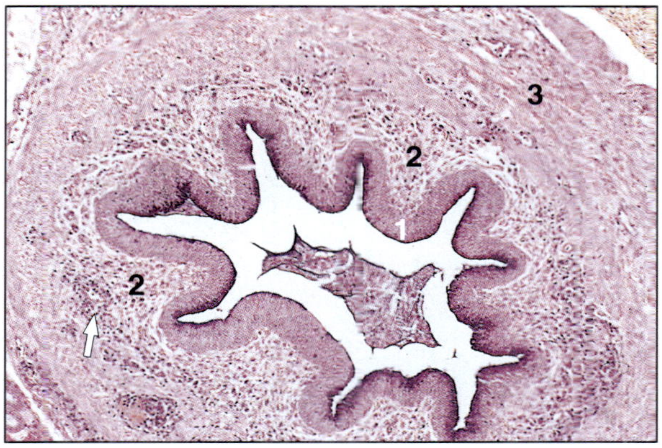

9.20 Ureter (bird). (1) Pseudostratified mucus-secreting epithelium lines the lumen. (2) Cellular lamina propria with groups of lymphocytes (arrowed). (3) Muscularis externa. H/PAS. ×125.

Reptilian urinary system

The renal tissues of reptiles are superficially very similar to those of birds and mammals, but there are some notable differences. In adult males of some species of squamate reptiles (snakes and lizards) there is an obvious and seasonal alteration in the size, shape, staining characteristics and cytoplasmic granularity of the cells comprising the DCTs. This change is termed the 'sexual segment' and is seen in sexually mature male crotalids (pit vipers), teiid and some iguanid lizards, to name but a few (**9.21**). The change is so striking that the sex of the animal from which the renal tissue was obtained is immediately apparent to the histologist. The epithelial cells of the DCTs of mature males become markedly hypertrophied and become packed with small, round and highly eosinophilic cytoplasmic granules that are extruded into the urinary wastes. They are believed to contribute a pheromone or similar chemical cue to the urates that are passed during periods of sexual courtship and mating activity. The sexual segment does not occur in females.

The histological characteristics of the amphibian and reptilian ureter and urinary bladder are similar to those of mammals. The lumen is lined by transitional epithelium (urethelium) that is several layers thick when the bladder is empty but becomes flatter and thinner when the bladder is distended. There is no submucosa; the bladder wall contains wispy strands of smooth muscle. Not all reptiles possess urinary bladders. Instead, the urinary wastes are passed from the twin ureters into the urodeum portion of the cloaca and thence out through the cloacal vent. In some reptiles, the urine is retained for a variable length of time, during which water is actively removed and 'recycled' before the now concentrated, urate-rich wastes are discharged as a pasty white, relatively water-insoluble microcrystalline substance.

9.21

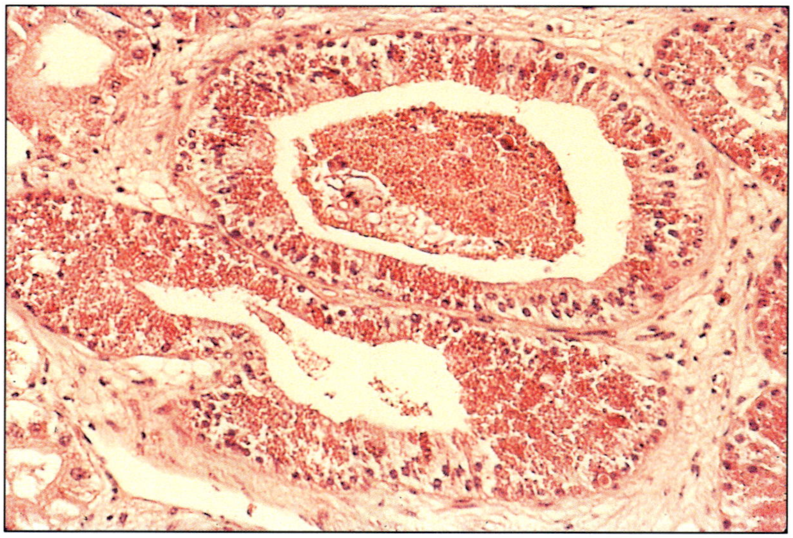

9.21 The kidneys of some species of sexually mature male snakes and lizards possess a characteristic 'sexual segment granulation' which is discerned by a marked hypertrophy and eosinophilic granularity of the distal convoluted tubules. This makes the kidneys of sexually mature males readily distinguishable from the kidneys of sexually mature females of the same species. Illustrated is a section of kidney from a mature male timber rattlesnake (*Crotalus horridus*). H & E. ×125.

Amphibian urinary system

There is a substantial change in the renal histology and function before, during and after metamorphosis in most amphibians. The pronephric kidney of early larval amphibians changes to become fully metanephric in the adult stage of most amphibians. However, in the caecilian amphibians, which are elongated, legless creatures, the kidneys are opisthonephric.

Some amphibians without tails (frogs and toads) excrete most of their nitrogenous wastes as toxic ammonia. Others excrete urea, yet others produce urate salts of uric acid similar to those produced by terrestrial reptiles. The mode of nitrogen excretion is dictated mainly by the living habits; aquatic forms tend to be more ammonotelic, whereas terrestrial amphibians tend towards ureotelism and uricotelism. In addition, season of the year and hydration affect the means by which these animals excrete their nitrogenous wastes.

The kidneys are one of the major sites of haematopoiesis in larval amphibians. During and after metamorphosis, the kidneys lose most of this ability and, as a result, assume a more familiar histological pattern consisting of nephrons that superficially resemble those of reptilian and avian species (9.21).

There is no loop interposed between the PCT and DCT and, therefore, the degree of concentration of the glomerular filtrate is variably limited.

Fish urinary system

Most fish excrete toxic ammonia-rich urinary wastes that are converted via nitrification by the bacteria *Nitrosomonas* spp. to nitrite and then by *Nitrobacter* spp. to nitrate, a less toxic ionic product that can be metabolized by aquatic plants. Thus the potential toxicity of water containing urinary wastes is prevented by the action of these two essential microbial organisms and aquatic flora which, in turn, yield oxygen via photosynthetic pathways.

The kidneys of fish are divided into a cranial pronephric (head) kidney and caudal mesonephric (tail) kidney. The cranial portion is the major site of erythropoiesis. Erythropoietic tissue occupies the interstitial spaces between adjacent glomeruli and renal tubules. The histology of fish kidneys varies widely between species and between marine and freshwater fish: the kidneys of some marine teleosts lack glomeruli. Structurally, the renal tissue of freshwater fish is readily recognizable as kidney at low magnification, but the intervening erythropoietic component may seem to be a cellular inflammatory infiltrate to histologists unfamiliar with fish kidneys.

The caudal portion functions in conventional renal manner as a site of proteinaceous waste filtration and removal. The glomerulus is easily recognizable by the tuft of capillaries and its parietal and visceral capsule. The renal tubules are composed of cuboidal to low columnar epithelial cells, similar to those seen in other vertebrates. In teleosts the kidney also plays a role in osmoregulation of sodium and chloride. The gills also participate in osmoregulation.

Clinical correlates

In all animals the main role of the kidney is the homeostatic control of extracellular fluid composition. This involves maintenance of normal concentrations of salt and water in the body, control of acid–base balance and excretion of waste products.

To function normally, the kidney requires adequate perfusion with blood, sufficient functional renal tissue and unimpeded urinary outflow. Failure of kidney function can therefore be related to inadequate perfusion (pre-renal), to inadequate processing in the kidney (renal) or to blockage of urinary outflow (post-renal).

Each of the four main contributing tissues in

the kidney, the blood vessels, glomeruli, tubules and interstitium can be a primary target of disease.

In animals, renal disease is often subclinical. Clinical disease may be divided into acute and chronic renal failure. Acute renal failure involves a sudden onset of oliguria or anuria and azotaemia and is often the result of acute glomerular, interstitial damage or acute tubular necrosis. This form of renal disease is often reversible. Once the kidney is fully developed, new nephrons (functional units) are not produced and chronic renal failure with progressive destruction of functional tissue, regardless of initiating cause, leads to a syndrome of salt and water imbalance, acid–base disturbance and accumulation of wastes. Chronic renal failure results in irreversible changes that produce shrunken, fibrosed 'end-stage' kidneys.

A wide variety of developmental, circulatory, metabolic, inflammatory and neoplastic conditions can affect the kidneys. Familial nephropathies are recognized in several dog breeds and renal cysts are quite common in pigs and cattle. Glomerulonephritis, often of immune origin, is a common cause of chronic renal failure in both dogs and cats (9.22–9.25). As glomerular damage leads to significant protein loss this can result in the development of nephrotic syndrome, characterized by hypoalbuminaemia, generalized oedema and hypercholesterolaemia. Primary renal neoplasms are uncommon in domestic animals, with renal carcinoma the most commonly recognized tumour in dogs, sheep and cattle, while in pigs, nephroblastomas (true embryonal tumours which arise in primitive nephrogenic tissue) are more frequently seen, especially in younger animals.

Renal tumours are common in salmonid fish and some amphibians, particularly leopard frogs (*Rana pipiens*) in which a specific virally induced adenocarcinoma (of Lucke) is found.

9.22

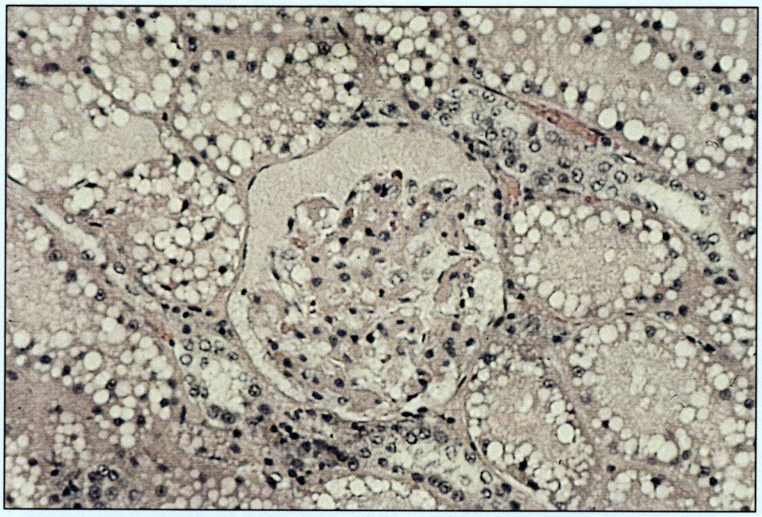

9.22 Feline infectious fibrinoperitonitis is caused by a feline coronavirus and can produce an immune mediated glomerulonephritis with severe proteinaemia. The glomerular space and tubular lumina contain eosinophilic proteinaceous material. The numerous intracytoplasmic lipid vacuoles seen in the tubular epithelial cells are normal in the feline kidney. H & E. ×250.

9.23 Severe chronic interstitial nephritis in an adult male neutered cat. A dense multifocal accumulation of mononuclear, mostly lymphoid, inflammatory cells is present in the interstitial tissue, especially in the subcapsular regions. The capsular outline is irregular and there is interstitial fibrosis with distortion of the tubules. H & E. ×25.

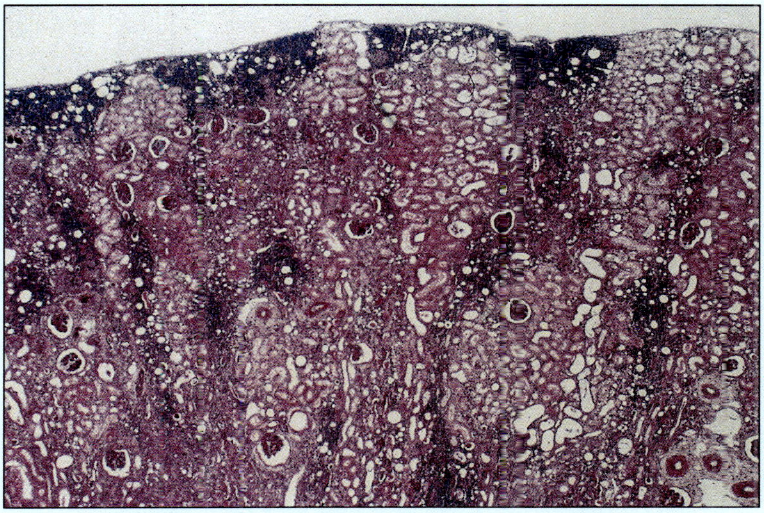

9.23

9.24 Chronic glomerulonephritis (dog). This high power micrograph shows thickening of the glomerular capillary loops, fine interstitial fibrosis and accumulation of proteinaceous fluid in the tubules. This disease ` is usually of immune origin and is a common precursor to the 'end-stage' kidney of renal failure. Masson's Trichrome & Orange G. ×250.

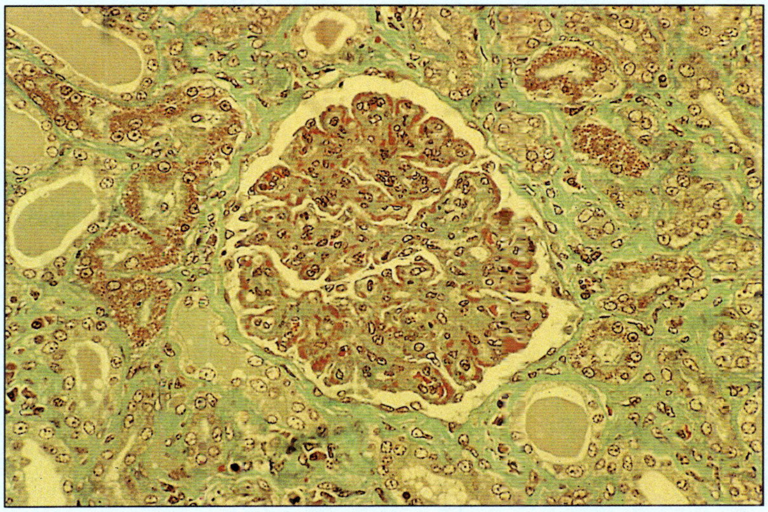

9.24

9.25 Acute interstitial nephritis (dog). This micrograph is of a kidney section from a dog with acute interstitial nephritis. Large numbers of inflammatory cells, mostly lymphocytes, are present between the tubules and around glomeruli. The disease in this dog was caused by infection with *Leptospira canicola* which can cause death through renal failure. H&E. ×62.5.

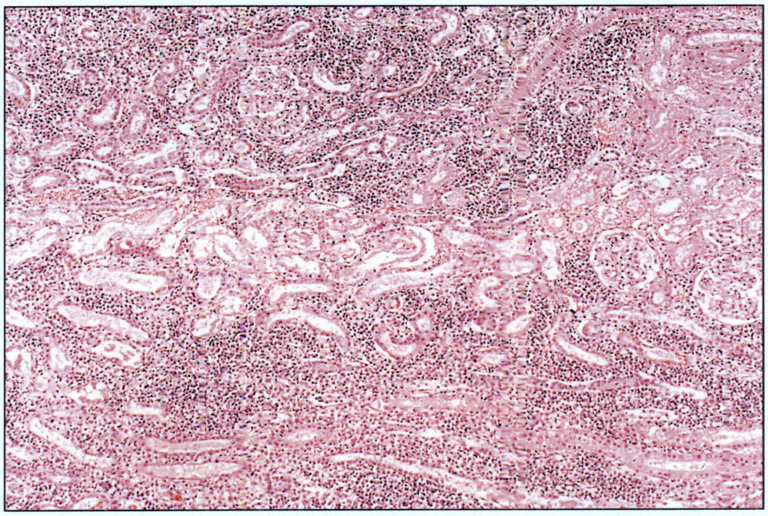

9.25

Histopathologically, similar renal tumours have been described in the Argentine horned frog (*Ceratophrys ornata*). Renal tubular adenoma and carcinoma are relatively frequently recognized in captive snakes and lizards.

Purulent interstitial glomerulonephritis in a kingsnake (**9.26**), renal gout in a boa constrictor (**9.27**), cholesterol nephrosis in a Galapagos tortoise (**9.28**) and renal trematodiasis in an Argentine horned frog (**9.29**) are shown.

9.26

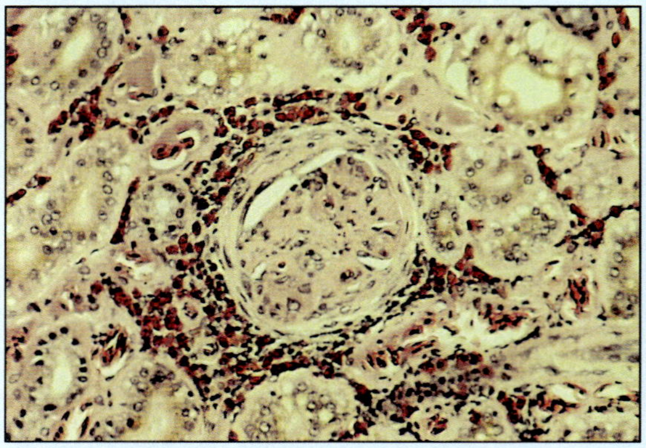

9.26 Purulent interstitial glomerulonephritis in a kingsnake (*Lampropeltis getulus*). The glomerular capsule and glomerular tuft are thickened. The renal interstitial connective tissue is infiltrated by heterophil granulocytic and mixed small mononuclear leucocytes. H & E. ×180.

9.27

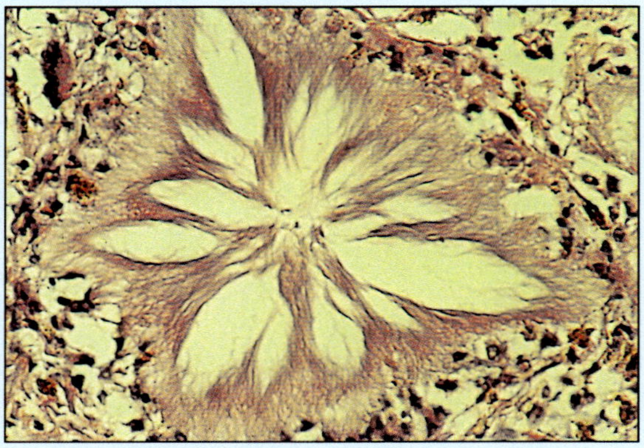

9.27 Renal gout. Illustrated is a section from the kidney of a boa constrictor that had been treated with several aminoglycoside antibiotic drugs without receiving adequate parenteral fluid therapy. A large 'star-burst'-shaped tophus has replaced the glomerulus and the periglomerular interstitial connective tissue is infiltrated by mixed small mononuclear leucocytes. H & E. ×180.

9.28

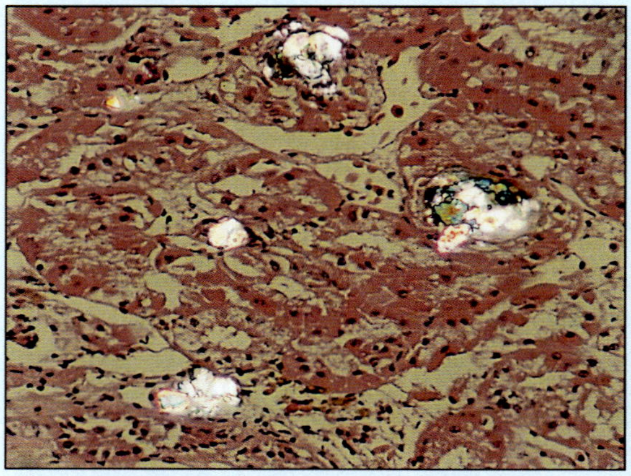

9.28 Cholesterol nephrosis. Illustrated is a section of kidney from a Galapagos tortoise (*Geochelone elephantopus*), which displays multifocal deposits of cholesterol crystals that are obstructing some glomeruli and renal tubules. This condition is seen in captive herbivorous reptiles that have been fed abnormal diets such as commercial dog and cat food. H & E, photographed with cross-polarized illumination. ×48.5.

9.29

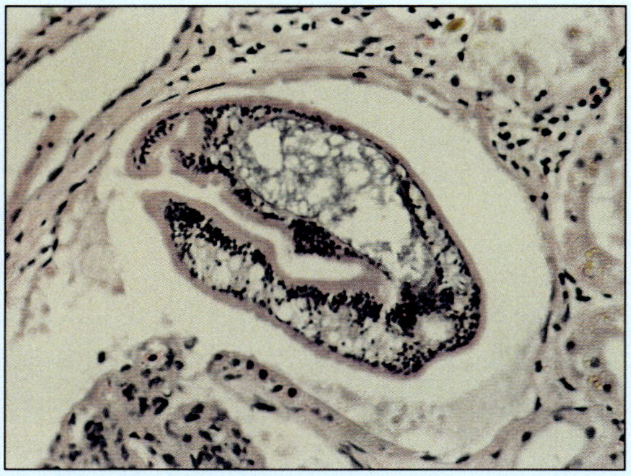

9.29 Renal trematodiasis. The renal pelvis of this Argentine horned frog (*Ceratophrys ornata*) is dilated and contains a large fluke. H & E. ×98.

10. ENDOCRINE SYSTEM

Endocrine tissue

Endocrine tissue is derived from epithelioid parenchymal cells and may form discrete glands, such as hypophysis cerebri (pituitary), thyroid, parathyroid, adrenal and epiphysis cerebri (pineal). Groups of endocrine cells are also active in the interstitial cells of the testes, the granulosa and luteal cells of the ovary, the pancreatic islets (of Langerhans) which are responsible for insulin production and release (see 8.92), the juxtaglomerular apparatus of the kidney and individual amine–precursor–uptake–decarboxylation (APUD) cells acting locally (paracrine). Endocrine cells secrete chemical messengers called hormones directly into a blood or a lymphatic vessel or tissue fluid to influence the activity of target organs. Endocrine tissue is characteristically ductless.

Clinical correlates

Diabetes mellitus, one of the most common endocrinopathies of the dog, may be asssociated with degenerative change and fibrosis in the pancreas (10.1). However, the diagnosis of this condition rests on clinical testing rather than biopsy, as the pancreas of non-diabetic elderly dogs may appear similar and, conversely, some diabetic dogs will have a histologically normal pancreas.

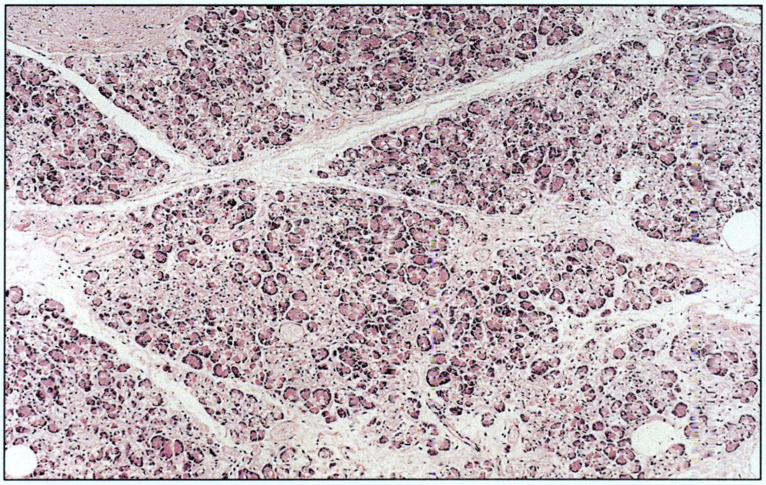

10.1

10.1 Diabetus mellitus (dog) The section of pancreas shown here was taken from an 11-year-old, neutered female English Springer Spaniel with a 2 year history of diabetus mellitus. There are pale eosinophilic areas of replacement fibrosis and the remaining epithelial cells of the exocrine pancreas, with their dark basal nuclei and strongly eosinophilic cytoplasm, can be seen. No islet tissue is discernible. H & E. ×62.5.

Hypophysis cerebri (pituitary gland)

The hypophysis cerebri consists of a glandular lobe, the adenohypophysis, and a fibrous lobe, the neurohypophysis (10.2 and 10.3).

Adenohypophysis

The adenohypophysis is derived from an outpocketing of the ectoderm of the dorsal portion of the oral cavity, the hypophyseal (Rathke's) pouch. It has three sub-divisions: the pars distalis, the pars intermedia and the pars tuberalis.

Pars distalis

The pars distalis is the major constituent of the glandular pituitary. The dense connective tissue capsule is continuous with a fine network of reticular fibres supporting the cords and clusters of parenchymal cells and the capillary/sinusoidal blood vessels. There are two broad categories of cells based on staining affinity: the chromophobes and the chromophils (10.4–10.8). The chromophobe cytoplasm has a few granules that are non-reactive to dyes. These may be reserve cells or exhausted degranulated cells. The

10.2

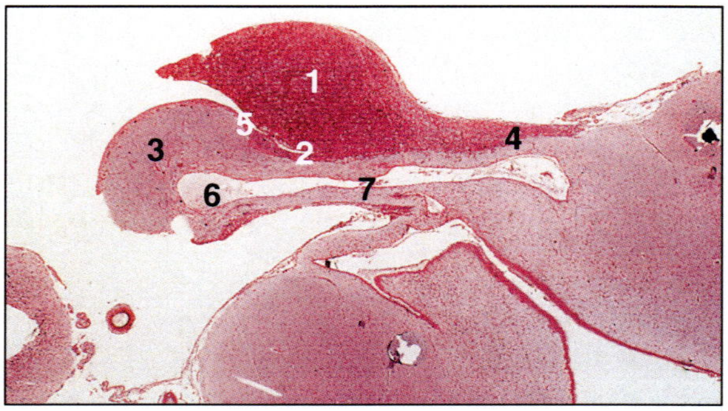

10.2 Hypophysis cerebri (cat). (1) Pars distalis. (2) Pars intermedia. (3) Pars nervosa. (4) Pars tuberalis. (5) Residual lumen (Rathke's pouch). (6) Infundibular recess (third ventricle). (7) Infundibular stalk. H & E. ×5.

10.3

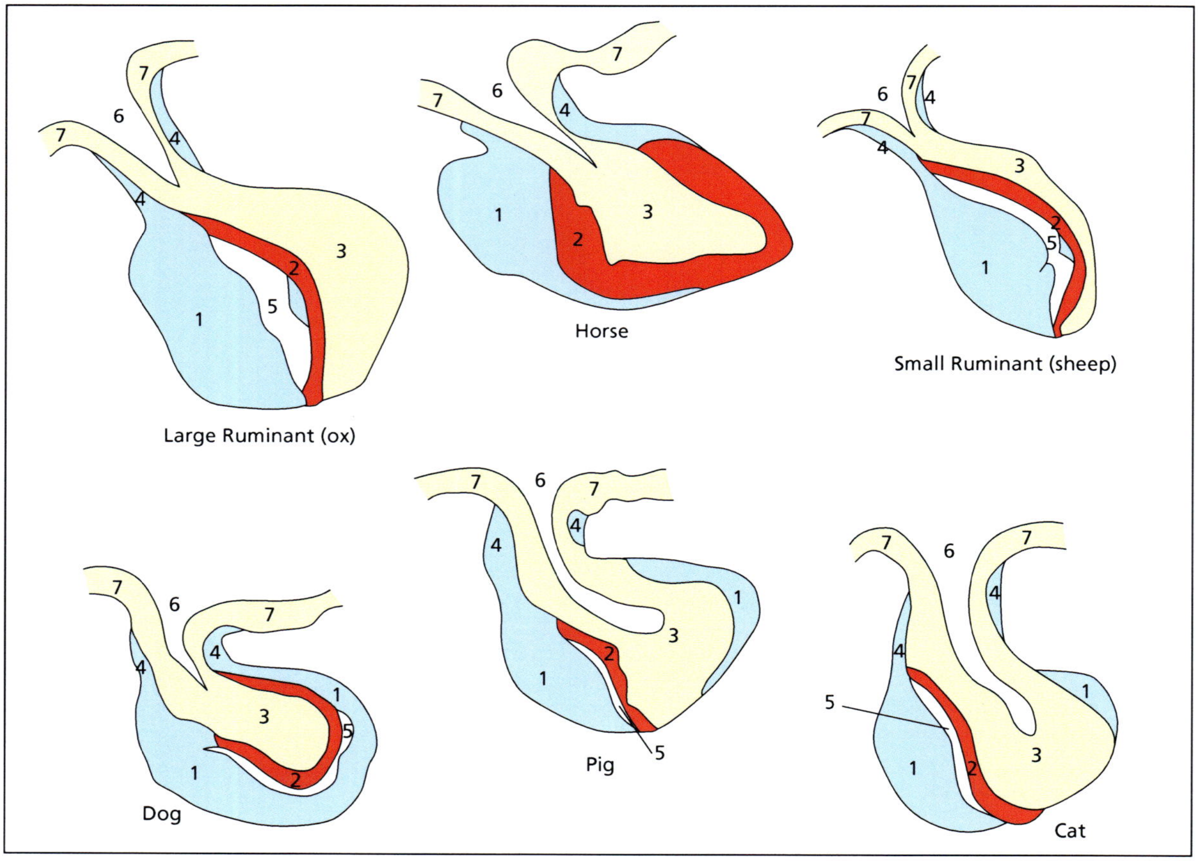

10.3 Diagram of the hypophysis cerebri (pituitary) in some domestic species. (1) Pars distalis. (2) Pars intermedia. (3) Pars nervosa. (4) Pars tuberalis. (5) Hypophyseal cleft (residual lumen of Rathke's pouch). (6) Infundibular recess (third ventricle). (7) Infundibular stalk.

chromophils have a strong affinity for dyes and are divided into acidophils (alpha cells) and basophils (beta cells) in H & E stained sections. The acidophils can be further subdivided using special dyes such as orange G (A cells, orangeophils) or azocarmine (B cells, carminophils). Basophils are larger than acidophils, fewer in number and the cytoplasmic granules stain strongly with PAS. The cells of the pars distalis secrete hormones controlling the other endocrine glands and also factors such as growth hormone.

0.4

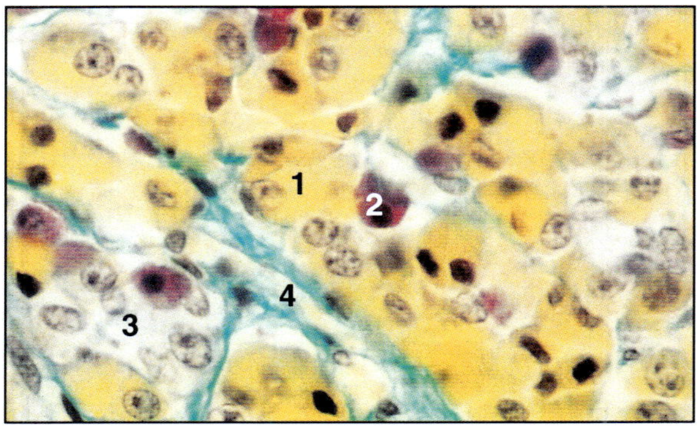

10.4 Pars distalis (cat). (1) Eosinophilic alpha cells. (2) Basophilic beta cells. (3) Chromophobes. (4) Sinusoidal blood vessels lie along the cords and clusters of secretory cells. Orange G/acid fuchsin. ×250.

10.5

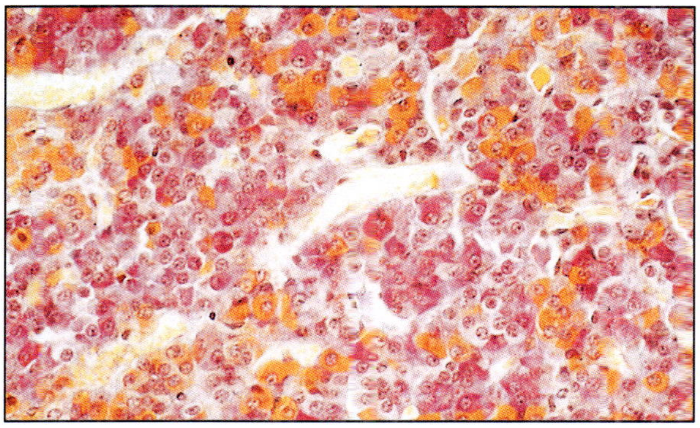

10.5 Pars distalis (horse). The orange staining A cells are easily distinguished from the deep pink staining B cells. Orange G/PAS. ×125.

10.6

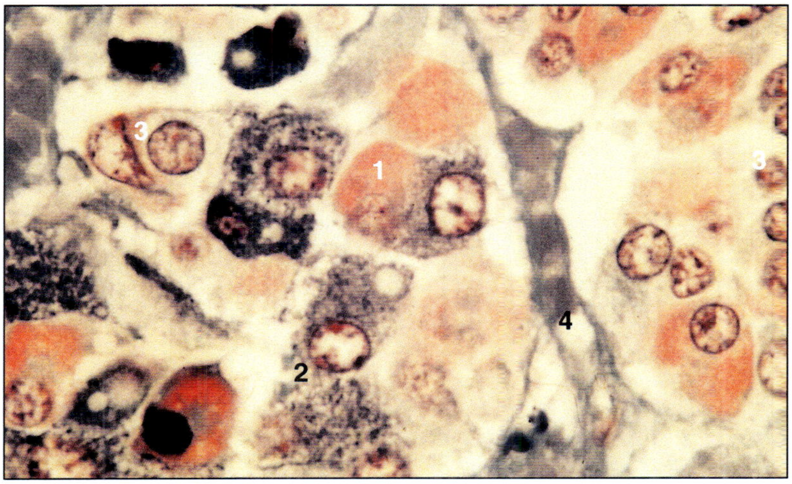

10.6 Pars distalis (cow). (1) Eosinophilic alpha cells. (2) Basophilic beta cells. (3) Chromophobe. (4) Sinusoid. H & E. ×500.

0.7

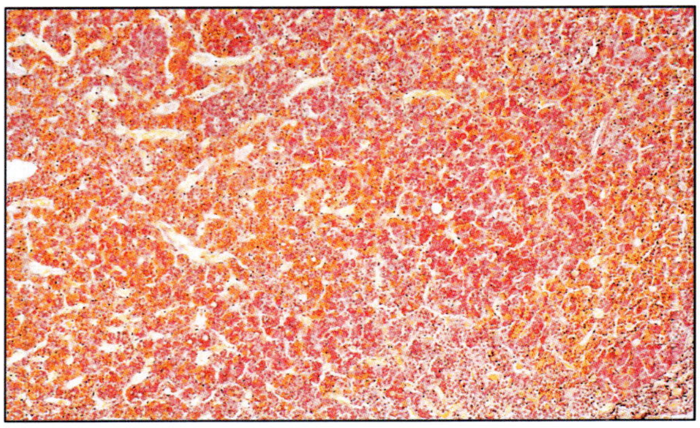

10.7 Pars distalis (dog). A cells stain with orange G and the B cells with acid fuchsin. Orange G/acid fuchsin. ×100.

10.8

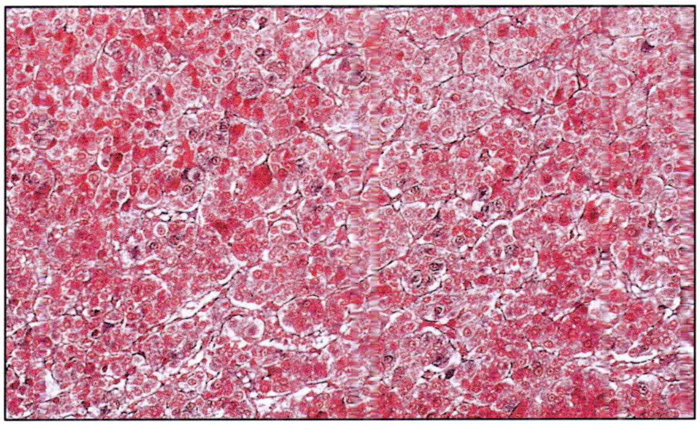

10.8 Pars distalis (horse). A cells stain with orange G and the B cells with acid fuchsin; the supporting connective tissue is green. Orange G/acid fuchsin/light green. ×100.

Pars intermedia

The pars intermedia is well developed in domestic animals and lies between the distalis and the nervosa. In the horse these regions lie closely together. In other domestic animals the pars intermedia and pars distalis are partially separated by the hypophyseal cavity. The parenchymal cells are basophilic with a few acidophilic cells and are arranged in columns or in follicles (10.9). The hormone secreted by these cells stimulates melanocytes and controls the degree of skin pigmentation.

Pars tuberalis

The pars tuberalis surrounds the infundibular stalk, and together they form the hypophyseal stalk (10.10). It is very vascular. The major blood vessels of the hypothalamic–hypophyseal portal system lie in the stalk, and allow the transfer of releasing factors secreted in the brain to the target cells in the distalis. The tuberalis cells are small and basophilic (10.11).

10.9
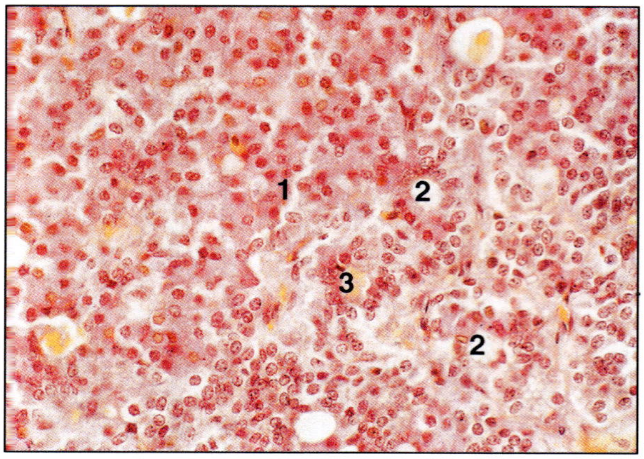

10.9 Pars intermedia (cat). The parenchymal cells are arranged in (1) columns or in (2) follicles. (3) Blood vessels. PAS/orange G/haematoxylin. ×250.

10.10
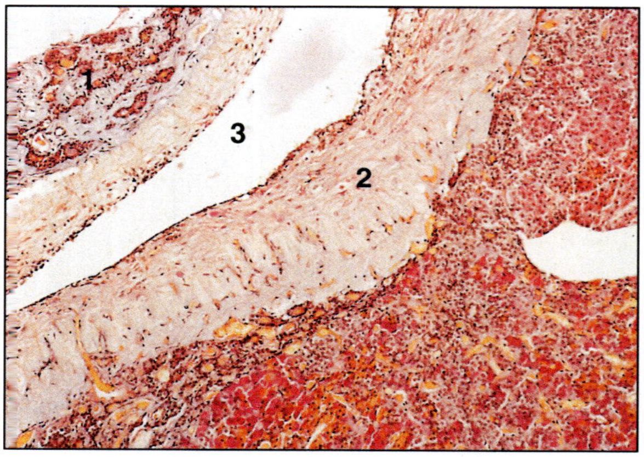

10.10 Pars intermedia/infundibular stalk (horse). (1) The parenchymal cells are separated by blood vessels (orange-staining erythrocytes). (2) The infundibular stalk is fibrous in appearance with small blood vessels of the portal system. (3) The third ventricle lined by ependyma. PAS/orange G/haematoxylin. ×50.

10.11
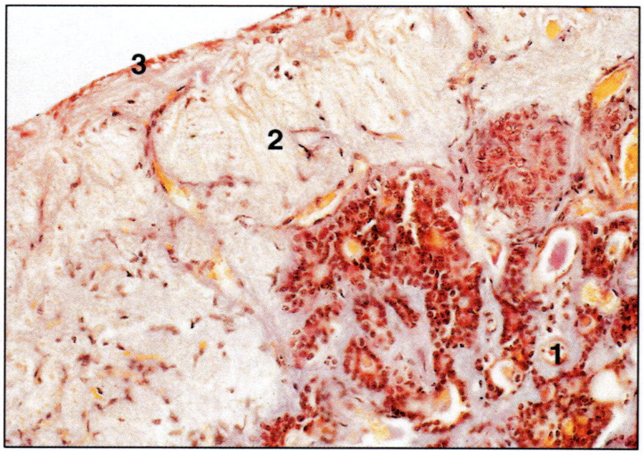

10.11 Pars nervosa/infundibular stalk (horse). (1) Pars tuberalis. (2) Infundibular stalk with portal vessels. (3) Ependyma lining the third ventricle. PAS/orange G/haematoxylin. ×125.

Neurohypophysis

The neurohypophysis is derived from a ventral outpocketing of the diencephalon (the caudal part of the forebrain) and is divisible into a pars nervosa, median eminence and infundibular stalk. The neurohypophysis is composed of numerous unmyelinated nerve fibres with cell bodies that are located in the supraoptic and paraventricular nuclei of the hypothalamus. The axons converge at the median eminence to form the hypothalamic–hypophyseal tract and pass through the infundibular stalk to terminate on the endothelial lining of the capillaries of the pars nervosa (10.12 and 10.13). The neurosecretions of these cells pass down the axons and accumulate at the terminal regions of the nerve fibres as neurosecretory (Herring) bodies (10.14). The axons are supported by pituicytes (neuroglial cells). Oxytocin (a stimulant to the pregnant uterus and lactiferous ducts) and vasopressin (antidiuretic) are the major hormones produced by the nervosa.

10.12

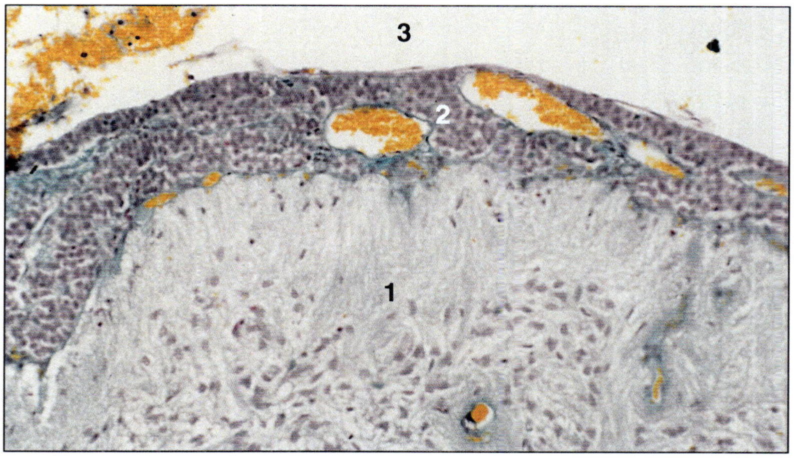

10.12 Pars nervosa (cat). (1) Pars nervosa. (2) Pars intermedia. (3) Infundibular recess. H & E. ×100.

10.13

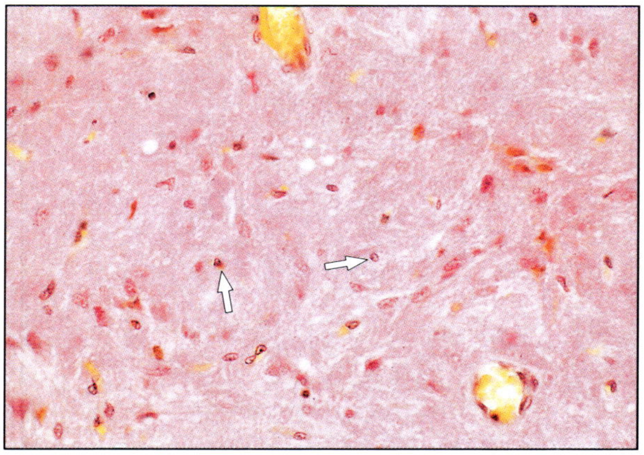

10.13 Pars nervosa (cat). The pars nervosa has a distinctive fibrous appearance; the nuclei of the pituicytes are arrowed. H & E. ×125.

10.14

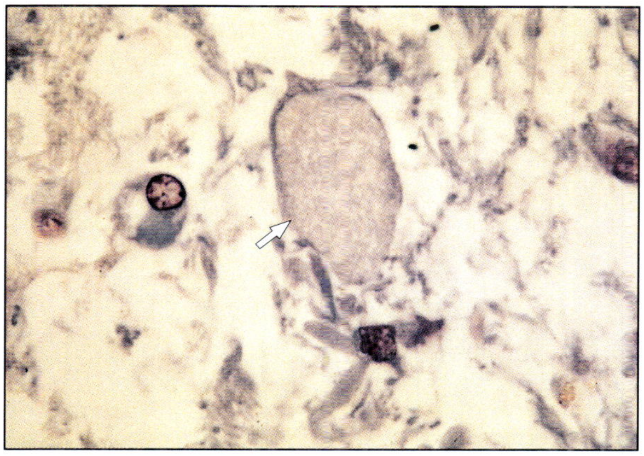

10.14 Pars nervosa (cat). The neurosecretion accumulates in the terminal part of the axons of the hypothalamic–hypophyseal tract to form neurosecretory bodies (arrowed). H & E. ×250.

Clinical correlates

Spontaneous haemorrhage and subsequent necrosis of the pituitary during late pregnancy and parturition occur infrequently in humans and rarely in domestic animals. Neoplasms involving one or more lobes of the pituitary are more common. Because of the location of the pituitary gland and the limited space available for an expanding lesion to occupy within the skull, the clinical signs that attend pituitary tumours are usually referable to pressure on adjacent structures. If the optic chiasm is affected, deterioration of vision extending to blindness will ensue. More specifically, the signs manifested by an animal with a hypophyseal neoplasm refer to hyper- or hyposecretion of one or more pituitary tropic hormones.

Hormonally active tumours of the adenohypophysis result in a clinical picture of corticosteroid excess known as Cushing's disease, while neoplasms of the neurohypophisis often result in abnormalities of antidiuretic hormone or oxytocin secretion. Neoplasms involving the neurohypophisis usually result in either the hypo- or hypersecretion of antidiuretic hormone or oxytocin. Therefore, the first clinical signs may be substantial changes in renal function, water loss or retention, and electrolyte regulation.

Thyroid gland

The thyroid gland is derived from an endodermal outgrowth from the floor of the embryonic pharynx. The thin capsule of dense irregular connective tissue is continuous with the fine reticular fibres of the vascular stroma. It is partially divided into lobules by thin trabeculae. Each lobule consists of numerous follicles lined with simple cuboidal epithelium; the principal follicular cells secrete the thyroid hormones (**10.15** and **10.16**). The secretion is stored in the follicles as homogenous eosinophilic colloid. The hormones cross back through the follicular cells as required and enter the capillaries as tri-iodothryonine and thyroxine (tetra-iodothyronine). These regulate the metabolic activity of all of the body cells and tissues. Large pale cells with an eosinophilic cytoplasm, the parafollicular cells, lie between the follicular cells (**10.17**). These cells produce thyrocalcitonin, an antagonist of parathyroid hormone controlling blood–calcium concentrations. The secretory activity of the thyroid is controlled by thyrotrophin secreted by the pars distalis of the pituitary gland.

10.15

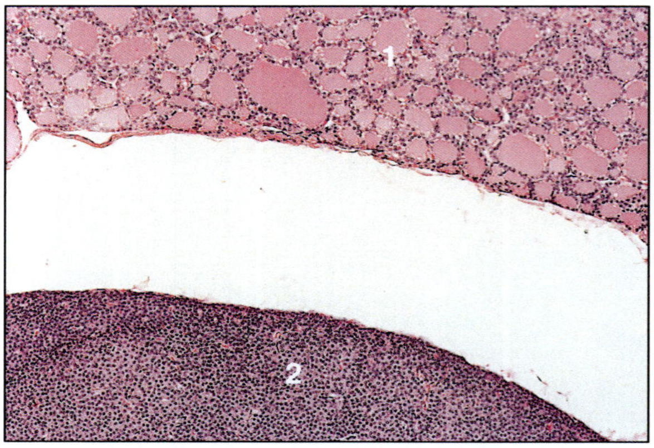

10.15 Thyroid/parathyroid gland (cat). (1) The thyroid follicles are filled with colloid. (2) Densely basophilic cords of parathyroid chief cells lie in the thyroid capsule. H & E. ×20.

10.16

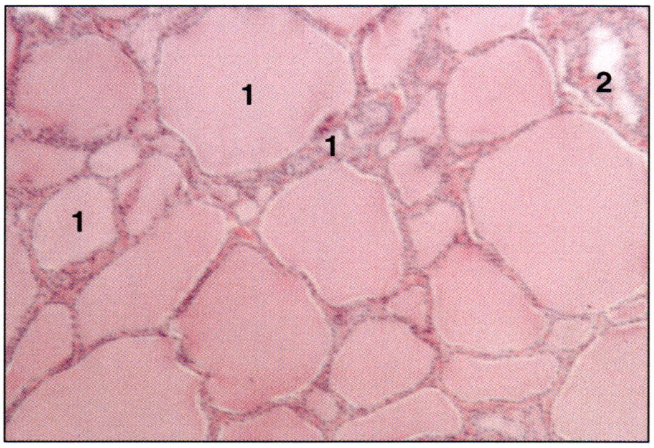

10.16 Thyroid gland (dog). (1) The thyroid follicles show considerable variation in size. (2) Vascular supporting connective tissue. H & E. ×50.

10.17

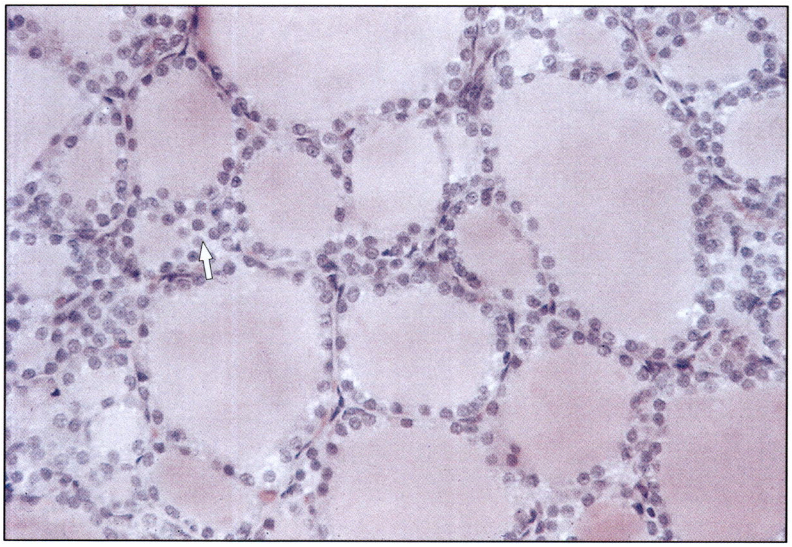

10.17 Thyroid gland (sheep). The thyroid follicle is lined by a simple cuboidal epithelium. The clear parafollicular cells are arrowed. H & E. ×160.

Clinical correlates

Feline hyperthyroidism (10.18) is one of the most common endocrine diseases encountered in veterinary practice. Typically, an elderly cat presents with weight loss and polyphagia. Vomiting and diarrhoea are also often reported. Hyperthyroidism results from hypersecretion of thyroid hormone by a hyperplastic or adenomatous thyroid gland which is often palpably enlarged (goitre).

10.18

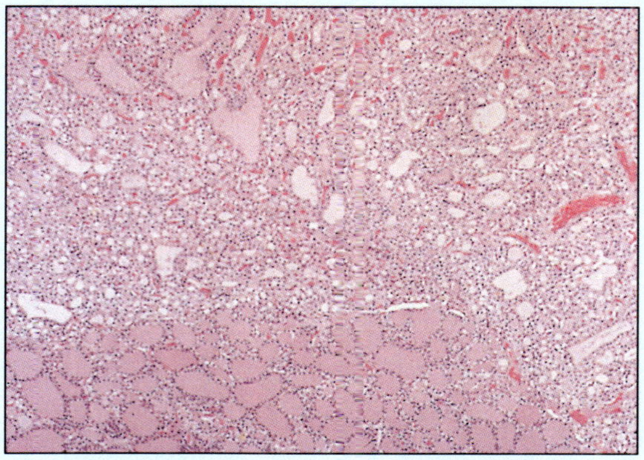

10.18 Thyroid adenoma (cat). Normal thyroid tissue, at the base of the micrograph, is compressed by an adenomatous growth that is more cellular and has less colloid production. The cells are quite uniform in appearance and form recognizable acinar patterns. The mitotic rate is low. H & E. ×50.

Parathyroid gland

The parathyroids are derived from the endoderm of the third and fourth pharyngeal pouches and are either internal (embedded in the capsule of the thyroid) or external (lying a variable distance away). A fine reticular framework supports the cells and the blood vessels. Cords of densely packed basophilic epithelial cells range along the rich capillary bed (10.15 and 10.19).

They are of two types: chief cells and oxyphil cells. Chief cells are the major source of parathyroid hormone regulating calcium homeostasis. Oxyphil cells are large cells with an acidophilic cytoplasm and a pyknotic nucleus (10.20). They are found in the horse and large ruminants but are rare in the other domestic animals. Their function is unknown.

.19

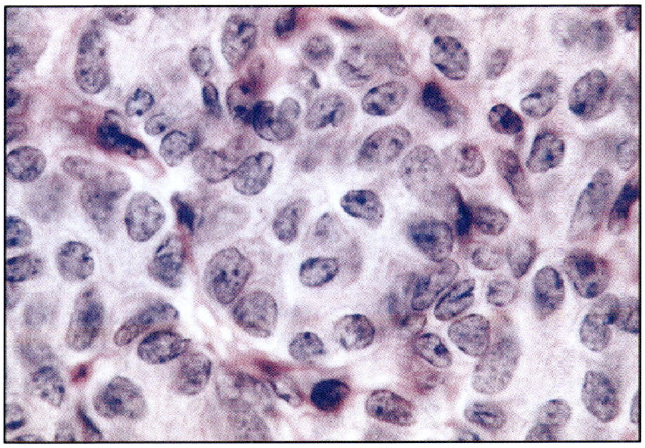

10.19 Parathyroid gland (dog). Darkly staining basophilic principal/chief cells are ranged along the capillary bed. H & E. ×250.

10.20

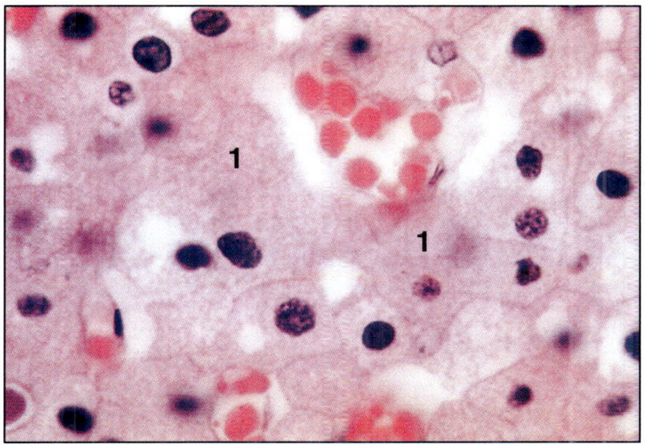

10.20 Parathyroid gland (cow). Clumps of oxyphil cells (1) are present in the parenchyma associated with small blood vessels. H & E. ×500.

Adrenal gland

The adrenal glands are paired and lie in the abdominal cavity close to the craniomedial border of the kidneys. The connective tissue capsule extends into the gland as thin trabeculae of loose vascular reticular connective tissue. The adrenal is divided into an outer cortex derived from mesenchyme and an inner medulla derived from neural crest cells (10.21).

The adrenal cortex produces three main groups of hormones: glucocorticoids, which regulate carbohydrate metabolism; mineralocorticoids, which maintain electrolyte concentrations in the extracellular fluid; and androgens, which possess the same masculinizing effect as testosterone. It is divided into four zones: the zona glomerulosa, the zona intermedia, the zona fasciculata and the zona reticularis.

The zona glomerulosa (arcuata, multiformis) is the outer layer immediately beneath the capsule. It consists of curved cords or arcades of columnar cells in the horses, carnivores and pigs (10.22 and 10.23), and as clusters of polyhedral cells in ruminants. The cellular cytoplasm is acidophilic with a small dark nucleus and secretes mineralocorticoids.

The zona intermedia (more common in the horse and carnivores than in other domestic animals) lies between the zona glomerulosa and the zona fasciculata. The cells appear undifferentiated.

The zona fasciculata, the most extensive zone, is formed of cuboidal or polyhedral cells arranged in radial cords separated by a sinusoidal network of blood vessels. The cytoplasm of these cells (also called spongiocytes) may appear foamy after routine processing and staining because of the loss of the steroid glucocorticoid hormones (10.22–10.25).

The zona reticularis is the innermost zone next to the medulla (10.26 and 10.27). The cells are small, darkly staining anastomosing cords surrounded by sinusoids. They secrete sex hormones.

The adrenal medulla produces adrenalin (epinephrine). This hormone is a powerful vasopressor, increasing cardiac output when the animal is distressed. It also regulates the sympathetic branch of the autonomic nervous system and stimulates the release of glucose from the liver. The medulla is composed mostly of columnar or polyhedral APUD cells, modified postganglionic sympathetic neurons that take up and stain strongly with chromium salts and have numerous brown granules in the cytoplasm. (The chromaffin reaction demonstrates the presence of adrenalin and noradrenalin.) In domestic mammals an outer and inner zone of the medulla can often be distinguished.

Other glands, such as the carotid and aortic bodies, also demonstrate the chromaffin staining reaction. Together with the adrenal medulla they are known as the chromaffin system.

10.21

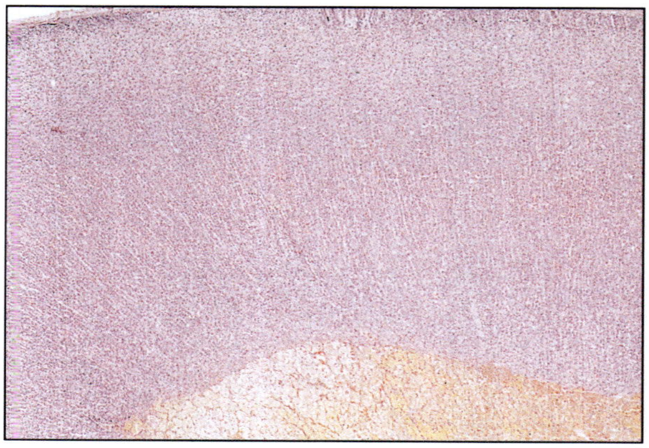

10.21 Adrenal gland (cat). The adrenal gland is divided into an outer cortex and an inner medulla. H & E. ×5.

10.2

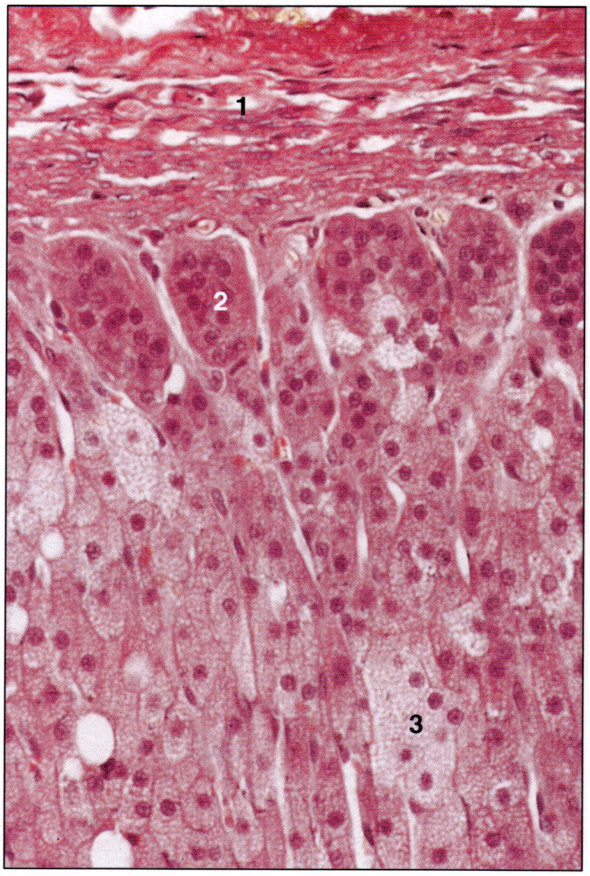

10.22 Adrenal cortex (cat). (1) Connective tissue capsule. (2) Zona glomerulosa. (3) Zona fasciculata cells are vacuolated spongiocytes. H & E. ×200.

10.23

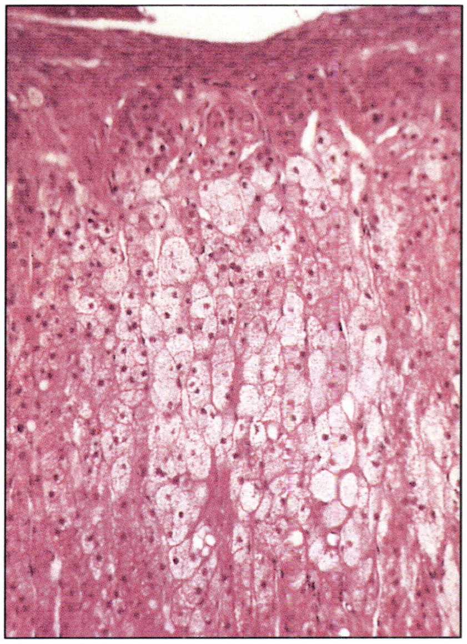

10.24

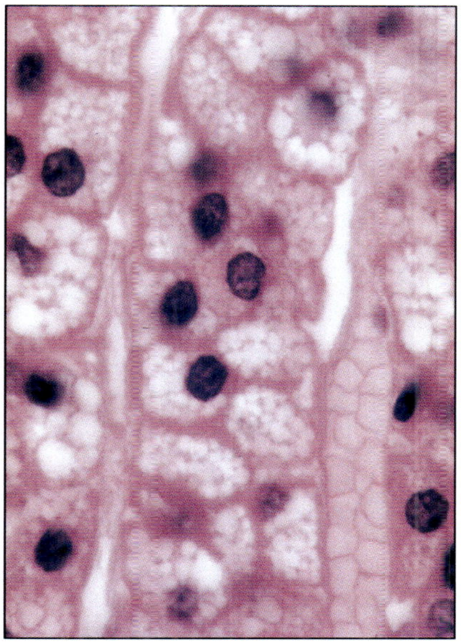

10.23 Adrenal cortex (pig). The vacuolated appearance of the zona fasciculata cells (spongiocytes) is evident. H & E. ×250.

10.24 Adrenal gland (pig). Spongiocytes line the sinusoids. H & E. ×50.

.25

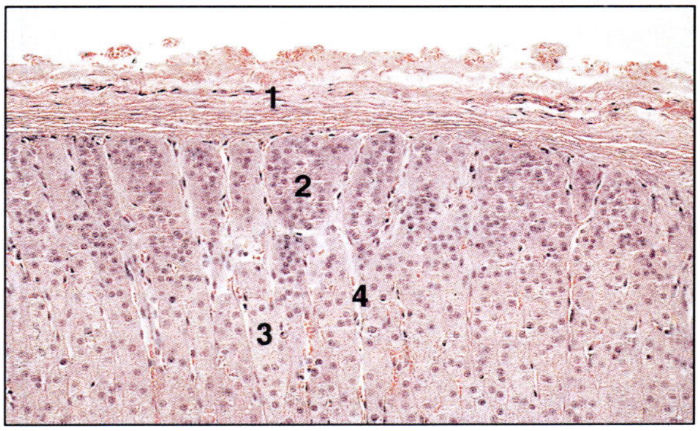

10.25 Adrenal cortex (cat). (1) Connective tissue capsule. (2) Zona glomerulosa cells are arranged in curved cords. (3) Zona fasciculata cells are polyhedral arranged in long radial cords. (4) Sinusoids. H & E. ×50.

.26

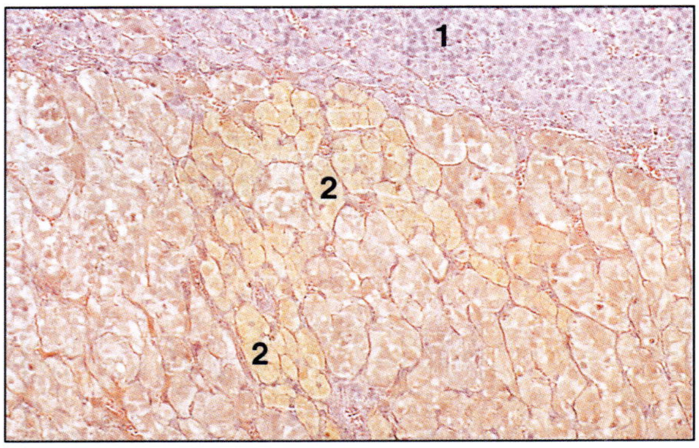

10.26 Adrenal cortex/medulla (cat). (1) Zona reticularis cells are arranged in anastomosing cords. (2) Adrenal medulla sympathetic neuron cell bodies. The cytoplasm is filled with golden brown granules, the chromaffin reaction. Bouin's fixation. ×100.

10.27

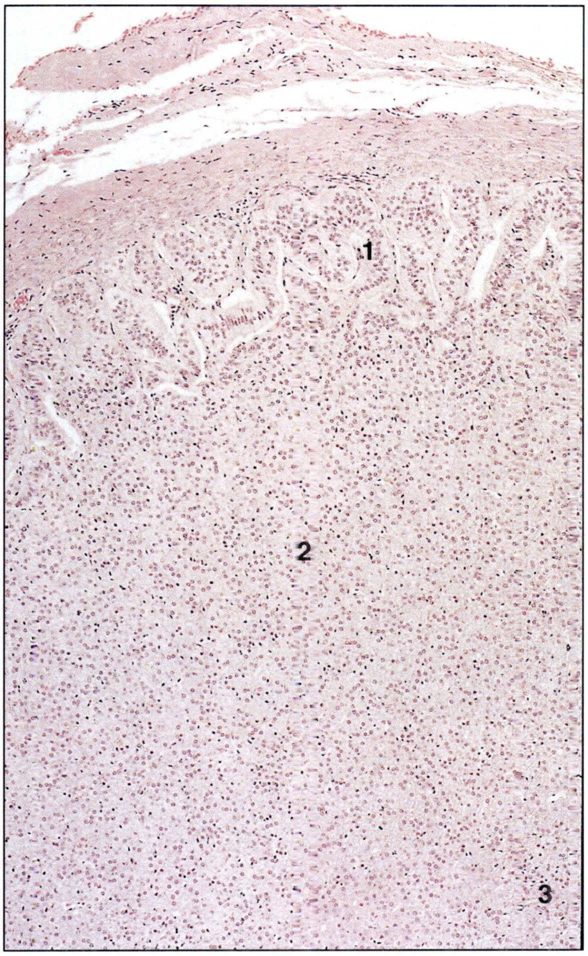

10.27 Adrenal gland (horse). (1) Zona glomerulosa. (2) Zona fasciculata. (3) Zona reticularis. H & E. ×62.5.

Clinical correlates

Clinical manifestations of adrenal disease depend on which cellular populations within the gland are affected and to what extent. Function of the adrenal cortex can be insufficient, leading to hypoadrenocorticism (Addison's disease). In dogs the most common lesion of this type is idiopathic bilateral adrenocortical atrophy in which all layers of the cortex are reduced in thickness and there is reduced production of all classes of corticosteroids. Inflammation of the adrenal cortex caused by a variety of microbial infections can also lead to insufficiency. Clinically, a patient often exhibits progressive loss of condition, weakness and gastrointestinal signs but presentation in a shock-like state of circulatory collapse is also possible.

Hypersecretion of adrenal corticosteroids produces hypoadrenocorticism (Cushing's syndrome), a clinical syndrome of steroid excess characterized by skin and hair changes, polydipsia, polyphagia and weight gain with muscle weakness. Causes include a functional adrenal tumour or may be referable to a pituitary tumour that overstimulates the adrenal glands. The typical skin biopsy changes in canine hyperadrenocorticism are illustrated by **10.28**. A primary adrenal tumour from a Syrian hamster is shown in **10.29**, and is accompanied by a skin section (**10.30**) from the same animal. In addition to the expected findings of adnexal atrophy the skin shows marked secondary hyperplastic changes, possibly associated with self trauma.

Disorders of the adrenal medulla are less commonly described but phaeochromocytomas (**10.31**), tumours of the chromaffin cells, are the most prevalent. These are usually recognized in dogs or cattle. In dogs, around half of these show malignant behaviour with metastasis to regional lymph nodes and beyond. The majority of phaeochromocytomas are not functionally active but an occasional tumour secretes catecholamines.

10.28

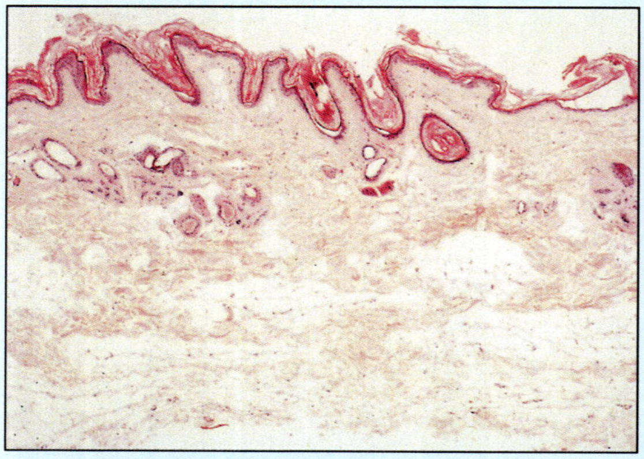

10.28 Hyperadrenocorticism (dog). This skin section is from an 8-year-old Whippet with hyperadrenocorticism. The epidermis is thin, the hair follicles inactive and their associated sebaceous glands atrophic. There is dermal atrophy with reduction in the number and thickness of the collagen bundles in the deep dermis. No inflammatory reaction is present. H & E. ×20.

10.29

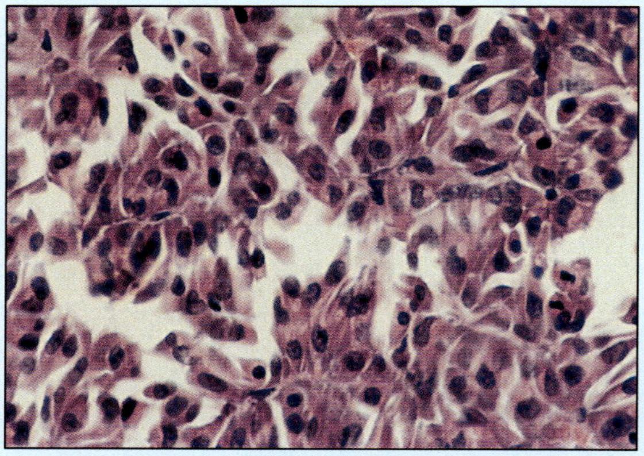

10.29 Adrenal cortical adenoma in a Syrian hamster (*Mesocricetus aurutus*). The corticosteroid-secreting cells are moderately pleomorphic, and a few mitotic figures are seen. H & E. ×125.

.30

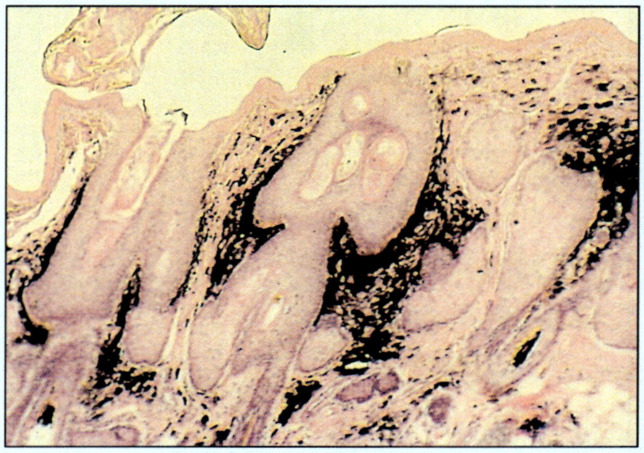

10.31

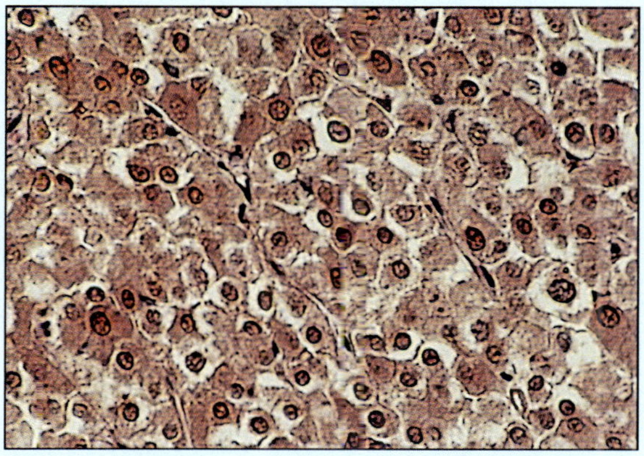

10.30 A section of skin from the hamster illustrated in **10.29**. The epidermis is hyperplastic, hyperkeratotic, acanthotic and heavily pigmented. There is a generalized atrophy of hairs and their precursors. H & E. ×20.

10.31 Phaeochromocytoma in a dog. The tumour cells contain abundant red–brown granules and their nuclei bear prominent nucleoli. Bouin's fixation; H & E. ×200.

Epiphysis cerebri (pineal gland)

The pineal gland (epiphysis cerebri) is a dorsal evagination of the diencephalon, attached by a stalk to the dorsal wall of the third ventricle of the cerebrum. It is covered by a capsule and trabeculae of the pia mater and is divided into lobules by connective tissue septa. The parenchyma is composed primarily of pinealocytes, small epithelioid cells with round nuclei and acidophilic cytoplasm, supported by neuroglial cells. Corpora arenacea are local calcified deposits present in the gland. These are more numerous in older animals (10.32 and 10.33). This gland secretes melatonin and serotonin, and responds to changes in daylight patterns to influence the sexual rhythm of seasonal breeders.

.32

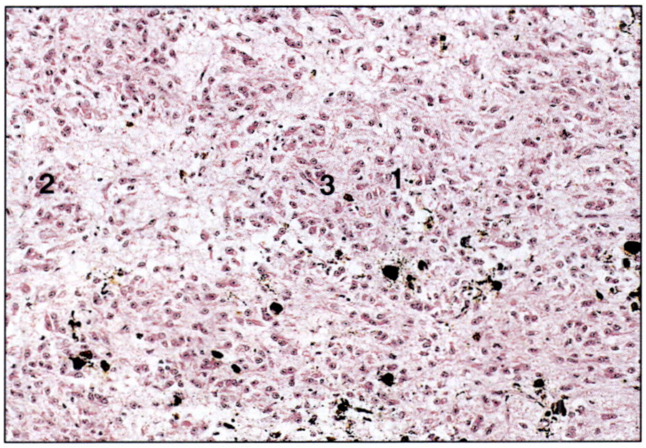

10.33

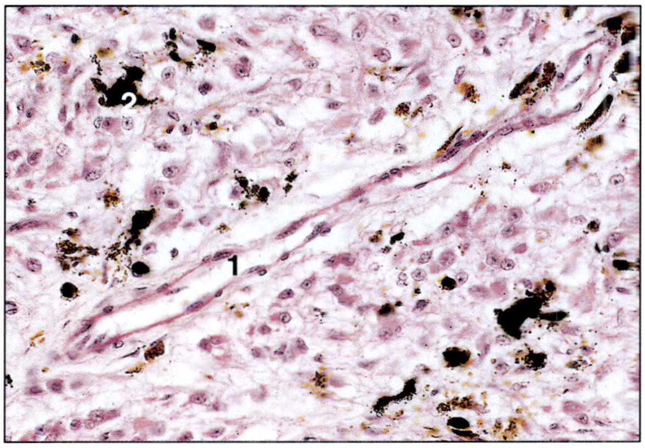

10.32 Epiphysis cerebri (pineal gland; ox). The pinealocytes are small epithelioid cells arranged in (1) cords, (2) clusters or (3) follicles. Corpora arenaceae (brain sand) are a feature of this gland. H & E. ×125.

10.33 Epiphysis cerebri (pineal gland; ox). (1) The pia mater extends into the gland. (2) Corpoa arenaceae. H & E. ×250.

10.34

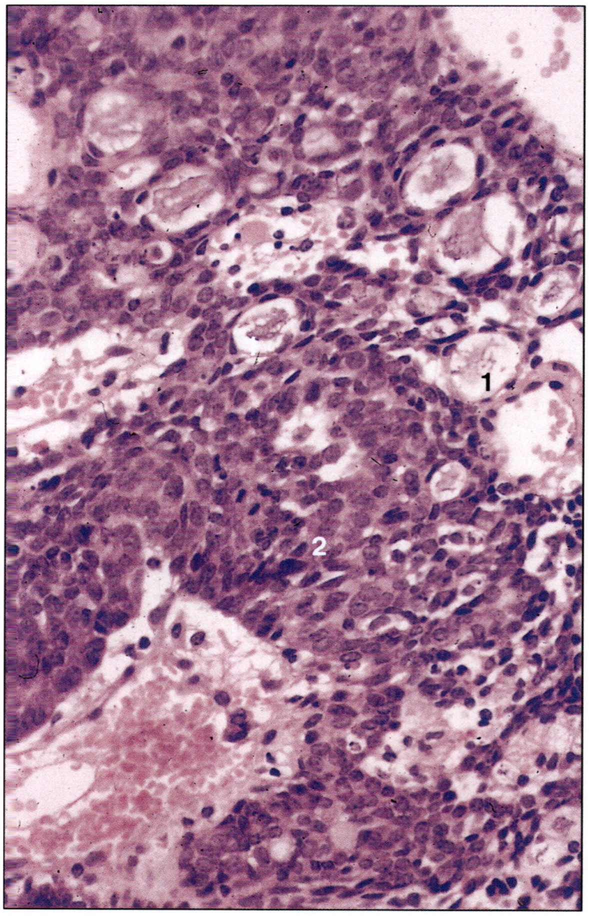

10.34 Ultimobranchial body (bird). The basophilic cells are arranged in (1) vesicles or in (2) cords in the connective tissue surrounding the carotid artery. H & E. ×125.

Avian endocrine system

The avian pituitary gland is similar to that of other mammals except for the absence of the pars intermedia. In the thyroid gland follicles are identical to those of mammals, but the parafollicular cells are located in a separate gland, the ultimobranchial body (10.34), which is located close to the origin of the carotid artery. There is no capsule. Vesicles or cords of round basophilic cells lie in the connective tissue surrounding the carotid artery. This is the source of calcitonin in the bird and together with parathyroid hormone it regulates calcium metabolism.

In the parathyroid gland the parenchyma is composed of irregular cords of principal/chief cells, separated by connective tissue and numerous sinusoids.

The adrenal gland has no clear division into cortex and medulla. Instead, the parenchyma is composed of intermingled cortical tissue and medullary (chromaffin) tissue. The cortical cells are arranged as anastomosing cords and are steroid-secreting. The chromaffin cells are polygonal (10.35).

10.35

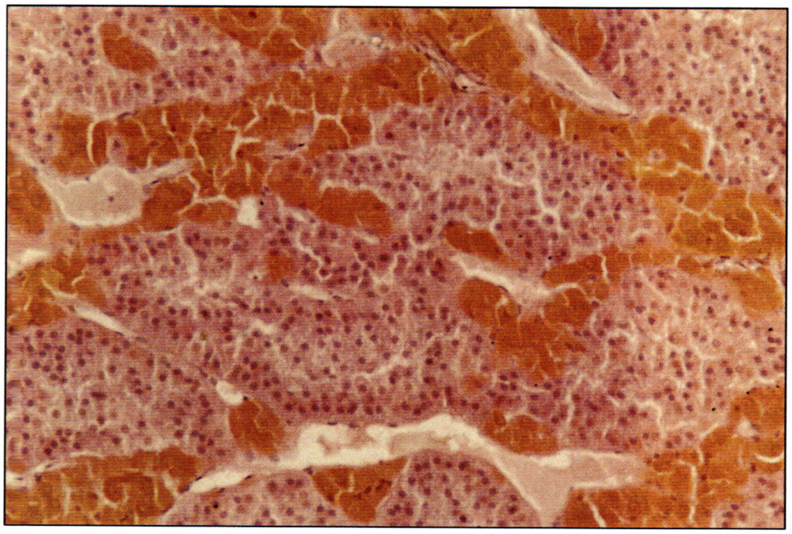

10.35 Adrenal (inter-renal) gland (bird). The chromaffin cells are filled with golden brown granules and lie in islands between the anastomosing cords of steroid-secreting cells. Bouin's fixation. ×125.

Reptilian, amphibian and fish endocrine system

Pituitary gland

The pituitary gland of amphibians and reptiles is similar to that in mammals and birds, but there are substantial differences between disparate families of reptiles. It is beyond the scope of this text to delineate each of them.

The adenohypophysis is composed of the intermediate lobe (pars intermedia) and distal lobe (pars distalis); the neurohypophysis is composed of the median eminence and neural lobe (pars nervosa).

Neurosecretory perikarya of the supraoptic and paraventricular nuclei form the hypothalamoneurohypophyseal tract.

The intermediate lobe is closely juxtaposed to the neural lobe and is joined to the distal lobe by a narrow band of glandular tissue. The distal lobe of most amphibians and reptiles tends to be flattened and lies ventral to the pars nervosa and is caudoventeral to the median eminence. It is composed of cellular cords of cuboidal or prismatic cells that are surrounded by a thin fibrovascular connective tissue. This forms fine septa separating adjacent cords of chromophilic cells that are situated peripherally from chromophobic ('principal') cells that are situated more centrally. Capillaries and thin-walled venous sinuses are a variable feature, depending upon the taxon of animal being studied.

The pars tuberalis (if it is present) consists of small groups of cells forming follicle- or duct-like structures on the ventral surface of the infundibular recess, in the region of the median eminence.

The pars nervosa forms a pit-like depression in the infundibular recess in some reptiles. In others, it lies more lateral or dorsolateral to the distal lobe. It may or may not be divided into lobules by thin connective tissue septa. The cells comprising the pars nervosa tend to be finely granular and stain paler than the pars distalis or pars intermedia (**10.36**).

The staining characteristics of amphibian and reptilian pituitary glands are generally comparable with those observed in higher vertebrates. Depending upon species and the laboratory staining protocols employed, acidophilic, basophilic, amphophilic (the secretory granules staining both erythrophilic and cyanophilic), chromophilic or erythrophilic glandular cells can be discerned. The pituitary cells of some reptiles are strongly PAS-positive, whereas they are not in reptiles of different families. In addition, seasonal, age and sex differences may further complicate the situation.

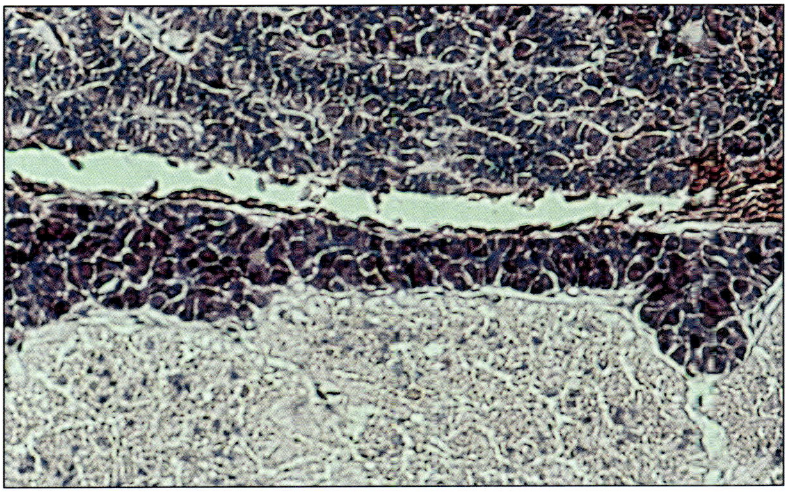

10.36

10.36 Whole mount sagittal section of the pituitary gland of a Children's python (*Liasis childreni*). The pars distalis is at the top; the pars intermedia is represented as a variably narrow band of eosinophilic cells; the pars nervosa is in the lower half. H & E. ×50.

Thyroid gland

The thyroid glands of most amphibians and reptiles are located just cranial to the cardiac outflow tract, often lying between or immediately adjacent to the twin aortic arches, cranial vena cava and pulmonary vasculature (10.37). In amphibians the thyroid is present as paired lobes. In reptiles it is usually a single organ, although bilobed glands with a thin isthmus joining the two lobes have been observed. The colloid-filled follicles are highly variable in size and are separated by a fine fibrovascular connective tissue (10.38). The thyroid often displays a marked seasonal change in the shape and height of the follicular epithelial cells and amount of colloid. They are usually flattened and decidedly squamous or may be tall columnar and pallisaded into a parallel 'picket-fence'-like pattern and contain scanty colloid during times of hypoiodine-induced hypothyroidism. Interfollicular 'C' cells are located in the interstitial connective tissue that separates adjacent follicles (10.39). Usually, the intrafollicular colloid is amorphous and agranular, but it can also be distinctly granular.

10.37

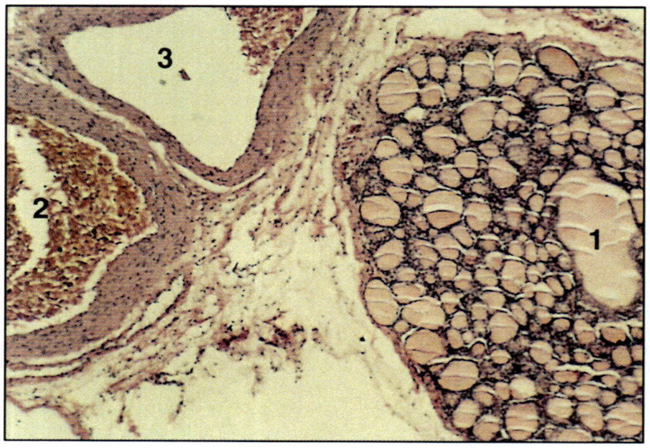

10.37 Whole mount section of the thyroid (1) of a Central American rattlesnake (*Crotalus durissus bicolor*). The thyroid lies immediately adjacent to the the heart base and is readily identified by its characteristic pink, colloid filled follicles. One aortic arch (2) and a jugular vein (3) are immediately to the left of the thyroid. H & E. ×20.

10.3

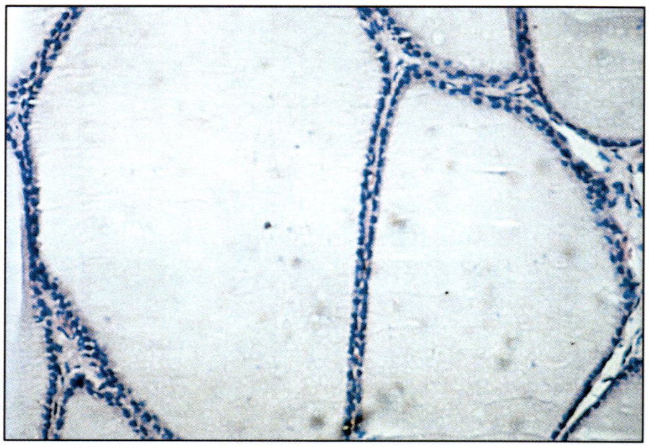

10.38 Thyroid from a red-eared slider turtle (*Trachemys scripta elegans*). The histological characteristics of the reptilian gland change seasonally and may range from follicles lined by cuboidal to a much flattened squamous epithelium. H & E. ×125.

10.39

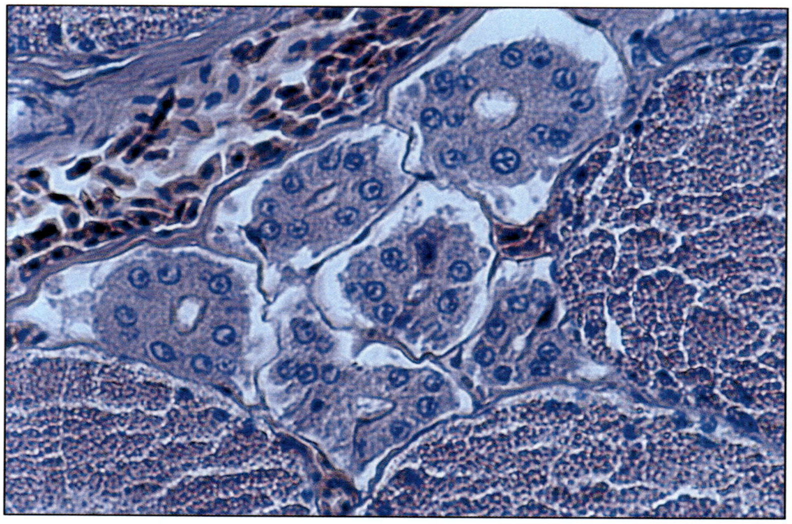

10.39 Interfollicular ('C') cells in the thyroid of a hog-nosed snake (*Heterodon platyrhinos*). These endocrine cells are arranged into small diameter tubuloacinar follicles with tiny central lumens. The thyroidal follicular colloid in this section is unusually granular. H & E. ×200.

Parathyroid gland

Fish lack a parathyroid gland. Rather, the ultimobranchial body is highly developed and serves as the major regulator of calcium and phosphorus metabolism. The parathyroid glands of most amphibians and reptiles are present as one or (usually) two pairs of lobes that are located in the caudal cervical region, often adjacent to the thymus or jugular veins. The cells may be cuboidal to prismatic or polyhedral and contain small intracytoplasmic granules that usually stain pale pink with H & E. They are formed into small lobules by thin fibrovascular connective tissue septa that penetrate the gland from the surrounding capsule (10.40). Under some conditions, clear or foamy appearing spaces may be scattered throughout the glandular tissue.

10.40

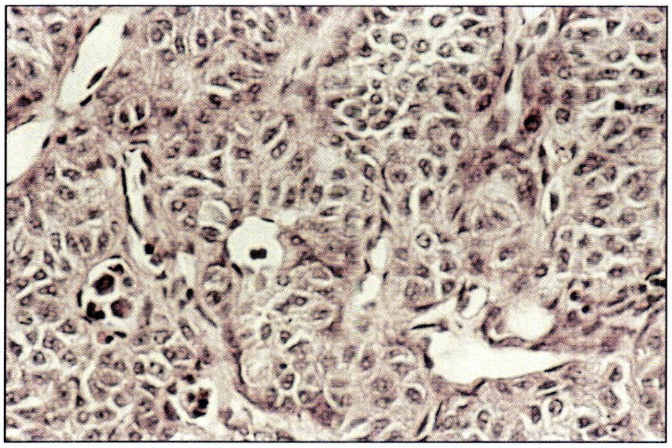

10.40 Parathryoid gland of a desert tortoise (*Xerobates agassizi*). The secretory cells are formed into small lobules bound by thin fibrovascular connective tissue septa H & E. ×125.

Adrenal glands

The adrenal tissues of fish, amphibians and many reptiles are significantly different. The adrenal glands (sometimes referred to as inter-renal or intrarenal tissue) of most fish are embedded in the cranial kidneys, where they surround the larger blood vessels and may be intermixed with haematopoietic tissue. There are two kinds of adrenal cells: medullary or chromaffin cells and sympathetic nerve-like paraganglion cells. Amphibians possess discrete paired adrenals composed of three major cell types: chromaffin 'medullary' cells that are of neurectodermal origin; 'cortical' cells; and Stilling cells that are of mesodermal origin. Although it is known that the cortical cells secrete adrenal corticosteroids, the function of Stilling cells is not known. Some investigators consider the Stilling cell to be a distinct glandular organ.

In reptiles the paired adrenals usually lie immediately adjacent to the kidneys or, in some instances where the kidneys are located within the pelvic canal, they lie medial to the gonads. Two major cell types are found: dark staining chromaffin or medullary cells that secrete catacholamines; and pale staining cortical steroidogenic cells. In mammals, these cells are confined to the cortical and medullary zones. In reptiles, the location of the cells tends to be less circumscribed; the chromaffin cells are in islands or nests scattered throughout the steroidogenic cortical cells. The cytoplasm of cortical cells often contains small clear lipid-like vacuoles (10.41).

10.41

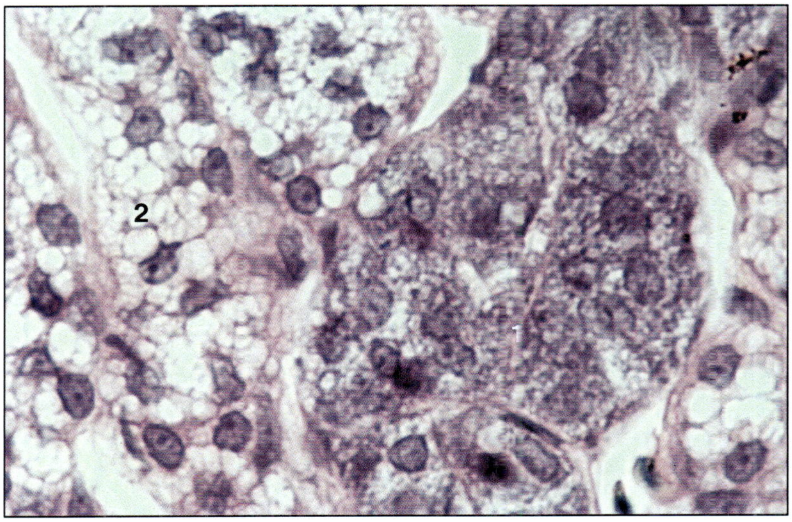

10.41 Adrenal gland of a desert tortoise (*Xerobates agassizi*). The kidney is in the lower right; the adrenal is on the left. Rather than being confined to a discrete cortex and medulla, the deeply staining chromaffin cells (1) and the pale spongiocytes (2) are grouped into nest-like aggregates that are admixed throughout the gland. H & E. ×200.

Pineal gland

In teleost fish the pineal gland is hollow and consists of columnar epithelial cells of three types: sensory, sustentacular and ganglion-like. It resembles a sensory organ; some primitive cyclostomes actually possess a pineal covered by a relatively clear lens-like structure that admits light.

In amphibians the pineal gland is more solid than in fish and arises as a median outgrowth on the dorsal surface of the brain. Like the gland in fish, it is photosensitive. In response to darkness it secretes melatonin, which causes peripheral melanophages to aggregate, thus lightening the integument's colour.

In reptiles the pineal gland is solid and composed of glandular secretory cuboidal to low columnar epithelial cells that are arranged into lobules separated by delicate fibrovascular septa that are extensions from the surrounding capsule (10.42). Preliminary investigations have revealed at least some inter-relationships between the pineal and other endocrine glands, especially the thyroid. The pineal gland of lizards lies slightly rostral to the parietal foramen. Whether sufficient light can enter the skull through the parietal eye and the parietal foramen (in those species that possess them) is conjectural, but appears to be possible.

10.42

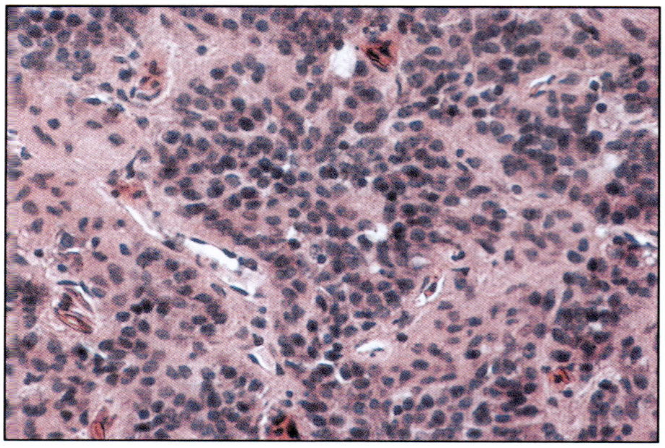

10.42 Pineal gland of a Burmese python (*Python molurus bivittatus*). The cuboidal epithelial cells have indistinct cell membranes and large round nuclei. They are arranged into lobule-like groups that are separated from each other by delicate fibrovascular septa. H & E. ×125.

Ultimobranchial body

In the lower vertebrates the ultimobranchial bodies play an important role that is shared in the higher vertebrates by the parathyroid and thyroid. In teleost fish the ultimobranchial body is well developed and lies in the transverse septum between the ventral surface of the oesophagus and liver, immediately caudal to the heart. The glandular tissue consists of tall columnar or pseudostratified columnar epithelium formed into spherical vesicle-like structures. They are paired in some amphibians, single in some salamanders, and absent in some frogs and in caecilians.

In reptiles the ultimobranchial bodies are paired and function in calcium and phosphorus regulation. They also have a relationship to thyroid function in some reptilian species. They are believed to secrete calcitonin in response to blood calcium concentrations. Reptilian ultimobranchial bodies are composed of cuboidal to low columnar glandular epithelial cells with finely granular pink staining cytoplasm, often containing clear lipid-like vacuoles (10.43).

10.43

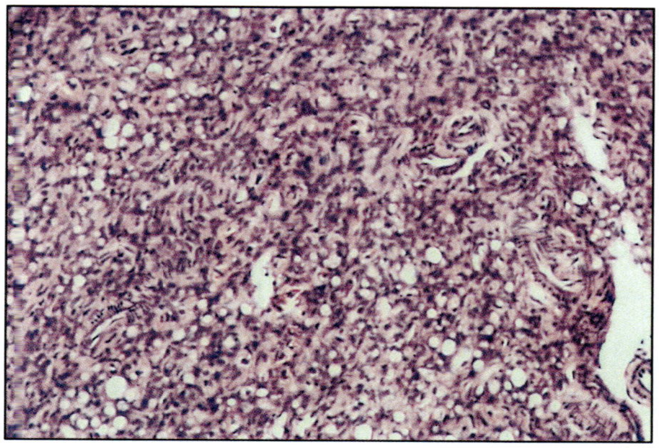

10.43 Ultimobranchial body of a boa constrictor (*Boa c. constrictor*). Many of the secretory epithelial cells that comprise this glandular organ contain large, clear, lipid vacuoles. Typically, these glands are formed from solid sheets of cells with little separation by connective tissue septa. Small blood vessels penetrate the tissue. H & E. ×50.

Clinical correlates

Thyroid gland

As is the case with the higher vertebrates, hypothyroidism, goitre, thyroid inflammation and neoplasia occur occasionally in the lower vertebrates. Clinical hyperthyroidism is relatively common in domestic cats. Dietary hypothyroidism is relatively common in semiaquatic turtles, especially those kept as pets by persons living in so-called 'goitre belts' where humans suffer from chronic hypothyroidism unless they receive supplemental iodine. Herbivorous chelonians, especially those originating from oceanic volcanic islands, appear to be particularly prone to dietary hypothyroidism.

Parathyroid gland

Captive reptiles often display the clinical signs of secondary hypoparathyroidism that are induced by being fed either food containing insufficient available calcium or, more commonly, food containing an improperly low calcium : high phosphorus ratio. The parathyroid glands from these animals become hyperplastic and hypertrophied. With chronicity, changes consistent with adenomatous hyperplasia are seen: the glandular cells become pleomorphic, distorted and may lose their normal granularity. Sometimes, actual primary hyperparathyroidism occurs. The cells then assume frankly pleomorphic shapes, their nuclear chromatin becomes more dense, occasional bipolar cells and mitotic figures may be observed, and the lobules become distorted or break through their septal confines and coalesce (10.44).

Adrenal gland

For discussion of this, see pages 158–9.

Pineal gland

One benign pinealoma has been reported in a green iguana (*Iguana iguana*). It was found at necropsy and was grossly and microscopically pigmented. It was composed of branching papillary fronds of streamer-like, very elongated columnar epithelial cells borne on thin stalks of fibrovascular connective tissue that projected into the lumen of cystic spaces within the mass.

Destruction of the pineal gland might be expected to disrupt the normal diurnal–nocturnal behaviour pattern, and perhaps the colour, of an animal subjected to this experimental protocol.

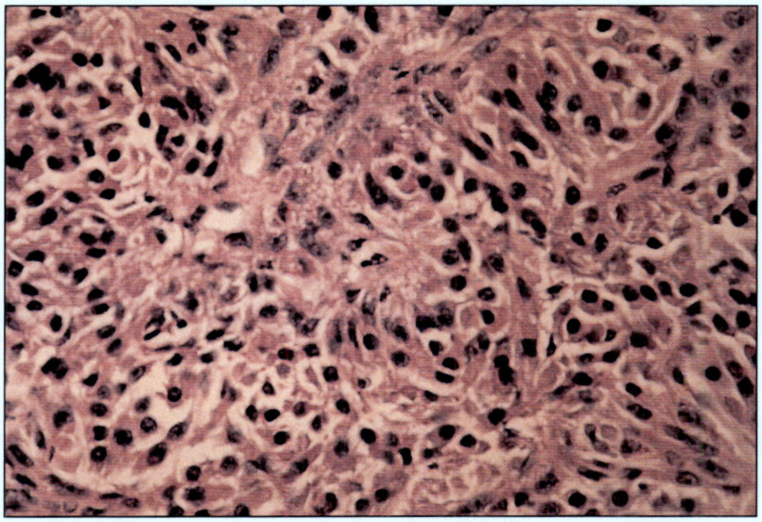

10.44

10.44 Parathyroid adenoma from a desert tortoise that was displaying clinical manifestations of primary hyperparathyroidism, including severe osteopenia. The tumour cells are pleomorphic, hyperchromatic and arranged irregularly. H & E. ×160.

Ultimobranchial body

The paired ultimobranchial bodies of reptiles undergo hypertrophy as a consequence of chronic hypocalcaemia. They have been reported to involute spontaneously with ageing in some normal lizards. Functional hyperplasia (or adenomata) of the ultimobranchial bodies can cause excessive mobilization of calcium from skeletal stores. Hypersecretion of calcitonin, with subsequent hypercalcaemia, may result in osteopenia and, occasionally, renal tubular calcium urolithiasis.

11. MALE REPRODUCTIVE SYSTEM

The male reproductive system consists of the paired testes suspended in the scrotal sacs, a continuous duct system for the storage and transport of the male gamete, the spermatozoon, and an ejaculatory organ, the penis. The accessory sex glands secrete into the urethra and provide a suitable fluid medium to transport the spermatozoa during ejaculation and in the female reproductive tract.

Testis

The testis is a compound tubular gland with an exocrine and an endocrine function. The exocrine function is the production of spermatozoa by the lining epithelium of the seminiferous tubules. The endocrine function is the production of the male sex hormone, testosterone, by the specific interstitial (Leydig) cells in the intertubular connective tissue. The testis is covered by mesothelium continuous with the visceral layer of the tunica vaginalis. A thick dense connective tissue capsule, the tunica albuginea, encloses the testis. A variable amount of smooth muscle may be present. The tunica vasculosa is the inner vascular layer of the tunica albuginea.

The capsule is reflected into the median plane of the testis to form a partition, the mediastinum, and gives off loose vascular connective tissue, the septula testis, to divide the testis into lobules to support the seminiferous tubules (**11.1** and **11.2**). The coiled seminiferous tubules are lined with a multilayered seminiferous epithelium of spermatogenic cells and sustentacular (Sertoli) cells. They rest on a basement membrane and are surrounded by a lamellated connective tissue with myoid elements. The specific interstitial (Leydig) cells are found in the loose vascular connective tissue separating the tubule.

11.1

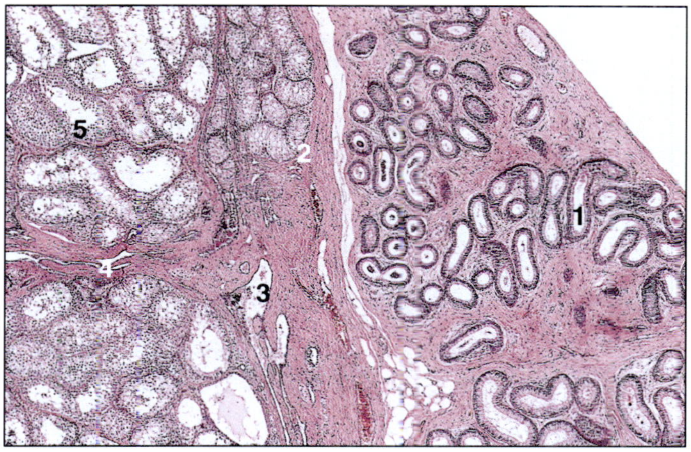

11.1 Testis (cat). (1) Efferent ducts invested by connective tissue. (2) Tunica albuginea. (3) Rete testis. (4) Mediastinum testis. (5) Seminiferous tubules. H & E. ×20.

11.2

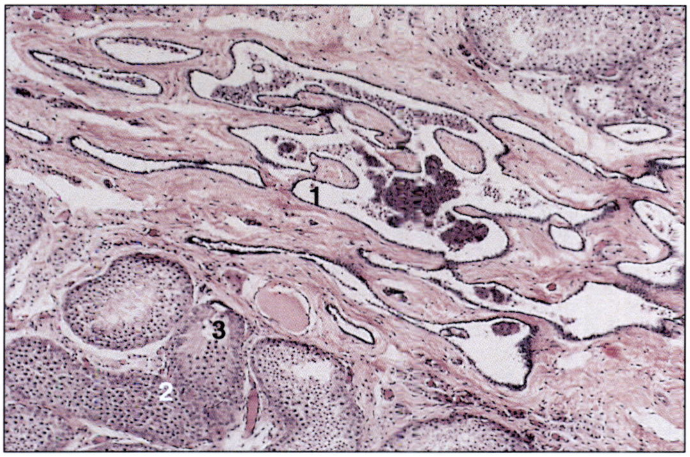

11.2 Testis (cat). (1) Rete testis lying in the mediastinum. (2) Seminiferous tubules leading into (3) tubuli recti lined by sustentacular cells. H & E. ×50.

Production of spermatozoa

In the prepubertal male there are two cell types: the sustentacular cell and the spermatogonium, the immature male germ cell. The sustentacular cells are tall columnar, extending from the basement membrane to the lumen of the tubule, with a pale vesicular basal nucleus and a prominent nucleolus. As the name suggests, the sustentacular cells support the later stages in the development of spermatozoa. Spermatogonia lie next to the basement membrane and are small round cells with a dark staining nucleus. At puberty they move away from the membrane and undergo mitotic divisions. When these cease the cells go through a period of growth, the deoxyribonucleic acid is replicated and the cells become tetraploid primary spermatocytes. The nucleus is granular and the coiled chromosomes give a dense staining reaction. The primary spermatocyte divides meiotically to form two secondary spermatocytes, which each divide immediately to form two haploid spermatids. These are small cells with a spherical nucleus and lie close to the lumen of the tubule. The spermatids move into recesses in the sustentacular cells and metamorphose into spermatozoa, shedding the excess cytoplasm into the lumen of the tubule (**11.3–11.5**).

11.3

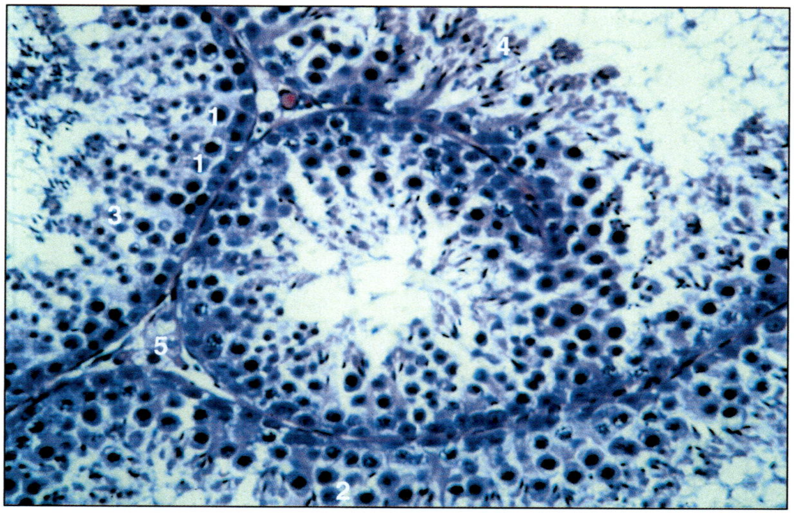

11.3 Testis (bull). The seminiferous tubules are lined by a multilayered epithelium. (1) Spermatogonia. (2) Primary spermatocytes. (3) Spermatids. (4) Developing spermatozoa. (5) Interstitial tissue separates the tubules. H & E. ×160.

11.4

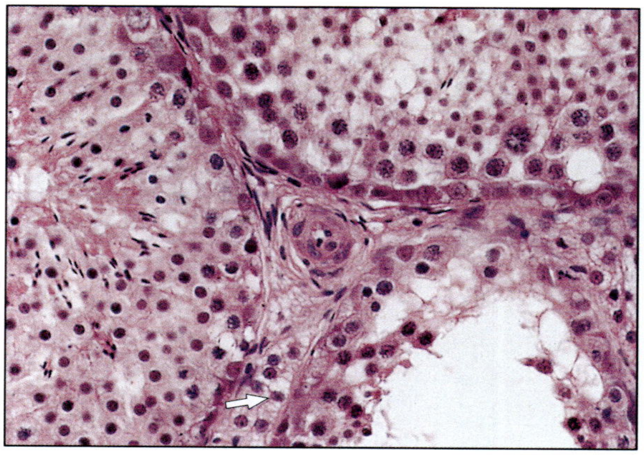

11.4 Testis (bull). Vascular interstitial tissue lies between the seminiferous tubules; specific interstitial cells are vacuolated (arrowed). H & E. ×200.

11.5

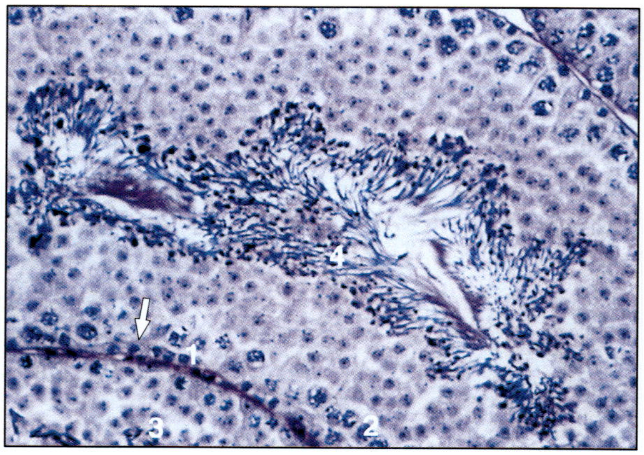

11.5 Testis (dog). All the stages of spermatogenesis are seen in the lining epithelium. (1) Spermatogonia. (2) Primary spermatocytes. (3) Spermatids. (4) Developing spermatozoa. The sustentacular cells are arrowed. H & E. ×200.

Structure of spermatozoa

The mature spermatozoon consists of a head and a tail (**11.6**). The head contains the condensed haploid nucleus. The anterior two-thirds is covered by the acrosomal cap, a derivative of the Golgi apparatus containing the enzyme hyaluronidase, which is required for penetration of the ovum at fertilization. The tail (a flagellum) has the characteristic structure of flagellae and cilia, with two central microtubules and more peripheral doublets making up the axial filament complex. The proximal part is surrounded by an end-to-end helix of mitochondria to provide the energy during movement. Sperm are non-motile and immature at this stage. The peritubular myoid elements push the mixture of sperm and debris down the seminiferous tubule towards the mediastinum.

11.6 Spermatozoa (bull). The spermatozoa consist of a head and a tail (flagellum). Unstained spermatozoa were live and stained spermatozoa were dead at the time of staining. Nigrosin–eosin. ×625.

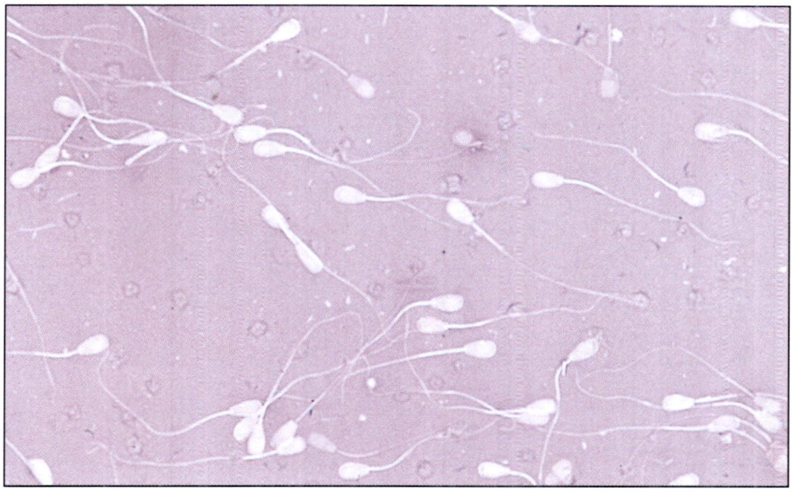

11.6

Tubuli recti rete testis, efferent ducts

The seminiferous tubules, at their terminal segments, are joined by a transitional zone, lined by sustentacular cells, to straight tubules (tubuli recti), which are continuous with a network of anastomosing channels that form the rete testis (**11.7**). The rete testis has a simple squamous or cuboidal epithelium. It is surrounded by the loose connective tissue of the mediastinum and is drained by between seven and 20 efferent ducts (see **11.1**). The ducts are lined with simple columnar or pseudostratified epithelium, and some of the cells are ciliated. The lumen of each duct is wide and the lamina propria is sparse connective tissue (with some smooth muscle in the stallion).

11.7 Testis (cat). (1) Seminiferous tubules. (2) Straight tubules. (3) Rete testis. H.& E. ×50.

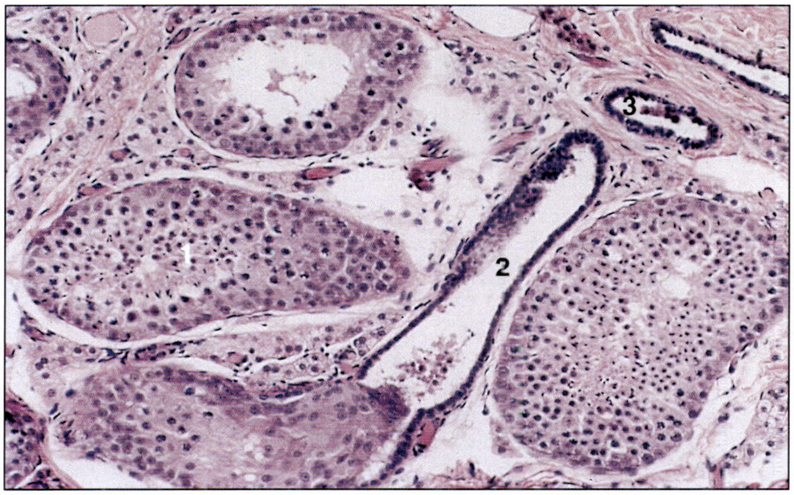

11.7

Epididymis and ductus deferens

The epididymis, where sperm mature and become motile (**11.8–11.10**), is a single, long coiled duct lined with pseudostratified epithelium. Long cytoplasmic processes, the stereocilia, project into the lumen. The epithelium rests on a connective tissue lamina propria and there is a variable amount of circular smooth muscle. The latter increases in volume as the tail of the epididymis approaches the ductus deferens.

The ductus deferens has a very thick muscular wall and a small lumen, and it is lined with pseudostratified columnar epithelium resting on a delicate lamina propria containing collagen and elastic fibres. The mucosa is arranged in longitudinal folds, and the muscularis is composed of smooth muscle fibres, presenting a variety of arrangements. In the domestic animals it is often difficult to determine specific layers of muscle. Circularly arranged fibres predominate, and a fibrous adventitial coat is present (**11.11** and **11.12**). The ductus deferens terminates at the colliculus seminalis of the proximal urethra. Near to this junction it dilates to form an ampulla in the stallion, bull, ram and dog. In the boar and tomcat, simple tubular glands are present in the lamina propria. The lamina propria and submucosa are tall columnar and lined with glandular secretory units. The secretion may calcify in the lumen to form cor-

11.8

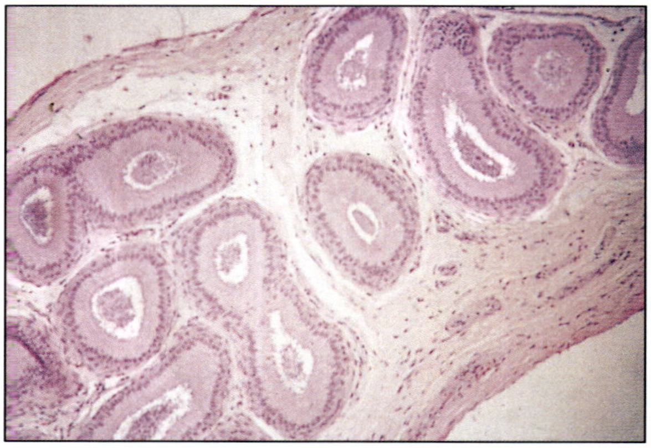

11.8 Epididymis (bull). The single coiled ductus epididymis is lined by a pseudostratified columnar epithelium resting on a vascular lamina propria continuous with the supporting connective tissue of the head of the epididymis. Spermatozoa are present in the lumen of the tubule. H & E. ×50.

11.

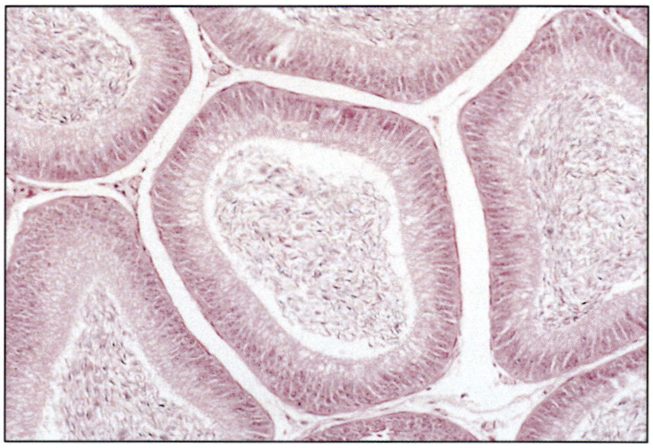

11.9 Epidiymis (bull). Pseudostratified columnar epithelium lines the tubule; the lumen is filled with spermatozoa. H & E. ×100.

11.10

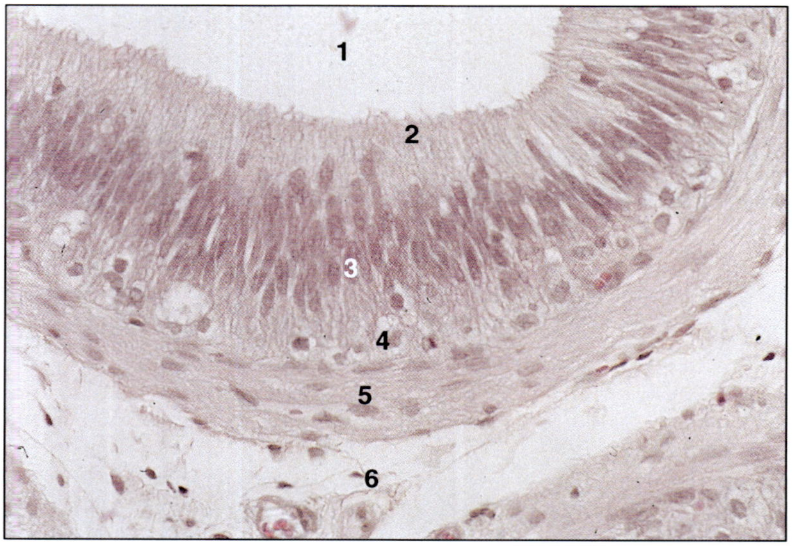

11.10 Epidiymis (bull). (1) Lumen of the tubule. (2) Luminal cytoplasm extends into the lumen as stereocilia. (3) Nuclear layer of the epithelial cells. (4) Vascular lamina propria. (5) Muscularis. (6) Vascular connective tissue. H & E. ×250.

pora arenaceae. The mucosa is arranged in complex folds and assumes a glandular appearance to become one of the accessory sex glands (**11.13**).

Urethra

The urethra is the terminal part of the male duct system and has both a urinary and a reproductive function. A long mucous tube extending from the bladder to the glans penis, it is divided into a pelvic and an extrapelvic or spongiose part. The epithelial lining varies from urethelium proximal to the bladder, to stratified columnar or cuboidal along the greater part of the urethra, to stratified squamous at the tip of the penis. Simple tubular mucosal glands open into the pelvic urethra. These are numerous in the horse, bull, boar and ram (**11.14**),

.11

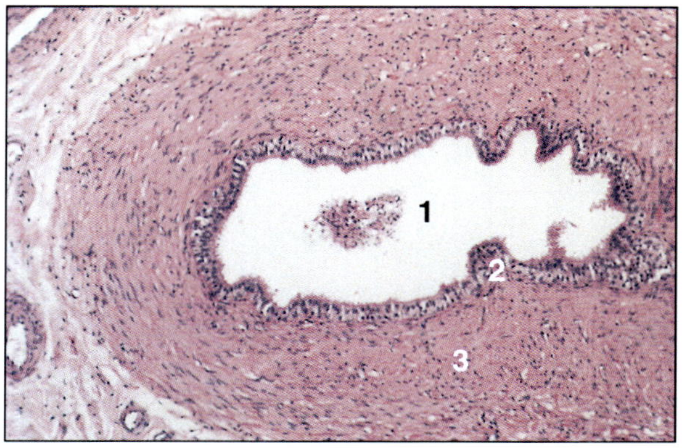

11.11 Ductus deferens (dog). (1) Lumen of the ductus deferens. (2) Mucosal folds. (3) Thick layer of smooth muscle of the muscularis externa. H & E. ×20.

11.12

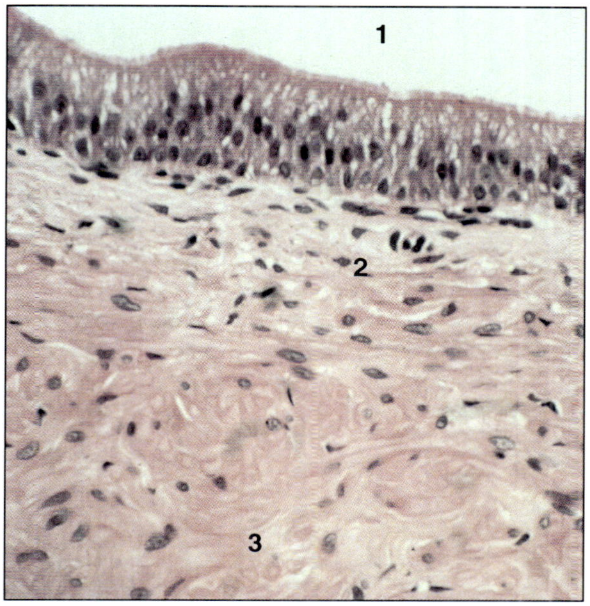

11.12 Ductus deferens (dog). (1) The lumen is lined by a pseudostratified ciliated epithelium. (2) Mucosal connective tissue. (3) Smooth muscle of the muscularis externa. H & E. ×125.

.13

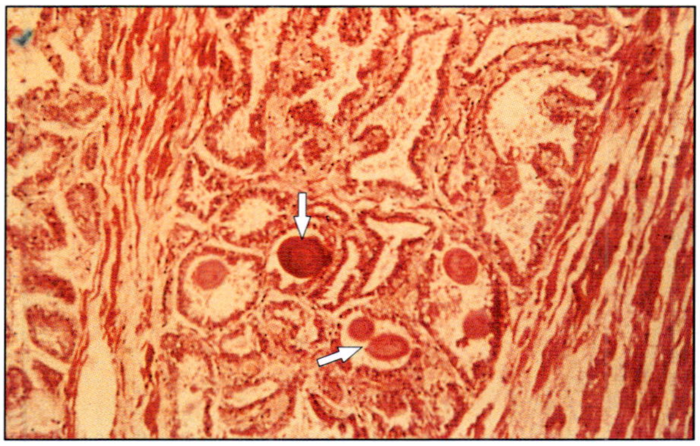

11.13 Ampulla (bull). The lining epithelium is simple columnar secretory; the mucosal folds create a glandular appearance. Corpora arenaceae are arrowed. H & E. ×62.5.

11.14

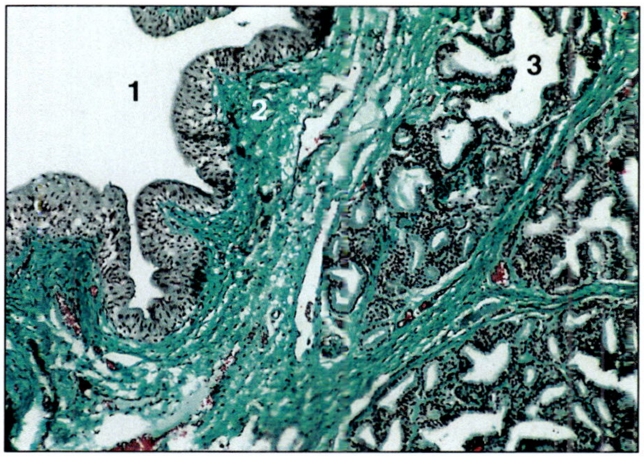

11.14 Cranial urethra (ram). (1) Lumen of the urethra lined by urethelium. (2) Vascular connective tissue of the lamina propria. (3) Simple tubular glands lined by a columnar secretory epithelium: the disseminate prostate. Masson's trichrome. ×125.

but sparse in the dog and cat (**11.15**). Circular smooth muscle is present in the proximal urethra, but the main mass of the muscularis is formed by the thick striated muscle of the m. bulbourethralis. The adventitia is loose connective tissue carrying blood vessels and nerves; nerve endings are a constant feature. Cavernous blood spaces are present in the lamina propria of the pelvic urethra and increase markedly in the penile region to become the corpus spongiosum urethrae (**11.16**). This is part of the erectile tissue of the penis, with little or no muscle. In the stallion and ruminants the urethra extends beyond the tip of the penis as the processus urethrae and is covered by a cutaneous membrane lined with transitional or stratified squamous epithelium.

Penis

The male copulatory organ consists of an outer fibroelastic connective tissue capsule, the tunica albuginea, extending into the body of the penis to form trabeculae supporting a network of endothelial lined spaces: the corpora cavernosa (**11.17**, **11.18**). With the corpus spongiosum urethra, these spaces fill with blood from the coiled helicine arteries during erection. Intimal cushions prevent back-flow of blood in these arteries and help to maintain the erection. In the stallion, smooth muscle predominates in the vascular penis (**11.19**); in the boar and ruminants fibroelastic connective tissue forms the bulk of the organ. In

11.15

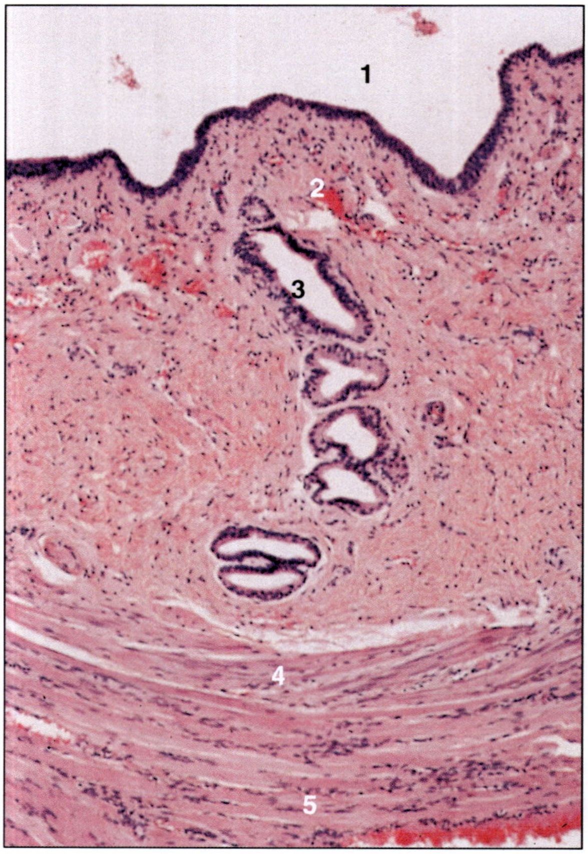

11.15 Cranial urethra (cat). (1) Lumen of the urethra lined by urethelium. (2) Vascular lamina propria. (3) Simple tubular gland of the disseminate prostate. (4) Inner layer of smooth muscle. (5) Outer layer of skeletal muscle. H & E. ×20.

11.16

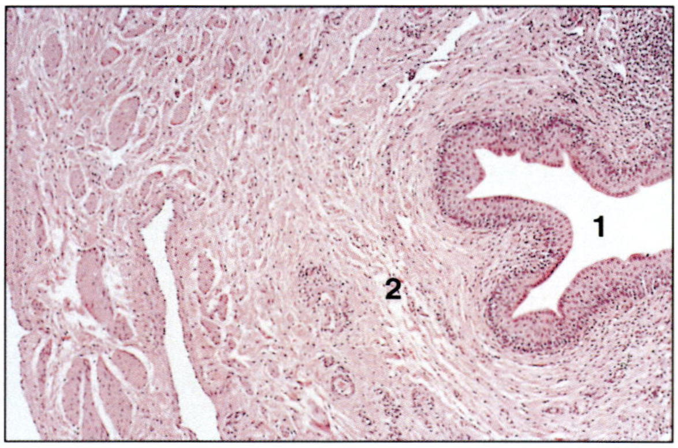

11.16 Penile urethra (dog). (1) Lumen of the urethra lined by urethelium. (2) Vascular lamina propria: the corpus spongiosum. H & E. ×62.5.

11.17

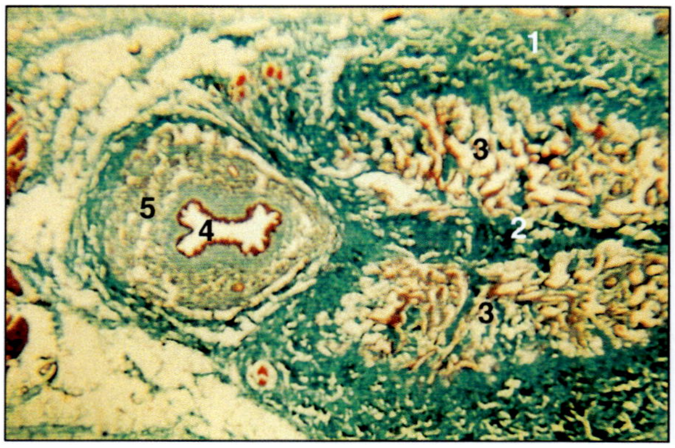

11.17 Penis (dog). (1) Tunica albuginea. (2) Medial connective tissue septum. (3) Vascular spaces of the corpus cavernosum penis. (4) Lumen of the urethra. (5) Corpus spongiosum urethrae. Masson's trichrome. ×5.

carnivores the terminal part of the corpus cavernosum ossifies to become the os penis (baculum) and contributes to the rigidity of the penis. Small keratinized epidermal spines are present on the glans penis of the tomcat (**11.20**) and are sometimes seen in the stallion and billy goat.

The prepuce is a double reflection of skin that covers the distal, free portion of the penis. It is composed of an external, parietal and visceral layer. Hair, sebaceous and sweat glands occur over a variable distance from the external layer to the parietal prepuce. This area is extremely sensitive, with many nerve endings (**11.21**).

.18

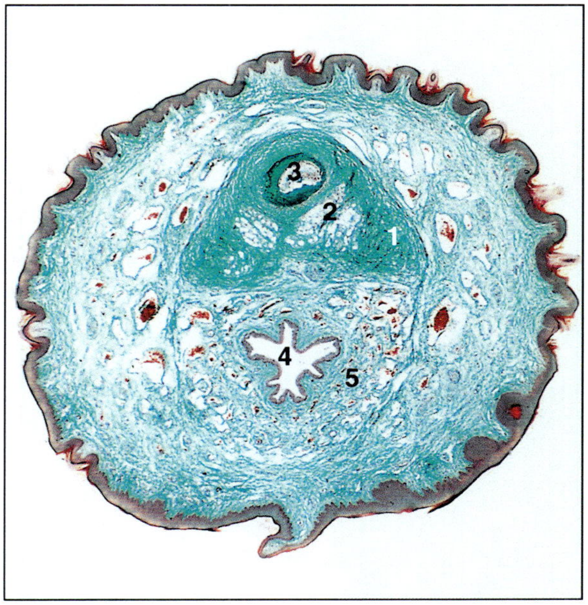

11.18 Penis (cat). (1) Tunica albuginea. (2) Corpus cavernosum penis. (3) Os penis. (4) Lumen of the urethra. (5) Corpus spongiosum urethrae. Masson's trichrome. ×125.

11.19

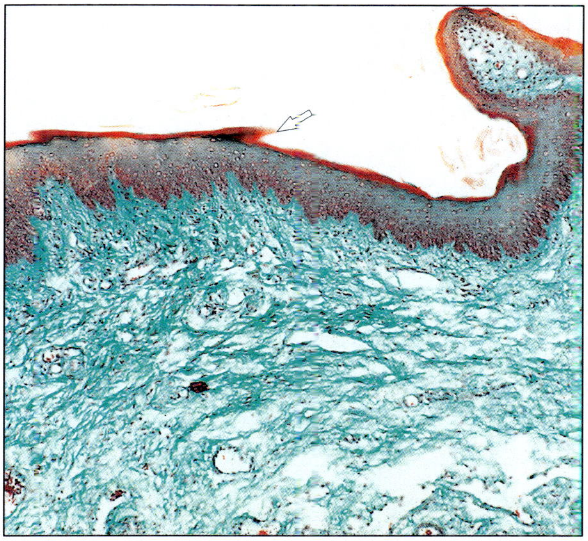

11.19 Penis (cat). A penile spine is arrowed. Masson's trichrome. ×125.

.20

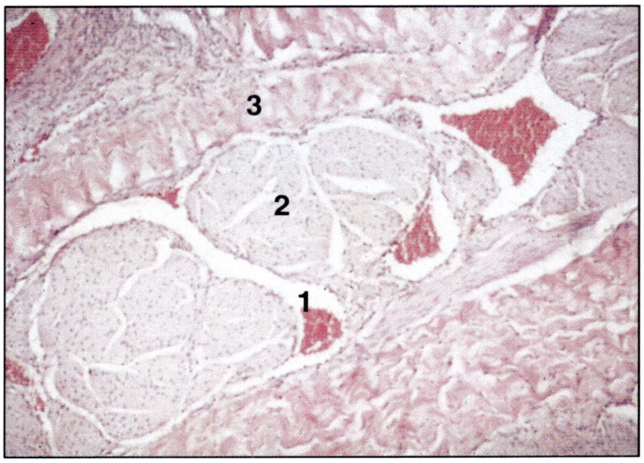

11.20 Penis (horse). (1) Vascular space. (2) Smooth muscle. (3) Connective tissue. H & E. ×20.

11.21

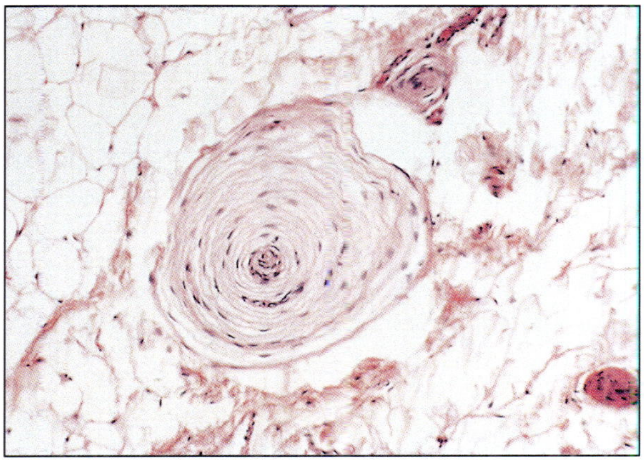

11.21 Penis (bull). A Pacinian corpuscle lies in the lamina propria of the penile urethra. H & E. ×125.

Male accessory genital glands

The male accessory genital glands include the prostate gland, the glands of the ampulla (*see* 'Epididymis and ductus deferens', above), the vesicular glands and the bulbourethral glands (**Table 11.1**). These glands are androgen dependent and exhibit pronounced regressive change after castration, generally resulting finally in loss of function.

Prostate glands

The prostate glands are androgen-dependent and exhibit profound regressive changes after castration, with a reduction in the secretory epithelium, deposition of fat and an increase in the connective tissue stroma. In the boar and ruminants, the prostate gland consists mostly of a disseminate portion in the form of a glandular layer in the submucosa of the proximal (prostatic) urethra. In the stallion and carnivores, the disseminate portion is represented only by scattered glands. The compact prostate (well developed in the stallion and carnivore and absent in the ram and goat) is a discrete compound tubular gland with a thick fibromuscular capsule extending into the gland to form the supporting framework. The epithelium is pseudostratified with tall columnar secretory cells and small basal reserve cells. In the dog the secretion is serous (**11.22** and **11.23**); in other animals it is seromucous.

Glands of the ampulla

Ampulla is described in 'Epididymis and ductus deferens', above.

Table 11.1
Male accessory genital glands, species variation

Species	Prostate		Ampulla	Bulbourethral	Seminal vesicles
	Compact	Disseminate			
Stallion	+	–	+	+	+
Bull	+	+	+	+	+
Ram	–	+	+	+	+
Boar	+	+	–	+	+
Dog	+	–	–	–	–
Tomcat	+	–	–	–	–

+. gland is present; – gland is absent.

11.22

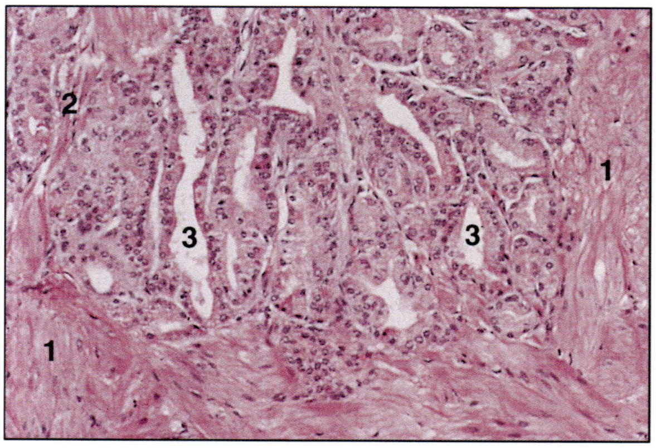

11.22 Prostate (dog). (1) Fibromuscular capsule. (2) Fibromuscular trabeculae. (3) Lumen of the secretory acinus lined by simple columnar epithelium. H & E. ×62.5.

11.2

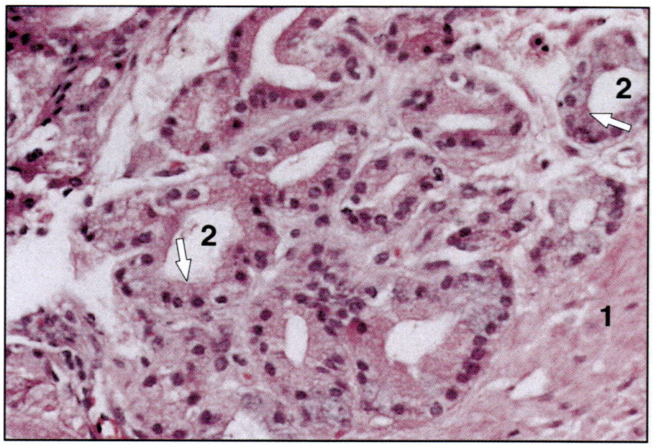

11.23 Prostate (dog). (1) Fibromuscular trabecula. (2) Lumen of the secretory acinus lined by tall columnar secretory epithelium (arrowed). H & E. ×125.

Seminal vesicles

The seminal vesicles are compound tubular glands with a fibromuscular capsule and elastic fibres in the connective tissue stroma. They are absent in carnivores and are true vesicles in the stallion (**11.24**). In the boar and ruminants they are compact with a lobulated surface. The secretory epithelium is tall columnar with surface blebs (large flaccid vesicles) giving a ragged appearance to the cells (**11.25** and **11.26**).

11.24

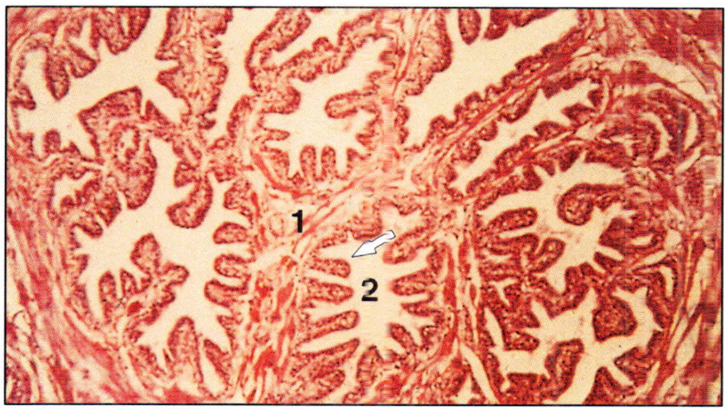

11.24 Seminal vesicle (stallion). (1) Connective tissue. (2) Lumen is lined by a tall columnar secretory epithelium (arrowed). H & E. ×100.

.25

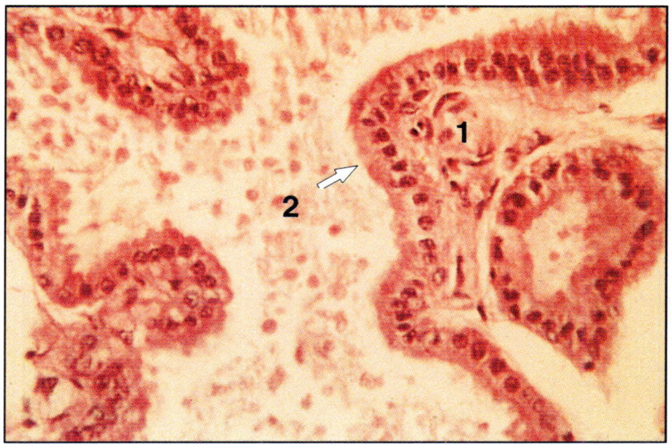

11.25 Seminal vesicle (stallion). (1) Connective tissue of the capsule. (2) Lumen lined by tall columnar secretory epithelium (arrowed). H & E. ×160.

11.26

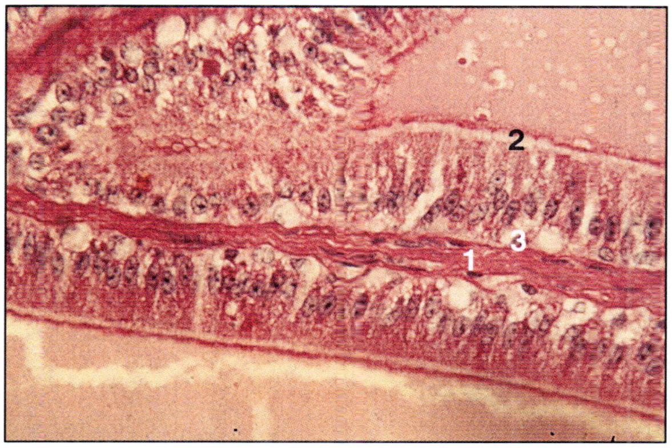

11.26 Seminal vesicle (bull). (1) Trabecular connective tissue. (2) Tall columnar secretory epithelium with apical blebs. (3) Basal replacement cells. H & E. ×250.

Bulbourethral glands

Bulbourethral glands are compound tubular and mucus secreting. A connective tissue capsule sends fine trabeculae into the gland, and the outer layer of striated muscle on the dorsal and lateral aspect is the m. bulbourethralis (**11.27** and **11.28**).

.27

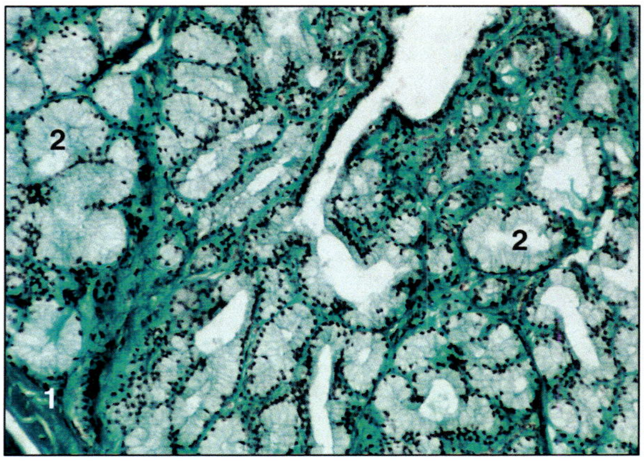

11.27 Bulbourethral gland (boar). (1) Striated muscle capsule. (2) Mucus-secreting secretory epithelium lines the acini. Light green/haematoxylin. ×50.

11.28

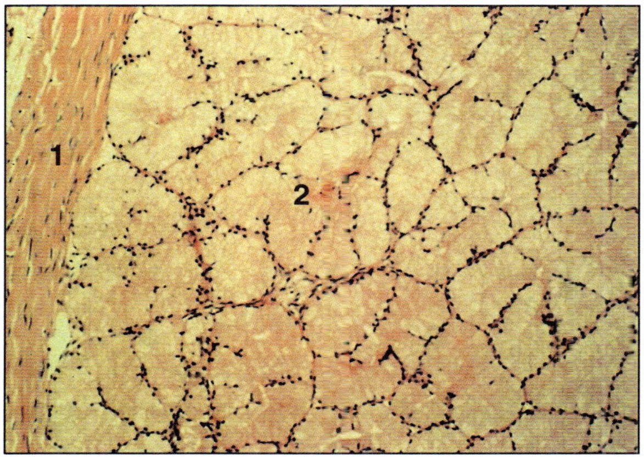

11.28 Bulbourethral gland (goat). (1) Striated muscle capsule. (2) Mucus-secreting secretory epithelium lines the acini. H & E. ×100.

Clinical correlates

Developmental problems are important in the pathology of the male reproductive tract (not surprisingly given the complex embryology of this system), but inflammatory, degenerative and neoplastic conditions are also recognized. These problems can be inter-related (e.g. retained testicles, which can be located at any level along the path of descent, are more susceptible to the development of tumours than are normally descended scrotal testicles). These internally retained testicles also undergo degenerative changes.

Bilateral cryptorchidism leads to infertility since normal spermatogenesis requires the testis to be several degrees cooler than core body temperature. Cryptorchidism is important in the horse (**11.29**), because hormone production by the internally retained testicle maintains stallion-like behaviours. Thus an animal with a retained testicle may appear to be gelded, but it is more

11.29

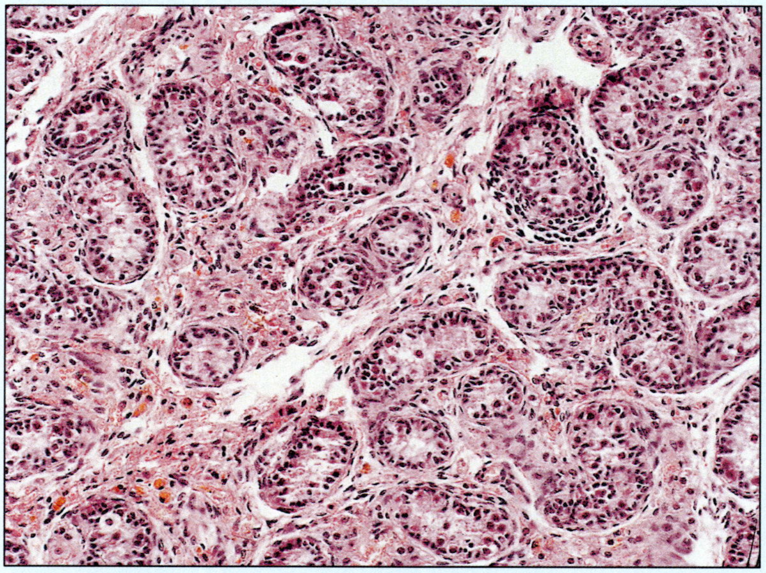

11.29 Cryptorchid (retained) testicle from a horse. The tubules are atrophic with absence of spermatogenesis. Fibrous tissue and interstitial cells lie between the tubules. H & E. ×125.

11.30

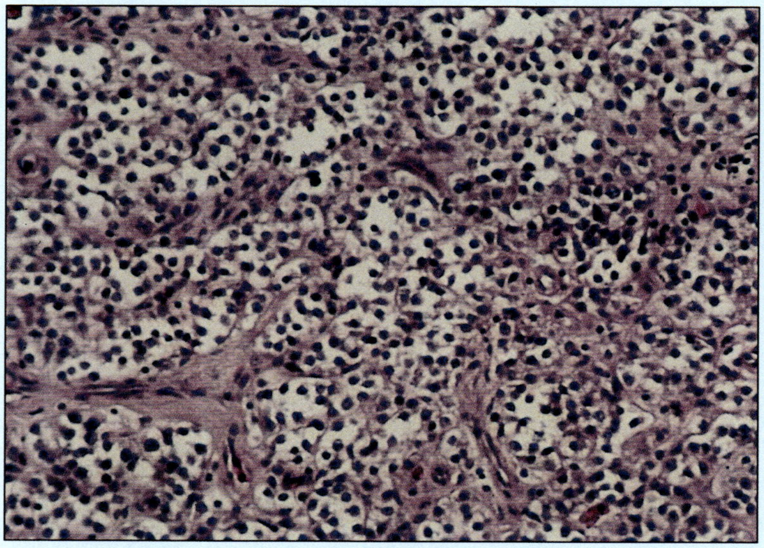

11.30 Sustentacular (Sertoli) cell tumour in a dog. In this intratubular example the seminiferous tubules are packed with and distorted by pale-staining neoplastic sustentacular cells with faintly vacuolated cytoplasm instead of normal spermatogenetic cells with an orderly pattern of maturation. H & E. ×200.

dangerous to handle. Blood testing can identify such animals.

Three major types of primary testicular tumours are identified. These are the sustentacular cell tumour (**11.30**), common in the dog, which can be associated with a feminization syndrome that results from oestrogen production by the tumour cells, the interstitial cell tumour, and the seminoma (**11.31**). A minority of sustentacular cell tumours and seminomas metastasize, but spread is very rare with interstitial cell tumours.

The pattern of accessory sex organs varies between different species. In the dog and cat the prostate gland is of primary importance. This gland is very sensitive to hormonal influence and prostatic hyperplasia is a common finding in older entire male dogs (**11.32**). Enlargement of the prostate, which may result from benign hyperplasia, prostatitis or neoplasia, can present with difficulty in defaecation, as this gland lies beneath the rectum.

11.31

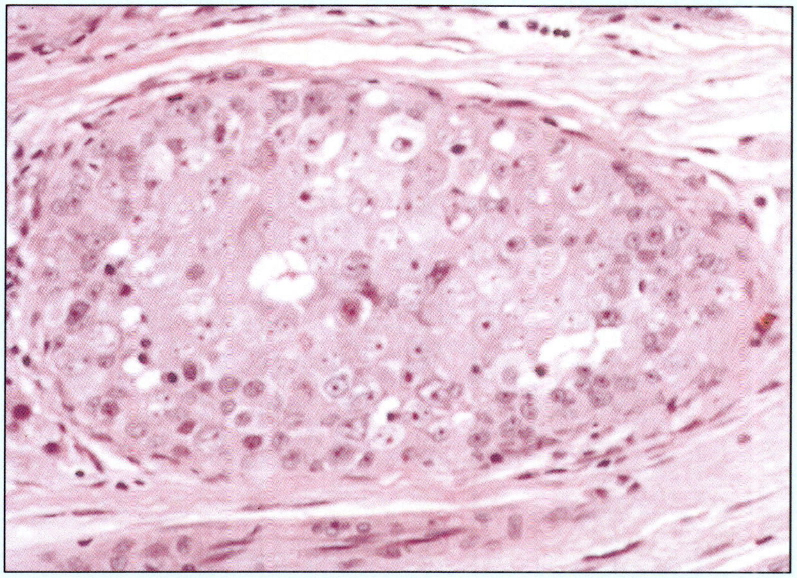

11.31 Seminoma in a 7-year-old dog. This intratubular example of a seminoma is composed of large polyhedral tumour cells with discrete cell borders and large, round, often vesicular nuclei. Seminomas do not produce hormones. H & E. ×200.

11.32

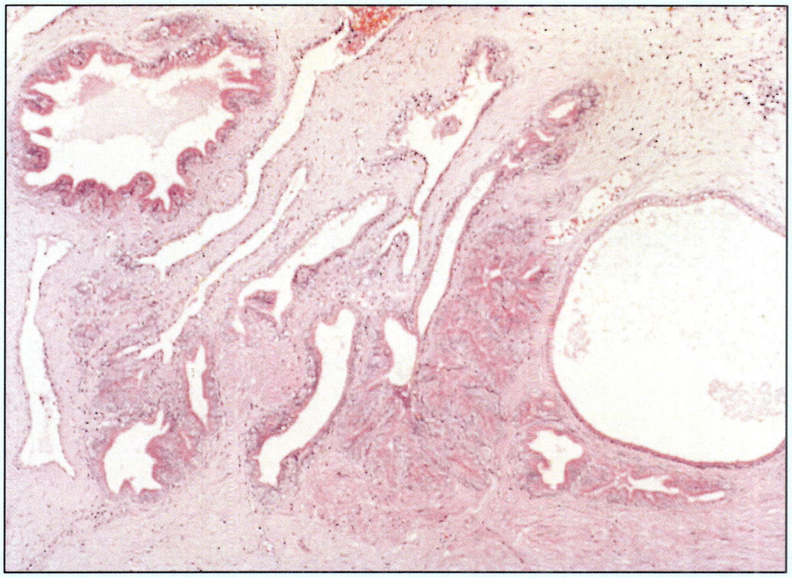

11.32 Prostatic hyperplasia in the dog. This micrograph shows dilated glandular structures and lymphatic ectasia within a hyperplastic fibrous stroma. H & E. ×20.

Avian testis

The avian testis has a fibrous tunica albuginea but no mediastinum or supporting connective tissue trabeculae. The seminiferous tubules form an anastomosing network, the interstices of which are occupied by blood vessels, fibroblasts and specific interstitial cells. The seminiferous epithelium is multilayered in the mature adult bird as in the mammal (**11.33**). The head of the spermatozoon

11.33

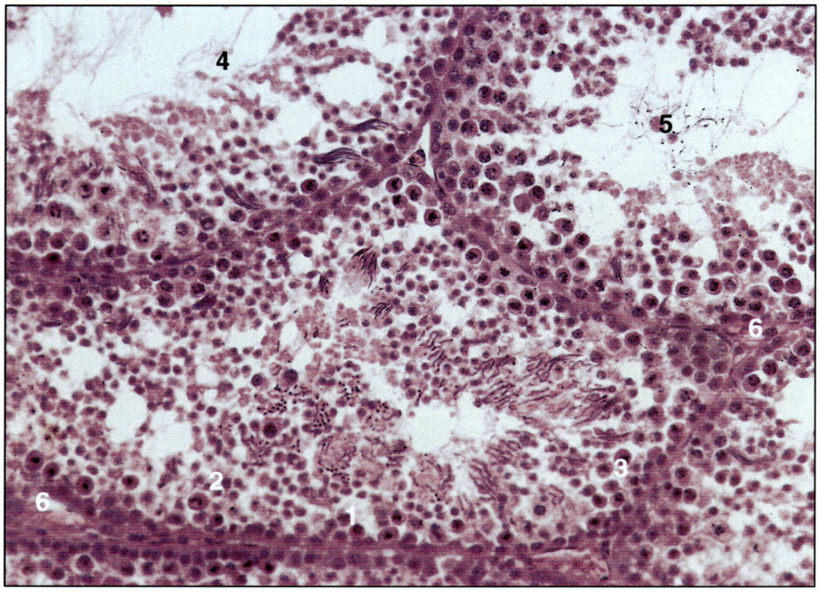

11.33 Testis (bird). (1) Spermatogonia. (2) Primary spermatocyte. (3) Spermatid. (4) Spermatozoa. (5) Lumen of the seminiferous tubule. (6) Interstitial tissue with specific interstitial cells. H & E. ×200.

11.34

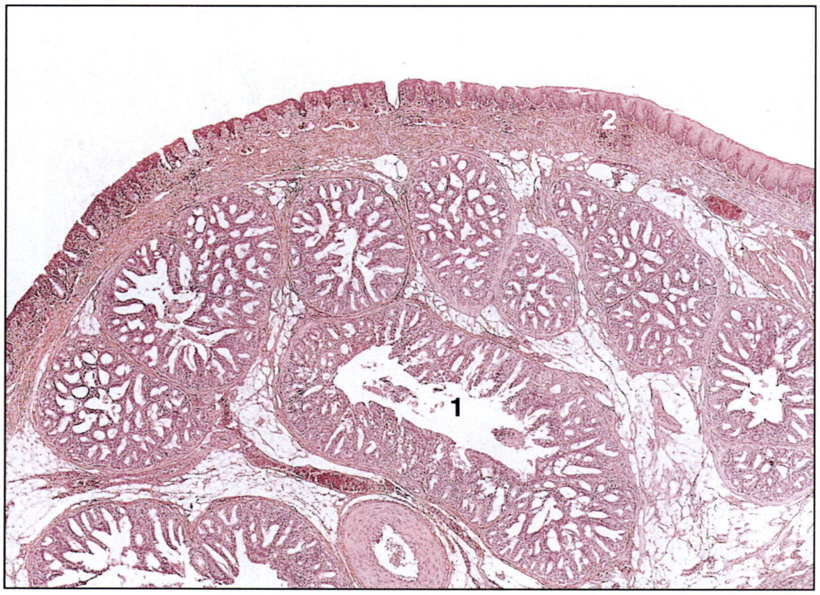

11.34 Urodeum (domestic fowl cockerel). (1) Simple tubular glands in the wall of the urodeum. (2) Lining epithelium of the urodeum. H & E. ×62.5.

is long, narrow and gently curved.

The ductus deferens traverses the wall of the urodeum (part of the cloaca; **11.34**) and is continued as the ejaculatory duct (**11.35**). Deep crypts are present with short tubular glands lying in the lamina propria of the urodeum (**11.36**). Lymphocytes are present in the subepithelial connective tissue.

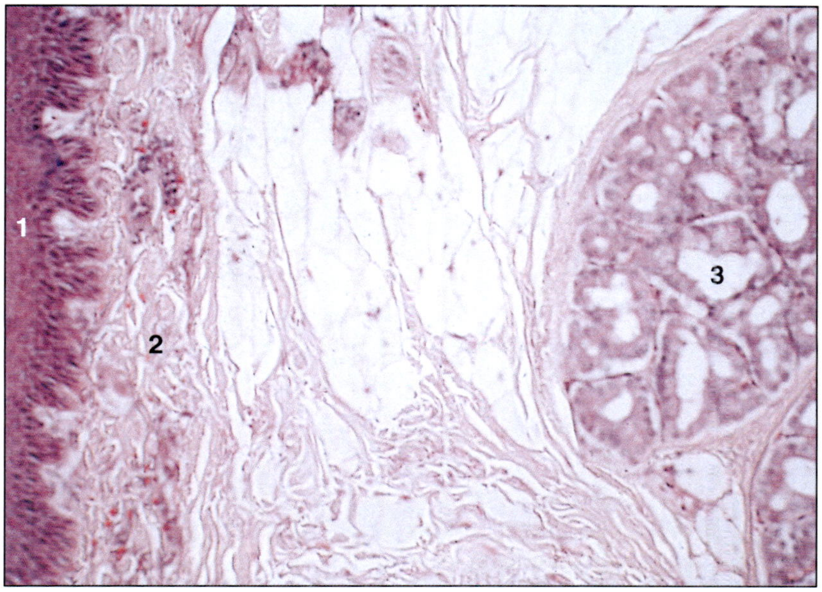

11.35

11.35 Ejaculatory duct (cock). (1) Stratified squamous epithelium. (2) Vascular lamina propria. (3) Simple tubular glands. H & E. ×160.

11.36 Ejaculatory duct (cock). (1) Stratified squamous epithelium. (2) Vascular erectile tissue. (3) Simple tubular gland. H & E. ×62.5.

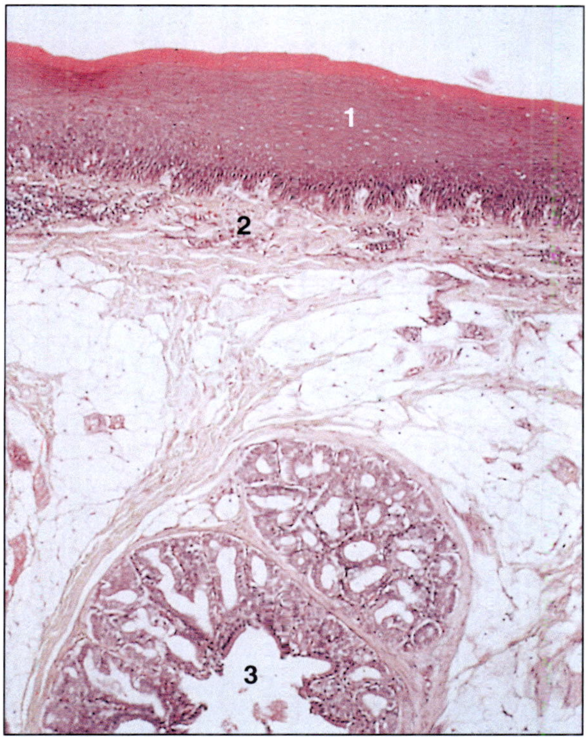

11.36

Reptilian, amphibian and fish male reproductive system

The histology of the testis and associated tubular post-testicular reproductive system of fish, amphibians and reptiles is sufficiently similar to that of mammals and birds (**11.37–11.39**) that only the differences need to be discussed here. Parallel to the situation that is observed in some mammals and birds that exhibit seasonal waxing and waning of spermatogenesis, the testes of many fish, most amphibians and many reptiles undergo seasonally induced testicular atrophy and recrudescence. The spermatozoa of these lower vertebrates are morphologically similar to those of higher vertebrates. During the quiescent portions of this cycle, the seminiferous tubules are devoid of active spermatogenesis. They are lined only by sustentacular cells and a few primary spermatogonia (**11.40**). The interstitial cells may or may not follow a parallel increase and decrease in activity, size or number. The epididymis and ductus deferents of reptiles are histologically similar to those of mammals.

Internal fertilization of ova is a rare exception in amphibian reproduction. Spermatozoa are usually discharged over the eggs as they are released by the female during amplexus, the term given to the 'nuptial clasp'. In many caudate amphibians the female is positioned during courtship over a packet consisting of sperm and accessory gelatinous secretions, called a spermatophore, that is released by a male. This structure is then taken up into the female's cloaca, where the sperm are released and fertilize ripe eggs. In a few species, females deposit their eggs directly upon a spermatophore. In caecilians, which are among the few amphibians in which internal fertilization occurs, the sperm are directed into the female's caudal genital tract with an eversible portion of the male's cloacal wall, called a phallodeum, which serves as an intromittant organ. One anuran (*Ascaphus truei*) possesses an intromittant organ that is actually a tail-like extension of the cloaca in which vascular erectile elements are located. The epithelium covering the cranial portion of this structure is mucous; distally, it is keratinized and bears horny spines near its orifice. In the few other species of amphibians in which internal fertilization occurs, the spermatozoa are introduced into the female by direct cloacal apposition without the intervention of an intromittant organ, or by the uptake of spermatophores that are deposited onto substrate. Once deposited into a female's body, spermatozoa are stored for a variably prolonged period in branched pouch-like spermathecae that are located in the wall of the roof of the cloaca. These crypt-like structures are lined by cuboidal to low columnar epithelial cells with eosinophilic granular cytoplasm.

11.37

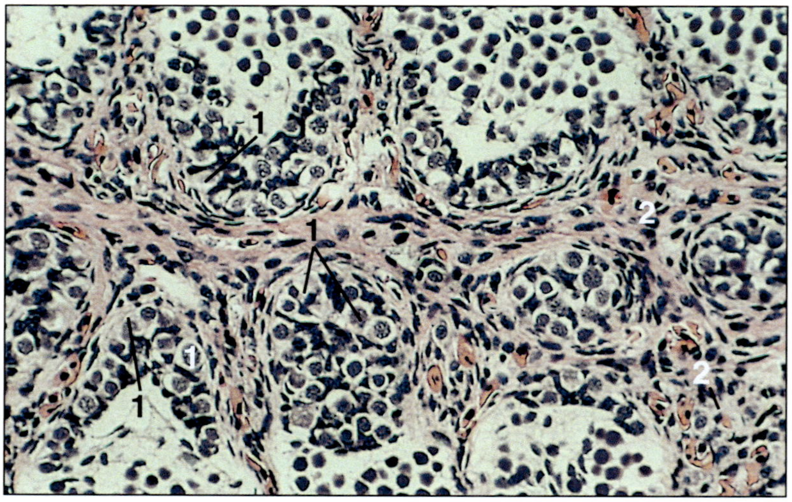

11.37 Section of the testis of an aquatic salamander (*Amphiuma tridactyla*). The paler staining sustentacular cells (1) are readily distinguished from the darker spermatogonia and spermatocytes. The interstitial cells (2) are contained within small lobules bound within concentric fibrovascular connective tissue stroma. H & E. ×125.

Reptiles utilize internal fertilization. Male chelonians possess a single erectile penis that is often heavily pigmented and is covered by lightly keratinized and mucous epithelium. Male snakes and lizards possess paired erectile intromittant organs, called hemipenes, that contain fibrovascular tissue that, when involuted, invaginates. When erect the outer surface is covered with keratinized epithelium. Additional flamboyant spines, flounces and other sexual adornments are species specific. The hemipenes receive lubrication from mucous glands that are located within the lumen of the hemipenial sheath. In some reptiles, modified sebaceous glands are associated with the hemipenes and their sheaths (11.41).

Male crocodilians possess a relatively small erectile penis that superficially resembles that of higher vertebrates; it even has a glans-like swelling at its distal end. The surface is covered with lightly keratinized epithelium without horny projections.

Male tuataras lack an erectile intromittant organ. Internal fertilization is accomplished by cloacal apposition during which semen is transferred to the female and enters the proctodeum portion of the cloaca.

11.38

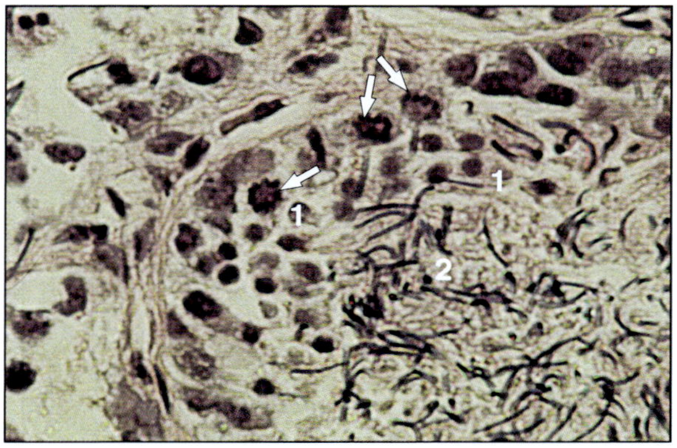

11.38 Section of a seminiferous tubule of a mature green iguana (*Iguana iguana*). Three spermatogonia are shown in mitosis (arrows). Primary spermatocytes (1) and many tailed spermatozoa (2) lie within the centre of the tubule. H & E. ×200.

11.39

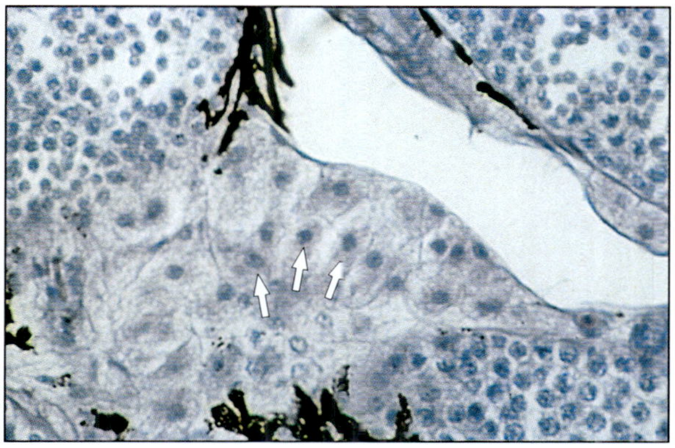

11.39 A section of the testis of a panther chameleon (*Chamaeleo pardalis*). A nest of large interstitial cells containing finely granular cytoplasm can be seen in the lower third of this image (arrows). H & E. ×200.

11.40

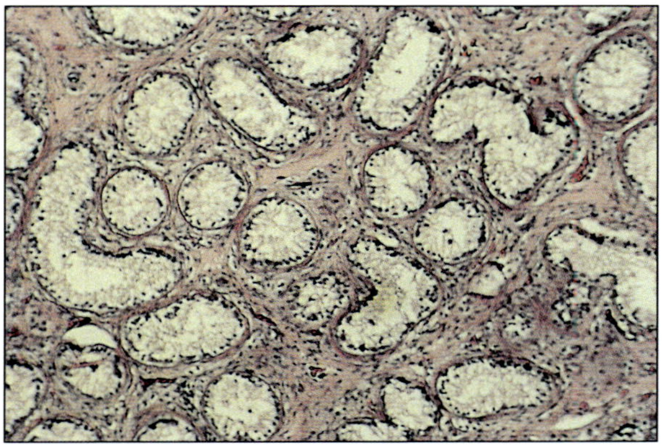

11.40 Inactive testis of a green sea turtle (*Chelonia mydas*). The seminiferous tubles are lined only by sustentacular cells and a few spermatogonia. H & E. ×100.

11.41

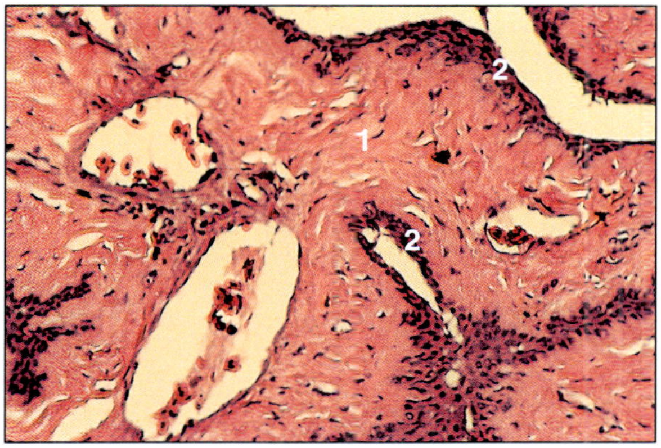

11.41 Inverted (detumescent) hemipenis of a Carolina anole lizard (*Anolis carolinensis*). The organ is composed of spongy fibrovascular tissues containing many arterial and venous channels (1), and stratified lightly cornified squamous epithelium (2). Lobules of glandular tissue, similar to sebaceous glands, lie at the base of each hemipenis and furnish lubrication and scent-rich secretions to the erectile intromittant organ. H & E. ×50.

Clinical correlates

True hermaphroditism occurs occasionally in reptiles but is usually only discovered at necropsy. The condition can involve one gonad of each sex, one or more ovotestes or separate masses of ovarian and testicular tissue.

A Bidder's organ is normally present in male bufonid toads. This interesting structure is a cap-like mass of ovarian tissue attached to the cranial pole of the testis (**11.42**). It is unclear why androgenic and ovarian hormone secretion do not each suppress their opposites.

As in domestic animals, the reptilian or amphibian testis can be the site of inflammatory disorders, atrophy and fibrosis (**11.43**), and neoplastic disease (**11.44**). Malignant tumours are more prevalent than benign variants.

11.42

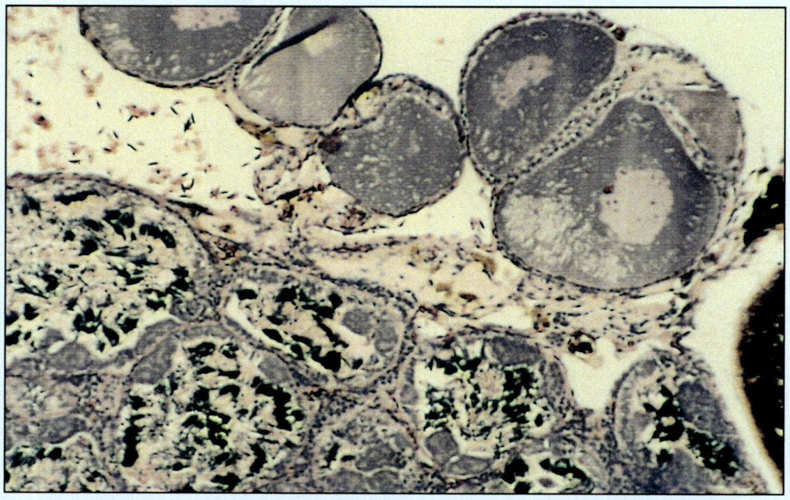

11.42 Bidder's organ in a western toad (*Bufo boreas*). Although similar to hermaphroditic gonadal tissue, Bidder's organ is a normal constituent found in some bufonid amphibians and consists of a cap-like assemblage of pigmented ovarian tissue, including yolked follicle-like structures attached to the cranial pole of each testis. The presence of ovarian tissue does not suppress spermatogenesis. H & E. ×50.

11.43

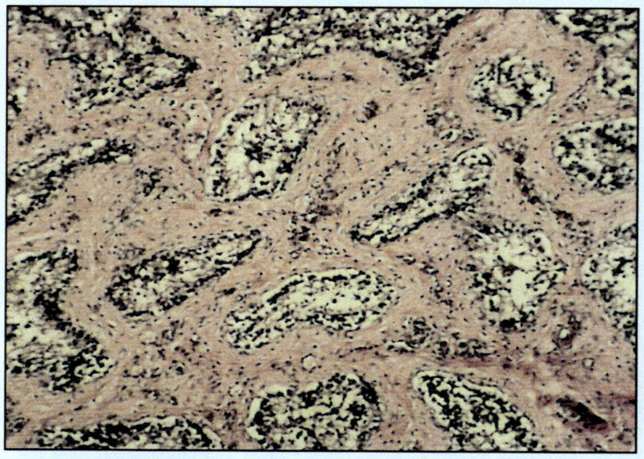

11.43 Testicular fibrosis in a blood python (*Python curtus*). The seminiferous tubules are atrophic and widely separated from each other by wide bands of mature fibrocollagenous connective tissue. H & E. ×20.

11.4

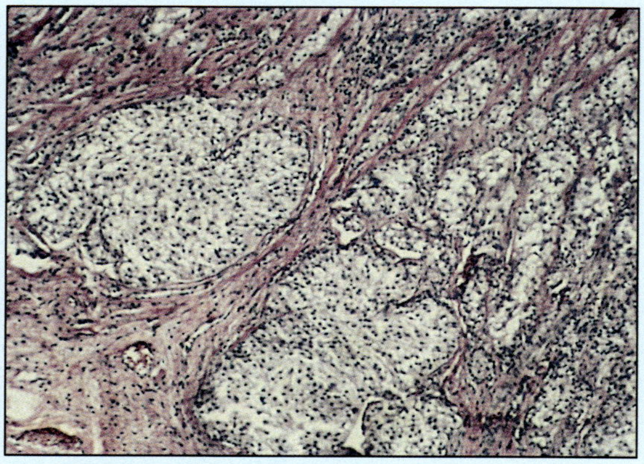

11.44 Sustentacular (Sertoli) cell tumour from a snake. Note large nests of pale-staining sustentacular cells. H & E. ×100.

12. FEMALE REPRODUCTIVE SYSTEM

The female reproductive system consists of the ovaries, uterine tubes (oviducts or Fallopian tubes), uterus, vagina and vestibule. The external genitalia are the vulva, labia, clitoris and external urethral orifice.

Ovaries

Cortex and medulla

The ovaries have an exocrine function, the production of the egg or female gamete, and an endocrine function, the production of female sex hormones. Each ovary is divided into an outer parenchymatous zone cortex and an inner vascular zone medulla (12.1), except in the mare where there is no zonal division. The cortex of each ovary is covered by a simple squamous or cuboidal epithelium that is continuous with the mesothelium of the visceral peritoneum (the germinal epithelium), except at the hilus where blood vessels and nerves enter and exit from the gland. Beneath the epithelium is a layer of dense connective tissue, the tunica albuginea. Deep to that is the ovarian or cortical stroma, containing ovarian follicles in various stages of development. The ovarian stroma consists of spindle-shaped cells arranged in whorls surrounding the ovarian follicles. In carnivores, particularly the cat, numerous specific interstitial cells are present in the stroma. They are small, round, epithelioid cells with a round nucleus and they stain poorly (12.2).

12.1

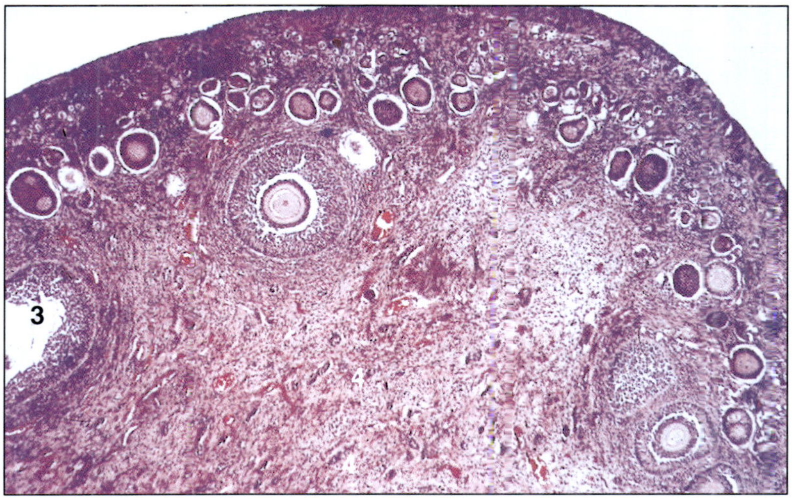

12.1 Ovary (cat). (1) Parenchymatous zone with primary follicles (2) and secondary follicles (3). (4) Vascular zone. H & E. ×7.5.

12.2

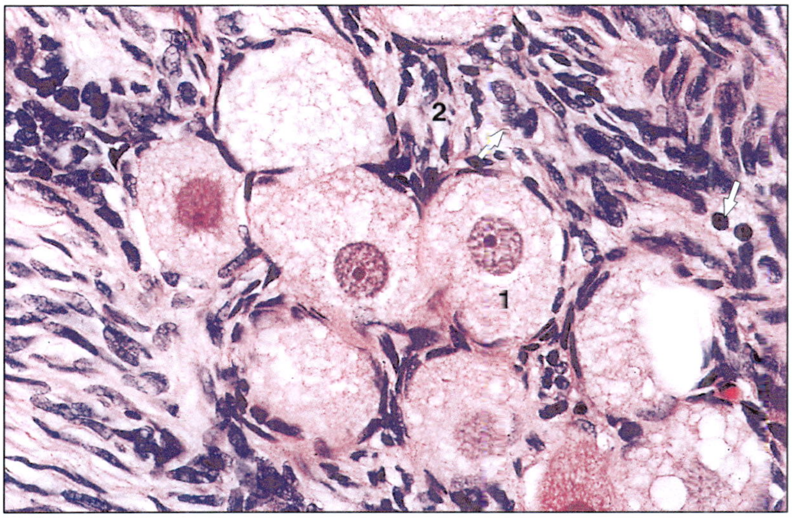

12.2 Ovary. Parenchymatous zone (cat). (1) Primary follicles; the large oocyte is surrounded by flattened nurse cells. (2) Cellular ovarian stroma. The specific interstitial cells are arrowed. H & E. ×250.

The medulla is highly vascularized and consists of fibroelastic connective tissue and some smooth muscle (12.3). Channels, lined with (densely staining) cuboidal epithelium and called the rete ovarii, are conspicuous components of the medulla in carnivores and ruminants (12.4). They are derived from the mesonephric tubules during embryogenesis.

Development of the follicles

Primordial follicles are the least developed and most numerous follicles of the ovary, lying just below the tunica albuginea. Each consists of a primary oocyte surrounded by a layer of simple squamous follicle (nurse) cells (see 12.2). The primary oocytes originate in the late embryonic/early postnatal ovary from oogonia and are surrounded by a flattened layer of nurse cells. Further development is arrested until puberty, when a regular cycle of events results in the passage of one or more follicles into the lumen of the uterine tube during reproductive cycles. A number of follicles begin to grow, and the primary oocyte accumulates yolk and enlarges from 60 µm to between 100 and 120 µm in diameter. Concomitantly, an acidophilic, translucent membrane, the zona pellucida, forms around the oocyte (12.5). The nurse cells become cuboidal, then columnar, then stratified and begin to accumulate fluid in the intercellular spaces. The follicle now comes under the influence of follicle-stimulating hormone from the pituitary gland and continues to grow to become a secondary follicle, with a C-shaped, fluid filled space, or antrum (12.6). Its cells are now called the granulosa layer. The follicle secretes oestradiol, the female sex hormone that prepares the endometrium to receive the fertilized egg. The ovarian stroma condenses around the developing follicle to form an inner layer, the theca interna, which is cellular and vascular, and an outer layer, the theca externa, which is composed of fibrous connective tissue.

The follicle continues to increase in size, moving to the surface of the ovary to become a vesicular [tertiary (mature) Graafian] follicle. The oocyte is surrounded by a multilayer of granulosa cells, the cumulus oophorus (12.7 and 12.8). Ordinarily, a mature vesicular follicle contains a single oocyte. The follicles of certain animals (carnivores, sows and ewes) may, however, contain up to six oocytes. Maximum size is reached just before ovulation.

12.3

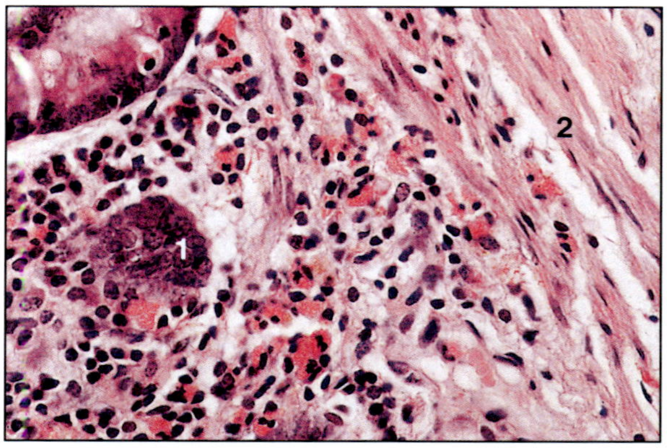

12.3 Ovary. Vascular zone (bitch). (1) The ovarian stroma is very vascular. (2) Smooth muscle cells. H & E. ×125.

12.4

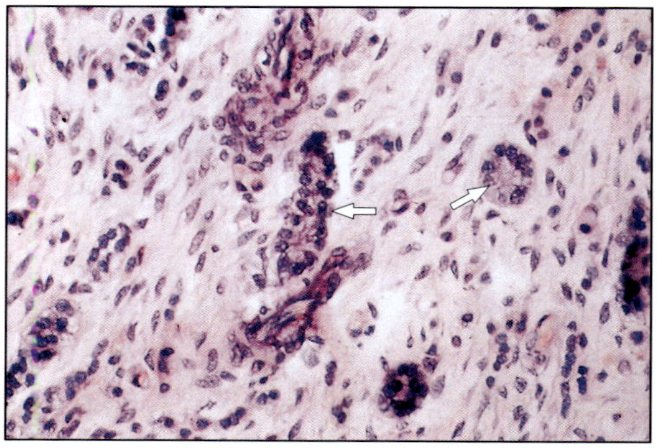

12.4 Ovary. Vascular zone (sheep). Tubules of the reti ovarii are arrowed. H & E. ×125.

12.5

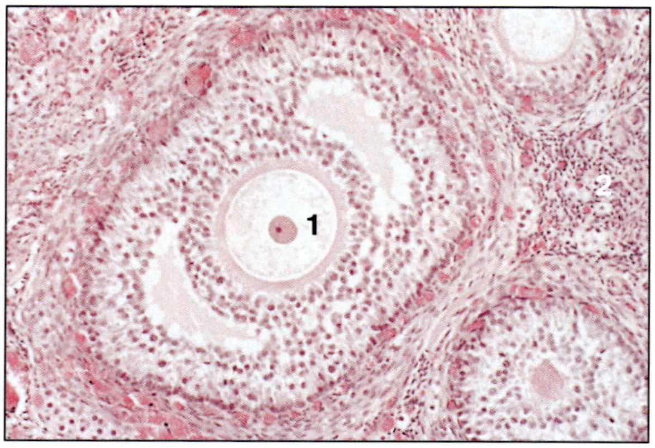

12.5 Ovary. Parenchymatous zone (sheep). (1) The oocyte is surrounded by the granulosa layer. (2) Ovarian stroma. H & E. ×125.

12.6 Ovary. Secondary follicle (bitch). (1) The oocyte is surrounded by the amorphous zona pellucida. (2) The granulosa cells are stratified. (3) Fluid accumulates to begin antrum formation. (4) Ovarian stroma concentrates around the follicle to form the theca. H & E. ×62.5.

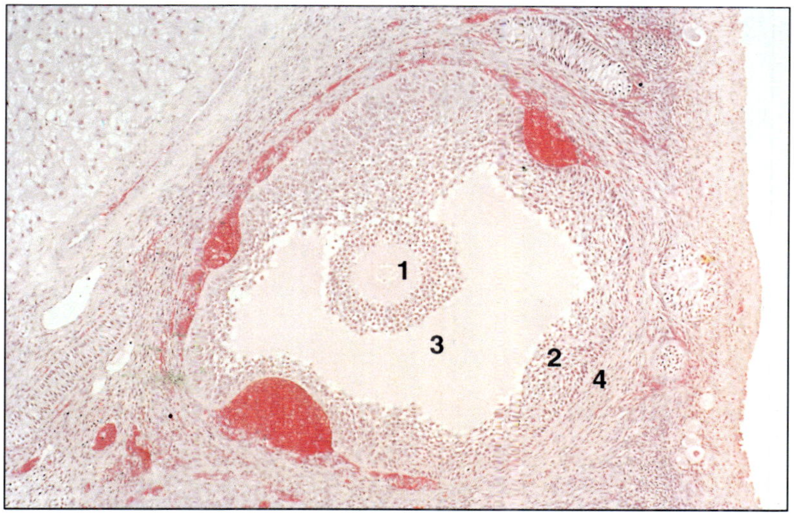

12.6

12.7 Ovary. Tertiary follicle (cow). (1) The oocyte surrounded by the zona pellucida is embedded in a mound of granulosa cells, the cumulus oophorous. (2) Theca or capsule of ovarian stroma. H & E. ×62.5.

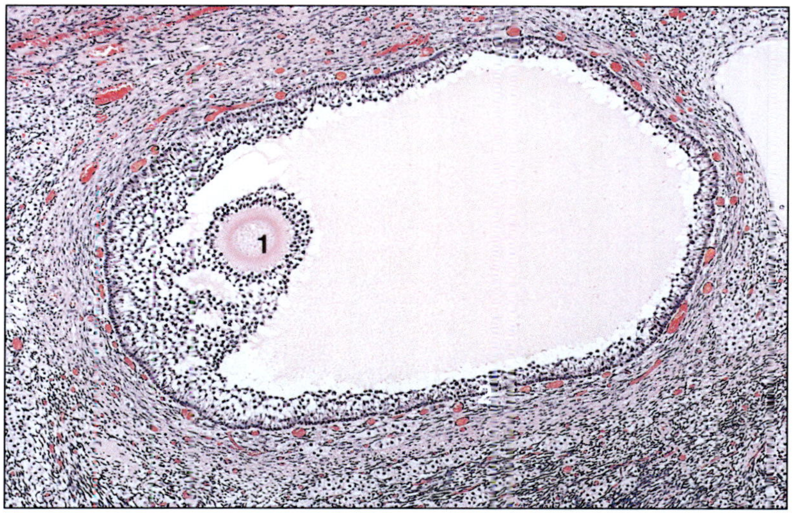

12.7

12.8 Ovary. Parenchymatous zone (cat). The cuboidal epithelium is arrowed. (1) Tunica albuginea is a thin layer of connective tissue. (2) Primary follicles. (3) Vescicular (tertiary) follicle with a large fluid filled antrum (4) lined by granulosa cells (5) and encapsulated by the vascular theca interna (6) and the fibrous theca externa (7). Gomori's trichrome. ×62.5.

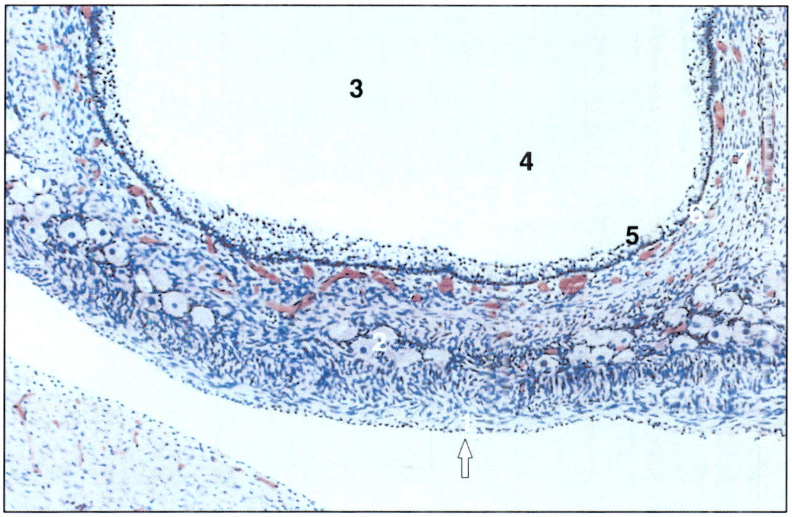

12.8

Ovulation

At ovulation the primary oocyte divides into secondary oocytes, one cell retaining most of the cytoplasm; completion of meiosis occurs at fertilization. The follicle breaks open, releasing the oocyte, which passes into the uterine tubes. The follicle collapses and the granulosa cells, together with those of the theca interna, hypertrophy, expanding into the cavity to form the granulosa lutein and theca lutein cells of the corpus luteum (**12.9** and **12.10**). They are arranged in long cords separated by vascular connective tissue. The luteal cells secrete progesterone which, with the oestradiol, prepares the uterus for possible conception. With regression of the corpus luteum, stromal elements move in and replace the dead cells with collagen to form a scar: the corpus albicans (**12.11** and **12.12**). Although many primordial follicles begin the process outlined above, few become mature. The majority undergo a degenerative regression. They are called anovular or atretic follicles and can be recognized by the irregular outline of the follicle and the separation of the granulosa cells (**12.13**). Cells of the theca interna hypertrophy and the zona pellucida becomes swollen. Eventually, the entire follicle is resorbed.

12.9

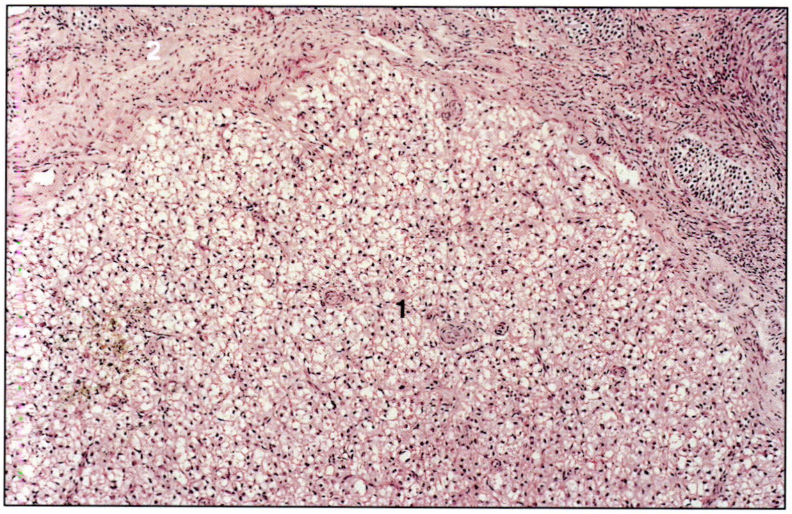

12.9 Ovary. Parenchymatous zone (sheep). (1) The pale vacuolated cells are part of the corpus luteum. (2) Ovarian stroma. H & E. ×62.5.

12.10

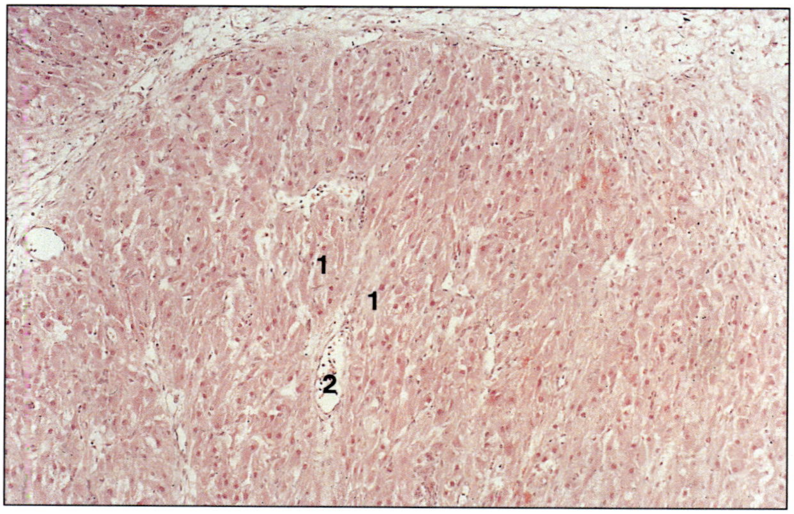

12.10 Ovary. Parenchymatous zone (sow). (1) Cords of large densely stained luteal cells are separated by (2) blood vessels. H & E. ×125.

12.11 Ovary. Parenchymatous zone (sheep). (1) Ovarian stroma. (2) Dense white connective tissue. (3) Active fibroblasts replacing degenerating luteal cells. H & E. ×125.

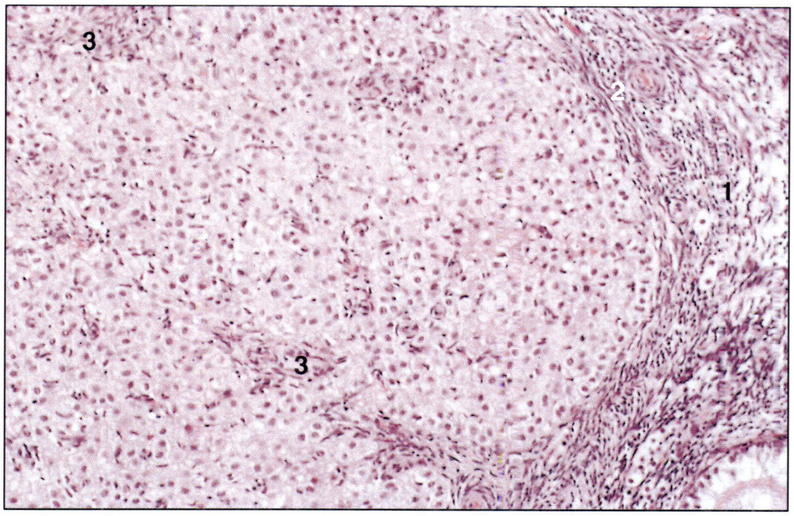

12.11

12.12 Sheep. Parenchymatous zone (sheep). The central pale staining area is dense white connective tissue (scar tissue) and represents a later stage in the development of a corpus albicans. H & E. ×250.

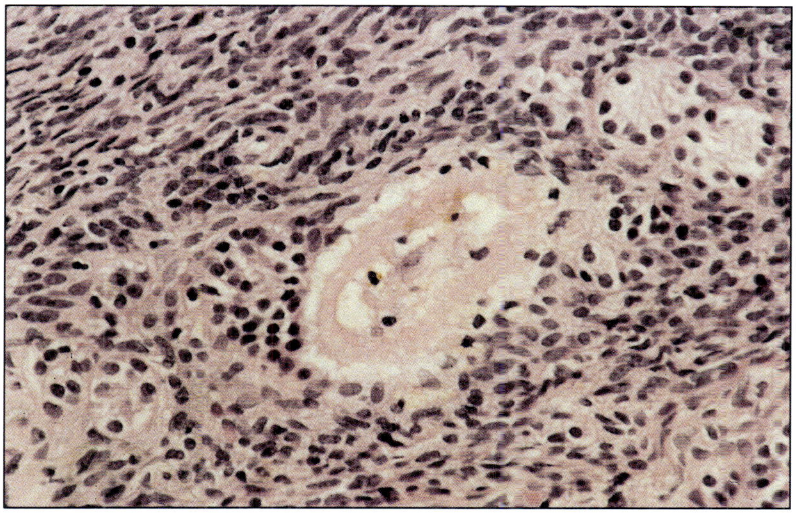

12.12

12.13 Ovary. Parenchymatous zone (bitch). Atretic follicle. (1) The granulosa cells are separating; spaces are present between them. (2) The oocyte is no longer in contact with the lining granulosa cells. H & E. ×125.

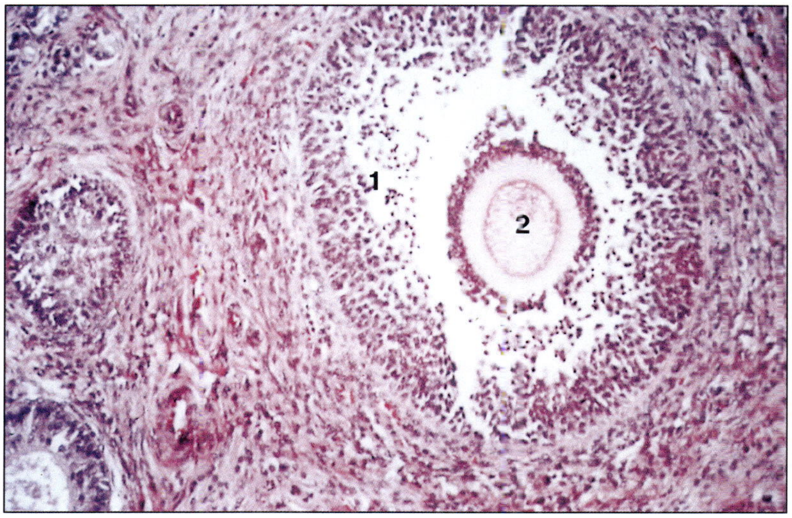

12 13

Uterine tubes (oviducts)

The uterine tubes are long flexuous musculomembranous tubes. They consist of an expanded cranial end, the infundibulum, which is close to the ovary; a middle segment, the ampulla; and a caudal narrow part or isthmus that opens into the ipsilateral horn of the uterus. The epithelium is simple or pseudostratified columnar with secretory and ciliated cells. The lamina propria has longitudinal folds giving it a glandular appearance. In some breeds of sheep (blackface and crosses), pigment cells are present. The muscularis is mainly a layer of circular smooth muscle, thickening at the junction with the uterine horn, with an outer layer of longitudinal muscle. The serosa is loose vascular connective tissue with prominent blood vessels (**12.14** and **12.15**).

12.14

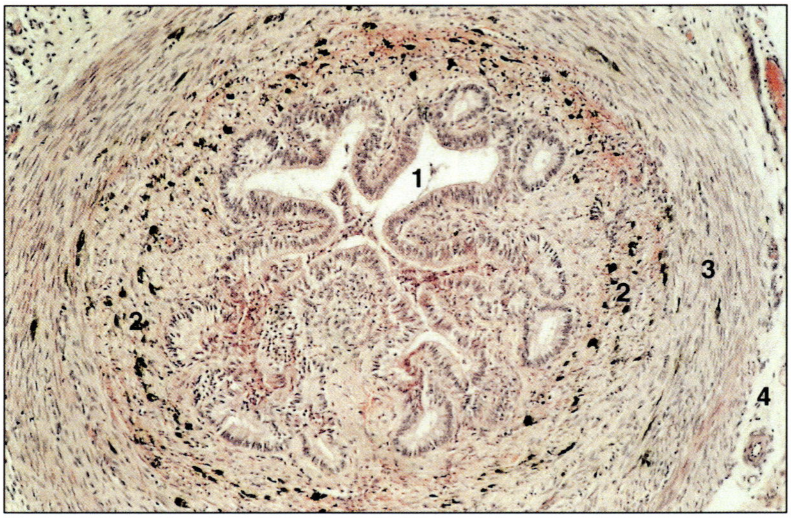

12.14 Transverse section (TS) uterine tube (sheep). (1) The lumen is lined by a pseudostratified epithelium thrown into deep folds. (2) The lamina propria has deposits of dark brown pigment. (3) The muscularis is for the most part circular smooth muscle fibres. (4) The serosa is loose vascular connective tissue with prominent blood vessels. H & E. ×62.5.

12.15

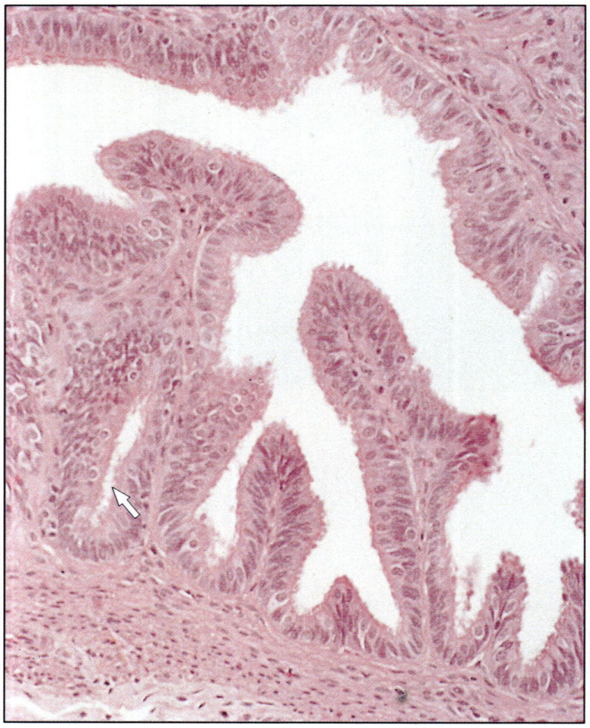

12.15 TS uterine tube (cow). The lining epithelium is pseudostratified columnar with ciliated and non-ciliated cells.The deep mucosal folds are cut in transverse section giving the appearance of mucosal glands (arrowed). H & E. ×125.

Uterus

The uterus is bicornuate, with right and left horns (cornua), a body (corpus) and a neck (cervix) (12.16–12.23, all illustrations in transverse section). The uterine wall in the cornua and corpus has three layers: an inner endometrium (mucosa), a middle myoemetrium (muscularis) and an outer perimetrium (serosa).

Endometrium

The epithelial lining of the endometrium is simple cuboidal or columnar in the mare and carnivores, and pseudostratified in the sow and ruminants. In ruminants, ciliated cells may be present. The lamina propria is a deep layer of vascular connective tissue, with simple tubular endometrial glands that open into the lumen of the uterus. These glands are

12.16

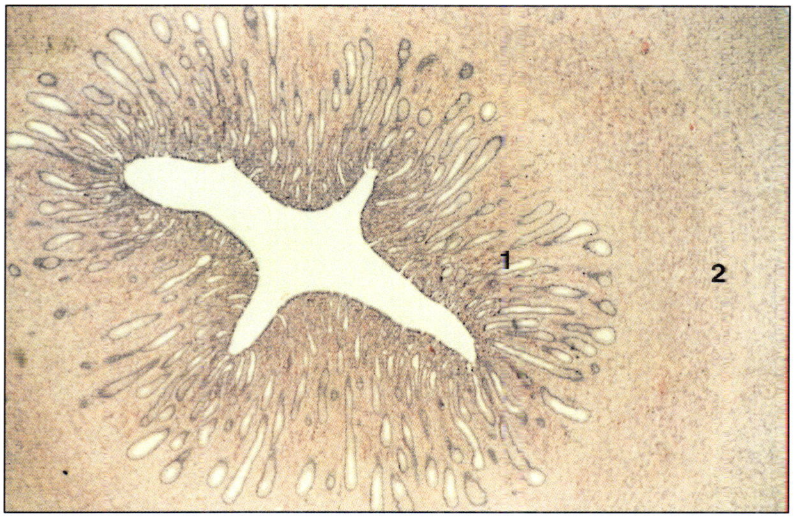

12.16 TS uterus (cat). (1) Endometrium with simple straight tubular glands. (2) Myometrium with circular and longitudinal smooth muscle. H & E. ×7.5.

.17

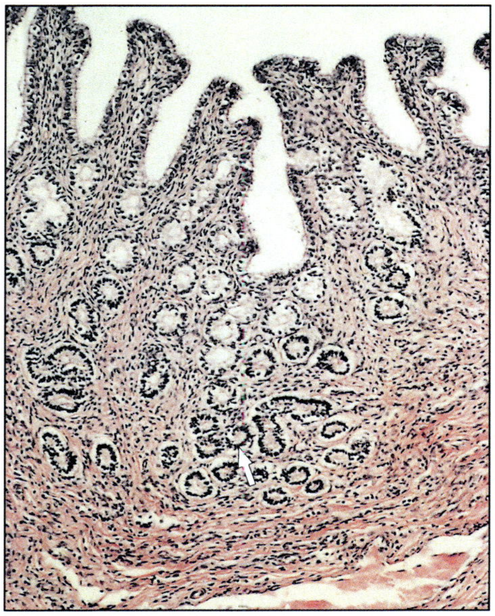

12.17 TS uterus (mare). Only the endometrium is present. The lining epithelium is simple columnar; the endometrial glands are slightly coiled at the base (arrowed). H & E. ×62.5.

12.18

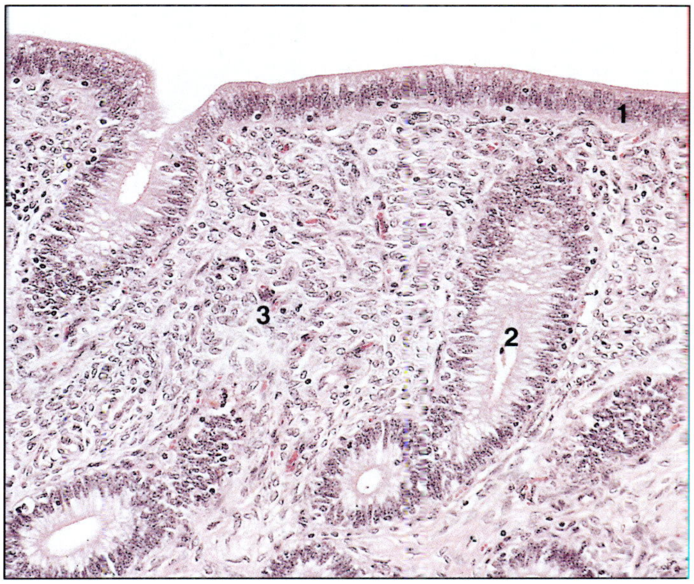

12.18 TS uterus (bitch). (1) The lining epithelium is simple columnar. (2) The endometrial glands are lined by tall columnar epithelial cells with a basal nucleus. (3) The lamina propria is very cellular with many small blood vessels. H & E. ×125.

12.19

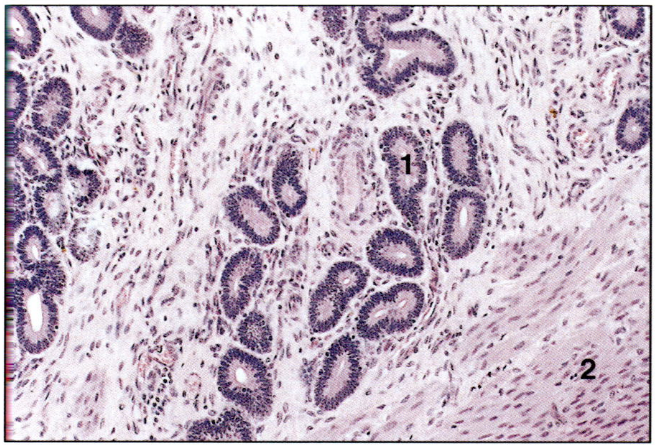

12.2

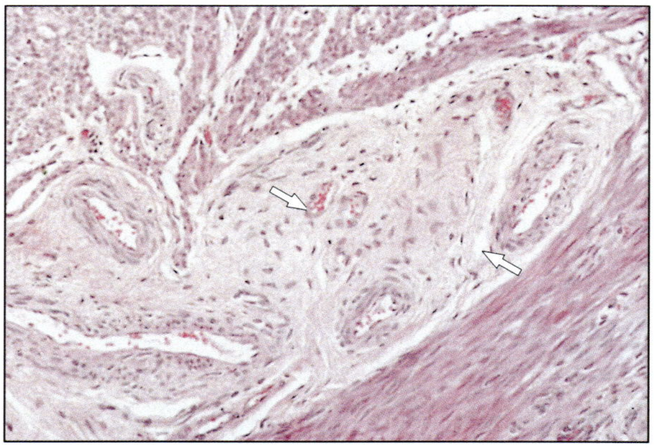

12.19 TS uterus (cow). (1) The endometrial glands are markedly coiled. (2) Thick layer of myometrium. H & E. ×100.

12.20 TS uterus (cow). The myometrium is split by the stratum vasculare (arrowed.). H & E. ×100.

12.21

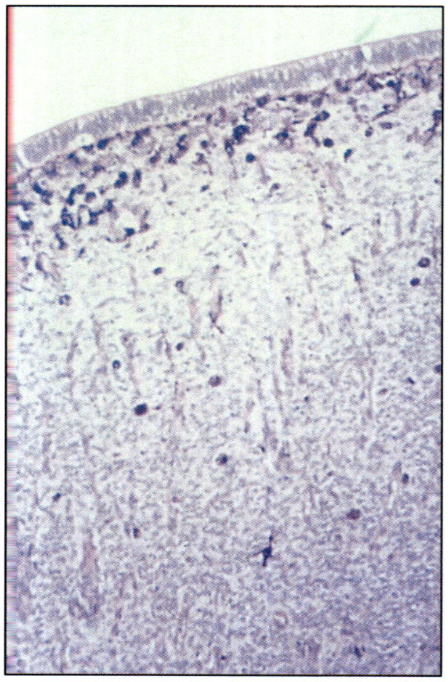

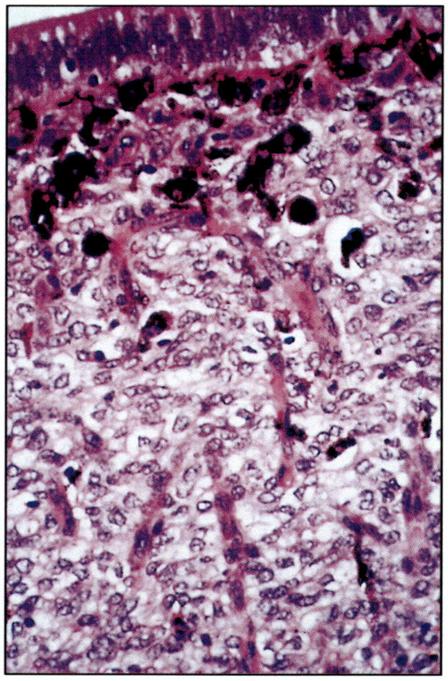

12.22

12.21 TS uterus (sheep). Only part of a caruncle is present; the connective tissue is very cellular and well vascularized. H & E. ×125.

12.22 TS uterus. Caruncle (sheep). Local deposits of pigment (melanin) are present in the connective tissue of some breeds of sheep. H & E. ×250.

12.23

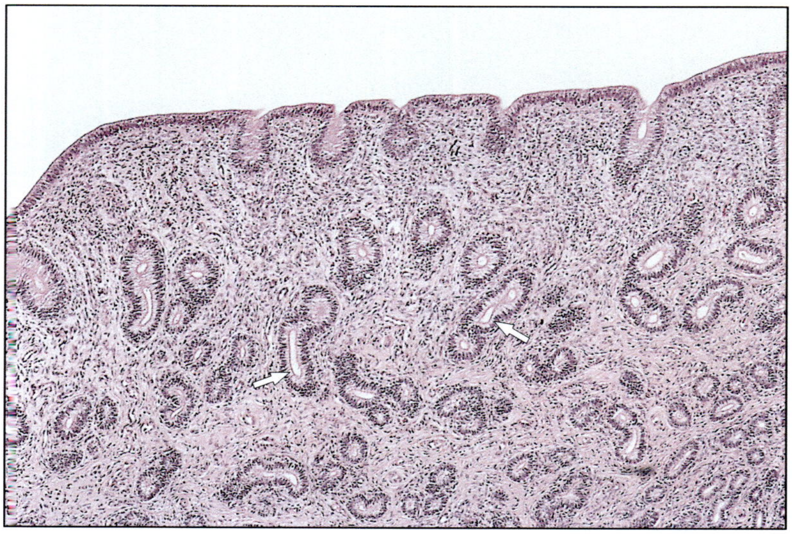

12.23 TS uterus. Intercaruncular area (sheep). The endometrial glands (arrowed) are confined to the intercaruncular area. H & E. ×100.

straight in carnivores and coiled in the mare, sow and ruminants. Caruncles are areas of non-glandular connective tissue and project into the lumen of the uterus in ruminants. They are larger when the animal is pregnant.

Myometrium

The myometrium (muscularis) is composed of a deep inner layer of circular smooth muscle and a less clearly defined outer layer of longitudinal smooth muscle. The stratum vasculare is a layer of connective tissue carrying large blood vessels to the uterus that divides the circular muscle into two layers in the cow, separates the inner and outer layers in carnivores, and forms an indistinct layer in the sow.

Perimetrium

This is the outer loose connective tissue layer or serosa, which is continuous with the broad ligament.

Cervix uteri

The mucosa appears as a series of longitudinal folds, which may become subdivided into secondary and tertiary folds (12.24). The epithelium is tall columnar with goblet cells (but areas of stratified squamous in the bitch and sow). The lamina propria is dense connective tissue, showing considerable variation according to the physiological status of the animal. The muscularis consists of an inner circular and outer longitudinal layer of smooth muscle. The serosa is loose connective tissue (12.25).

12.24 LS cervix (sheep). The mucosa has deep folds. The epithelium (1) is tall columnar mucus-secreting, and the lamina propria (2) is dense connective tissue. H & E. ×125.

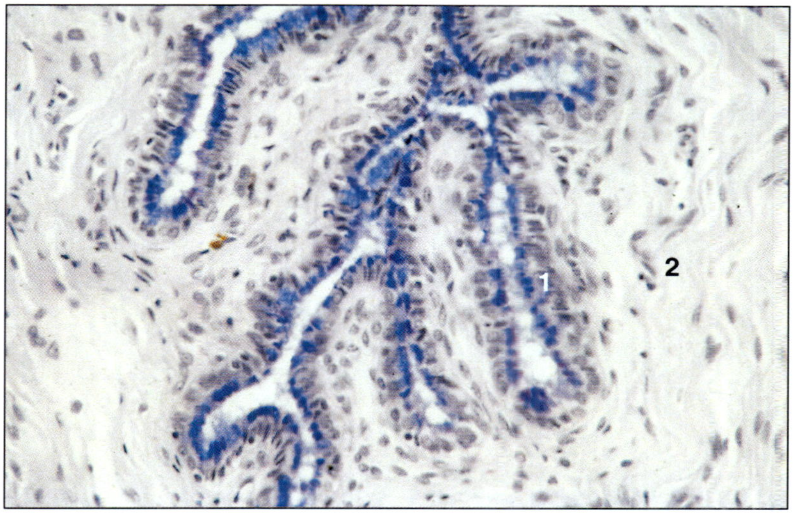

12.24

12.25 LS cervix. Sheep. The mucus is stained deep pink, and is present in the lumen and in the luminal cytoplasm of the columnar cells. H/PAS. ×250.

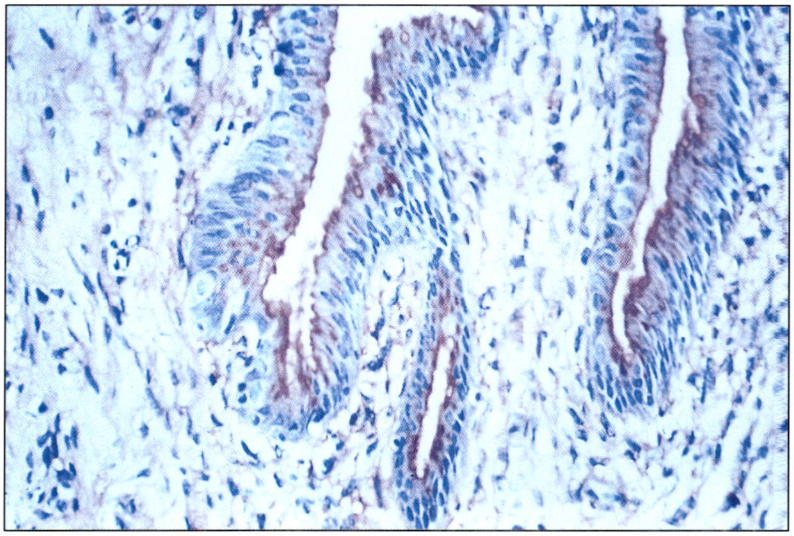

12.25

Vagina

The vaginal wall consists of three layers: mucosa, muscularis and adventitia or serosa.

The mucosa is lined with stratified squamous epithelium in all species except the cow, in which the cranial vagina is stratified columnar with goblet cells. The mucosa rests on a papillated lamina propria (12.26–12.28). The subepithelial connective tissue is very cellular, with a vascular and fibrous deeper layer. Elastic fibres are present and lymph nodules are uncommon.

The muscularis consists of inner circular and outer longitudinal smooth muscle. In the bitch, queen and sow, a thin layer of longitudinal muscle occurs internal to the circular layer.

During the breeding season, the vaginal epithelium undergoes cyclic changes. There is an oestrogen-determined proliferative stage in pro-oestrus. During oestrus in carnivores, cornification of the surface cells occurs. With development of the corpus luteum and secretion of progesterone, the surface cells desquamate and polymorphs migrate into and through the epithelium. These changes are clearly defined in the bitch and queen, and vaginal smears are used to indicate the stage of the cycle, with a high degree of accuracy (12.29–12.32). This has an important practical application in determining the exact time of mating. The vaginal changes are not well-defined in the other domestic species.

12.26

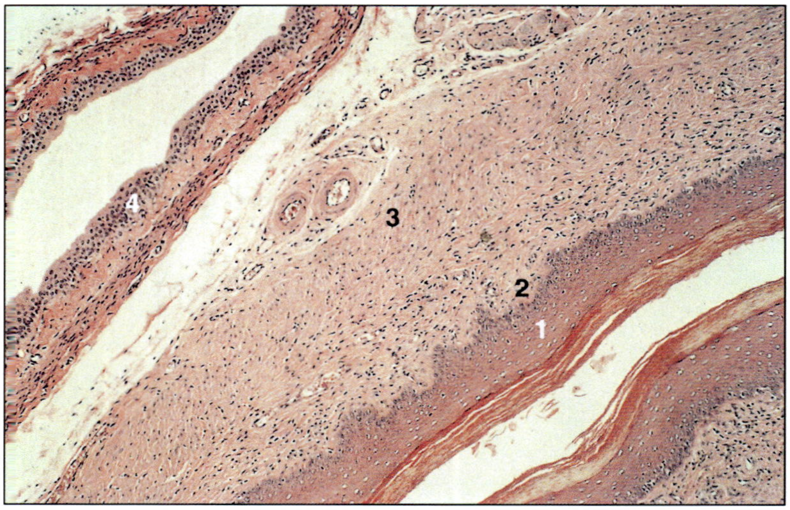

12.26 LS vagina and urethra (bitch). (1) Stratified squamous keratinized epithelium lining the vagina. (2) Papillated lamina propria. (3) Muscularis. (4) Urethelium of the urethra. H & E. ×62.5.

12.27

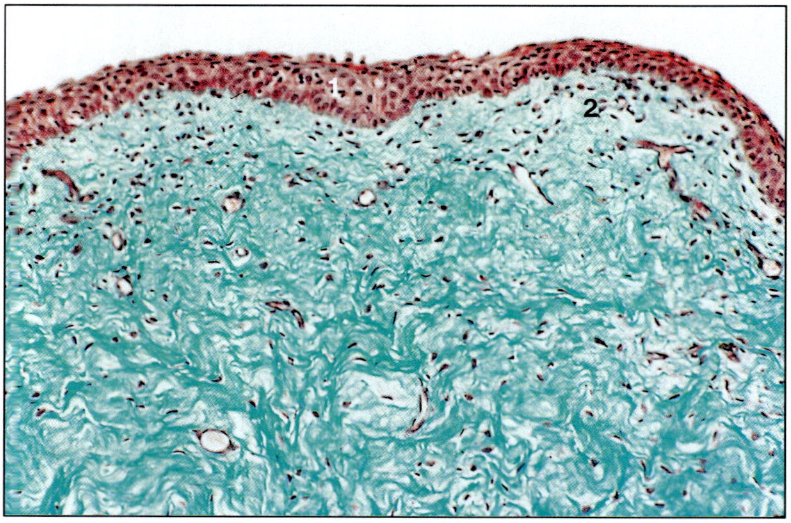

12.27 TS vagina (sheep). (1) Stratified squamous non-keratinized epithelium. (2) Lamina propria. Masson's trichrome. ×125.

12.28

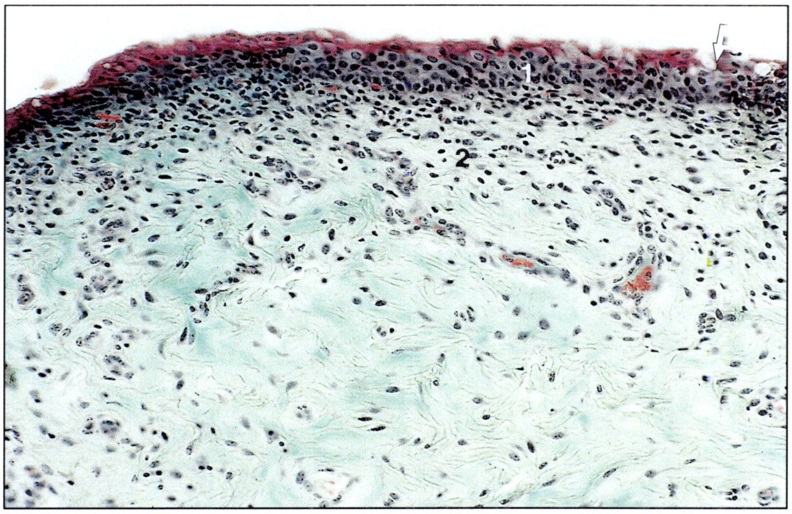

12.28 TS vagina (cow). (1) Pseudostratified epithelium with mucus-secreting cells (arrowed). (2) Cellular lamina propria. Masson's trichrome. ×125.

12.29

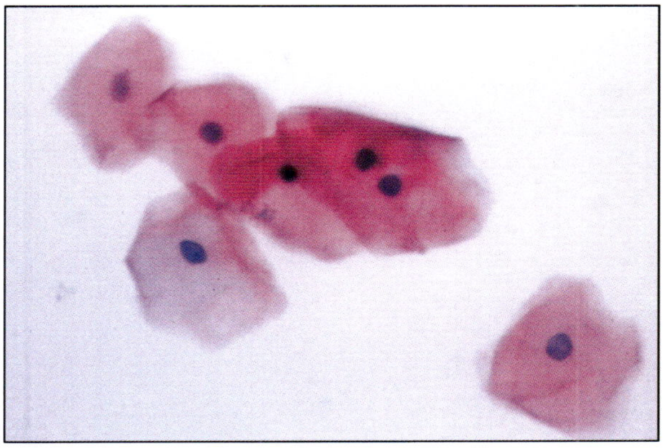

12.29 Vaginal smear. Bitch in anoestrus. This vaginal smear consists of typical nucleated epithelial cells from an anoestrus bitch. Papanicolaou. ×250.

12.30

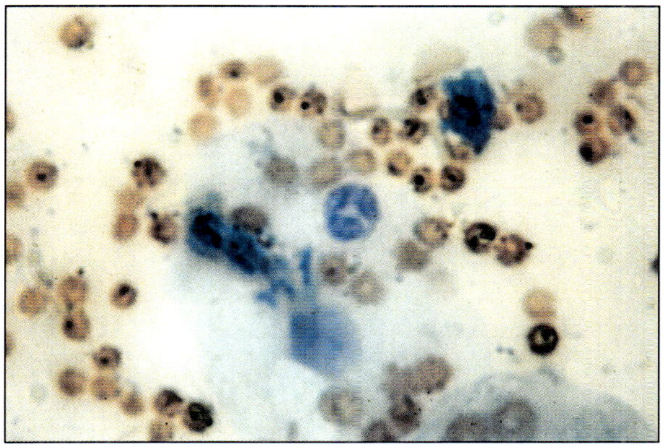

12.30 Vaginal smear. Bitch in pro-oestrus. Nucleated surface epithelial cells and erythrocytes are present. Papanicolaou. ×250.

12.31

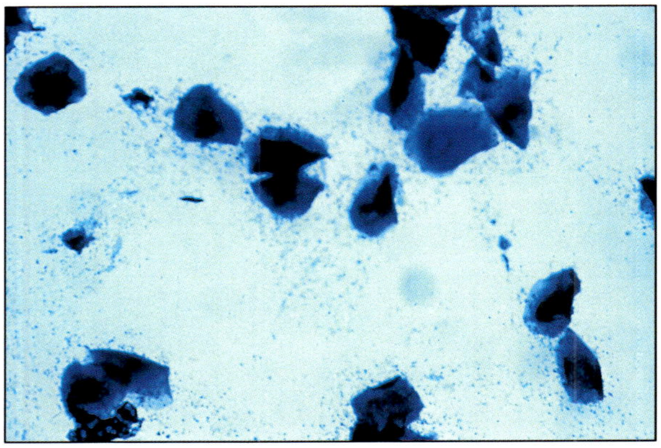

12.31 Vaginal smear. Bitch in oestrus. This is the typical 'dirty smear' of the oestrus phase of the cycle, with anucleate squames predominating. Papanicolaou. ×250.

12.32

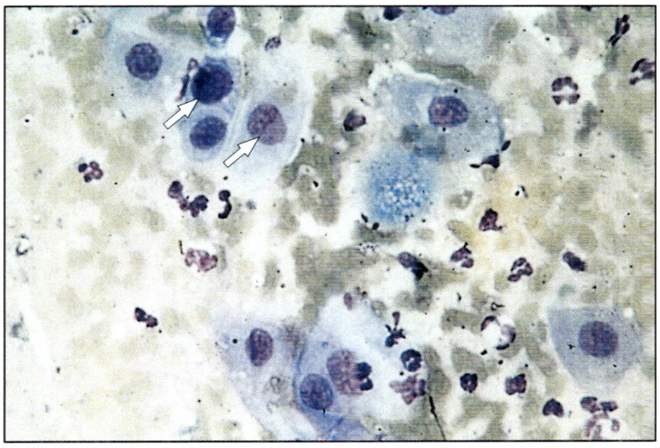

12.32 Vaginal smear. Bitch in metoestrus. Pale blue staining surface cells (arrowed) mingled with polymorphonuclear leucocytes. Papanicolaou. ×250.

Vestibule

The vestibule is lined with stratified squamous epithelium. Cyclic changes are less evident than in the vagina. The lamina propria is characterized by a plexus of large veins and vestibular bulbs, and by the major and minor mucus-secreting vestibular glands. The muscularis is a continuation of the vaginal smooth muscle. External to this is the striated muscle: the constrictor vestibuli.

Vulva, labia and clitoris

The stratified squamous epithelium of the vulva is continuous with the skin at the labia; sebaceous and sweat glands are present in the lamina propria. The clitoris, like the penis, consists of erectile tissue (corpus cavernosum clitoridis), a glans and a prepuce.

Mammary glands

The mammary glands are the distinguishing feature of the mammal and are modifed sweat glands that secrete milk. Each gland is enclosed in a muscular fibroelastic capsule extending into the substance of the gland and dividing it into lobes and lobules. In the non-lactating gland the lobules consist of a duct system surrounded by loose connective tissue, separated from the adjoining lobules by fatty interlobular tissue (**12.33**). During pregnancy the duct system expands at the expense of this tissue and it is reduced to thin strands of vascular connective tissue as parturition approaches.

The terminal parts of the ducts expand to form secretory saccules (alveoli) lined with cuboidal/low columnar epithelium (**12.34–12.36**). Myoepithelial cells lie between the secretory cells and the basement membrane. Plasma cells are numerous in the stroma immediately postpartum, and immunoglobulin is passed via the saccules into the colostrum (first milk) where it provides a passive immunity to the neonate. The saccules open onto the interlobular ducts that empty into the lactiferous ducts and lactiferous sinuses at the base of the teat. Initially, the epithelium is columnar, then bicolumnar then bistratified cuboidal. In the larger ducts some smooth muscle cells are present in the wall.

The papilla or teat contains the main excretory duct (or ducts depending on the species: one for the cow; two to three for the mare and sow; four to seven for the queen; seven to 16 for the bitch; **12.37** and **12.38**). The epithelium is bicolumnar, changing to stratified squamous at the external orifice. The lamina propria has abundant elastic fibres. The muscularis consists of inner and outer layers of smooth muscle with a middle circular layer, and condenses to form a sphincter in the cow, sow and bitch. In the cow, complex epithelial folds are present in the upper part of the papillary duct. In the cow and sow the skin covering the teat is hairless and non-glandular; in the mare, bitch and queen, abundant sebaceous glands and fine hairs are present.

12.33

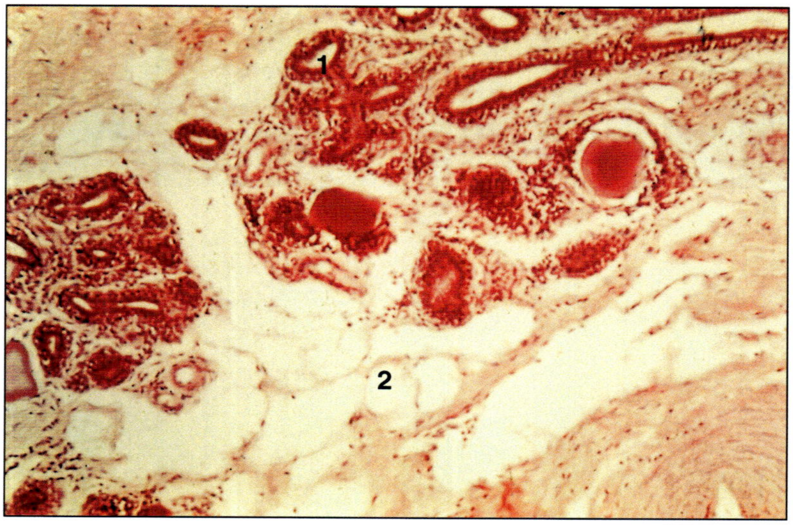

12.33 Non-lactating mammary gland (cow). (1) Only the densely staining remnants of the duct system are present. (2) Interlobular adipose connective tissue. H & E. ×62.5.

12.34

12.34 Lactating mammary gland (cow). (1) The duct system expands and terminates in (2) the secretory alveoli in the active gland. The connective tissue is reduced to a supporting role. H & E. ×62.5.

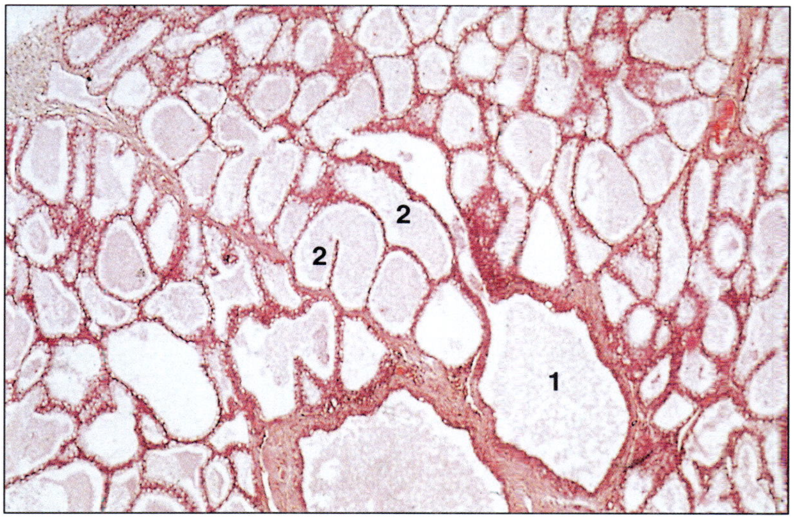

.35

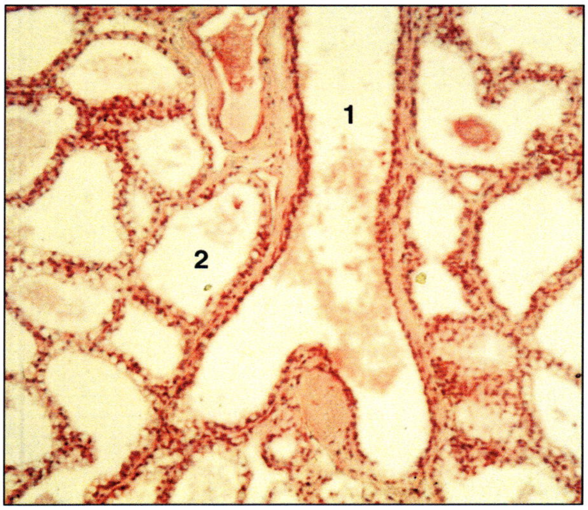

12.35 Lactating mammary gland (cow). (1) Large excretory lobular duct. (2) Secretory alveoli. H & E. ×125.

12.36

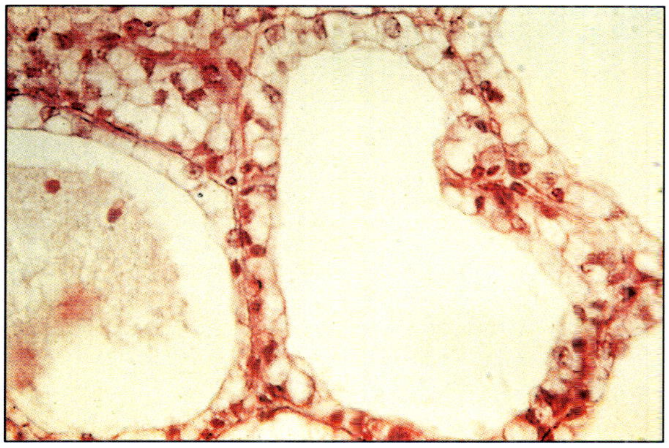

12.36 Lactating mammary gland (cow). The secretory alveoli are lined by a cuboidal epithelium. Loss of fat in processing causes the empty appearance of the cells. H & E. ×250.

.37

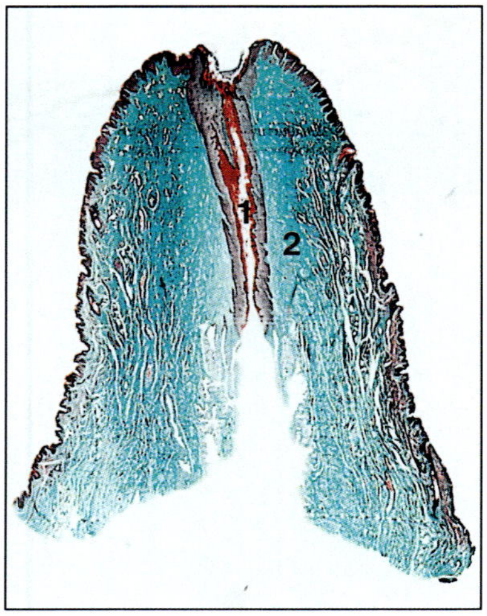

12.37 LS teat (sheep). (1) The teat canal is lined by stratified squamous epithelium. (2) The connective tissue of the lamina propria is continuous with that of the skin. Masson's trichrome. ×7.5.

12.38

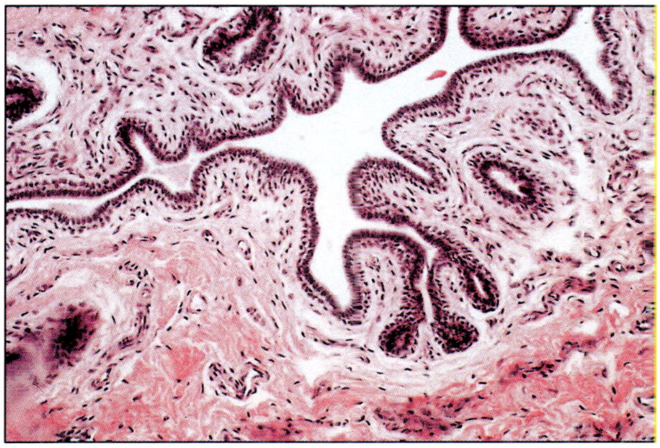

12.38 TS teat canal (cow). The columnar epithelium lining the canal is folded. H & E. ×25.

Placentation

The extra-embryonic fetal membranes are developed from the fertilized egg and are not part of the developing embryo, but establish an intimate apposition with the endometrium at implantation for the purpose of physiological exchange. This is the placenta. The fetal membranes are the amnion, the yolk sac, the allantois and the chorion, and these are derived from the three basic germ layers (ectoderm, mesoderm and endoderm) in a variety of combinations. This is illustrated diagrammatically in **12.39–12.43**, and a classification is given in Appendix Table 3.

The histological classification of the placenta is based on the concept that placental exchange during pregnancy is dependant on the approximation of the fetal and the maternal capillary bed: the interhaemal membrane. In **12.44** there are six layers separating the fetal and maternal bloods.

In the type of placenta where all six layers persist, the chorionic epithelium (trophectoderm/ trophoblast) is apposed to the maternal epithelium; this is an epitheliochorial placenta. There is no

12.39

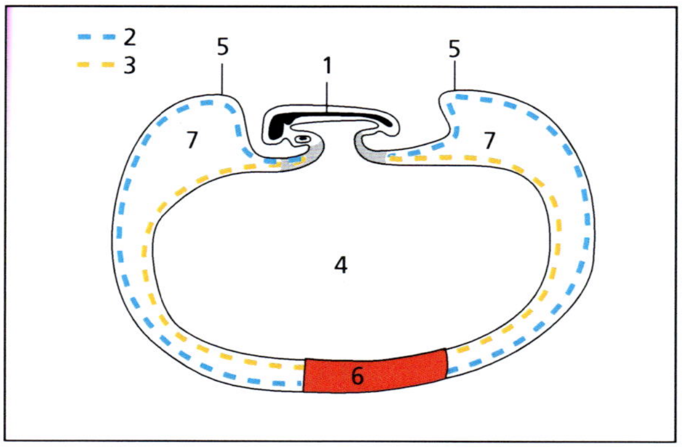

12.4

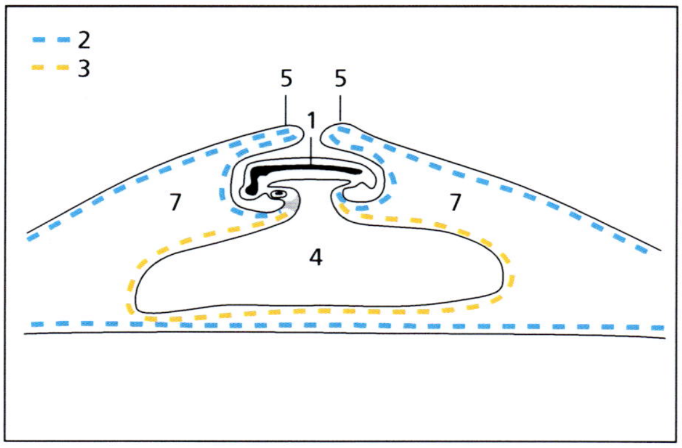

12.41

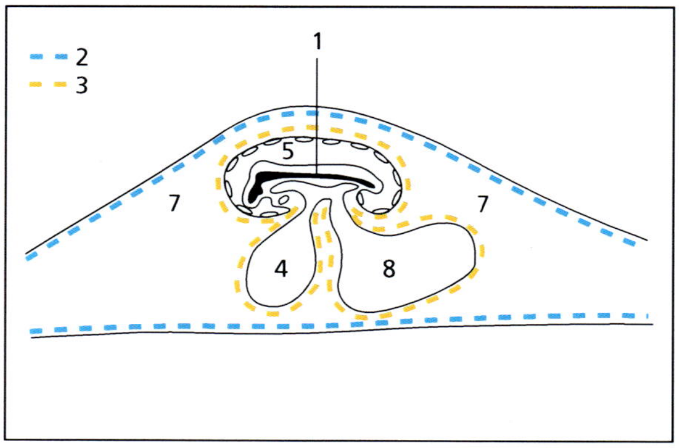

12.4

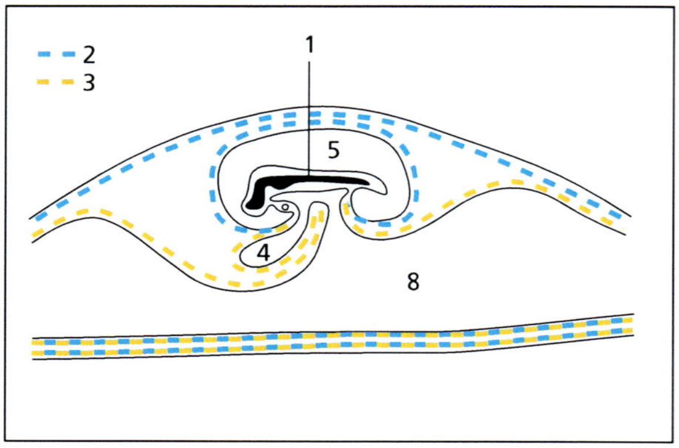

12.43

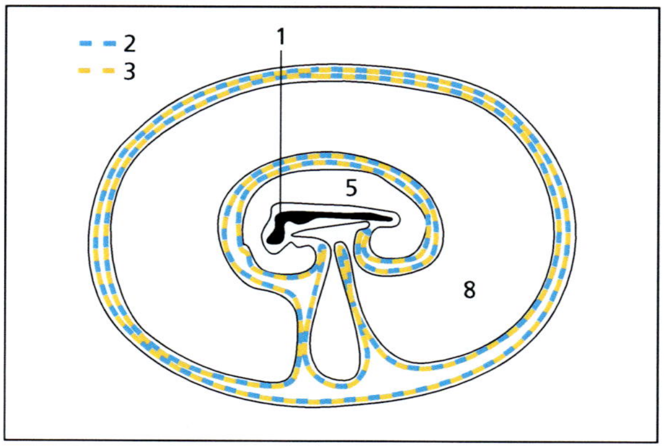

12.39–12.43 **12.39–12.41** illustrate the common early stages of development of the extra-embryonic membranes. **12.42** illustrates the cow, sheep and pig and **12.43** illustrates the mare and carnivore. (1) Embryo. (2) Somatopleure (ectoderm + somatic mesoderm) forms the lateral and ventral walls of the fetus. (3) Splanchnopleure (endoderm + splanchnic mesoderm) forms the digestive tube. (4) Yolk sac. (5) Amniotic folds. (6) Unsplit mesoderm. (7) Extra-embryonic coelom. (8) Allantois.

destruction of maternal tissue and no loss at parturition; therefore, it is non-deciduate. This type of placentation is seen in the sow, mare and ruminant. Apposition occurs over the extensive chorionic sac in the sow and mare, a diffuse placenta, and specifically at the caruncle–cotyledon interface in the ruminant, a cotyledonary placenta.

In the carnivore there is considerable destruction of the maternal tissues in the central band of the gestational sac and the chorionic epithelium (trophoblast/trophectoderm) is apposed to the endothelium of the maternal blood vessels. This is a zonary endotheliochorial placenta. In rodents, lagomorphs and primates the maternal tissue is destroyed over a limited discoidal area, and the trophoblast is bathed by maternal blood. Some maternal tissue is lost at parturition; therefore, the placenta is deciduate.

The placenta is a complex endocrine gland genetically programmed to remain for a species-specific period.

12.44

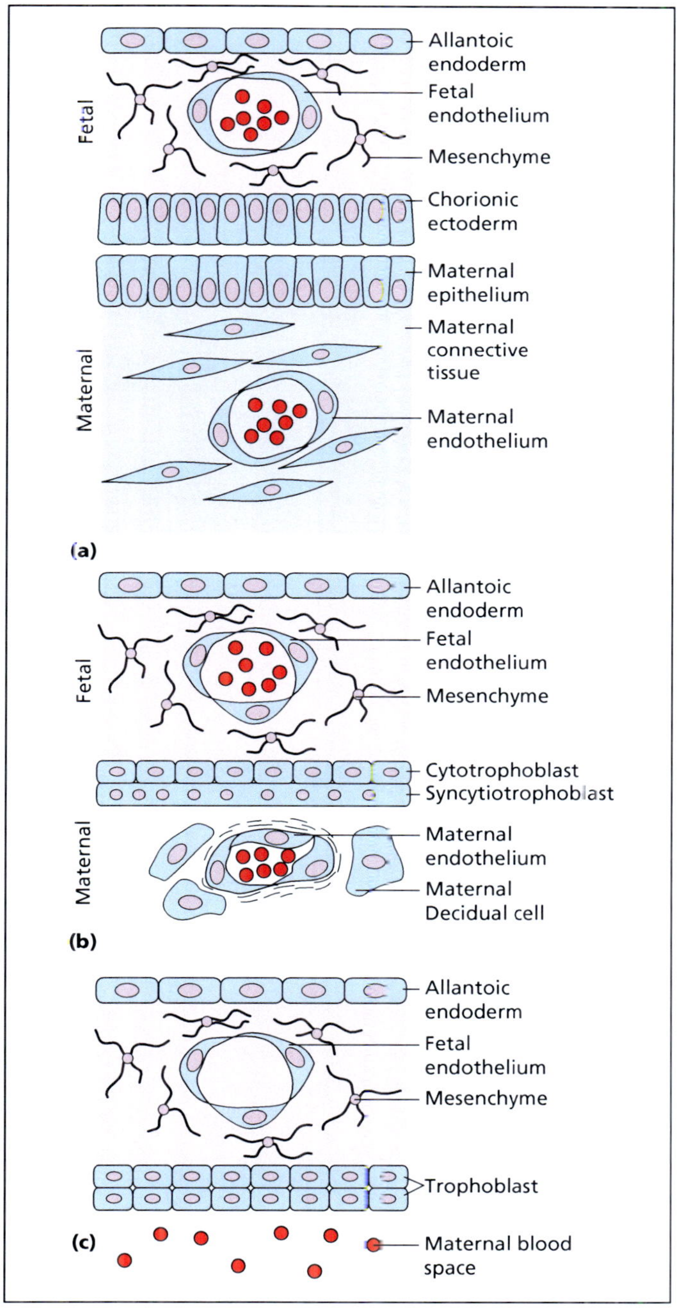

12.44 Histological classification of the placenta. (a) Sow, mare and ruminant; (b) endotheliochorial placenta, dog and cat; (c) haemochrial placenta, rodents, primates and man.

Sow

Sows have a diffuse, epitheliochorial, non-deciduate placenta, and a gestation period of 114 days.

In the early placenta the chorioallantois is folded and simply apposed to the endometrial folds. Both epithelia are columnar and the capillary bed is subepithelial. As pregnancy advances the membranes increase in volume, the epithelial surfaces become interlocked, the epithelium is reduced in height, the folds become more complex, and the capillaries on both sides in the immediate subepithelial tissue often project between the epithelial cells where they are known as intraepithelial capillaries (**12.45** and **12.46**). Specialized areas, the areolae, exist for the absorption of uterine milk. The endometrial glands secrete into a space between the chorion and the endometrium, and the trophoblast cells are tall columnar absorptive (**12.47** and **12.48**).

12.45

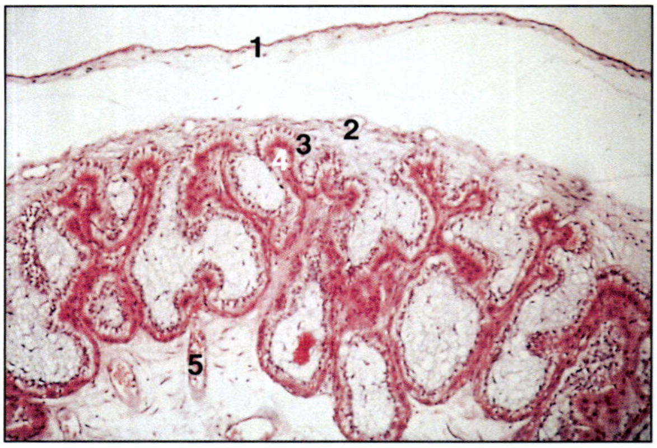

12.45 Epitheliochorial placenta (sow). (1) Allantoic endoderm lining the allantoic sac. (2) Mesenchyme. (3) Trophectoderm. (4) Maternal epithelium. (5) Maternal blood vessels in the endometrium. The simple folding of the early pig placenta is shown here. H & E. ×25.

12.4

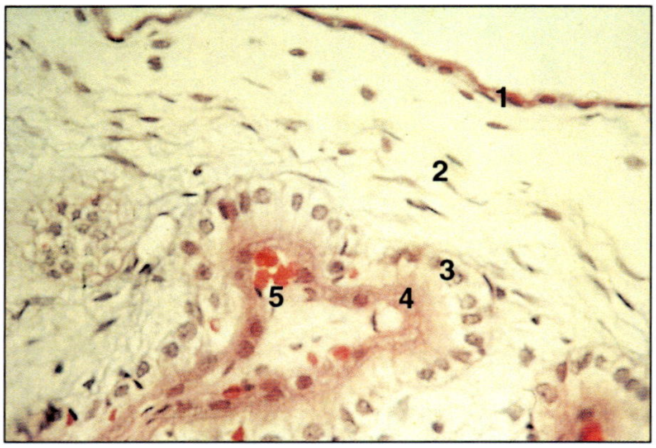

12.46 Epitheliochorial placenta (sow). (1) Allantoic endoderm. (2) Mesenchyme. (3) Trophectoderm. (4) Maternal epithelium. (5) Maternal blood vessels in the endometrium. H & E. ×100.

12.47

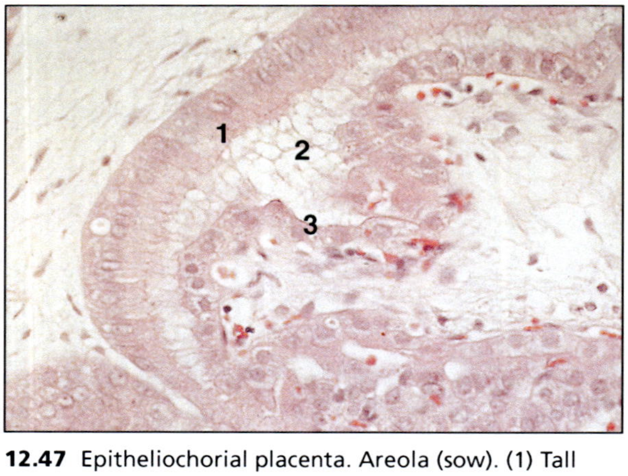

12.47 Epitheliochorial placenta. Areola (sow). (1) Tall columnar absorptive trophectodermal cells. (2) Endometrial gland secretion. (3) Maternal epithelium. H & E. ×100.

12.4

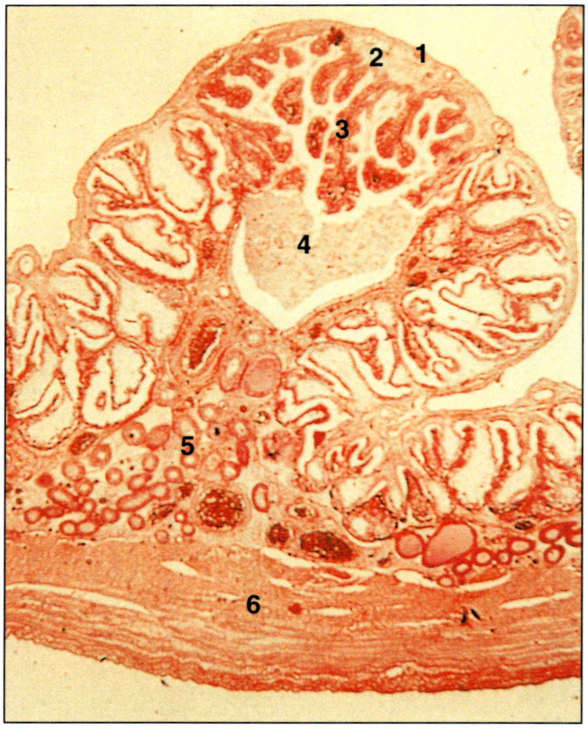

12.48 Epitheliochorial placenta. Areola of late gestation (sow). (1) Allantoic endoderm. (2) Mesenchyme. (3) Fetal villi covered by absorptive trophectoderm. (4) Endometrial gland secretion. (5) Endometrial glands. (6) Myometrium. H & E. ×25.

Mare

Mares have a diffuse, epitheliochorial, non-deciduate placenta, and a gestation period of 331–350 days.

The membranes develop slowly in the mare and a choriovitelline placenta is established in early pregnancy; simple folding very similar to that in the sow is seen. Short simple villi now appear over the chorionic sac with the development of the chorioallantois (**12.49**). As pregnancy advances, the villi branch repeatedly to form complex tufts embedded in the endometrium; these are called placental units or microcotyledons.

The chorionic epithelium between them is highly absorptive and the endometrial glands secrete into the space to form an areola (**12.50** and **12.51**).

Endometrial cups are peculiar to the mare and are only present from weeks 5–20 of gestation. The endometrial epithelium disappears over small areas, the endometrial glands hypertrophy and decidual cells (of fetal origin) migrate into the maternal tissue (**12.52**). A brown coagulum accumulates between the fetal and the maternal tissue, the richest known source of gonadotrophic hormone. This is responsible for the second wave of follicles and corpora lutea seen in the mare after the loss of the corpus luteum of pregnancy.

.49

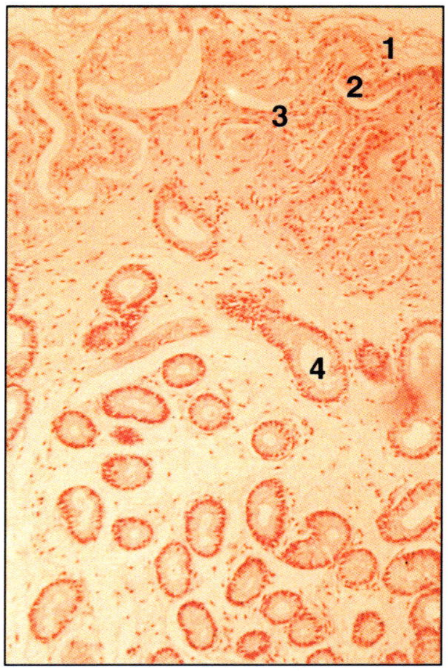

12.50

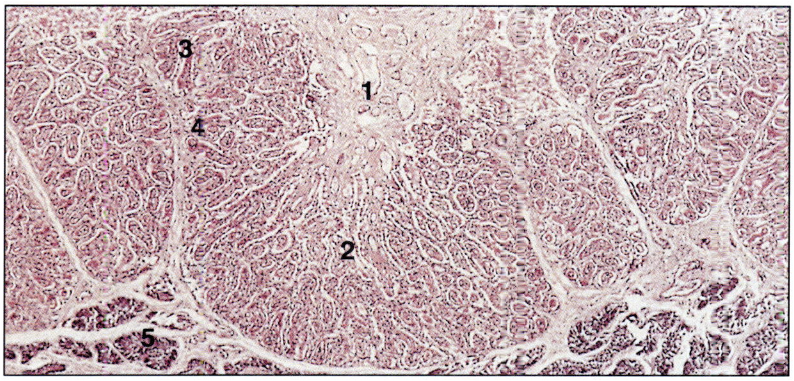

12.50 Epitheliochorial placenta (mare). (1) Main stem fetal villus. (2) Microcotyledon. (3) Absorptive trophectoderm, the areola. (4) Uterine milk. (5) Endometrial glands. H & E. ×25.

12.49 Epitheliochorial placenta (mare). In this early gestation example of the mare placenta, short simple villi indent the maternal tissue. (1) Mesenchyme. (2) Trophectoderm. (3) Maternal epithelium. (4) Endometrial glands. H & E. ×62.5

12.51

12.51 Epitheliochorial placenta. Mare in late gestation. (1) Main stem fetal villus. (2) Absorptive trophectoderm. (3) Interlocking fetal/maternal tissue of the microcotyledon. H & E. ×62.5.

12.52 Epitheliochorial placenta. Endometrial cup (mare). Only the endometrium is present. (1) Area of eroded maternal epithelium. (2) Distended endometrial glands. (3) Decidual cells. (4) Lymphocytes. H & E. ×62.5.

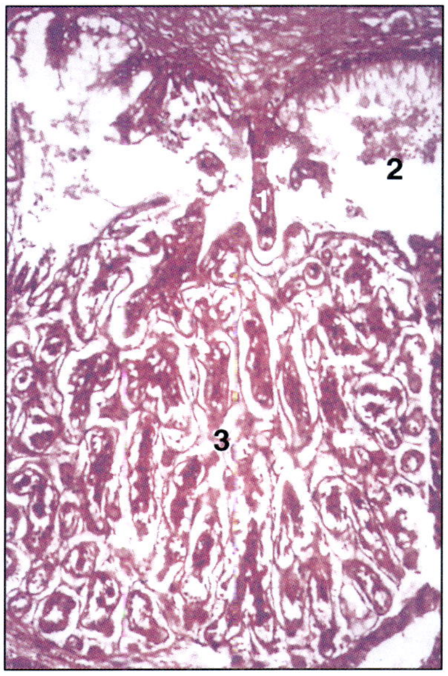

12 52

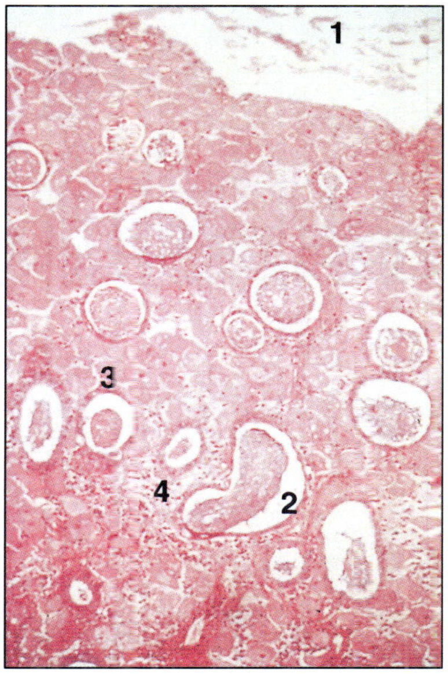

Ruminants

Ruminants have an epitheliochorial, cotyledonary, non-deciduate placenta, and the following gestation periods: cow, 279–282 days; ewe, 148–150 days; and goat, 150 days.

Apposition to the endometrium begins with the development of focal areas of short simple villi, called cotyledons, on the chorionic surface opposite the caruncle. Folding of the caruncle creates crypts and the villi project into these to form a complex arrangement of interlocking fetal/maternal tissue: the placentome. Binucleate giant cells are present in the trophoblast from day 16 of gestation. In the ewe the maternal epithelium is often so attenuated that it is difficult to see with the light microscope. In the cow the epithelium is cuboidal or even columnar through pregnancy. Maternal blood is released at the tips of the septae and absorbed by the trophoblast: arcade haemorrhages. The uterine glands secrete onto the uterine surface in the intercaruncular zone and areas of absorptive trophoblast form areolae (12.53–12.58).

12.53

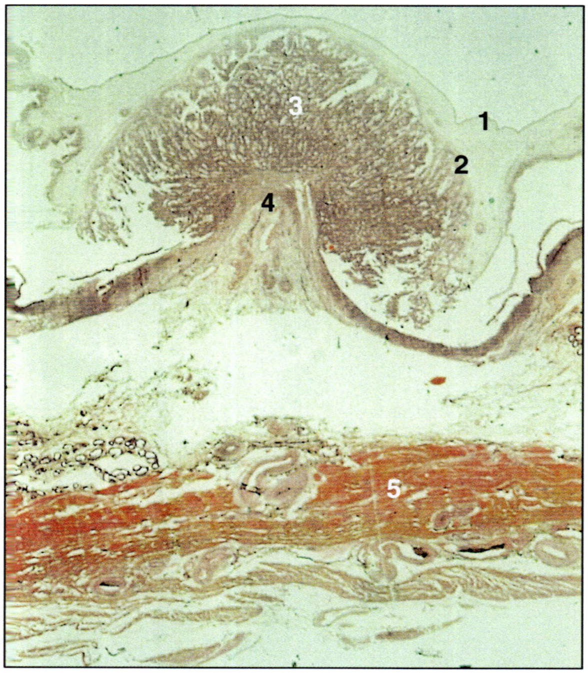

12.53 Epitheliochorial placenta (cow). This is an early bovine placentome; note the convex appearance. (1) Endoderm lining the allantois. (2) Chorioallantoic membrane. (3) Interlocked fetal/maternal tissue. (4) Endometrium at the caruncle. (5) Myometrium. H & E. ×17.5.

12.54

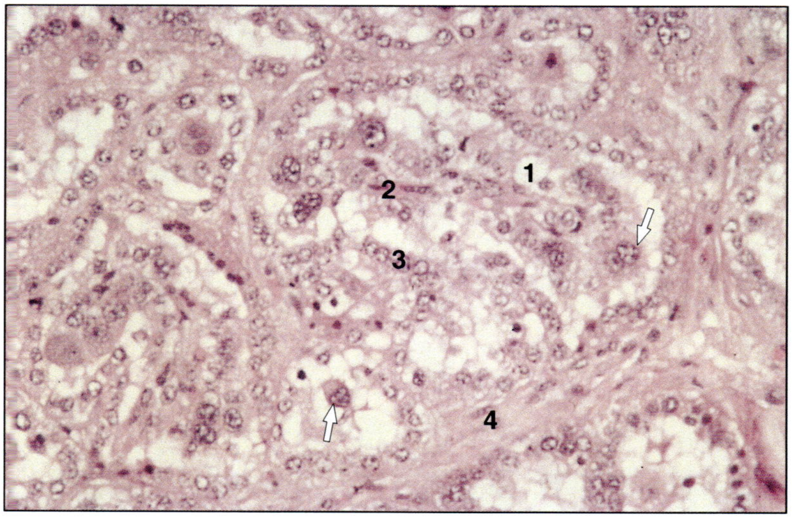

12.54 Epitheliochorial placenta (cow). (1) Mesenchyme. (2) Trophectoderm. (3) Maternal epithelium. (4) Maternal connective tissue. The binucleate giant cells are arrowed. H & E. ×125.

12.55 Epitheliochorial placenta (cow). (1) Dark strands of maternal connective tissue. (2) Maternal epithelium. (3) Trophectoderm with binucleate giant cells. (4) Mesenchyme. H & E. ×125.

12.55

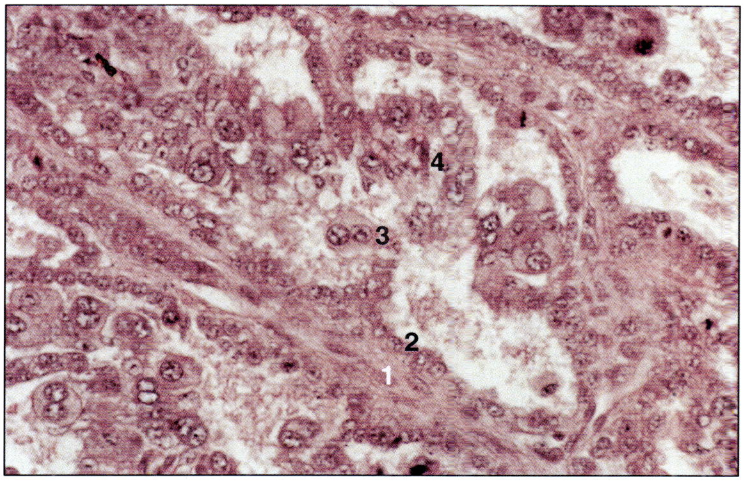

12.56 Epitheliochorial placenta. Placentome (sheep). Note the concave appearance of the placentome. (1) The chorioallantoic membrane projecting into the caruncle. (2) Endometrium of the caruncle surrounding the chorioallantois. (3) Myometrium. (4) Intercaruncular area. H & E. ×7.5.

12.56

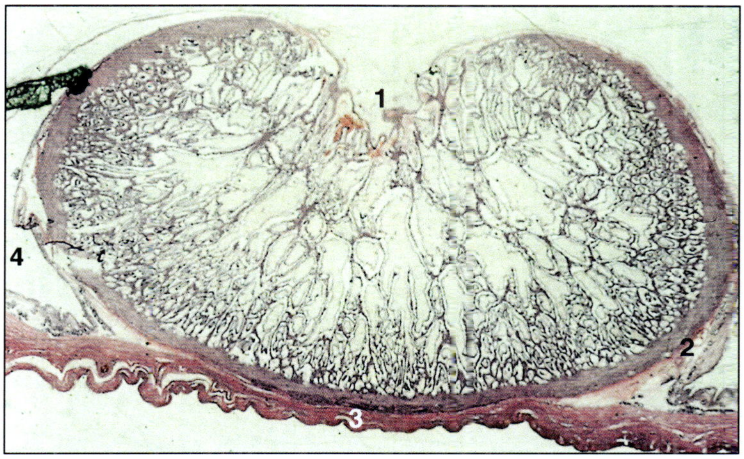

.57

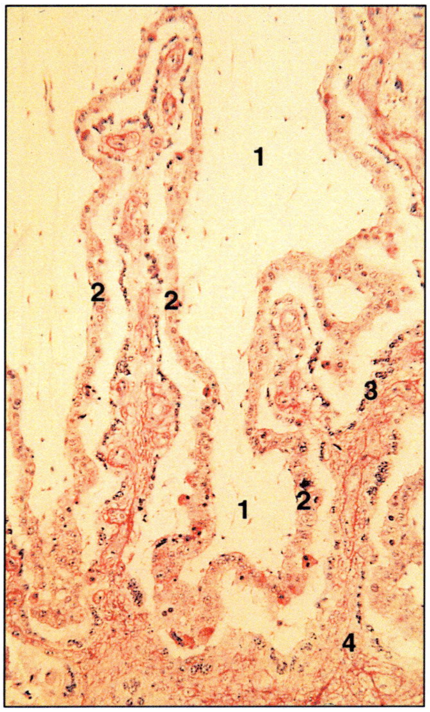

12.58

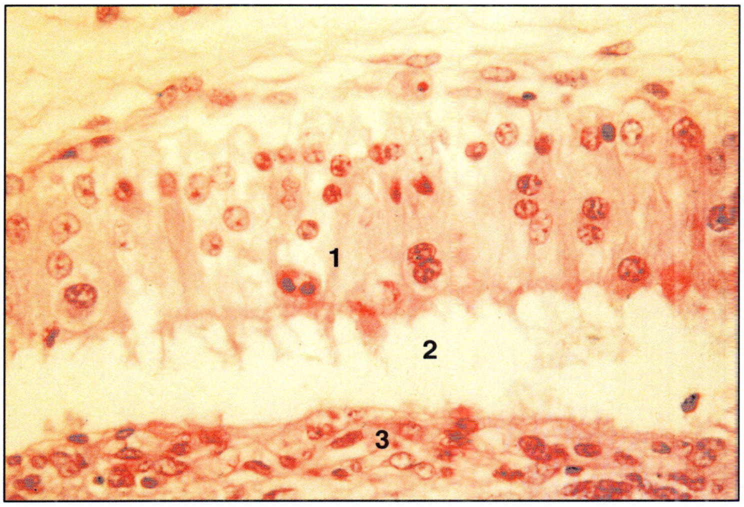

12.58 Epitheliochorial placenta. Intercaruncular area (sheep). (1) Absorptive trophectoderm with giant cells. (2) Uterine milk. (3) Endometrium, note the apparent absence of epithelium. H & E. ×160.

12.57 Epitheliochorial placenta. Placentome (sheep). (1) Mesenchyme of the chorioallantois. (2) Trophectoderm with giant cells. (3) Maternal epithelium. (4) Maternal connective tissue. H & E. ×62.5.

Carnivores

Carnivores have an endotheliochorial, zonary deciduate placenta, and the following gestation periods: bitch, 58–65 days; and queen, 60 days.

The trophoblast in the central zone of the choriovitelline placenta becomes two-layered, with an outer syncytial layer, the syncytiotrophoblast, and an inner cellular layer, the cytotrophoblast. Cords of trophoblast block the mouths of the uterine glands and secrete lytic enzymes, destroying the maternal tissue. With the development of the more invasive chorioallantois, the maternal tissue is further eroded and the trophoblast is apposed to the endothelium of the maternal blood vessels (**12.59** and **12.60**).

Decidual cells, probably fetal in origin, are also present. Haematomata are present on the margin of the zonary band (bitch) and centrally dispersed (queen). These are pools of maternal blood surrounded by absorptive trophoblast, where maternal erythrocytes have been destroyed; these are the haemophagous zones. A green deposit of uteroverdin occurs in the bitch and a brown deposit in the queen. Outside the zonary band there is simple apposition of chorion and endometrium with no loss of maternal tissue at parturition, as opposed to the zonary band where damage is considerable (**12.61, 12.62**).

12.59

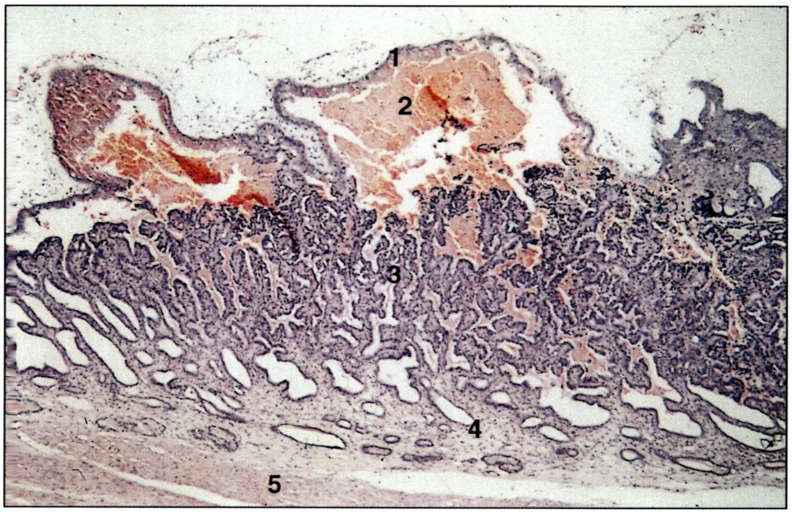

12.59 Endotheliochorial placenta. Cat placental band. (1) Absorptive trophectoderm. (2) Haematoma, pools of maternal blood. (3) Interlocking zone of fetal/maternal tissue. (4) Endometrium. (5) Myometrium. H & E. 7.5.

12.60

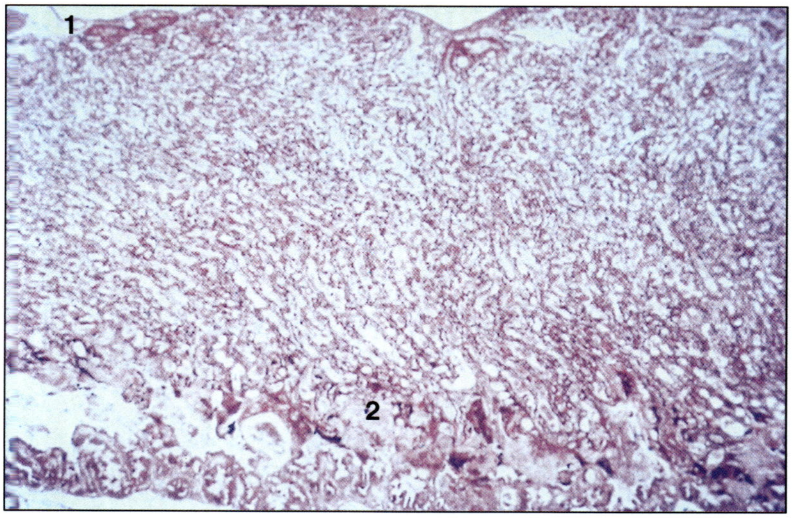

12.60 Endotheliochorial placenta. Placental band in the bitch. The lamellae are more regular than in the cat. (1) Chorioallantoic membrane. (2) Junctional zone marks the deep penetration of fetal tissue. H & E. ×25.

12.61

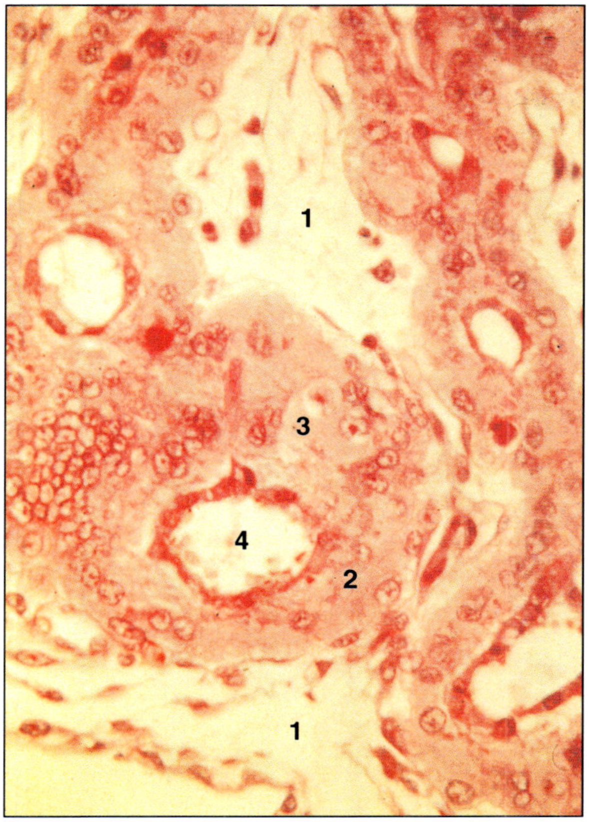

12.61 Endotheliochorial placenta (bitch). (1) Chorioallantoic mesenchyme. (2) Trophectoderm. (3) Decidual cell. (4) Maternal blood vessels lined by thickened endothelium. H & E. ×200.

12.62

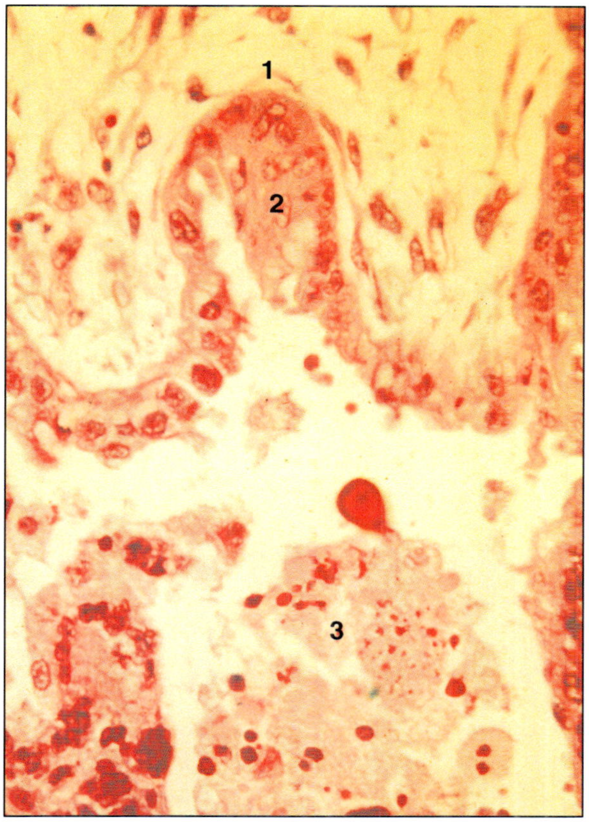

12.62 Endotheliochorial placenta (bitch). This represents the junctional zone, the limit of the fetal invasion (1) Chorioallantoic mesenchyme. (2) Trophectoderm. (3) Maternal tissue debris. H & E. ×200.

Umbilical cord

The umbilical cord is the communications link between the fetus and the placenta. The umbilical arteries leave the fetus and carry deoxygenated blood to the placenta. The umbilical veins carry nutrient blood to the fetus (these commonly fuse to form a single vein). The umbilical vesicle is the remnant of the yolk sac and the small canal is the lumen of the allantoic duct (12.63).

12.63

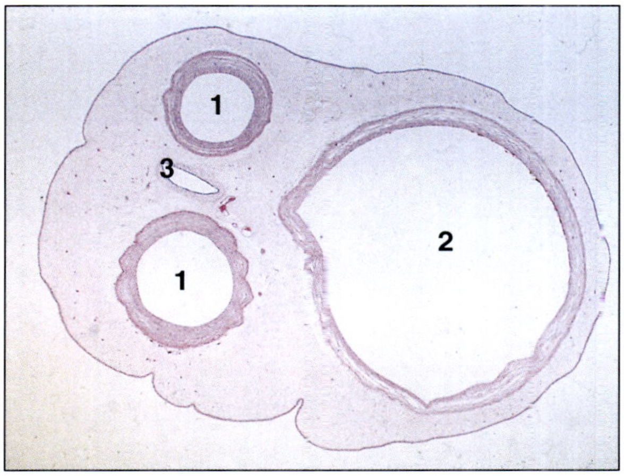

12.63 Umbilical cord (foal). (1) Umbilical arteries. (2) Umbilical vein. (3) Allantoic duct. H & E. ×7.5.

Clinical correlates

Mammary glands

Inflammation of the mammary glands, termed mastitis, can affect any mammal and is most common in the lactating mammary gland, where the moist, nutrient-rich secretions provide an ideal environment for growth of microorganisms.

A variety of mammary tumours are recognized and several classification schemes exist that divide the tumours according to the cell types and patterns of growth present. For example, a mixed mammary tumour (**12.64**) is derived from more than a single germ layer and includes epithelium, myoepithelium, cartilage and possibly bone. In the bitch, early ovariohysterectomy is known to reduce significantly the incidence of future mammary tumour development. True behavioural malignancy is recognized in a minority of canine mammary tumours, but is present in a higher proportion of mammary tumours in the cat (**12.65, 12.66**). Rats of both sexes have extensive mammary-type glandular tissue and may present with masses of this origin anywhere from the neck to the inguinal region. Most are benign fibroadenomas. Mammary tumours are also recognized in the rabbit (**12.67**).

12.64

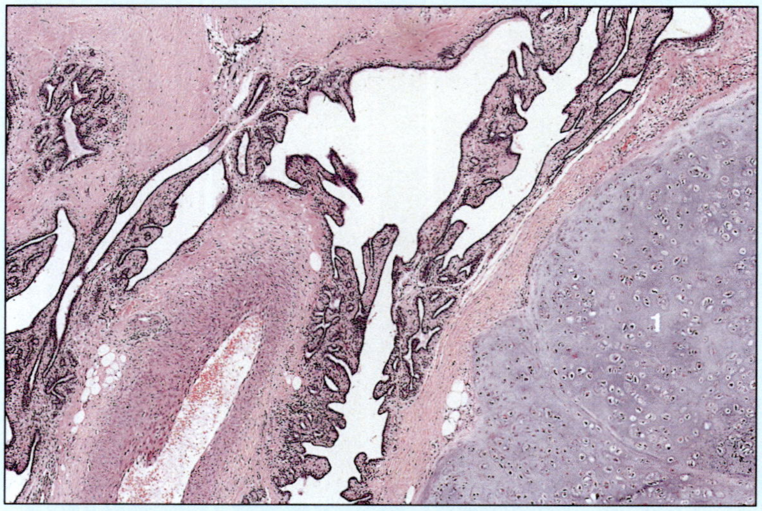

12.64 Mixed mammary tumour from an elderly bitch. In addition to glandular epithelial and stromal components, cartilage (1) is formed. The glandular lumina are dilated and the epithelium is arranged in a single layer. This tumour is benign. H & E. ×62.5.

12.65

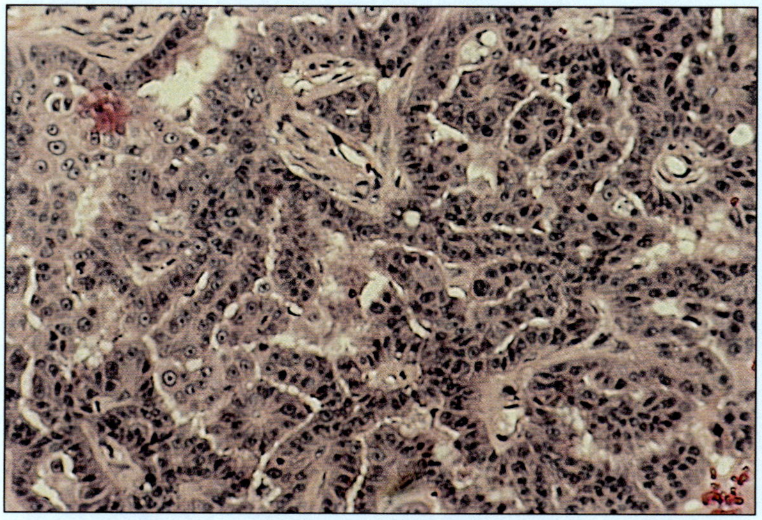

12.65 Feline mammary papillary cystadenocarcinoma. The cells in this malignant tumour form multiple frond-like papillae that extend into cystic spaces. H & E. ×125.

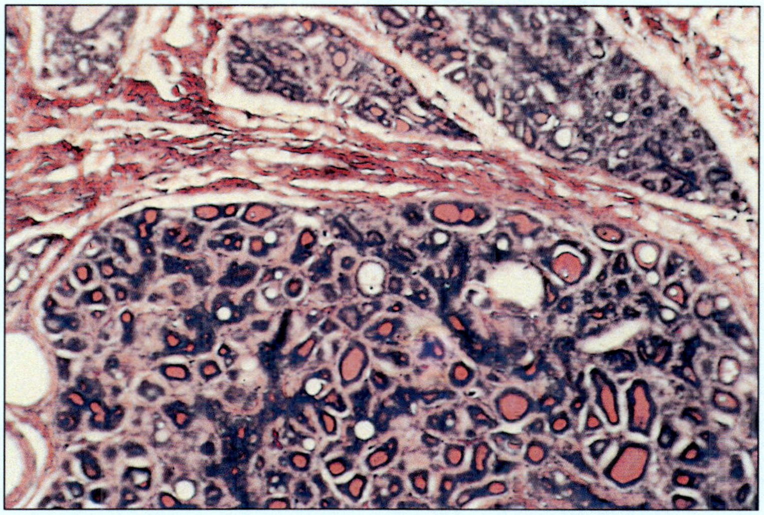

12.66

12.66 Feline ductal adenocarcinoma. The thin-walled ductal structures are filled with eosinophilic proteinaceous secretion and are divided by fibrocollagenous connective tissue. Invasion into surrounding tissue and lymphatic metastasis are common with this type of tumour. H & E. ×62.5.

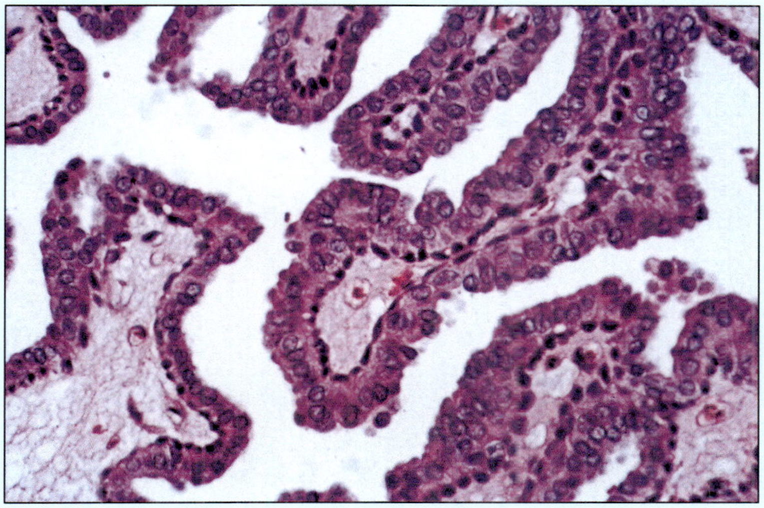

12.67

12.67 Mammary adenoma from an adult female rabbit. This high-power view shows frond-like papillary projections with fibrous cores overlain by well-differentiated columnar epithelium. H & E. ×250.

Female reproductive system

Developmental disorders of the genital system occur in all species of domestic animals, but are uncommon. These disorders are caused by abnormalities of genetic origin or by aberrant hormonal influences. Often, precise mechanisms have not been defined, but specific syndromes, such as freemartinism in cattle, are recognized. A freemartin is a genetically female calf twinned with a male. If, as is common, anastomoses form between the placental circulations, then factors passed between the twins lead to abnormalities in the female reproductive system, including inhibition of ovarian development or testis-like differentiation within the ovary and the absence of parts of the tubular tract. Effects on the male twin are minimal.

A spectrum of cystic changes are recognized in the mammalian ovary. Cystic ovarian disease in cows is important as a cause of reproductive failure and hence economic loss. Tumours that arise from tissues which are specifically ovarian can be divided into three broad categories: tumours of the surface coelomic epithelium, those of the gonadal stroma and those of the germ cells. Tumours of the surface epithelium are significant only in the bitch as papillary and cystic adenomas and rarely papillary adenocarcinomas. Tumours that arise from the gonadal stroma include granulosa (**12.68**) and thecal (**12.69**) cell tumours. These neoplasms can produce hormones and are rarely malignant in any species. Germ cell tumours include dysgerminomas (**12.70**) and teratomas (**12.71**). The dysgerminoma is morphologically similar to primordial germ cells and resembles its testicular homologue, the seminoma. In teratomas the totipotential germ cells have undergone somatic differentiation and a variety of tissues of different germ lines are present within the tumour.

Obstructive and inflammatory conditions are recognized in the uterine (Fallopian) tubes. A range of inflammatory, hyperplastic or cystic changes (**12.72**) that are under hormonal influence can affect the uterus itself. Hyperplastic change, which is usually focal within the uterus, does not appear to be preneoplastic in domestic animal species, but is an important precancerous indicator in humans. Uterine neoplasia is uncommon in most domestic species, although obviously many female domestic animals are neutered. In the rabbit, however, uterine adenocarcinoma occurs in a large percentage of adult females (**12.73**).

12.68

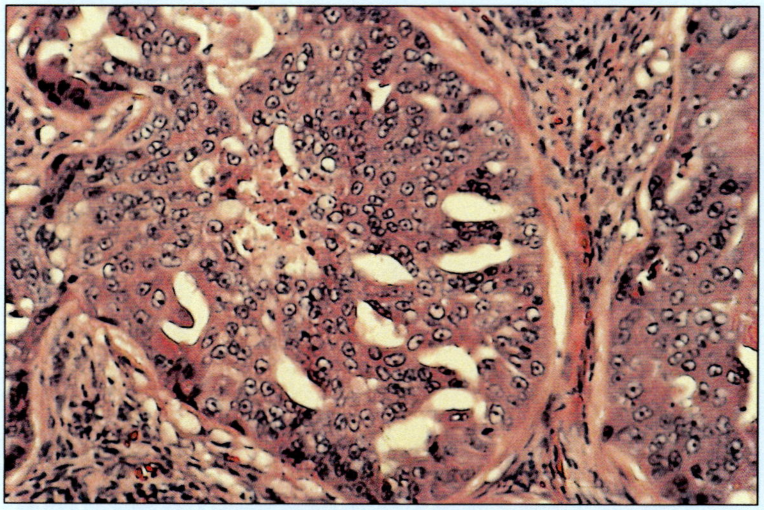

12.68 Canine ovarian granulosa cell tumour. This is the most common gonadostromal tumour in all species. Histological appearances vary. This section shows a lobular mass with clefting between the tumour cells. H & E. ×125.

12.69

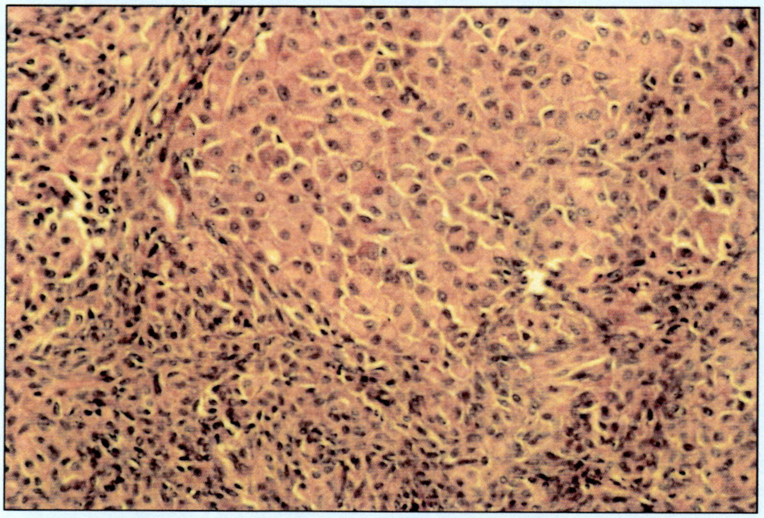

12.69 Canine ovarian thecoma in a 12-year-old Springer Spaniel bitch. The tumour cells are large and polyhedral, contain finely granular eosinophilic cytoplasm, and are arranged in solid lobules separated from each other by a fine fibrovascular stroma. H & E. ×125.

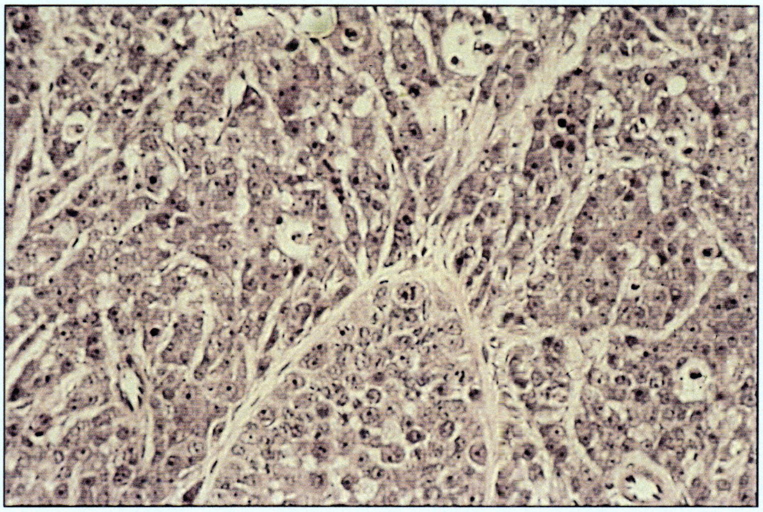

12.70

12.70 Canine ovarian dysgerminoma. The tumour is composed of lobular sheets of large cells with central nuclei and prominent nucleoli that resemble the testicular seminoma. Giant cells may be present. H & E. ×125.

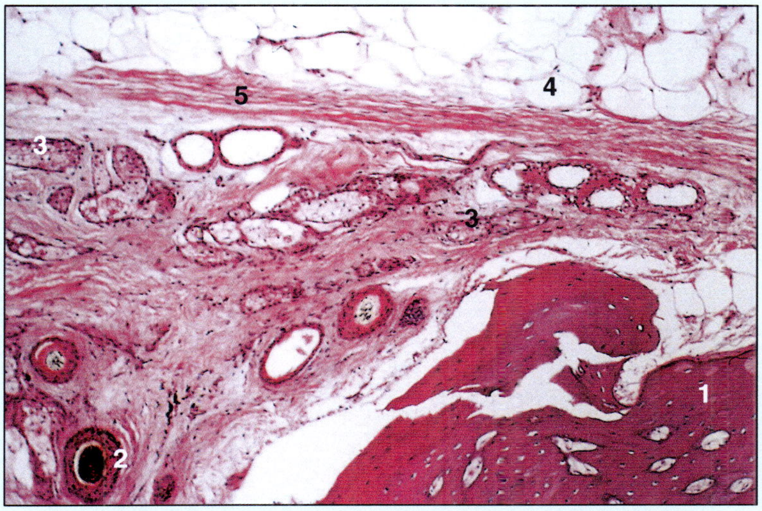

12.71

12.71 Teratoma from a 2-year-old bitch. Several germ lines are represented. Within this section, (1) dense bone, (2) well-developed hair follicles and (3) sebaceous glands, and (4) adipose and (5) collagenous connective tissue can be seen. H & E. ×62.5.

.72

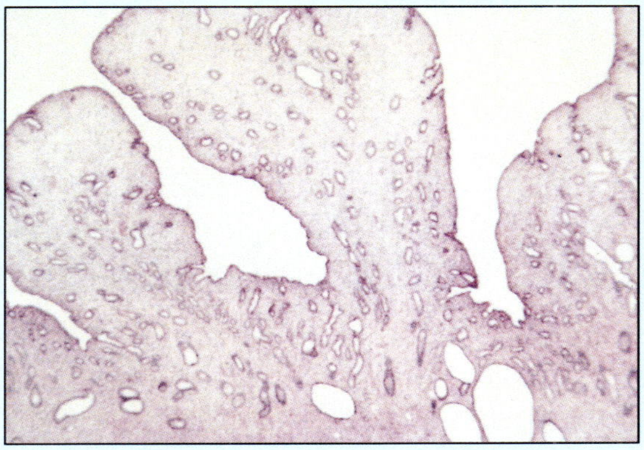

12.72 Cystic endometrial hyperplasia in a 13-year-old cat. Localized papillary outgrowths and cyst formation are present within the uterine lining. Hydrometra or mucometra may develop concurrently. Progestagen administration is the most common cause of this condition. H & E. ×44.

12.73

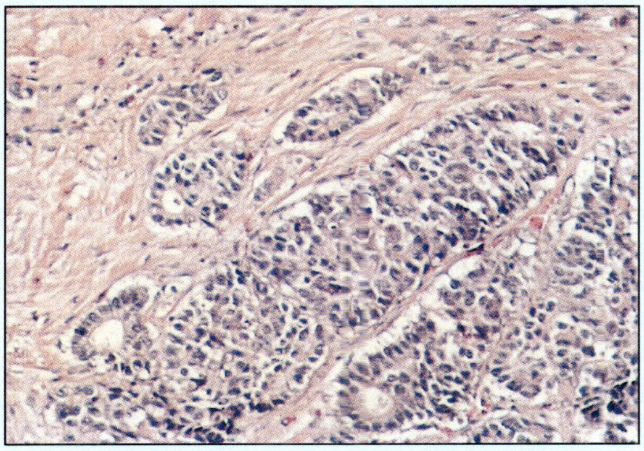

12.73 Uterine adenocarcinoma in a domestic rabbit. The myometrium is infiltrated by intersecting cords of neoplastic acini and distorted duct-like structures with hollow lumens filled with pink staining proteinaceous fluid. H & E. ×44.

Avian female reproductive system

Ovary

In the majority of birds only the left ovary and oviduct are functional. The ovary consists of an outer cortex that envelops a vascular medulla. The cortex is covered with cuboidal epithelium continuous with the mesothelium of the peritoneum. The underlying tunica albuginea is a thin layer of dense connective tissue. The stroma is very vascular loose connective tissue with sinusoidal blood vessels and follicles of varying sizes, postovulatory follicles and atretic follicles. Large follicles (the avian egg is megalethical or large yolked) are suspended from the surface of the ovary by stalks of cortical tissue (**12.74** and **12.75**). Each follicle consists of a growing yolk-laden oocyte with a rounded nucleus. The oocyte is surrounded by several layers: the theca externa, theca interna, membrana granulosa and perivitelline membrane (**12.76** and **12.77**).

12.74

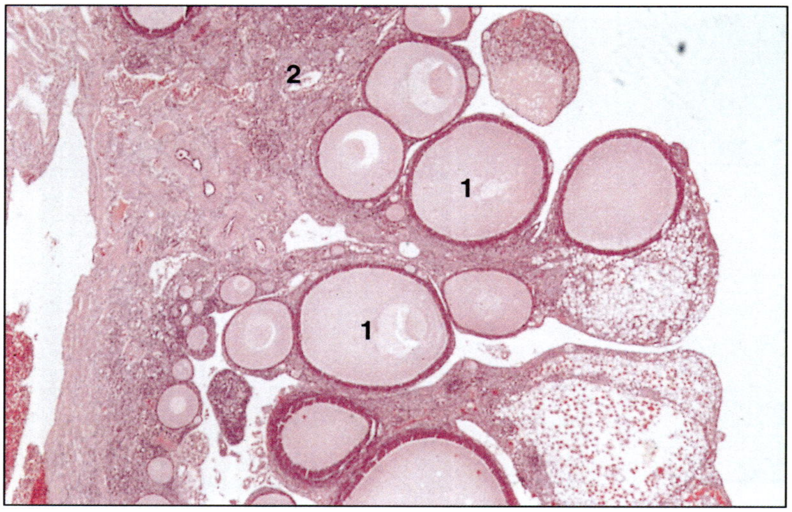

12.74 Ovary (bird). (1) The follicles consist of the megalethic ovum surrounded by a single layer of granulosa cells. (2) Vascular ovarian stroma. H & E. ×25.

12.75

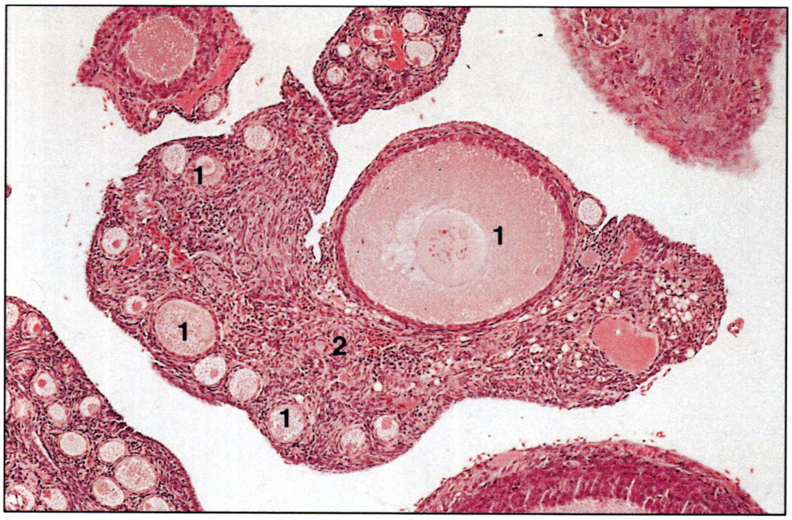

12.75 Ovary (bird). (1) The range of follicle sizes depends on the size of the ovum. (2) Vascular stroma. H & E. ×62.5.

.76

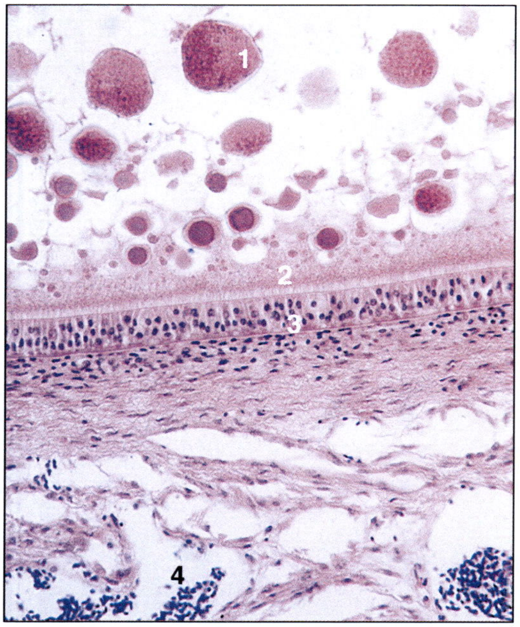

12.76 Ovary (bird). (1) Yolk granules. (2) Plasma membrane of the egg. (3) Granulosa cells. (4) Vascular ovarian stroma. H & E. ×200.

12.77

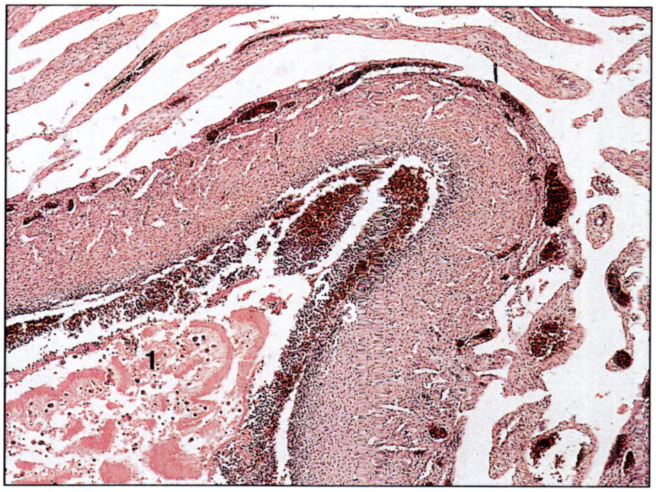

12.77 Ovary. Atretic follicle (bird). (1) Remnants of the yolk filled ovum. (2) Disrupted granulosa layer. (3) Theca formed from ovarian stroma. H & E. ×100.

Oviduct

In the domestic fowl the functional left oviduct consists of five regions: infundibulum, magnum, isthmus, uterus or shell gland, and vagina. The wall of the oviduct consists of a mucosa made up from pseudostratified epithelium and a glandular lamina propria. Longitudinal folds in the mucosa extend spirally down the length of the oviduct but vary in height and thickness. The muscularis is smooth muscle with inner circular and outer longitudinal layers increasing gradually in thickness. Loose connective tissue forms the serosa.

The infundibulum engulfs the shed oocyte and, after fertilization, lays down the first layer of albumen. The greatest proportion of albumen is produced by the next and longest part of the duct: the magnum. The mucosal glands of the magnum are lined with columnar cells packed with eosinophilic granules before the arrival of an egg and depleted after its passage (12.78 and 12.79). The shell membranes are formed in the next short, narrow

.78

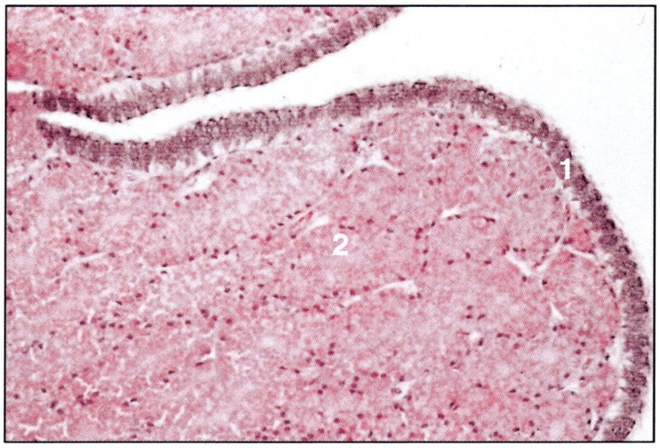

12.78 Oviduct. Magnum (bird). (1) The lining epithelium is pseudostratified columnar ciliated. (2) The lamina propria is filled with simple tubular glands lined by columnar cells packed with eosinophilic granules. H & E. ×100.

12 79

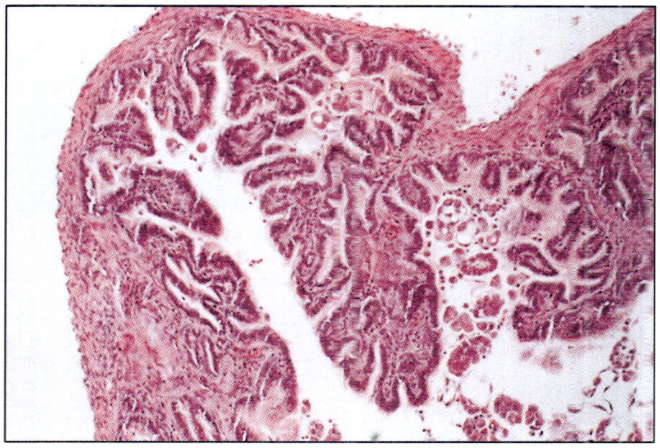

12.79 Oviduct. Magnum (bird). After passage of the egg the glands are empty and the deep mucosal folds project into the lumen. H & E. ×20.

region, the isthmus. Here the mucosal glands are lined with poorly staining vacuolated cells (12.80) that do not exhibit such marked secretory phases as those seen in the magnum. The mucosal folds of the isthmus are elongated and lie in leaf-shaped folds. Once received by the 'uterus' or shell gland (12.81), the egg remains in this region for about 20 hours, during which calcification of the shell and formation of the cuticle take place (12.82 and 12.83). Watery fluid is also added to the albumen. The uterine mucosa forms flat, leaf-shaped, longitudinal folds. The epithelium is a continuous layer of columnar cells with alternating basal and apical nuclei, and these have been named basal and apical cells. The basal cells have a restricted apical surface; the apical cells are ciliated. The tubular glands of the uterus are lined with cells that contain pale staining granules both before and during the phase of shell formation, but which are subsequently depleted.

The vagina is short and narrow and has a well-developed muscularis. Short simple tubular glands, the sperm host glands, are found near the junction of the vagina with the shell gland and lie within the mucosal tissue (12.84). As their name suggests, their function is to store sperm after insemination. The mucosal folds are long and slender at this point and bear short secondary folds.

The surface is lined with pseudostratified columnar epithelium and mucous cells. The vagina opens into the cloacal urodeum.

12.80

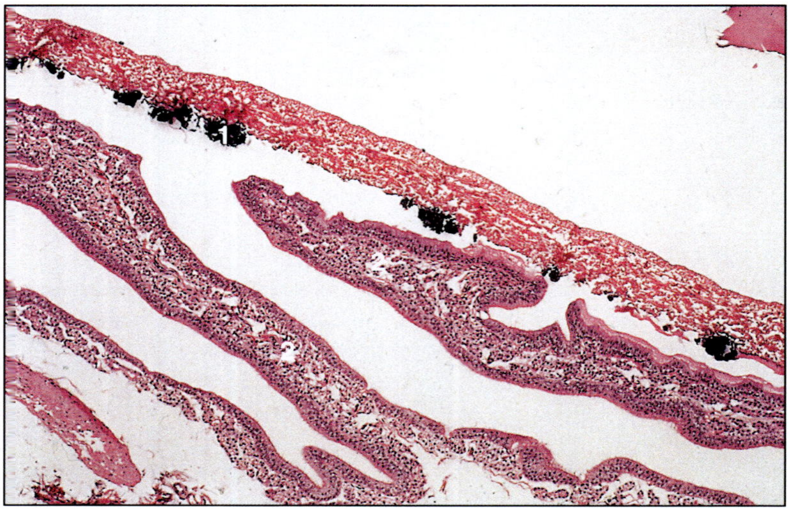

12.80 Oviduct. Shell gland/uterus (bird). (1) Shell membranes, the dark blue areas, are sites of calcification. (2) The long mucosal folds lie parallel to the developing shell. H & E. ×62.5.

12.81

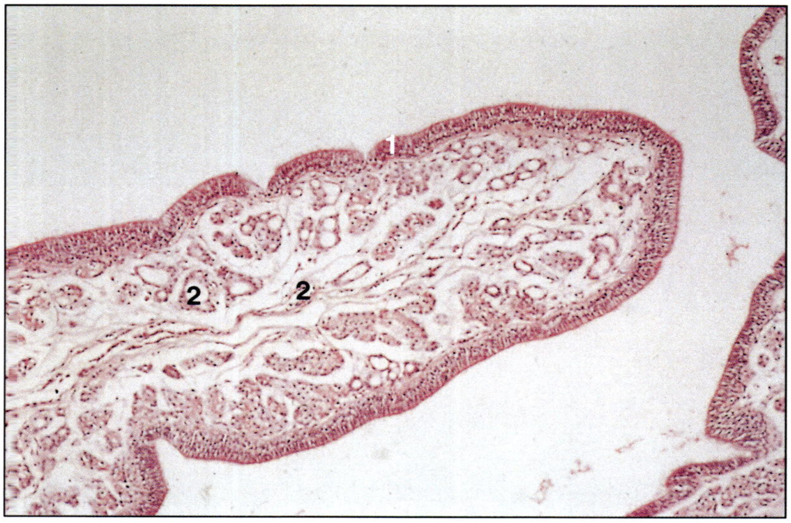

12.81 Oviduct. Shell gland/uterus (bird). (1) The lining epithelium is pseudostratified columnar with two distinct rows of nuclei. (2) The mucosal glands in the long folds appear empty. H & E. ×62.5.

12.82 TS eggshell with the membranes removed. (1) Gaseous pore. (2) Cuticle. (3) Multiple layers of calcite containing organic matrix. (4) Mammillary layer. Scanning electron micrograph. ×160.

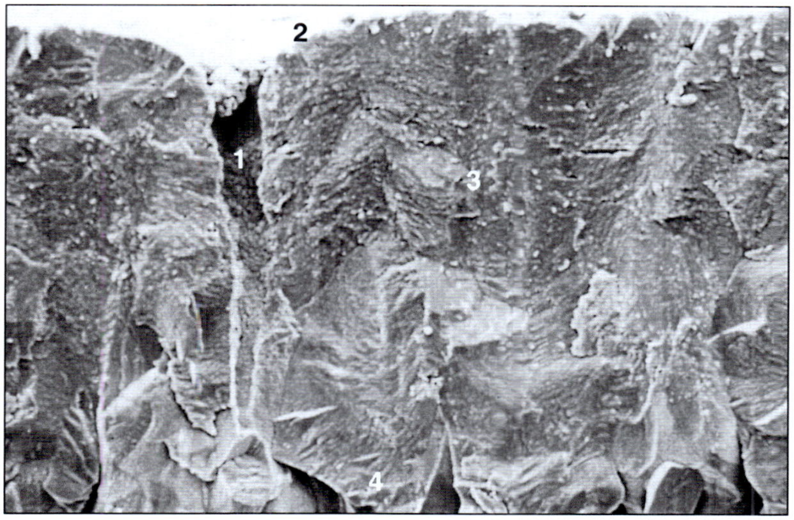

12.82

12.83 Mammillary layer of the eggshell. This is the organic component. The individual structural units are the mammillae arranged as (1) mammillary caps and (2) mammillary cones. Scanning electron micrograph. ×320.

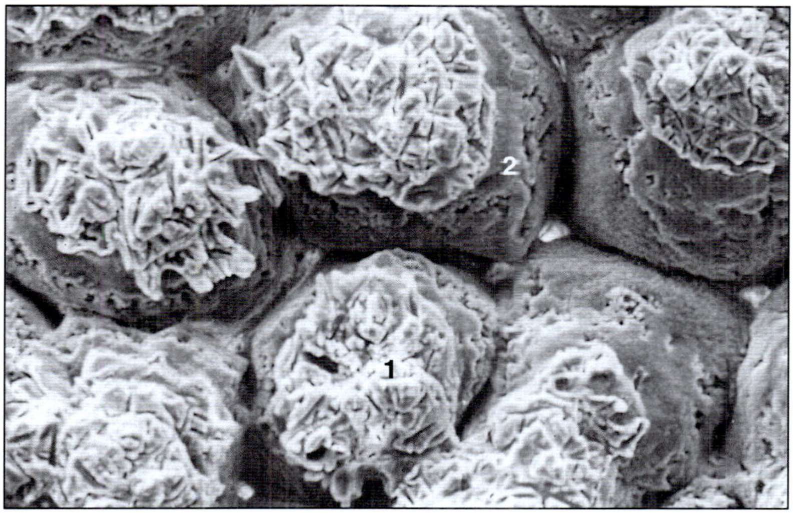

12.83

12.84 Vagina (bird). A pseudostratified columnar epithelium lines the vagina; small tubular glands (sperm-host glands) are found in the lamina propria (arrowed). H & E. ×62.5.

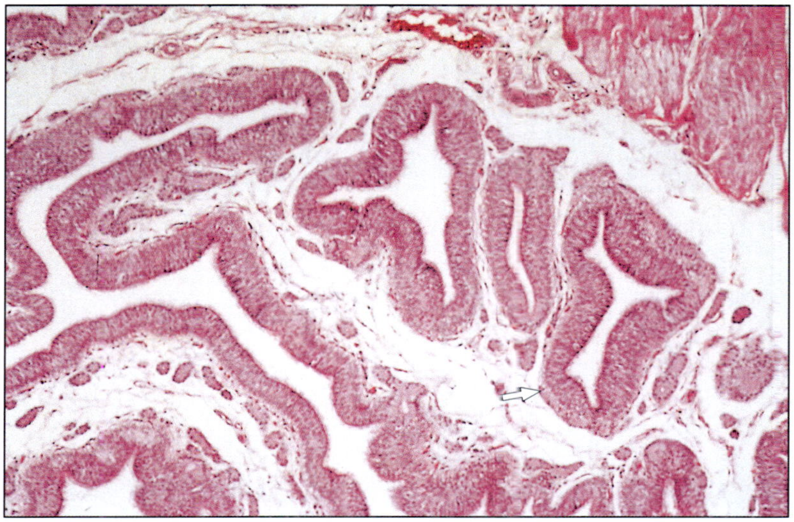

12.84

Reptilian, amphibian and fish female reproductive system

Paired ovaries are typical in fish, amphibians and reptiles, and the histology of oogenesis is similar to that in mammals (**12.85** and **12.86**). The ovaries are composed of germinative, stromal, vascular and nervous tissue. The ova begin their development as oogonia that are mitotically derived from successive generations of oocytes. Diploid primary oocytes then undergo meiotic division to become primary oocytes, and primary polar bodies that are discarded. Another reduction division yields haploid ova, and secondary polar bodies that also are discarded.

The ovum is encircled by a cell membrane, a variably narrow zona pellucida and a layer of follicle cells. During vitellogenesis, the yolk is added. This process occurs after a variable period of time after ovulation. Although the ova of most amphibians are uninuclear, some species are known to produce multinucleated ova. However, before fertilization all of the nuclei, except one, become inactivated. Reptile ova typically have a uninuclear ovum. However, binucleated ova are produced occasionally and, after being fertilized, may yield twin embryos.

After ovulation, the corpora lutea, then the corpora albicans and finally the corpora atretans replace the ovulated follicles.

The appearance of reptilian oviducts varies depending on the species and whether the female is egg laying (oviparous) or live bearing (ovoviviparous or viviparous). However, they are readily recognizable. The histological features of the tubular oviduct changes with each segment as it courses distally from the infundibulum. It is lined by ciliated, often mucus-secreting, glandular columnar epithelium for at least part of its length. The thin walls of the oviducts contain alveolar or tubuloalveolar glands that secrete albumin and shell substrate onto the yolked egg as it descends. The cuboidal to columnar epithelial cells comprising these glands tend to be characterized by their distinctive eosinophilic cytoplasmic granularity (**12.87** and **12.88**). The caudal oviduct of many reptiles also contains straight or branched crypt-like depressions that are surrounded by cuboidal epithelium with eosinophilic granular cytoplasm (**12.89**). In many species these glandular crypts serve as spermathecae in which spermatozoa are nourished and stored for prolonged periods of time. The oviducts of viviparous and ovoviviparous reptiles are thick-walled, muscular and vascular, and contain glands with secretions that help nourish the developing embryo(s). They often exhibit marked plaiting, which facilitates their distension during gravidity or pregnancy. These modified oviducts are called the 'uterus' by some authorities.

The embryos of some viviparous reptiles develop a primitive vascular placenta. In the lizard (*Xantusia vigilis)* it is disc-shaped; in others it is more diffuse. Although it was long thought that embryonic development did not occur in shelled eggs until they were deposited and exposed to atmospheric oxygen, it has been demonstrated that significant embryonic development can occur before egg deposition in some species.

12.85

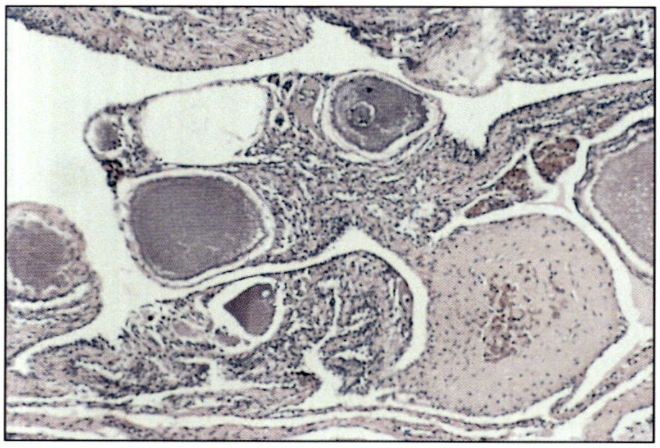

12.85 Ovary and proximal oviduct (fimbrium) of a desert tortoise (*Xerobates agassizi*). H & E. ×25.

12.86

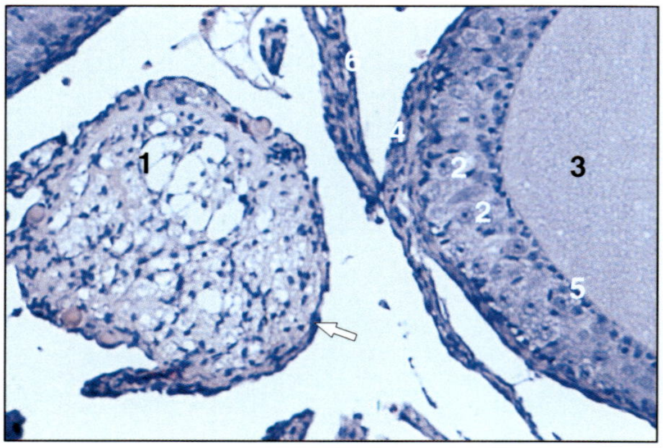

12.86 Corpus luteum (arrowed) of a leopard gecko (*Eublepharis macularius*). (1) Granulosa lutein cells. (2) Primordial follicles. (3) Oocyte cytoplasm. (4) Tunica albuginea. (5) Theca externa. (6) Stroma. H & E. ×62.5.

12.87 and **12.88** Shell gland portion of the oviduct of a Pacific pond turtle (*Clemmys marmorata*). The luminal lining epithelium is pseudostratified columnar and contains numerous goblet cells. Subjacent to the mucosa are lobules of shell-secreting glands with characteristic eosinophilic granule-containing cells. H & E. ×127.

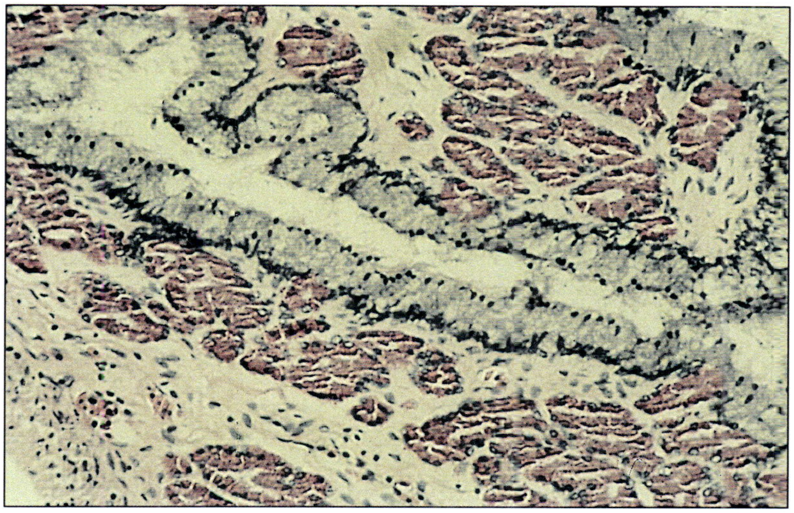

12.87

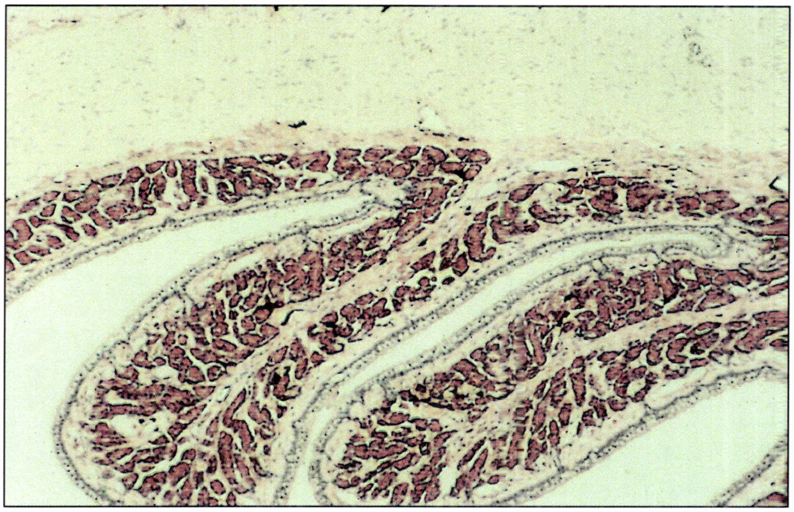

12.88

12.89 Caudal oviduct from a sexually mature female green iguana (*Iguana iguana*). This portion of the oviduct is characterized by numerous shallow crypts that connect with small lobules of glandular epithelial cells. These crypts are thought to be sites of sperm storage and nourishment that sustain spermatozoa for prolonged periods that may exceed 4–6 years in some reptiles. H & E. ×62.5.

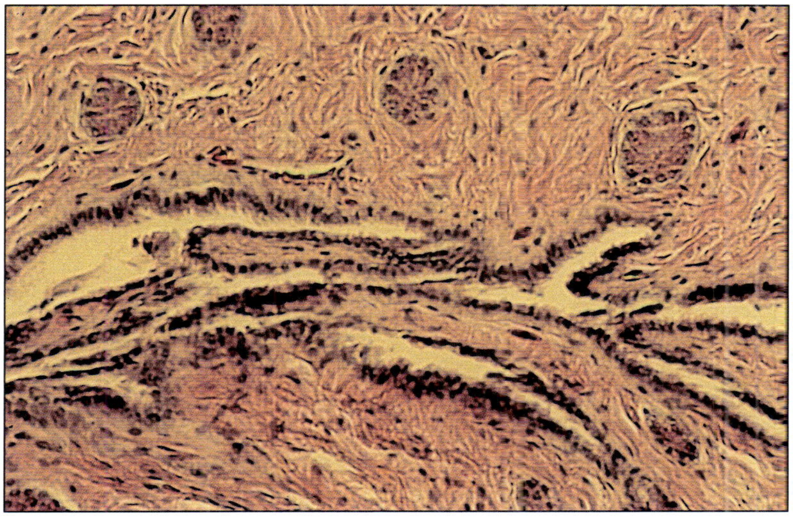

12.89

Clinical correlates

Ovarian and oviductal (or 'uterine') inflammation and infections are less common in fish, amphibians and reptiles than in mammals. Rupture of yolked eggs with subsequent leakage of yolk into the coelomic cavity is, however, a relatively frequent reproductive disorder in oviparous reptiles. Once lipid has gained entry into the vascular system, it is disseminated widely in the form of yolk-lipid emboli throughout the body (**12.90** and **12.91**).

Ovarian neoplasms have been observed in fish and amphibians, but are less prevalent than in mammals, birds and reptiles. As with mammals, relatively common reptilian ovarian neoplasms are granulosa cell tumours (see **12.68**), luteal tumours and thecal cell tumours (see **12.69**). Dysgerminoma (see **12.70**) and teratoma (**12.92**) occur less often. The teratoma is distinguished by usually having tissue from all three germ layers present: hair (or scales), bone, cartilage, teeth, muscle (of all three types), glandular tissue, nerve and brain-like structures, and so on.

12.90

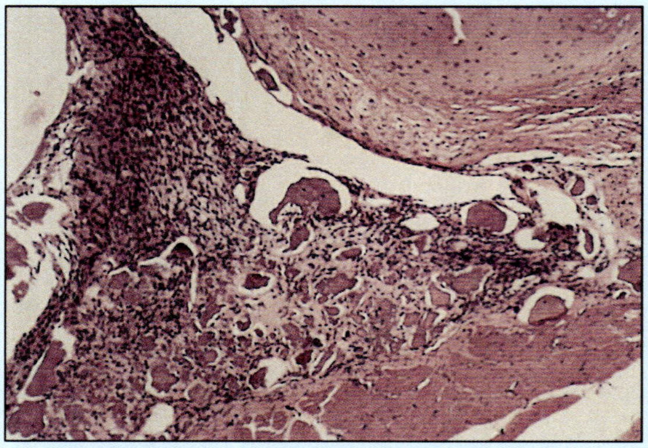

12.90 Egg-yolk serocoelomitis from an iguana. The intense exudative reaction to yolk characterized by numerous histiocytic macrophages with engulfed yolk lipid. H & E. ×62.5.

12.91

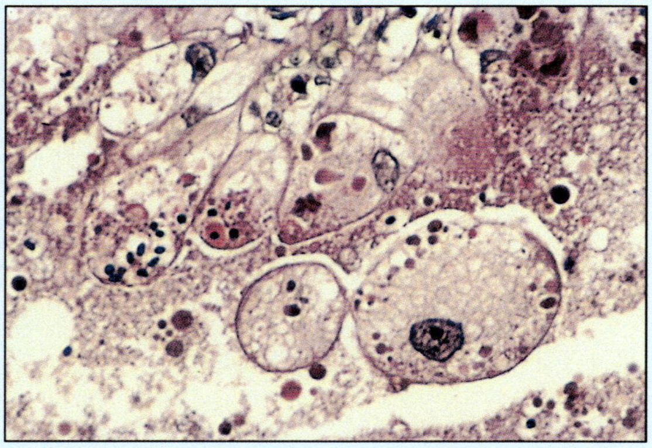

12.91 Yolk serocoelomitis in a green iguana (*Iguana iguana*). The smooth muscle tunic of the viscus organ is covered with yolk, and an inflammatory exudate is comprised of macrophages with engulfed lipid. H & E. ×125.

12.92

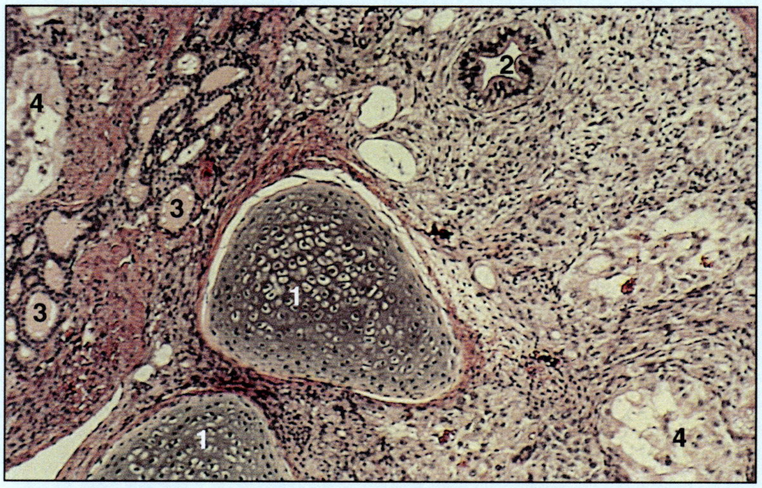

12.92 Ovarian teratoma from a green iguana (*Iguana iguana*). This section illustrates (1) two masses of cartilage, (2) a duct-like structure, (3) an aggregate of thyroid-like follicles filled with pink staining protein resembling colloid, and (4) nervous tissue. H & E. ×62.5.

13. NERVOUS SYSTEM

Two properties of cytoplasm are typified by nervous tissue: irritability – the ability to react; and conductivity – the ability to transmit the elicited response.

The nervous system is subdivided into the central nervous system (CNS), which comprises the brain and spinal cord, and the peripheral nervous system (PNS), which covers all other nervous tissue and acts to interconnect all the tissues of the body with the CNS. The nervous system is derived from a specialized region of surface ectoderm along the dorsal midline of the flat embryonic disc. The ectodermal cells thicken to become neural ectoderm. During flexion, the neural folds form and the lips fuse to become the neural tube. This is incorporated into the developing embryo to form the brain and spinal cord. A separate population of neural ectodermal cells remains separate from the neural tube. This is the neural crest and forms the PNS.

The basic cellular unit of nervous tissue is the neuron. This comprises a large cell body (from 0.4 to 12 μm in diameter) with a single nucleus and a prominent nucleolus. Basophilic granules (Nissl's granules) are present in the cytoplasm and represent rough endoplasmic reticulum (13.1). The function of the neuron is to receive and transmit impulses. The dendrites are branching processes at the receiving end, and the axon is the single, long process for onward transmission of the impulse. Information passed along a chain of neurons is transmitted from axon to dendrite at a specialized junction: the synapse.

Multipolar neurons are by far the most common type. The single axon arises from one pole at a granule-free area of the neuron body: the axon hillock. One or two dendrites arise from the opposite pole and branch extensively. Examples of these neurons are found in the CNS, in the cerebral and cerebellar cortex, and in the spinal cord (13.2). Bipolar neurons have one axon and one main dendrite, with

13.1

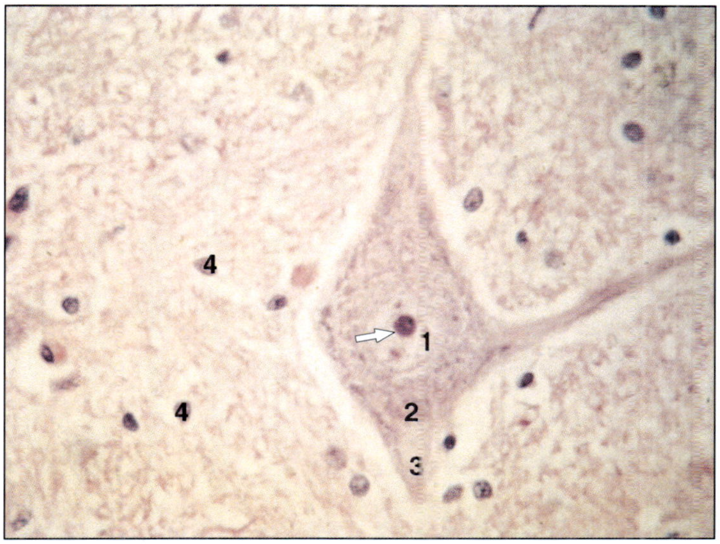

13.1 Motor neuron. Trigeminal nerve (dog). (1) Nucleus and nucleolus (arrow). (2) Basophilic granules (Nissl's granules). (3) Axon hillock. (4) Neuroglial cells. H & E. ×200.

13.2

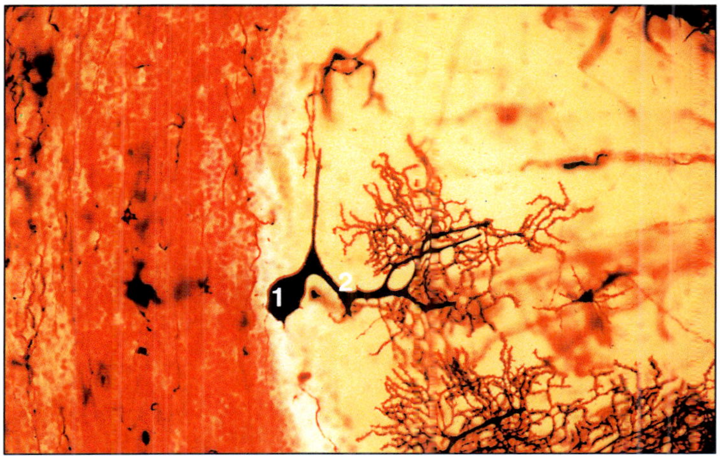

13.2 Multipolar neuron. Cerebellar cortex (dog). (1) Cell body. (2) Branching processes. Golgi's silver. ×125.

little branching, and are found in the retina. Pseudounipolar neurons are so-called because a single process arises from the cell body and divides into two. These cells are found in the dorsal root ganglia and in the sensory ganglia of the cranial nerves.

The axon with its covering myelin sheath, the neurilemma, constitutes the nerve fibre. The neurilemmal sheath is composed of individual cells that form a continuous investment from the origin of the axon almost to the peripheral termination (13.3). These cells produce a lamellar system of membranes with a high fat content. In the PNS the neurilemmal sheath is produced by neurolemmocytes, and in the CNS by neuroglial cells: oligodendrocytes. The degree of the investment varies; heavily invested fibres are known as myelinated and minimally invested fibres as non-myelinated. The axon has no sheath at the peripheral nerve endings; these are naked fibres. The individual sheaths divide the nerve fibre into segments. Where adjoining cells meet, a node (of Ranvier) is formed so that each internodal segment represents an investing neurilemmal cell. The high fat content of the sheath means that fat stains are best used to demonstrate the myelinated fibres (13.3).

Peripheral nervous system

The PNS is derived from the neural crest and is composed of nerves and ganglia. Nerves are composed of nerve fibres and ganglia are localized groups of nerve cells. The individual fibres are gathered into bundles or fascicles by a connective tissue sheath, the epineurium, and form an anatomical nerve. The epineurium extends into the

13.3

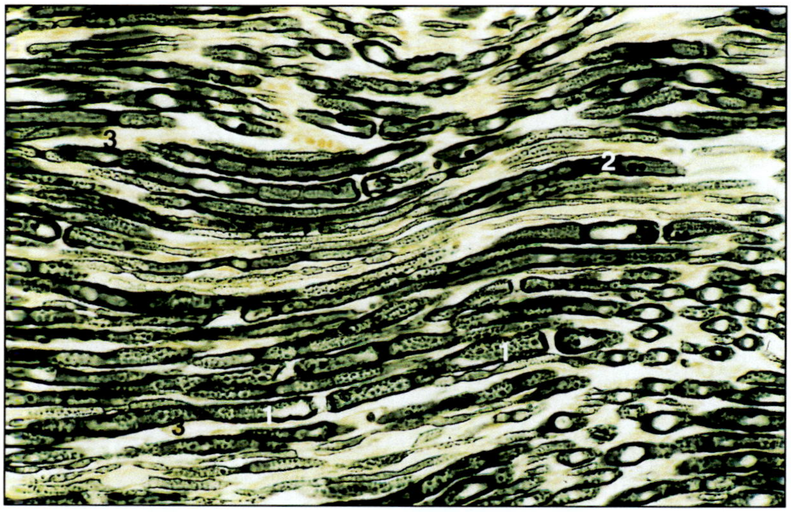

13.3 Longitudinal section (LS) peripheral nerve (cat). (1) Axon. (2) Neurilemmal sheath. (3) Node. Osmic acid. ×200.

13.4

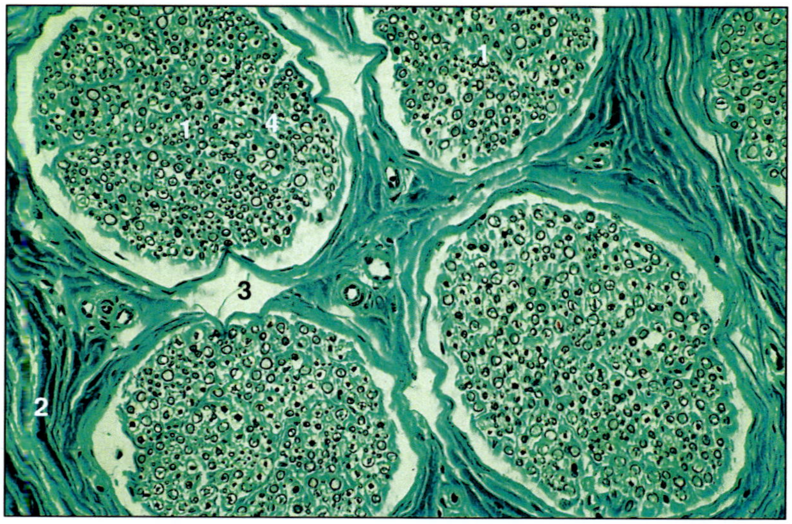

13.4 Transverse section (TS) peripheral nerve (dog). (1) Bundles of axons cut in transverse section, fascicles. (2) Epineurium. (3) Perineurium. (4) Endoneurium. Masson's trichrome. ×25.

nerve and subdivides the fascicles with a vascular connective tissue investment: the perineurium. This in turn surrounds each nerve fibre with fine vascular connective tissue: the endoneurium (13.4–13.7). In the dorsal root ganglion the neurons are peripherally arranged, with the nerve

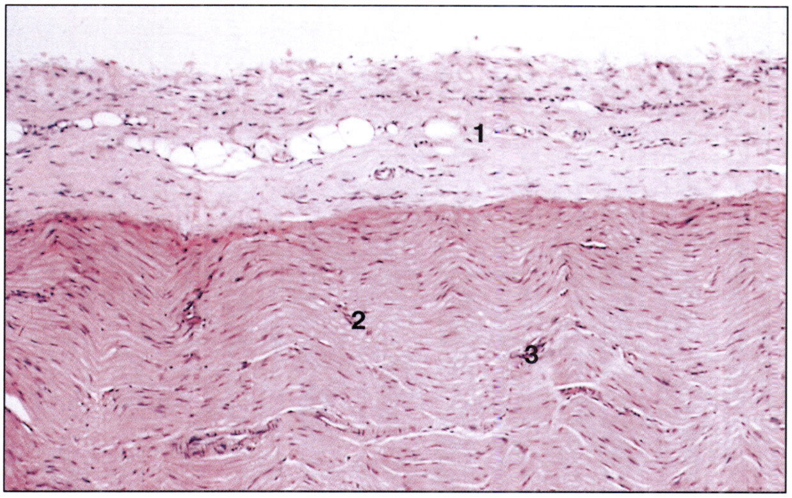

13.5

13.5 LS peripheral nerve (dog). (1) Epineurium with fat cells. (2) Nuclei of the neurilemmal cells. (3) Axons cut longitudinally; note the wavy appearance. H & E. ×62.5.

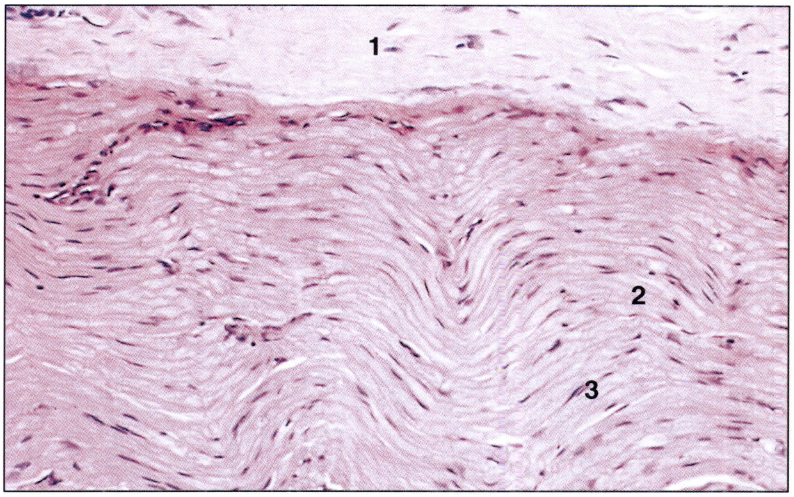

13.6

13.6 LS peripheral nerve (dog). (1) Epineurium. (2) Axons. (3) Neurilemmal cell nuclei. H & E. ×125.

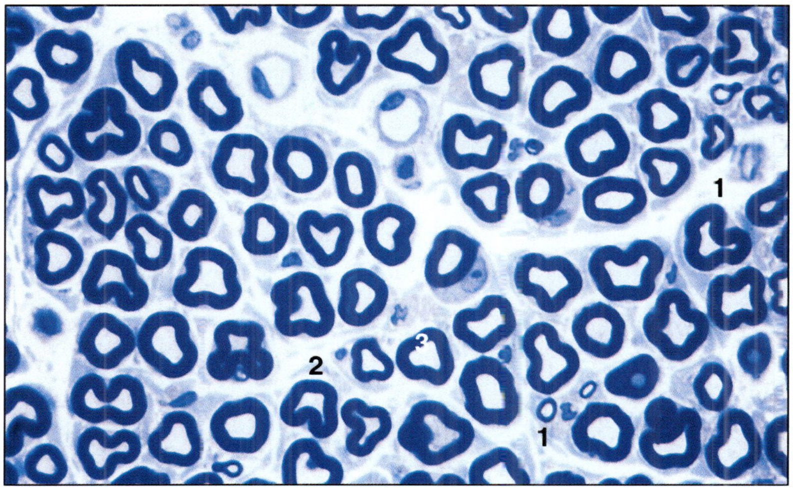

13.7

13.7 TS laryngeal nerve (horse). (1) Perineurium with blood vessels. (2) Endoneurium. (3) Axons. Toluidine blue. ×62.5.

fibres in the centre of the ganglion (13.8). The large neuron bodies are surrounded and supported by satellite cells (13.9). In the sympathetic ganglion the neurons are evenly distributed, the cell bodies are smaller and the nucleus is eccentrically placed in the cell (13.10). Parasympathetic ganglia are small groups of neurons within the terminal tissue (13.11).

13.8

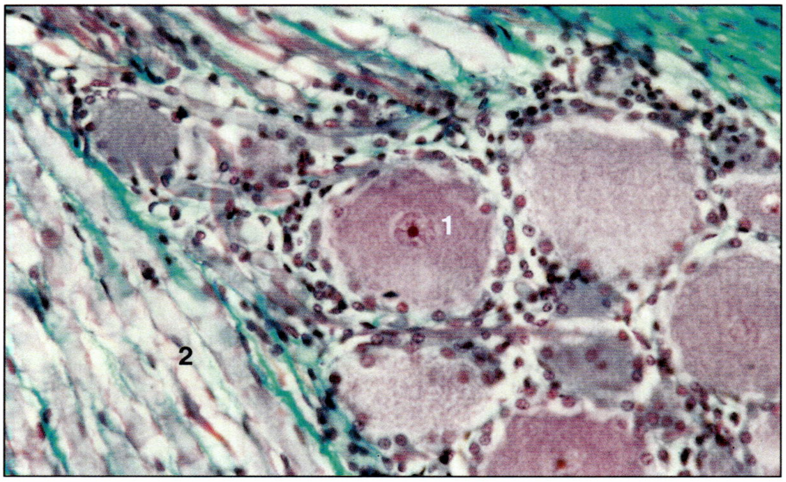

13.8 Dorsal root ganglion (cat). (1) Neuron bodies. (2) Nerve fibres and supporting neuroglial cells. Masson's trichrome. ×160.

13.9

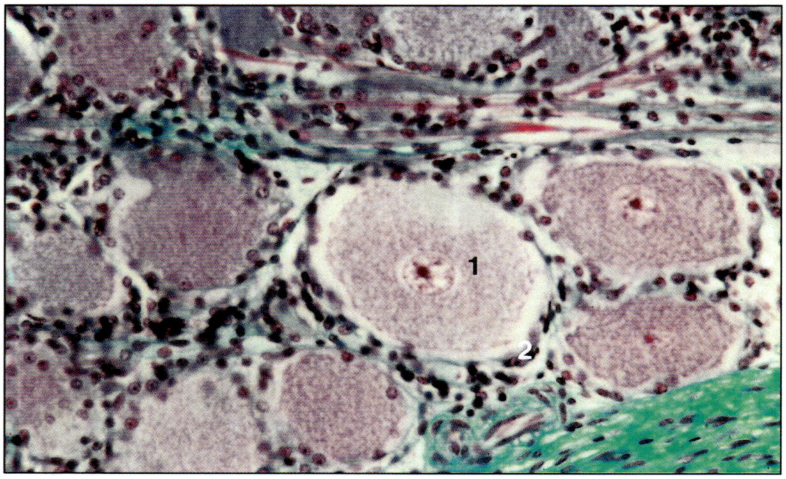

13.9 Dorsal root ganglion (cat). (1) Neuron body. (2) Satellite cells; these are supporting neuroglial cells. Masson's trichrome. ×160.

13.10

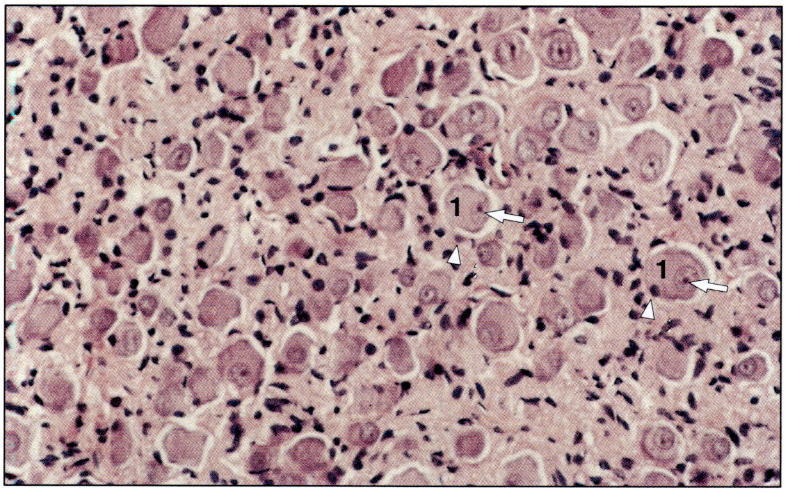

13.10 Sympathetic ganglion (dog). (1) Neuron body with eccentric nucleus (arrow) and satellite cells (arrowhead). H & E. ×125.

13.11

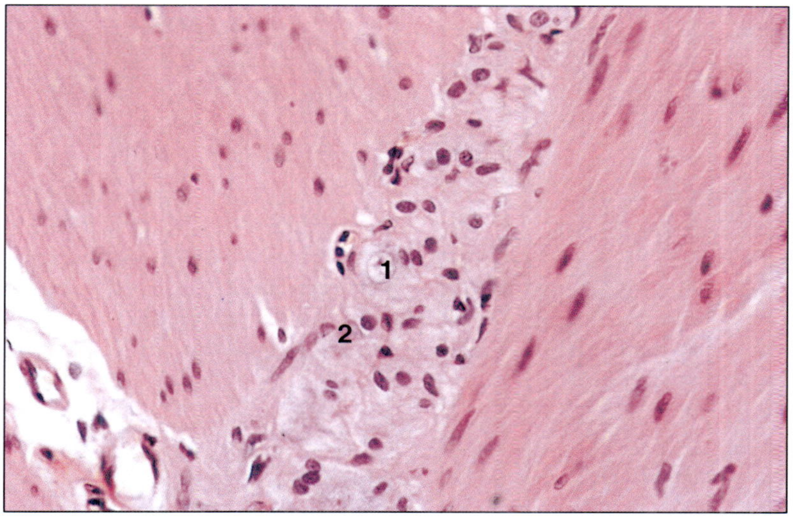

13.11 Parasympathetic ganglion. Stomach (pig). (1) Neuron body. (2) Nerve fibres and supporting neuroglial cells. H & E. ×250.

Central nervous system

The brain and spinal cord are enveloped in connective tissue membranes, the meninges. The outer dense membrane is the dura mater; the middle fine cobweb-like membrane is the arachnoid; and the inner, very vascular, areolar membrane is the pia mater. The arachnoid and pia mater are continuous and called the leptomeninges (**13.12**). The central fluid filled canal and the ventricles of the brain are lined with a columnar epithelium: the ependyma. The tela choroidea lies in the thin roof plate of the third and fourth ventricles. Its surface is covered with modified ependymal cells that secrete

13.12

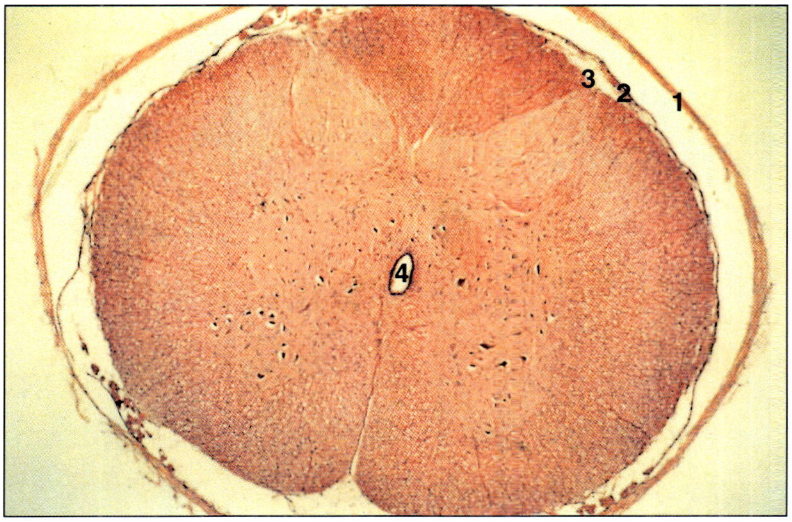

13.12 TS spinal cord (cat). (1) Dura mater. (2) Arachnoid. (3) Pia mater. (4) Spinal canal lined by ependyma. H & E. ×7.5.

cerebrospinal fluid (**13.13**). The pia mater coats the entire surface of the CNS, extends into the fissures and sulci and is separated from the ependyma only by the basal lamina.

In the CNS, collections of functionally related neurons are called nuclei and collections of nerve fibres are called tracts. The fibres have an investing sheath cell: the oligodendrocyte. The presence of fat gives a white glistening appearance and the fibres are called white matter. By contrast, the cell bodies appear grey and form the grey matter (**13.14**).

Neuroglial cells are the supporting cells of the CNS, taking the place of the connective tissue of other systems. Oligodendrocytes invest the axon, provide the myelin sheath and act as supporting satellite cells. Astrocytes are stellate cells with long processes. In fibrous astrocytes the processes are thin with minimal cytoplasm, whereas in protoplasmic astrocytes they are thick and fleshy (**13.15–13.18**). The cell processes extend to the blood vessels in the pia mater, acting as anchors and transferring nutrients. The blood vessels are

13.13

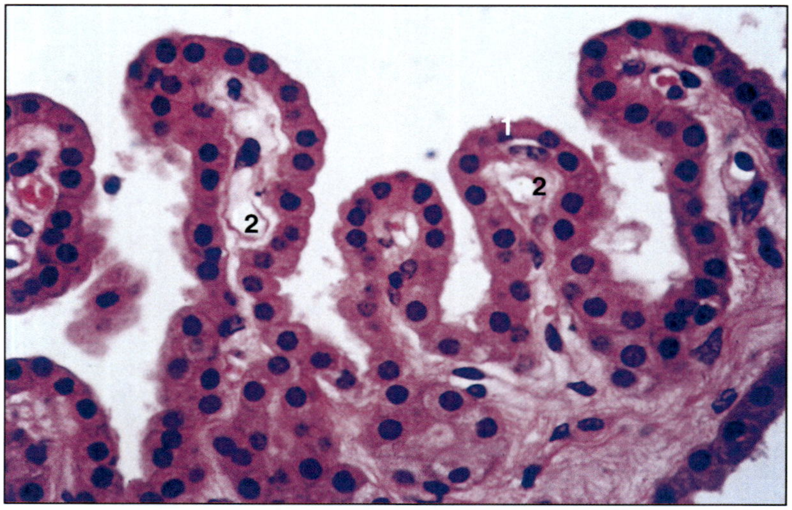

13.13 TS choroid plexus in the fourth ventricle (cat). (1) Ependyma. (2) Capillaries. H & E. ×160.

13.14

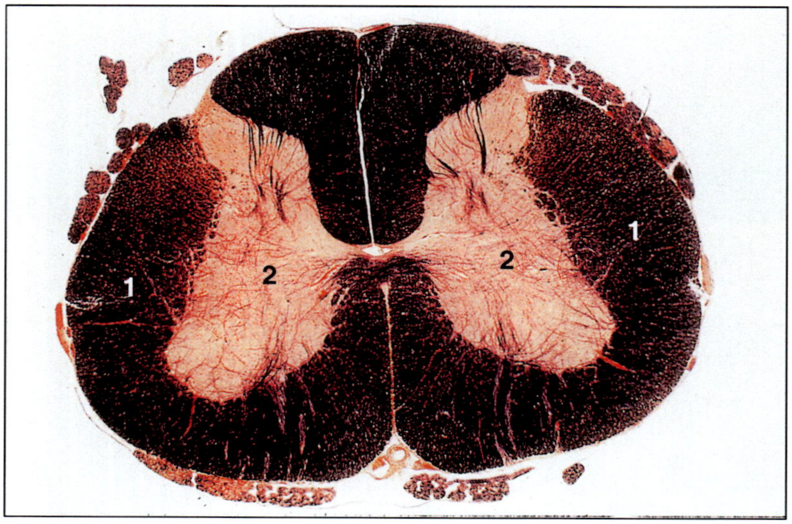

13.14 TS spinal cord (cat). (1) Black areas are the fat stained white matter. (2) Pink stained areas are the cellular grey matter. Osmic acid. ×7.5.

13.15

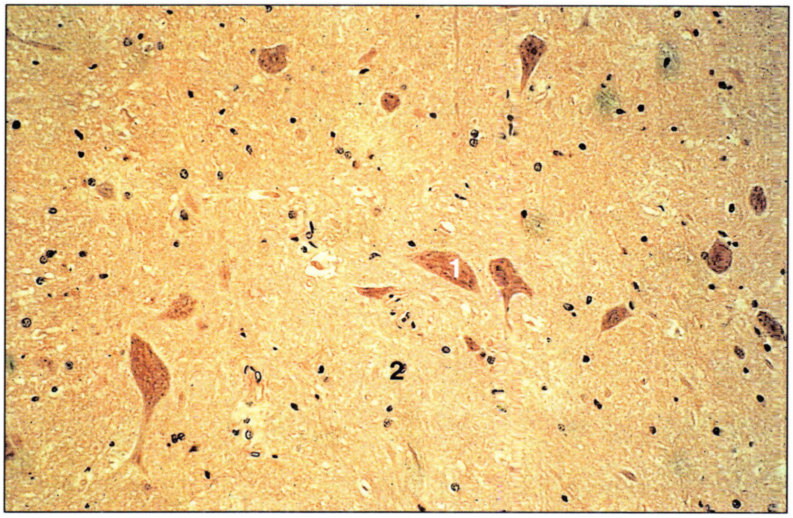

13.15 Spinal cord (dog). (1) Neuron. (2) Nuclei of protoplasmic astrocytes. H & E. ×125.

13.16

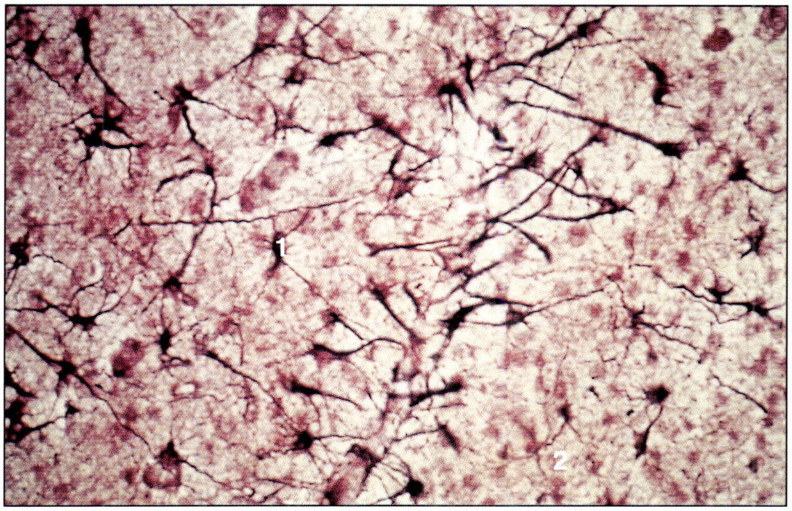

13.16 Spinal cord (dog). (1) Neuron. (2) Nuclei of protoplasmic astrocytes. H & E. ×125.

.17

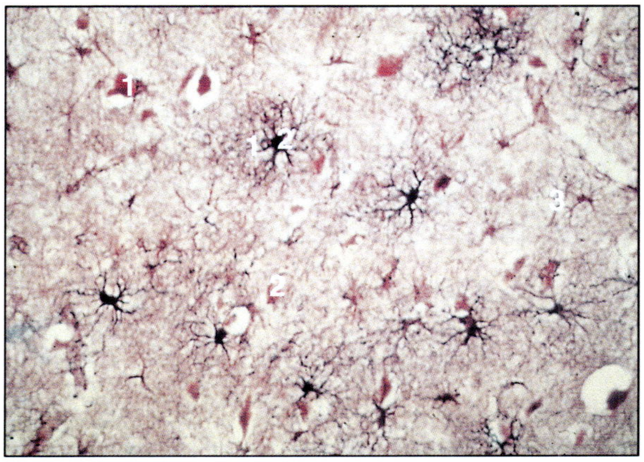

13.17 Spinal cord (dog). (1) Neuron. (2) Nuclei of protoplasmic astrocytes. (3) Fibrous astrocytes. H & E. ×125.

13.18

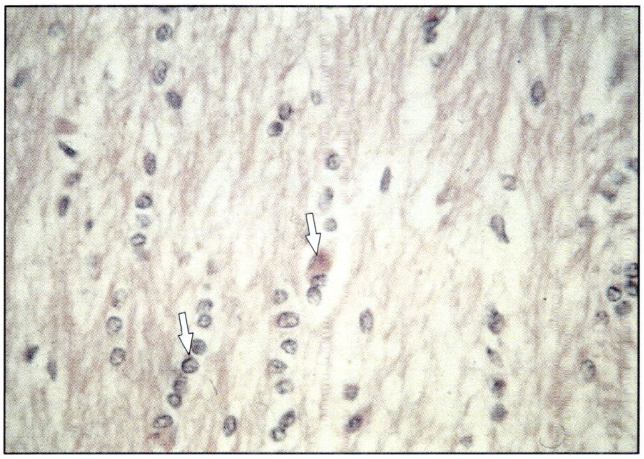

13.18 Corpus callosum (dog). Oligodendrocyte nuclei in orderly columns (arrowed) providing the neurilemmal sheath in the central nervous system. H & E. ×125.

lined by a continuous endothelium. There is a well-developed basal lamina that, with the protoplasmic astrocyte processes, forms the formidable blood–brain barrier. Microglia are the phagocytic, scavenging cells of the CNS (13.19).

The cerebral and cerebellar cortices are highly specialized folded areas of outer grey matter with layers of neurons of various sizes and supporting cells, as well as a central core of white matter (13.20–13.25).

13.19

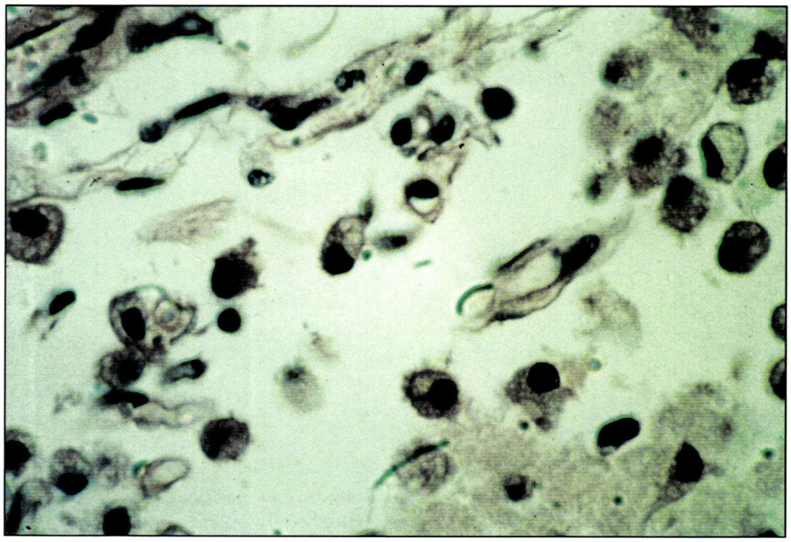

13.19 Microglial cells in the central nervous system (cat). H & E. ×256.

13.20

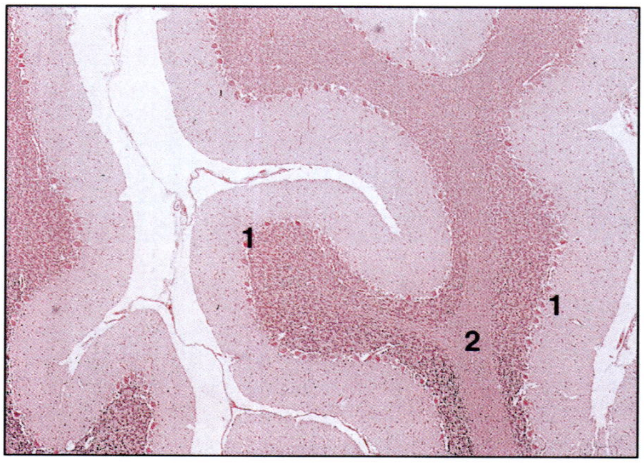

13.20 Cerebellum (cat). (1) Outer cellular layer of grey matter and (2) inner fibrous layer of white matter. H & E. ×25.

13.21

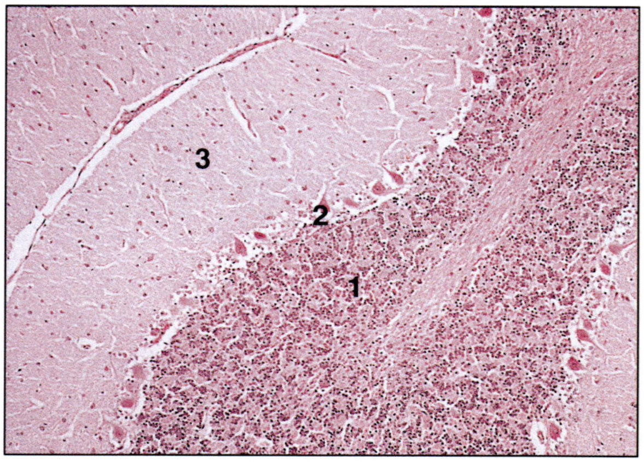

13.21 Cerebellum (cat). (1) Inner granular layer of small neurons. (2) Middle Purkinje layer of large neurons. (3) Outer molecular layer with few neurons and many branching processes. H & E. ×100.

13.22

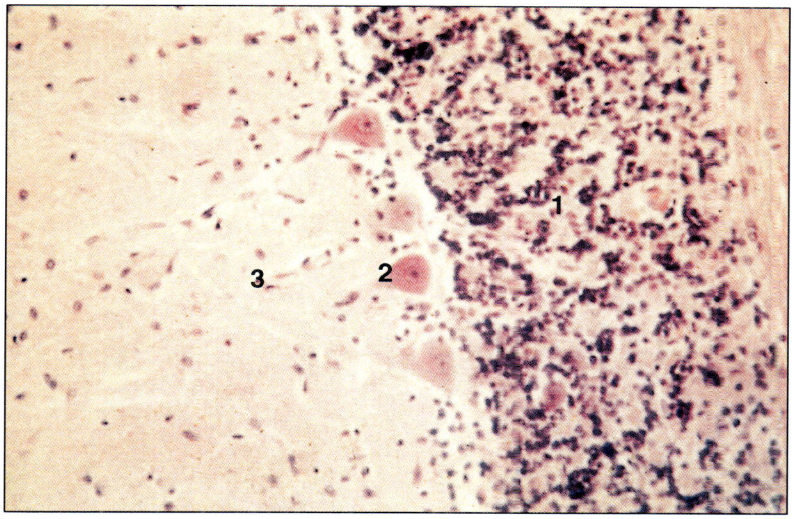

13.22 Cerebellum (sheep). (1) Granular layer. (2) Purkinje cell layer. (3) Molecular layer. H & E. ×125.

13.23

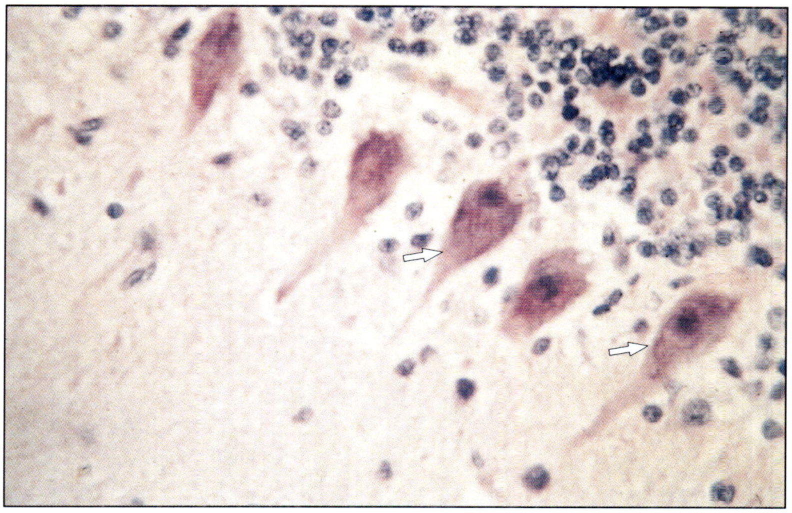

13.23 Cerebellum (dog). Large Purkinje cells are arrowed. H & E. ×250.

13.24

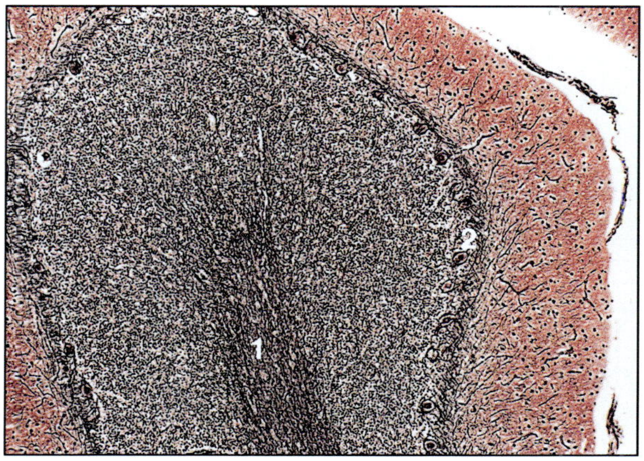

13.24 Cerebellum (cat). Each folium has (1) a central core of white matter, the nerve fibres and supporting cells, and (2) a surface cellular layer of grey matter. Cajal's silver. ×62.5.

13.25

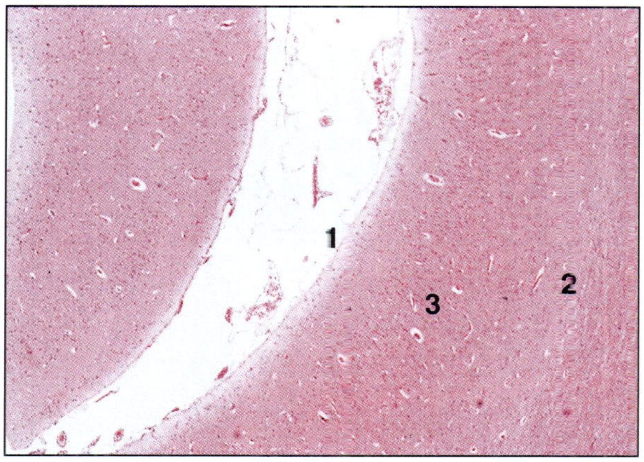

13.25 Cerebral cortex (cat). (1) Meninges. (2) White matter. (3) Grey matter. H & E. ×100.

13.26

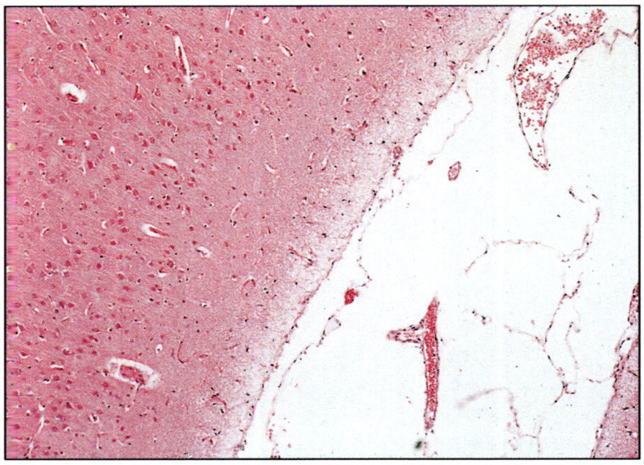

13.26 Cerebral cortex (cat). Cellular grey matter. H & E. ×25.

Nerve endings and receptors are specialized terminal parts of axons or dendrites. They include motor end plates, pressure receptors (such as Pacinian corpuscles) and taste buds (**13.26–13.31**).

Nerve tissue is so characteristic that it is readily identified, even in invertebrates.

13.27

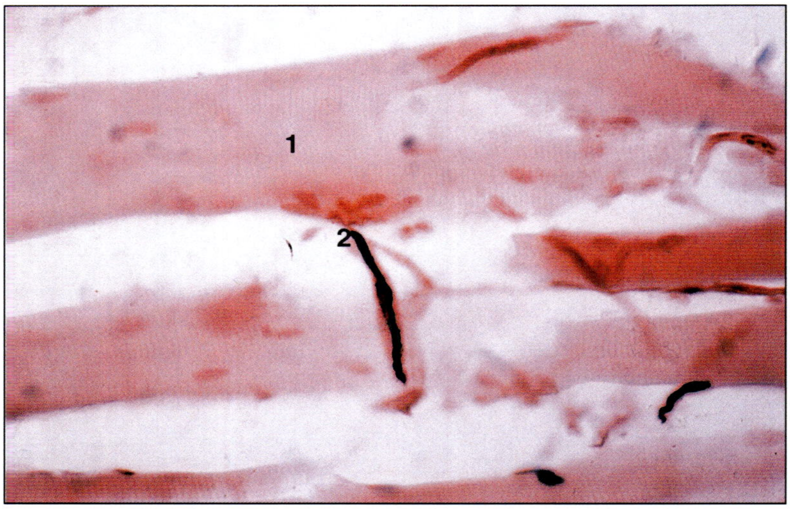

13.27 Motor end plate in striated muscle (dog). (1) Striated muscle fibre. (2) Terminal nerve fibre. Cajal's silver. ×250.

13.28

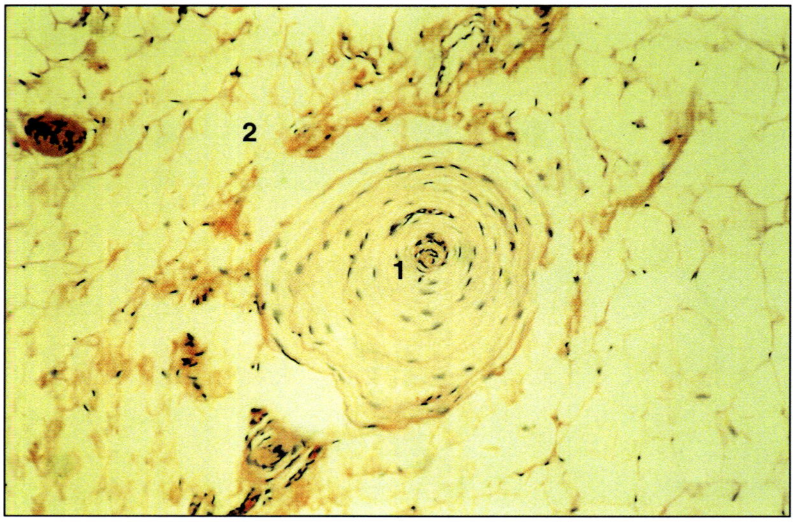

13.28 Pacinian corpuscle. Bladder (dog). (1) Pacinian corpuscle. (2) Loose areolar connective tissue. H & E. ×20.

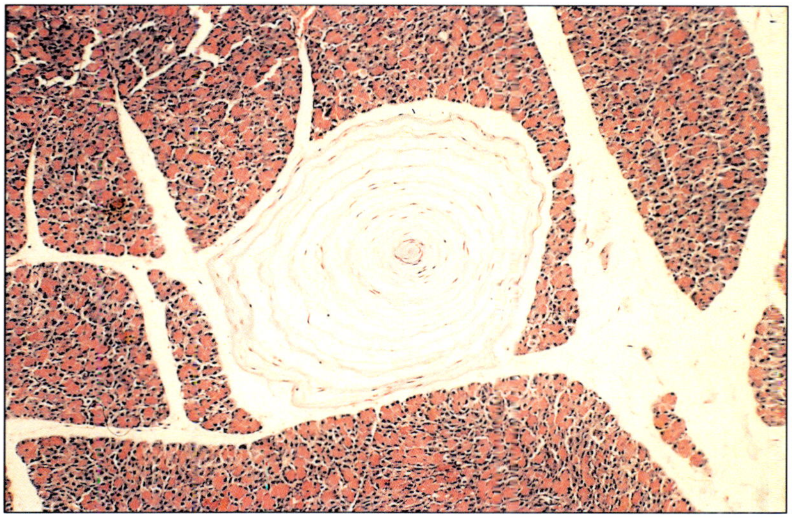

13.29

13.29 Lamellar (Pacinian) corpuscle in a serous gland (dog). H & E. ×20.

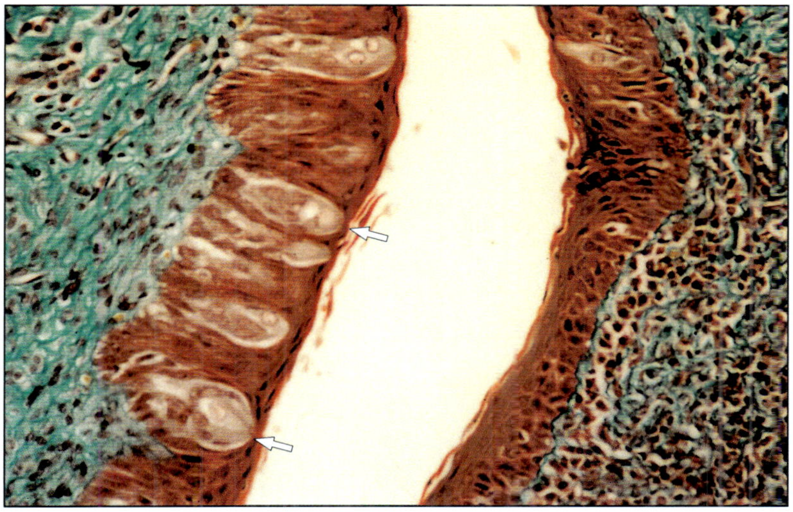

13.30

13.30 Circumvallate papilla. Tongue (cow). Taste buds are arrowed. Masson's trichrome. ×160.

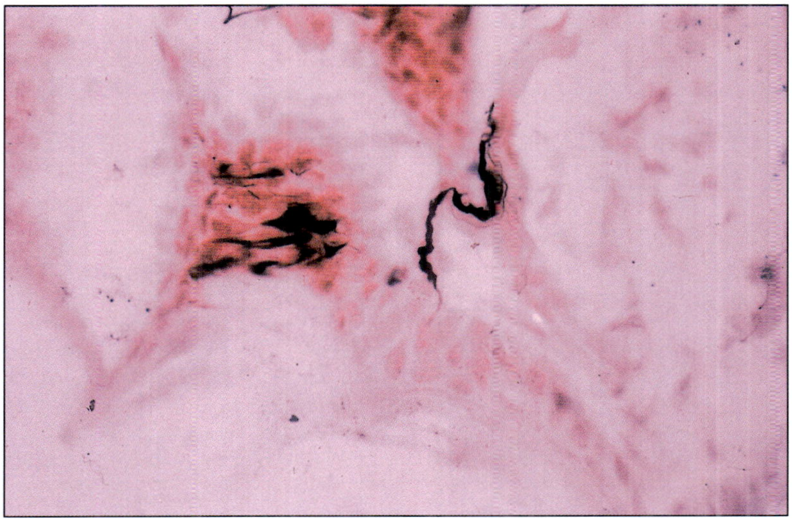

13.31

13.31 Cat skin to illustrate nerve endings stained black with Cajal's silver. ×250.

Clinical correlates

The CNS is affected by a variety of congenital disorders that occur with relatively high frequency, possibly because of the susceptibility of this complex system to teratogenic insult. Inherited CNS disease is also recognized and a heritable basis is suspected for conditions such as idiopathic epilepsy.

Inflammatory, neoplastic, metabolic and parasitic disorders are all recognized in the CNS, with certain specific entities appearing in particular species. For example, feline parvovirus, which is trophic for dividing cells, attacks the external germinal layer of the cerebellum in kittens when infection occurs before or shortly after birth. Primary CNS neoplasms are not uncommon in the dog and cat and tumours that arise from almost every type of cell within the nervous system have been recognized. The functional distinction between benign and malignant neoplasms within the CNS is not as significant as in other systems, as any space-occupying lesion, even the most biologically benign, has serious consequences. Even non-neoplastic lesions, such as equine cholesteatoma (**13.32**) in which a mass of cholesterol crystals surrounded by inflammatory cells located in the choroid plexuses can produce space-occupying effects, in particular hydrocephalus caused by obstruction of ventricular drainage.

Transmissible spongiform encephalopathies (TSE) are an unusual group of infectious central nervous disorders, although the nature of the infective agent, which differs from conventional agents like bacteria and viruses, is not precisely defined. The agent is believed to enter via the oral route and proliferate in lymphoid tissues and in the intestine, but no effects are observed until it reaches target areas of the CNS. The sheep TSE, scrapie (**13.33**), has been known for a very long time. This disease produces no significant gross pathology, although emaciation and self trauma are common, and provokes no immune response. The cattle variant, bovine spongiform encephalopathy (BSE; **13.34**) was recognized more recently and produces similar histological changes to those seen in scrapie in sheep.

13.32

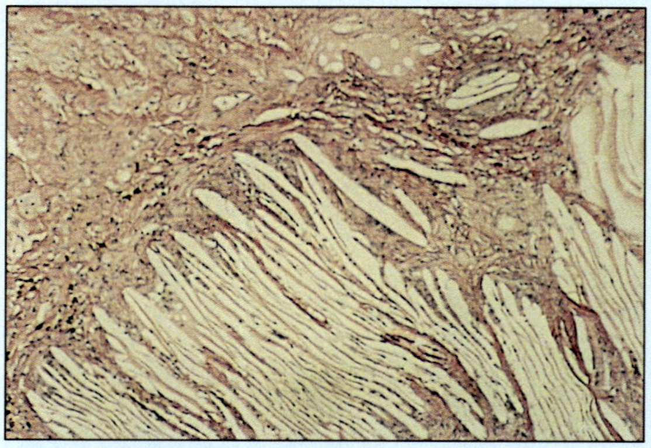

13.32 Cholesteatoma in the brain of a horse. Note the numerous clefts that previously held cholesterol deposits lost during the histological processing. H & E. ×20.

13.33

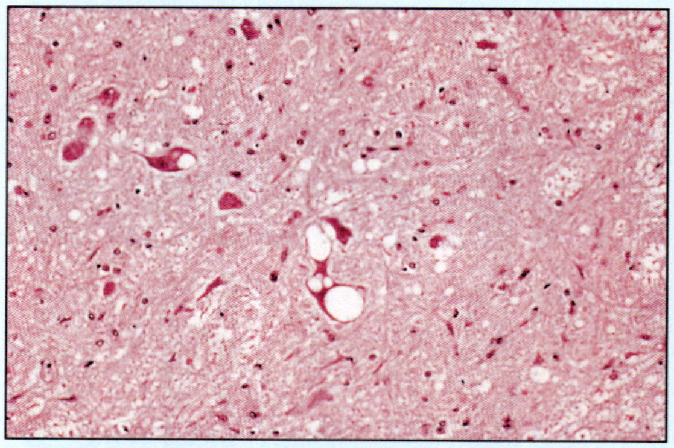

13.33 Scrapie (sheep). This is a section of midbrain from a sheep with scrapie. The characteristic large intraneuronal vacuoles and diffuse vacuolar change in the neuropil can be seen. No stainable material is present in the vacuoles. H & E. ×125.

13.34

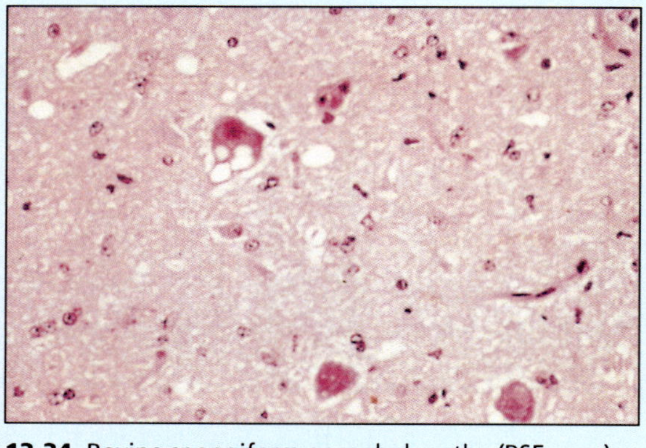

13.34 Bovine spongiform encephalopathy (BSE, cow). This section is taken from the midbrain of a cow with BSE. The histological changes are similar to those found in scrapie, with vacuolation of neuronal cell bodies in target areas of the brain, which include in particular the medullary nuclei. Some vacuolation of the neuropil is present in this section. The severity is variable between cases. Special precautions, including treating the tissues with formic acid to inactivate the BSE agent, are employed when processing these tissues. H & E. ×125.

14. SPECIAL SENSES

Eye

The eye is the organ of vision and comprises the eyeball or globe of the eye and the optic nerve. It is protected by the eyelids and lacrimal apparatus.

Eyelids

The eyelids are movable folds of skin in front of the eyeball protecting and lubricating the surface of the eye. The outer surface is covered with stratified squamous epithelium, tactile hairs, sebaceous glands (glands of Zeiss) and sweat glands (glands of Möll; **14.1**). The inner surface is lined with the palpebral conjunctiva, a thin transparent mucous membrane. The bulbar conjunctiva is continuous with the surface of the cornea at the limbus. The epithelium may be stratified columnar or stratified squamous, with goblet cells. Between the dermis of the skin and the lamina propria of the conjunctiva is a plate of dense connective tissue: the tarsal plate is surrounded by the multilobular tarsal glands (**14.2**). The nictitating membrane (third eyelid) is situated at the medial angle of the eye. It is a semi-

14.1 Eyelid (horse). Outer skin layer of the eyelid with a tactile hair (arrowed). H & E. ×7.5.

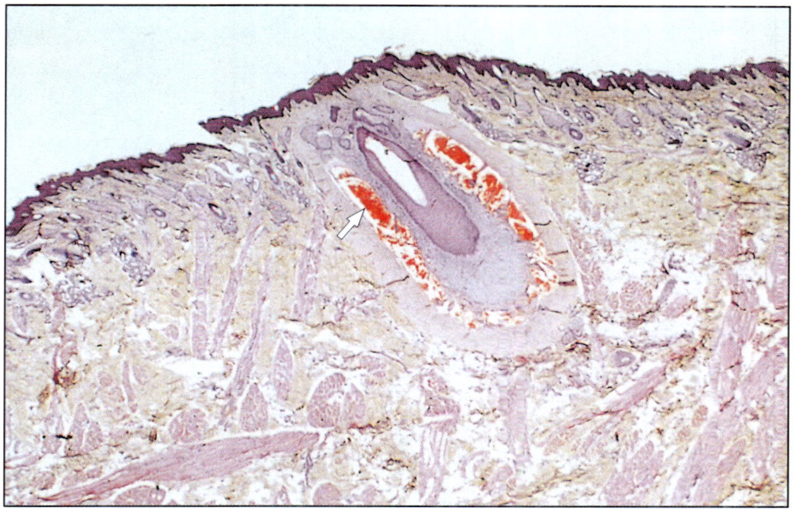

14.1

14.2 Eyelid (horse). (1) The conjunctiva, stratified columnar epithelium with mucus-secreting cells. (2) Sebaceous glands in the lamina propria. (3) Tarsal plate. H & E. ×25.

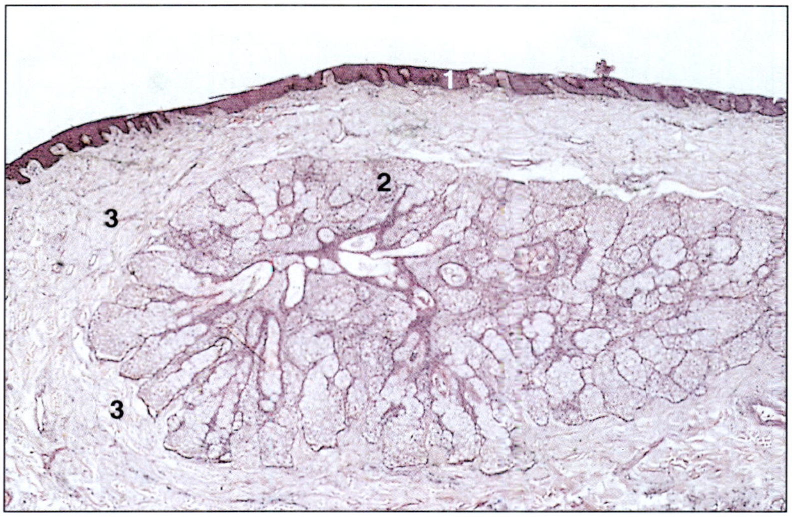

14.2

14.3
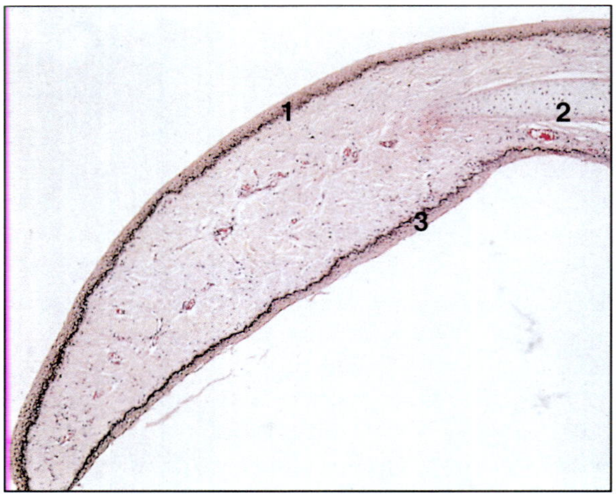

14.3 Nictitating membrane (membrana nictitans; horse). (1) Anterior surface is covered by conjunctiva. (2) Elastic cartilage plate in a central core of connective tissue. (3) Posterior plate covered by conjunctiva. H & E. ×7.5.

14.4
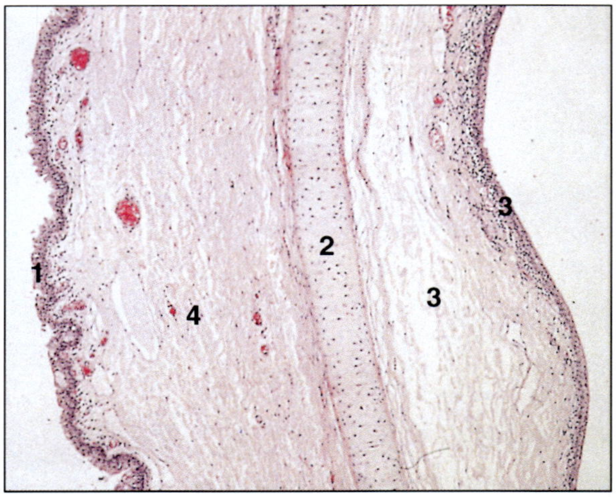

14.4 Nictitating membrane (horse). (1) Anterior conjunctival surface. (2) Elastic cartilage plate. (3) Posterior conjunctival surface. (4) Lamina propria. H & E. ×7.5.

14.5
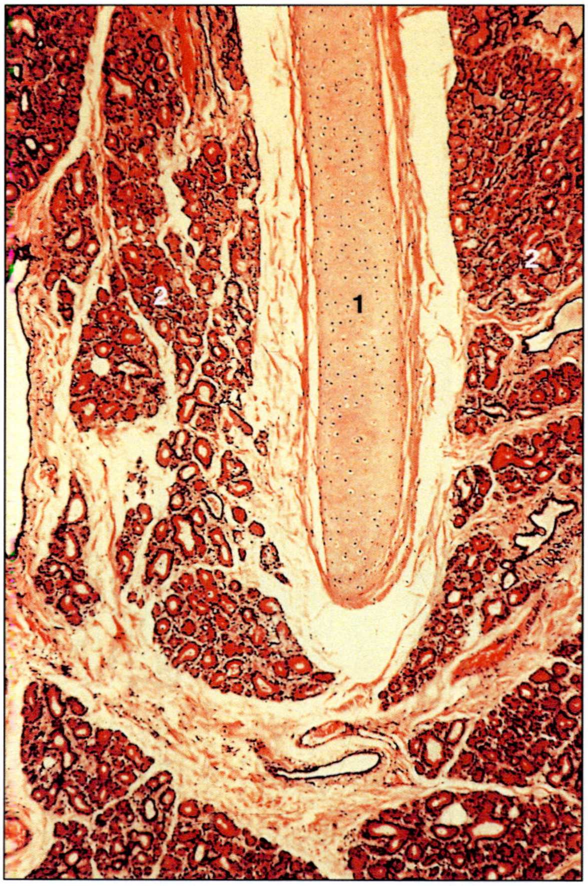

14.5 Nictitating membrane (dog). (1) Hyaline cartilage. (2) Seromucus-secreting glands in the lamina propria. H & E. ×50.

circular fold of conjunctiva enclosing a plate of cartilage (hyaline in ruminants and dog; elastic in the horse, pig and cat; **14.3–14.5**).

Lacrimal apparatus

The lacrimal glands are tubuloacinar: serous in the cat, seromucous in the horse, ruminant, dog and pig. (In the horse and ruminant they are predominantly serous, and in the pig predominantly mucous.) Lymph nodules are seen in the lamina propria (**14.6** and **14.7**). The pig and ox also have a deep gland (Harderin gland) of the nictitating membrane.

Development of the eye

The eyes are recognizable in the early embryo as lateral diverticulae of the diencephalon. As the diverticulum approaches the surface ectoderm, it invaginates to form the optic cup. The inner layer becomes the light-sensitive retina; the outer layer becomes the retinal pigment, pigmented ciliary and anterior iris epithelium. The surface ectoderm overlying the optic cup thickens and invaginates to form the lens. The reconstituted ectoderm and the local mesenchyme form the cornea; the surrounding mesoderm provides the connective tissue, blood vessels and ocular muscles (**14.8** and **4.9**).

14.6

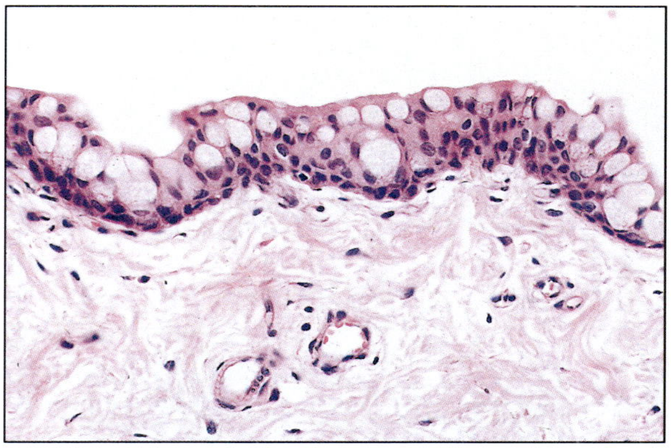

14.6 Nictitating membrane (pig). The mucus-secreting cells in the outer epithelium are stained pale pink. H/PAS. ×100.

14.7

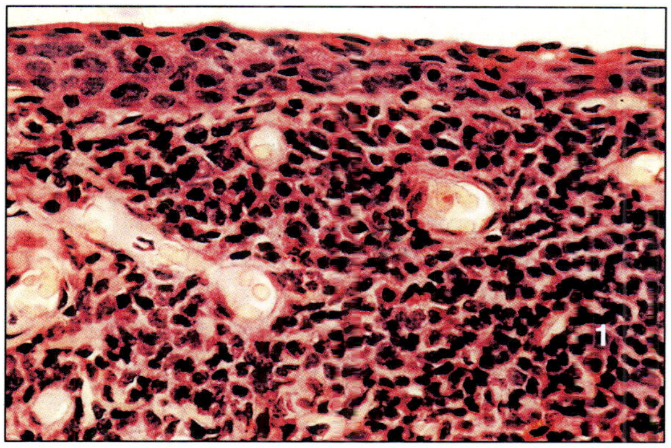

14.7 Nictitating membrane, posterior surface (dog). (1) Lymphoid cells in the lamina propria. H & E. ×125.

14.8

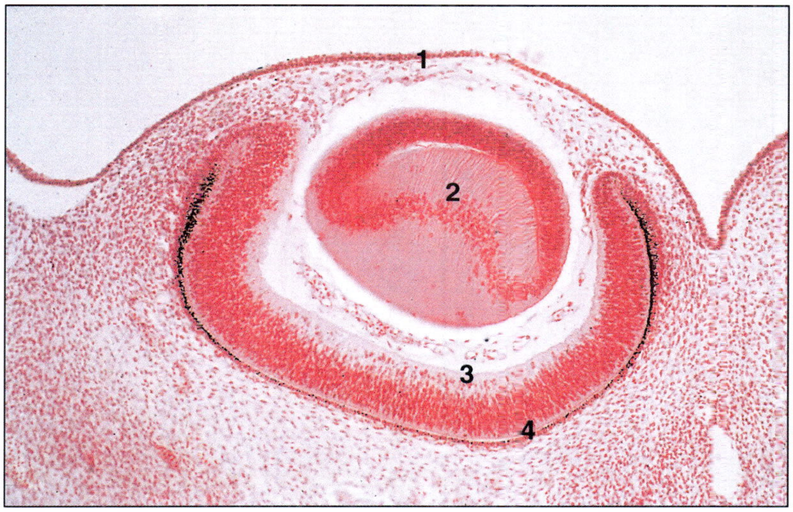

14.8 Developing eye in a 35-day cat embryo. (1) Surface ectoderm. (2) Developing lens. Optic cup has a thick inner layer (3) and a thin outer layer (4) with the pigment cells. H & E. ×7.5.

14.9

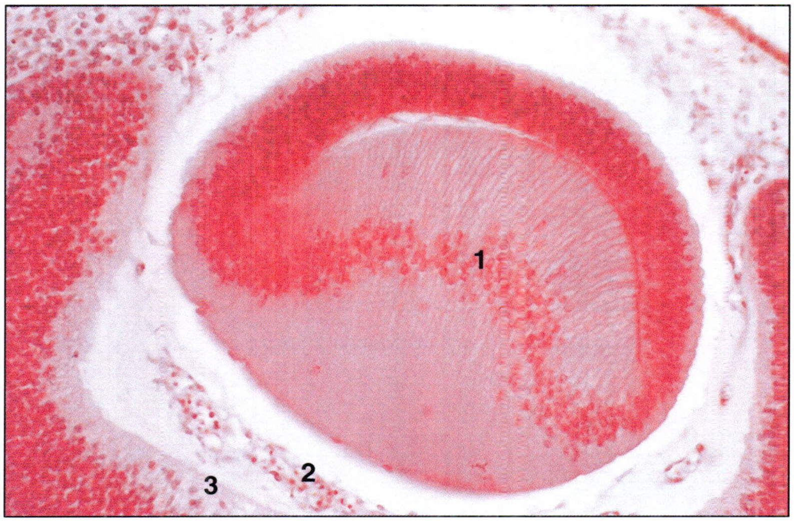

14.9 Developing eye in a 35-day cat embryo. (1) The lens fibres almost fill the lens vescicle. (2) Loose vascular mesenchyme. (3) Retina. H & E. ×25.

Structure of the eyeball

The eyeball (**14.10**) is spheroid and composed of a lens and a wall that is divided into three layers: an outer fibrous tunic (corneoscleral layer); a middle vascular tunic (uvea); and an inner retinal tunic, which consists of a 10-layered photosensitive retina and a bilayered non-photosensitive portion that covers the ciliary body and posterior surface of the iris.

The eye contains three fluid-filled regions: the anterior chamber, bordered by the cornea, iris and lens; the posterior chamber, located between the iris, lens, zonular fibres and ciliary processes; and the cavity of the vitreous humour, which lies behind the lens (**14.10**). The lens is a biconvex transparent body composed of epithelial cells within a homogeneous outer capsule. The anterior epithelial cells are cuboidal at the pole, and become elongated, prismatic and arranged in meridional rows at the equator where they form lens fibres (**14.11**). The aqueous humour circulates continuously, and is secreted and absorbed by the blood vessels in the sclera at the corneoscleral junction.

The corneoscleral layer is divided into a transparent anterior segment, the cornea, and an opaque posterior segment, the sclera. The avascular cornea is transparent, covered with non-keratinized stratified squamous epithelium resting on a basement membrane (Bowman's). The underlying stroma, the substantia propria, consists of thin lamellae of collagenous fibres and flattened fibroblasts running parallel to the corneal surface in a mucoid ground substance (**14.12** and **14.13**). The caudal limiting membrane (Descemet's) separates the connective tissue of the substantia propria from the simple squamous corneal endothelium (also called posterior epithelium; **14.14**).

The opaque sclera consists of interlacing bundles of white fibrous tissue with a few elastic fibres. The

14.10

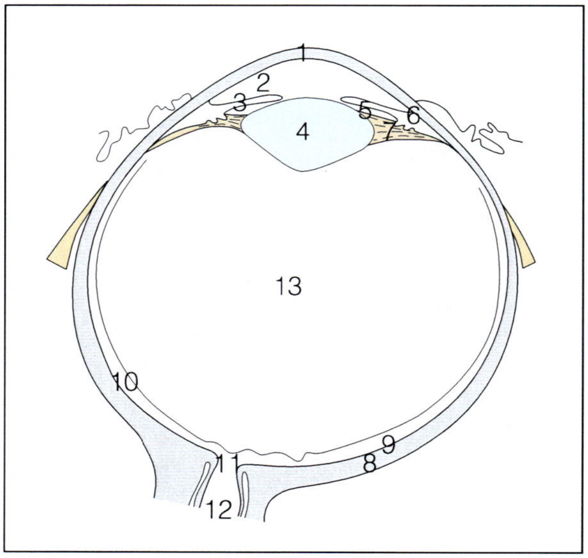

14.10 Diagram of the eye. (1) Cornea. (2) Anterior chamber. (3) Iris. (4) Lens. (5) Posterior chamber. (6) Ciliary body. (7) Ciliary processes. (8) Sclera. (9) Choroid. (10) Retina. (11) Optic papilla. (12) Optic nerve. (13) Vitreous humour.

14.11

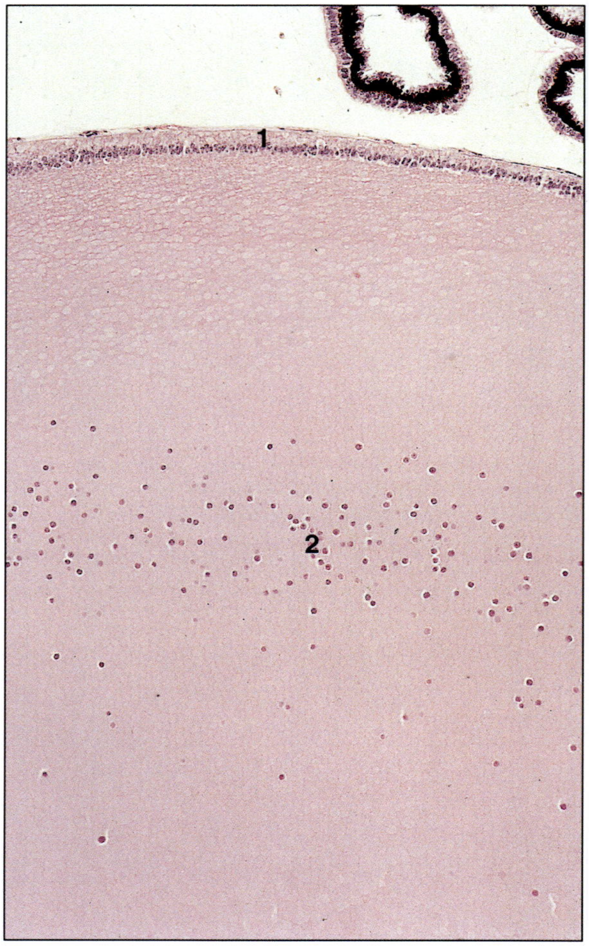

14.11 Lens (dog). (1) Anterior epithelium. (2) Nuclei of the lens fibres. H & E. ×62.5.

14.12

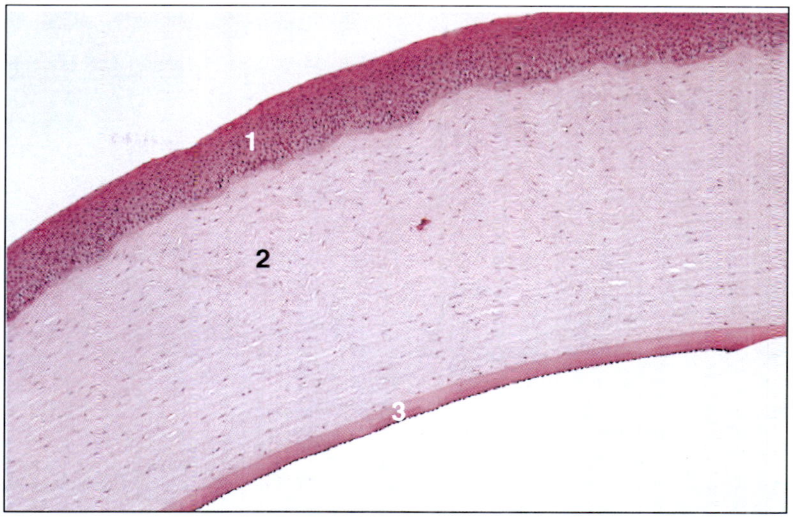

14.12 Cornea (horse). (1) Stratified squamous epithelium of the anterior surface. (2) Substantia propria. (3) Simple cuboidal endothelium of the posterior surface resting on a thick basement membrane (Descemet's). H & E. ×62.5.

14.13

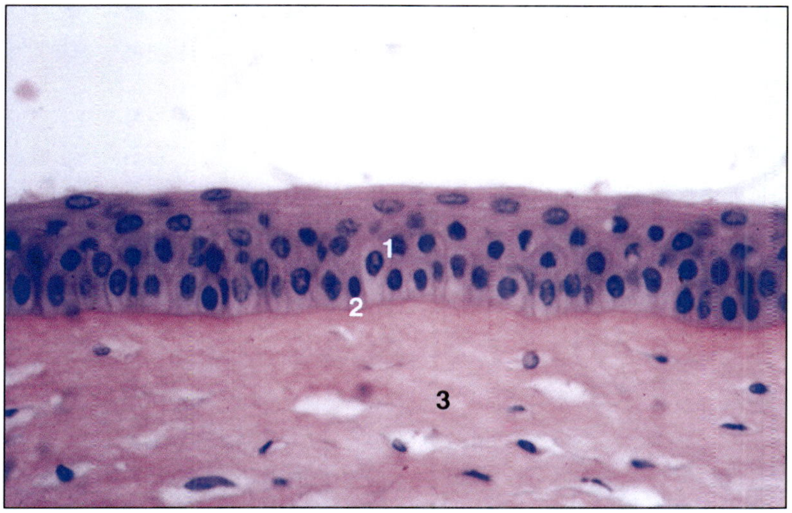

14.13 Cornea. Anterior surface (dog). (1) Stratified squamous epithelium of the anterior surface. (2) Basement membrane (Bowman's). (3) Substantia propria. H & E. ×125.

14.14

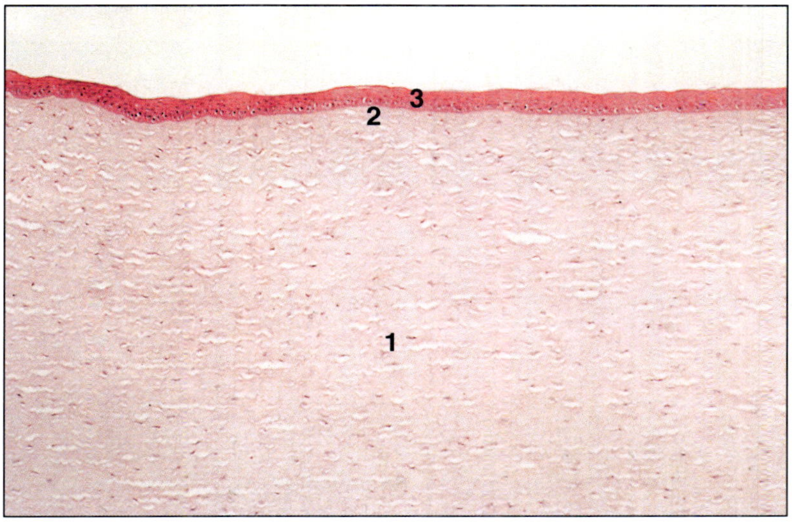

14.14 Cornea. Posterior surface (dog). (1) Substantia propria. (2) Basement membrane (Descemet's). (3) Simple squamous endothelium. H & E. ×62.5.

inner surface is attached to the middle tunic, the choroid, by a layer of delicately pigmented connective tissue, the lamina fusca (**14.15**). The optic nerve passes through the sclera at the lamina cribrosa (**14.16**).

The choroid is vascular and has numerous melanocytes. The ciliary body is an anterior continuation of the choroid that extends to the base of the iris. The inner surface is a continuation of a non-light-sensitive retina: the pars ciliaris retinae. The loose connective tissue of the stroma contains the ciliary muscle, bundles of smooth muscle fibres. An inner non-pigmented choriocapillary layer contains a capillary network that supplies the retina (**14.17–14.20**). The choroid of some species has an iridescent reflecting tissue layer: the *tapetum lucidum* (dog, **14.15**; cat, **14.19**). This gives their

14.15

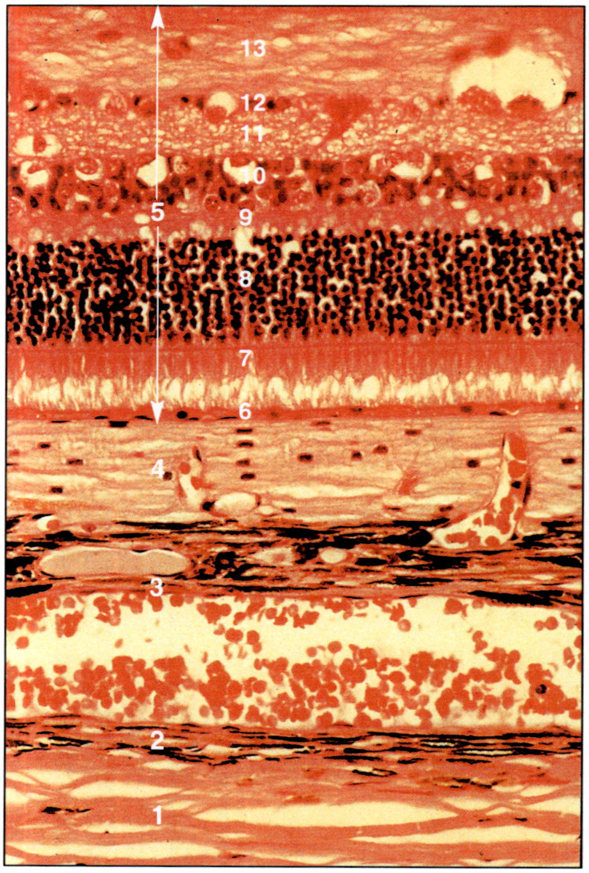

14.15 Eye. Tapetum fundus (dog). (1) Sclera composed of dense white fibrous tissue. (2) Lamina fusca. (3) Chorioid with capillaries. (4) Tapetum cellulosum. (5) The photosensitive retinal layers are (6) pigment layer, (7) rods and cones, (8) nuclei of the rods and cones, (9) outer synaptic layer, (10) bipolar nerve cell nuclei, (11) inner synaptic layer, (12) optic nerve cells, (13) optic nerve fibres. H & E. ×160.

14.

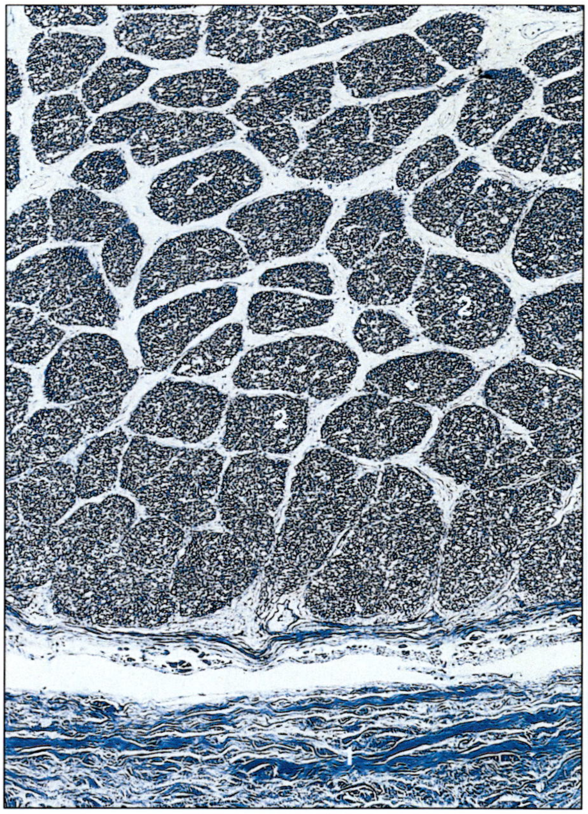

14.16 Optic disc (horse). (1) Scleral connective tissue. (2) Optic nerve bundles. H.& E. ×25.

14.1

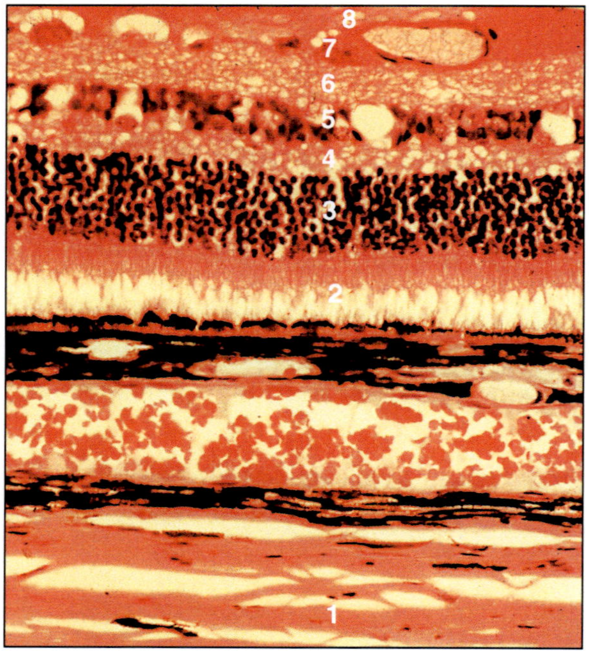

14.17 Eye. Non-tapetum fundus (dog). The retinal layers are (1) pigment layer, (2) rods and cones, (3) nuclei of the rods and cones, (4) outer synaptic layer, (5) bipolar nerve cell nuclei, (6) inner synaptic layer, (7) optic nerve cells, (8) optic nerve fibres. H & E. ×160.

14.18

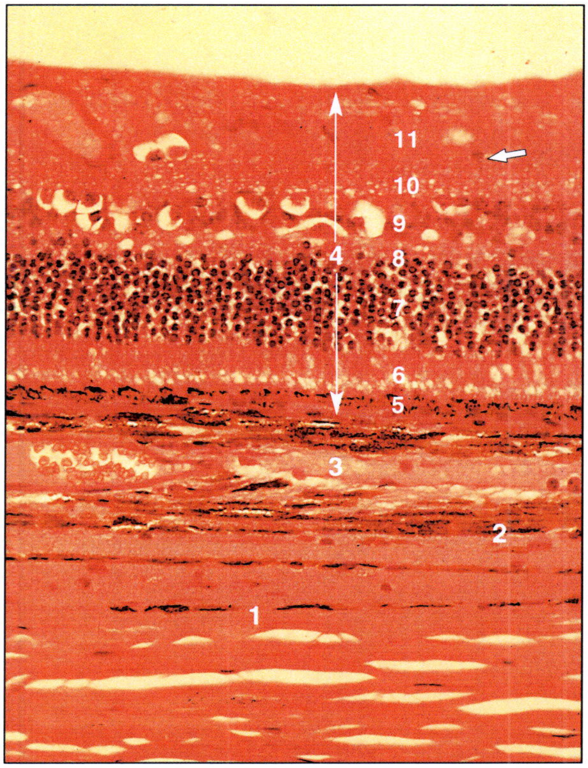

14.19

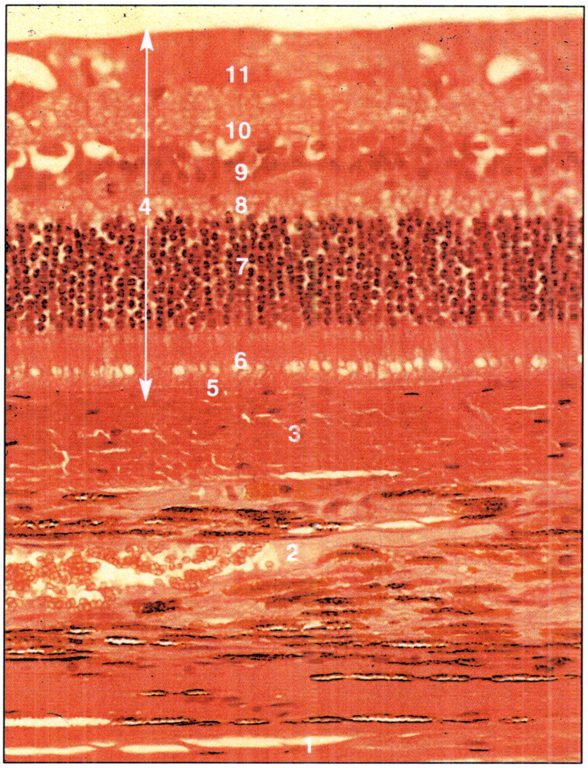

14.18 Eye. Non-tapetum fundus (cat). (1) Sclera composed of dense white fibrous tissue. (2) Lamina fusca. (3) Choroid with capillaries. (4) The photosensitive retinal layers are (5) pigment layer, (6) rods and cones, (7) nuclei of the rods and cones, (8) outer synaptic layer, (9) bipolar nerve cell nuclei, (10) inner synaptic layer, (11) optic nerve fibres. Optic nerve cells are arrowed. H & E. ×160.

14.19 Eye. Tapetum fundus (cat). (1) Sclera. (2) Choriocapillaris. (3) Non-pigmented tapetum cellulosum. (4) The photosensitive retinal layers are (5) pigment layer, (6) rods and cones, (7) nuclei of the rods and cones, (8) outer synaptic layer, (9) bipolar nerve cell nuclei, (10) inner synaptic layer, (11) optic nerve fibres. H & E. ×160.

14.20

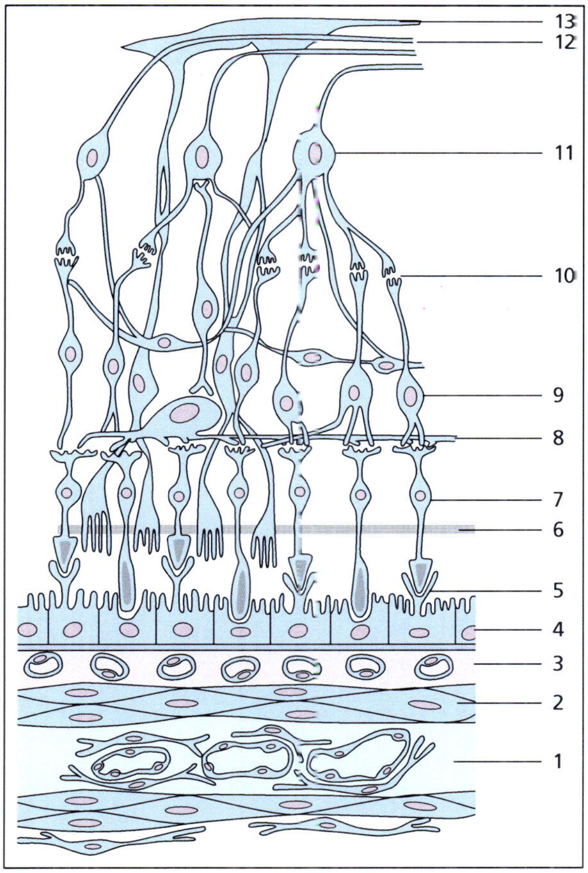

14.20 Eye. Layers of the retina. (1) Vessel layer of the choroid. (2) Connective tissue/tapetum lucidum. (3) Choriocapillaris. (4) Pigment epithelium. (5) Photoreceptors, layers of rods and cones. (6) External limiting membrane. (7) Outer nuclear layer. (8) Outer plexiform layer. (9) Inner nuclear layer. (10) Inner plexiform layer. (11) Ganglion cell layer. (12) Nerve fibre layer. (13) Internal limiting membrane.

eyes the property of shining in the dark, and allows incident light two opportunities to stimulate the retinal receptors. It is located between the choriocapillary and vascular layers of the choroid in the dorsal portion of the eye. In ungulates and the horse a fibrous area of the choroid forms the tapetum fibrosum (**14.21**). In carnivores, a cellular layer forms the tapetum cellulosum (**14.19**).

The ciliary processes form a circle of radial folds surrounding the lens. This epithelial basal layer consists of pigmented columnar cells and the surface layer of non-pigmented columnar cells (**14.22**).

The iris, the most anterior part of the uveal layer, is a muscular diaphragm rostral to the lens and pierced centrally by an opening: the pupil. The base of the iris is attached to the ciliary body. The connective tissue stroma supports many blood vessels and contains pigment cells. The epithelium is confined to the posterior surface, and is the most anterior part of the non-light-sensitive retina: the pars iridica retinae. Both layers of epithelial cells are pigmented. The anterior surface is non-epithelial, and is covered with fibrocytes and melanocytes (**14.23** and **14.24**).

The retina is the innermost layer of the wall of the eye. The photosensitive portion lines the inner surface of the eye posteriorly from the ora ciliaris retinae, the point of transition between the photosensitive and non-photosensitive areas of the retina. The latter consists of two layers of non-light-sensitive epithelium beginning at the ora serrata forming the pars iridica retinae and the *pars ciliaris retinae*. From the choroid to the cavity of vitreous humour the 10 layers (**14.15**) of the photosensitive area are as follows:

- pigment epithelium (the inner layer of the embryonic cup);
- layer of rods and cones (modified dendrites that act as photoreceptors);
- outer limiting membrane, formed by neuroglial processes;
- outer nuclear layer (nuclei in the cell bodies of the rods and cones);
- outer synaptic (plexiform) layer (connecting the rod and cone neurons with the dendrites of the bipolar neurons);
- inner nuclear layer of bipolar neurons relaying the impulses received at layers 2 to 8.
- inner synaptic (plexiform) layer (linking the axons of the bipolar neurons and the dendrites of the optic nerve cells);
- ganglion cell layer (optic nerve cells);
- nerve fibre layer (the axonal processes of the optic nerve cells converge at the optic disc and become myelinated to form the optic nerve; this sieve-like part of the sclera is the lamina cribrosa);
- inner limiting membrane, the expanded extremity of the neuroglial cells in layer 3.

Layers 2 to 10 are derived from the outer layer of the embryonic optic cup.

14.21

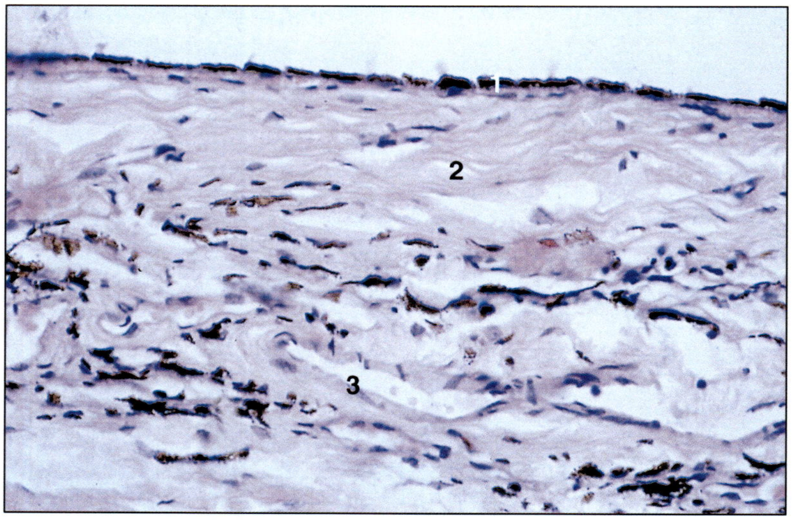

14.21 Eye. Tapetum fibrosum (horse). (1) Pigment layer of the retina. (2) Compact layer of fibrous connective tissue, the tapetum fibrosum. (3) Choroid with blood vessels and some pigment cells. H & E. ×100.

14.22 Ciliary processes (dog). (1) The long ciliary processes extend from the ciliary body, a localized expansion of the vascular coat. The epithelium is arrowed. (2) Ciliary muscle. H & E. ×62.5.

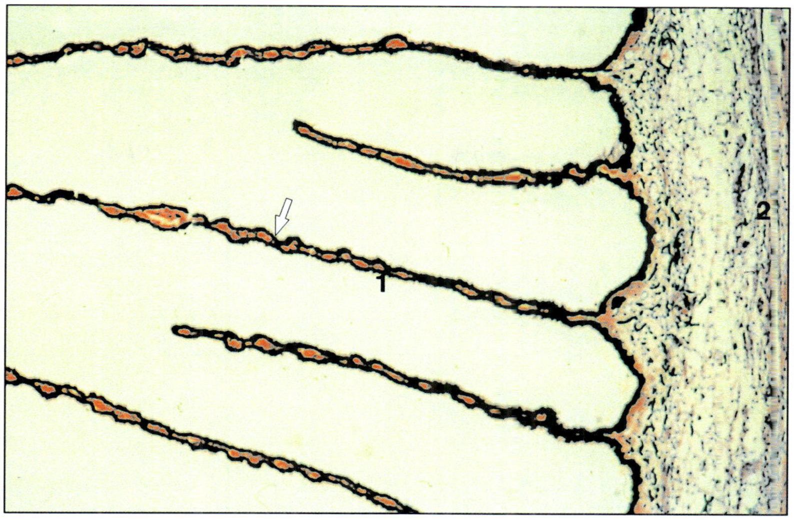

14.22

14.23 Iris (dog). (1) The anterior surface is covered by flattened fibrocytes. (2) The core of the iris is vascular connective tissue. (3) The posterior surface epithelium is two layers of cells and part of the retina. Pigment is present. H & E. ×62.5.

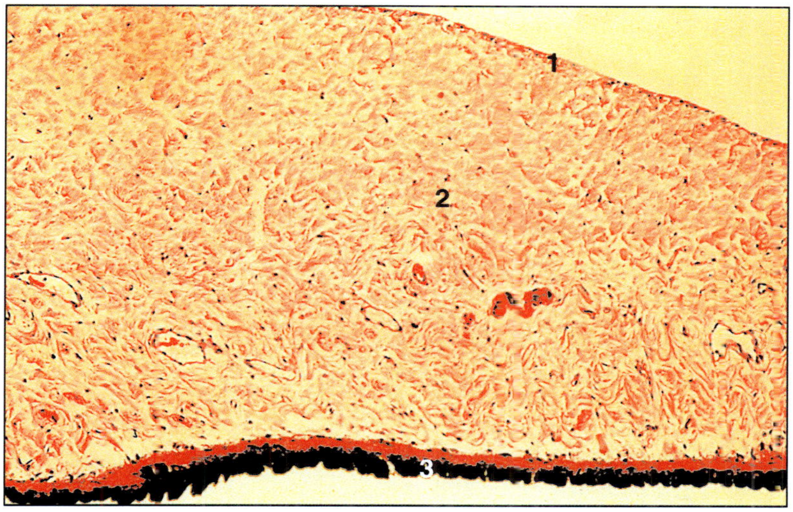

14.23

14.24 Iris (dog). Compare this with **14.23** and note the pigment; this eye will be much darker. H & E. ×62.5.

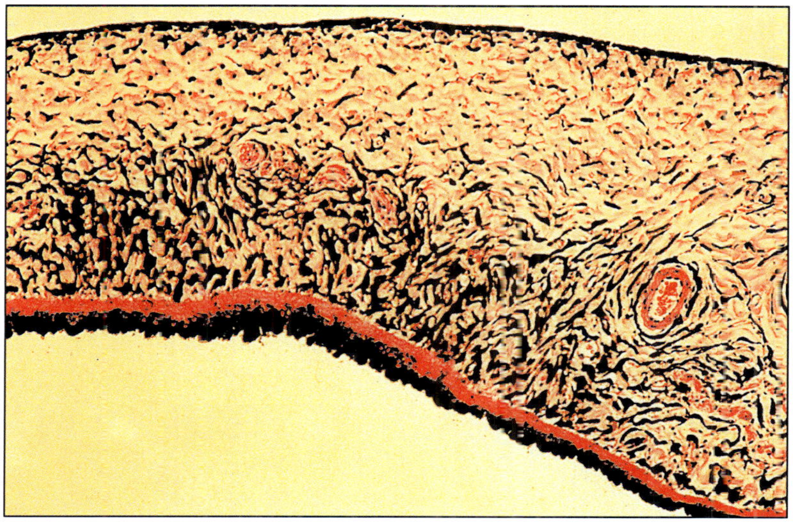

14.24

Clinical correlates

Numerous inherited ocular abnormalities are recognized in purebred dogs. In some cases control or monitoring schemes exist. Such defects may affect structures of the globe or associated tissues, such as the eyelids. Some dog breeds have exaggerated palpebral fissure shapes which can predispose to entropion and may require surgical correction. Dermoids, foci of cutaneous-type differentiation on the cornea or conjunctiva that may produce hair and other adnexal structures, are recognized in all species.

Inflammatory lesions of the eyes are named according to the structures affected and may result from infectious agents, chemical irritation or trauma. Ocular lesions may be part of a generalized disease syndrome, as in keratitis associated with malignant catarrhal fever (MCF) in cattle (**14.25**). Migrating parasitic larvae can reach the eye with potentially damaging consequences, and occasional incidents of human visceral larva migrans caused by infections with intermediate stages of ascarid parasites (*Toxocara canis*) occur. Thelazia species of spiuroid worms inhabit the conjuctival sacs and lacrimal glands of horses, cattle and in North America dogs and cats also.

Important primary neoplasms of the ocular structures include squamous cell carcinoma, tarsal gland tumours and melanomas. The eye may also be affected in cases of multicentric lymphosarcoma in several species and may be affected by metastatic tumour spread.

14.25

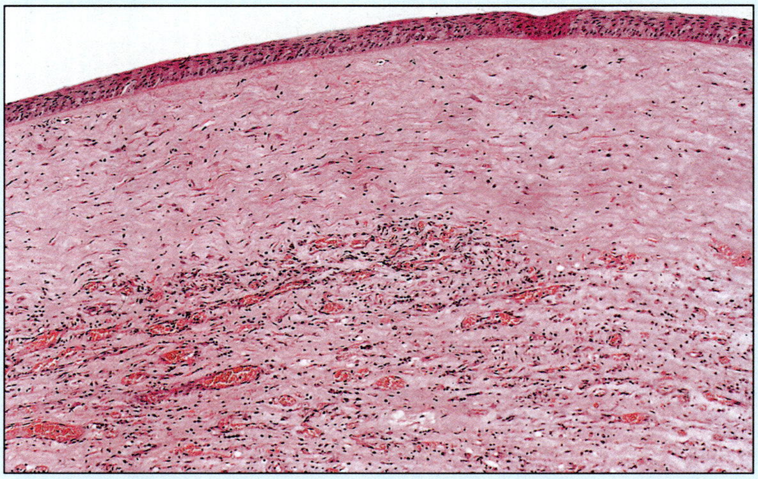

14.25 Keratitis (cow). This section, illustrating keratitis, or inflammation of the cornea, is from a cow with MCF. The effects of this highly fatal, sporadic herpes virus infection of ruminants are multisystemic and characterized by vasculitis. The normally avascular cornea shows neovascularization – the production of a capillary network, fibroplasia, oedema and infiltration by mononuclear inflammatory cells around the vessels. H & E. ×62.5.

Avian eye

The avian sclera has a ring of overlapping scleral ossicles enclosed in dense connective tissue (**14.26** and **14.27**). The avian cornea is similar to the mammalian but has a more prominent basement membrane. The choroid is thick and well-vascularized with numerous pigment cells; there is no tapetum. The avian retina has the same number of layers as the mammalian, but is avascular. The cones contain oil droplets, thought to enhance colour vision. The pecten oculi is a thin, folded, heavily pigmented membrane projecting into the vitreous humour from the optic disc (**14.28**). The lens is composed of a body and an annular pad forming a ring around the equator of the lens. The lens fibres of the annular pad are arranged radially, but in the lens body the fibres run parallel to the optical axis.

Deep (Harderian) gland

This gland lies on the ventral caudomedial aspect of the eyeball. The gland cells are vacuolated. Large numbers of plasma cells are present seeded from the cloacal bursa. These cells discharge antibodies mixed with the gland secretion into the conjunctival sac, thus providing local immunity. Lacrimal glands are also present.

.26

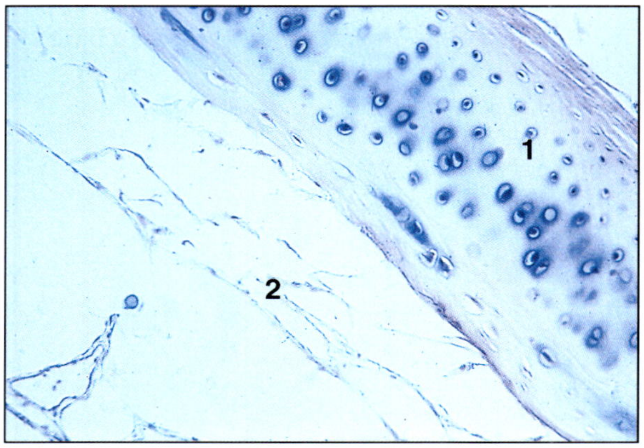

14.26 Avian eye. (1) Sclera with hyaline cartilage. (2) Choroid. H.& E. ×62.5.

14.27

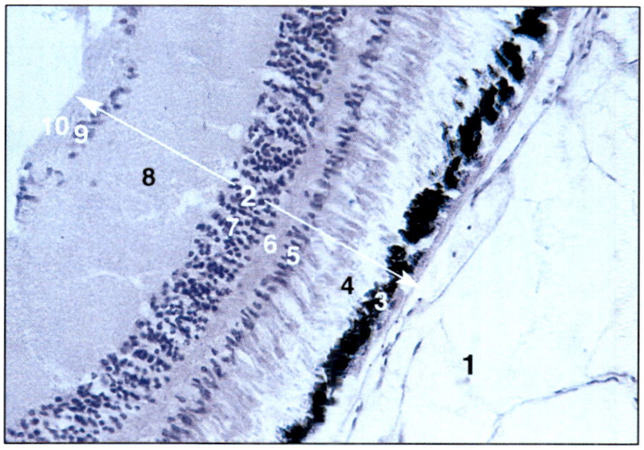

14.27 Avian eye. (1) Choroid. (2) Retinal layers are (3) pigment layer, (4) rods and cones, (5) nuclei of the rods and cones, (6) outer synaptic layer, (7) bipolar nerve cell nuclei, (8) inner synaptic layer, (9) optic nerve cells, (10) optic nerve fibres. H.& E. ×125.

14.28 Avian eye. The pecten (arrowed) is a heavily folded,vascular pigmented membrane projecting into the vitrous humour from the posteroventral surface of the eye. (1) Optic nerve. (2) Retina. (3) Choroid. H.& E. ×12.5.

14.28

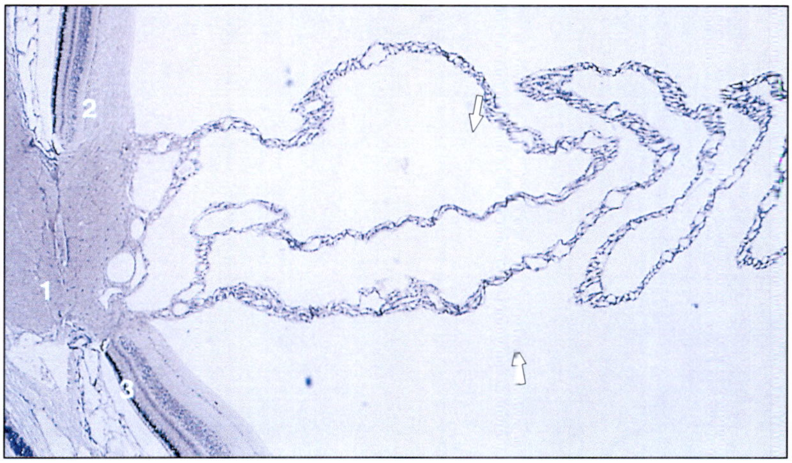

Reptilian, amphibian and fish eyes

Fish, amphibians, reptiles and birds are relatively close phylogenetically to each other. Generally, the histological features of their eyes are similar, but there are some notable exceptions.

The pupillary shapes in fish, amphibian and some reptilian eyes vary considerably between families within a given class.

Some species possess nictitating membranes; others do not. Snakes and some lizards lack moveable eyelids, and their corneas are covered with a tertiary spectacle, an optically clear keratinized epidermal tunic that is derived from the integument. This structure is shed and renewed with each moult of the epidermis (14.29). Like many

14.29

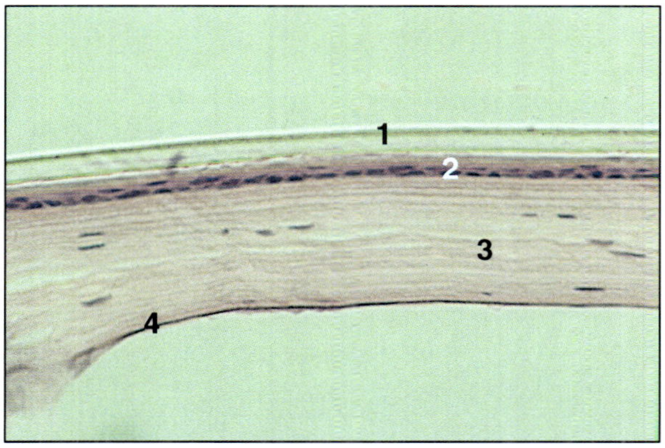

14.29 Cornea and tertiary spectacle of a regal (ball) python (*Python regius*). The thin keratinized spectacle (1) is contiguous with the periorbital integument, and it is shed and renewed with each moult. (2) Anterior epithelium. (3) Descemet's membrane. (4) Cornea stroma. H & E. ×125.

birds, numerous reptiles have eyes supported in part by scleral ossicles. The crystalline lens in the eyes of fish, amphibians and reptiles is histologically similar to that in mammals. The posterior segment of the eye, particularly the visual epithelium, varies markedly within each class. The layers of the retina and choroid are similar to those in mammals (**14.30** and **14.31**). In many reptiles, particularly diurnal species, a vascular and heavily pigmented conus papillaris projects anteriorly into the globe from the head of the optic nerve (**14.31**).

14.30

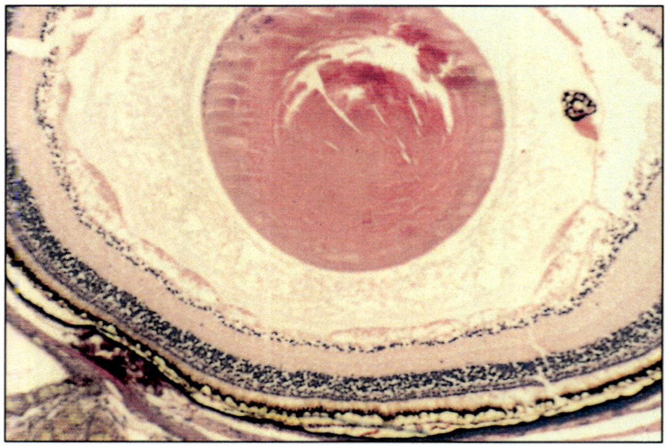

14.30 Whole mount section of the eye of a small yucca night lizard (*Xantusia vigilis*), a species that lacks moveable eyelids. H & E. ×7.5.

14.31

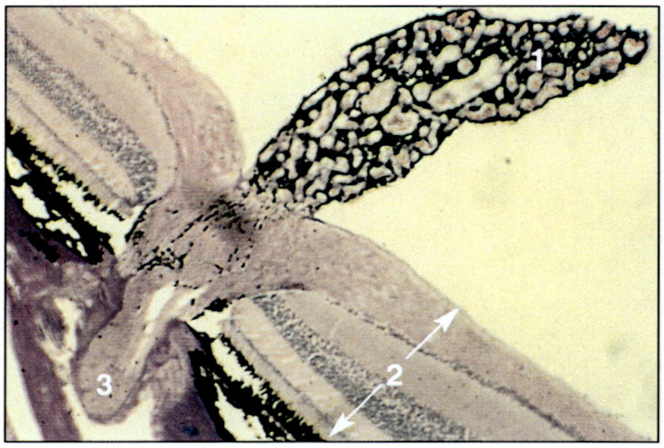

14.31 Visual epithelium of a panther chameleon (*Chamaeleon pardalis*). (1) Conus papillaris. (2) Retina. (3) Optic nerve. H & E. ×20.

Clinical correlates

Essentially, all of the clinically significant ophthalmic disorders affecting mammalian eyes can affect the eyes of lower vertebrates. However, some conditions are unique to some lower vertebrates because their eyes are characterized by structures that are lacking in the mammalian eye; for example, inflammation of the tertiary spectacle and the subspectacular space could only occur in an animal whose eyes are lidless and covered with an epidermally derived spectacle (**14.32**). Some species are more prone to certain ophthalmic disorders induced by their incorrect captive diets. Examples of such lesions are the lipid and calcified corneal opacities of some frogs. Cholesterol deposits occasionally develop in the corneas of some reptiles.

14.32

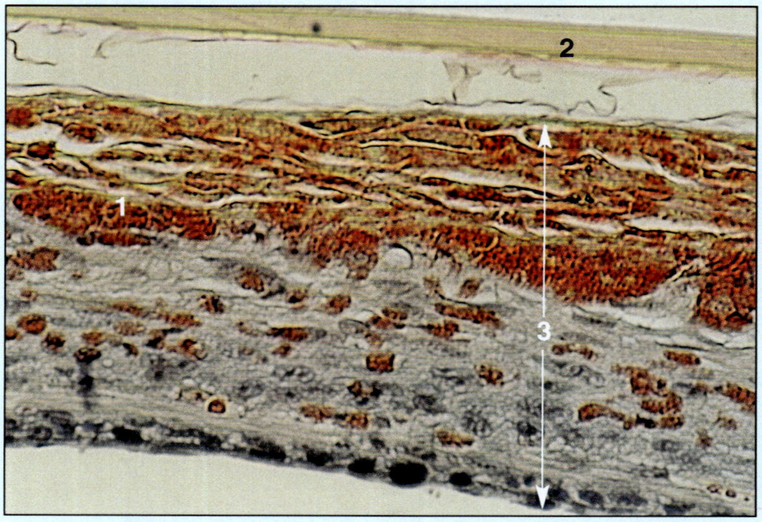

14.32 Suppurative keratitis in a mountain kingsnake (*Lampropeltis zonata*). The corneal stroma (1) contains numerous heterophilic granulocytic leucocytes. (2) Tertiary spectacle. (3) Cornea. Congo Red. ×160.

Ear

The ear has three divisions: external, middle and internal.

External ear

The external ear comprises the auricle (pinna), the auditory canal and the tympanic membrane. The auricle consists of a central plate of elastic cartilage covered by skin rich in sebaceous glands. There are also some sweat glands and a variable amount of hair (**14.33**). The auditory canal is a rigid tunnel lined with thin skin; the upper portion is supported by elastic cartilage, the remainder by bone. It contains large coiled sweat glands, some fine hair and a few sebaceous glands that secrete cerumen (ear wax; **14.34**).

Middle ear

The auditory canal ends at the tympanic membrane, which separates the external ear from the middle ear. The external surface of the membrane is covered by skin and the internal surface by a simple squamous or cuboidal epithelium. The centre consists of dense collagen bundles (**14.35**).

Three auditory ossicles, the malleus, the incus and the stapes, form a chain of small bones from the tympanic membrane to the oval window in the petrous part of the temporal bone. Sound is transmitted by the ossicles to the fluids of the internal ear and generate movement of the delicate basilar membrane of the cochlea. The expanded rostral part of the tympanic cavity forms the auditory (Eustacian) tube and connects the middle ear and the pharynx [*see* also Chapter 7, Gutteral pouch (**7.6**)].

14.33 External ear canal (dog). (1) Stratified squamous keratinized epithelium lines the canal. (2) Hair follicles. (3) Sebaceous glands. (4) Sweat glands. (5) Elastic cartilage. Masson's trichrome. ×20.

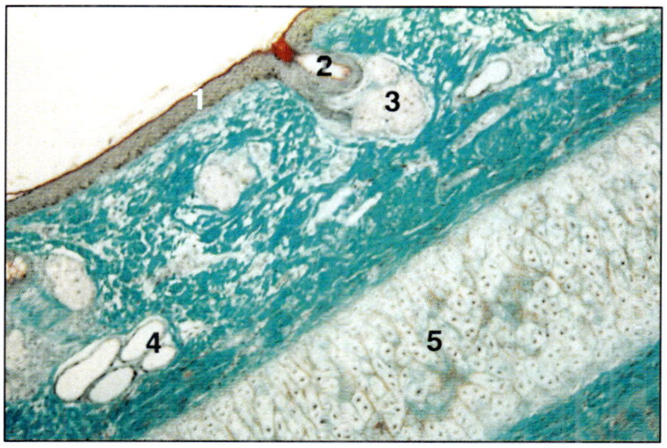

14.33

.34

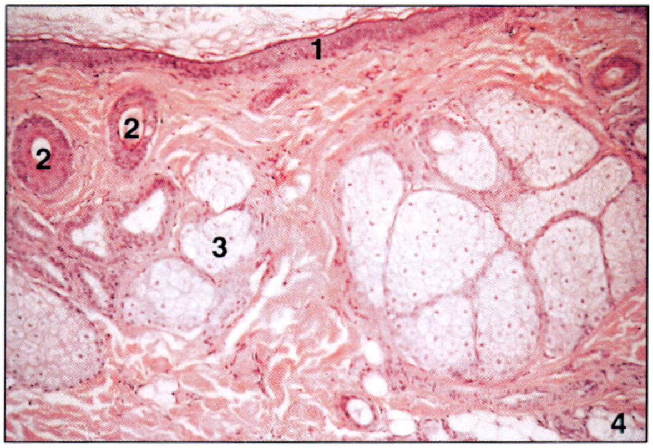

14.34 Ear canal (dog). (1) Stratified squamous keratinized epithelium. (2) Hair follicles. (3) Special sebaceous glands secreting cerumen. (4) Sweat glands. H & E. ×50.

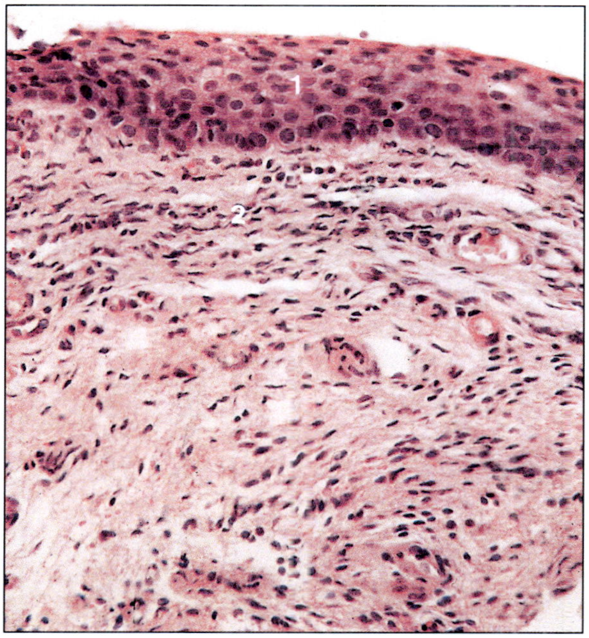

14.35

14.35 Tympanic membrane (goat). (1) External surface covered by stratified squamous epithelium. (2) Dense connective tissue. H & E. ×125.

Internal ear

The internal ear consists of the osseous (bony) labyrinth and the membranous labyrinth. The osseous labyrinth is a space within the temporal bone and consists of the vestibule, semicircular canals and cochlea. The membranous labyrinth is inside the osseous labyrinth and consists of the utricle and saccule (within the vestibule), the semicircular ducts (within the semicircular canals) and the cochlear duct (within the cochlea). It contains endolymph and is separated from the walls of the osseous labyrinth by perilymph. It adheres to the wall of the osseous labyrinth by means of fine connective tissue strands derived from the connective tissue lamina propria of the lining endothelium. This endothelium is replaced at certain points by neuroepithelial cells (**14.36**). In the semicircular canals, local expansions of the ampullae house sensory structures: the cristae ampullaris. The neuroepithelial sensory hair cells and supporting (sustentacular) cells of each crista are covered by a gelatinous cupola (**14.37**). When the latter is deflected during rotational movements of the head, the sensory cells are stimulated and impulses sent to the brain.

Both the utricle and saccule are lined in part by maculae, patch-like collections of sensory hair cells and supporting cells. Maculae are lined with mesothelium and covered with a gelatinous otolithic membrane, in which are embedded calcium carbonate crystals: the otoliths. As the membrane shifts in response to gravity acting upon the otoliths, sensory cells of the maculae are stimulated. They enable the animal to determine the position of its head in space and to assess linear acceleration and deceleration (**14.38**). The sensory cells are surrounded by terminals of the vestibular nerve.

The osseous cochlea surrounding the cochlear canal in a spiral around a central pillar of bone, the modiolus, contains in turn the spiral lamina, a thin shelf of bone that travels up the modiolus. The canal is divided into three compartments: the dorsal scala vestibuli and ventral scala tympani, which contain perilymph and are lined with squamous epithelium, and the cochlear duct between them (**14.39**). The floor of the duct is formed from the fibrous basilar membrane and the roof from the vestibular (Reissner's) membrane, and consists of two layers of simple squamous epithelium. The acoustically sensitive spiral organ (of Corti) rests on the basilar membrane and is composed of uroepithelial hair cells and sustentacular cells. The lower surface of the membrane, facing the ventral scala tympani, is lined with simple squamous epithelium. The bases of the cells are widely separated and the apices enclose to form a triangular space, the inner tunnel, containing a gelatinous substance and the cochlear nerve fibres. Overlying the spiral organ and extending from the spiral limbus (an elevation of protective tissue above the spiral lamina) is the tectorial membrane, resting on the cilia of the hair cells. The cilia are displaced when the basilar membrane vibrates in response to sound waves passing through the fluid-filled scalas. Nerve terminals form a web around the bases of the hair cells and transmit stimuli to the spiral ganglion of bipolar neurons. The axons form the cochlear division of the eighth cranial nerve (**14.40**).

14.36

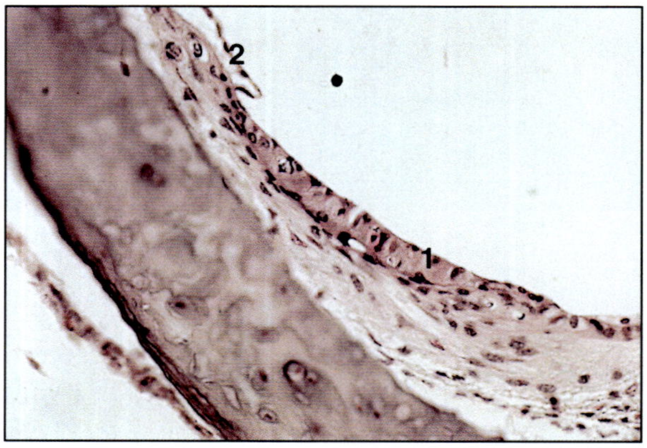

14.36 Inner ear (cat). (1) Specialized neuroepithelial cells in the vestibule continuous with (2) endothelial cells lining the labyrinth. H & E. ×125.

14.3

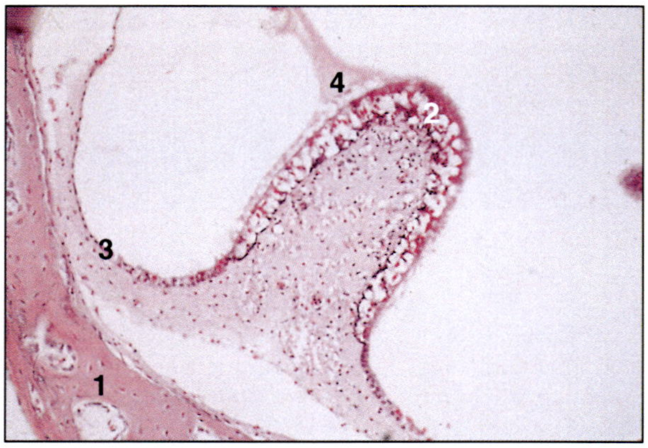

14.37 Inner ear. Crista (cat). (1) Bone of the osseous labyrinth. (2) Neuroepithelial (hair) cells and supporting cells of the crista continuous with (3) endothelium lining the membraneous labyrinth. (4) Cupula. H & E. ×125.

14.38

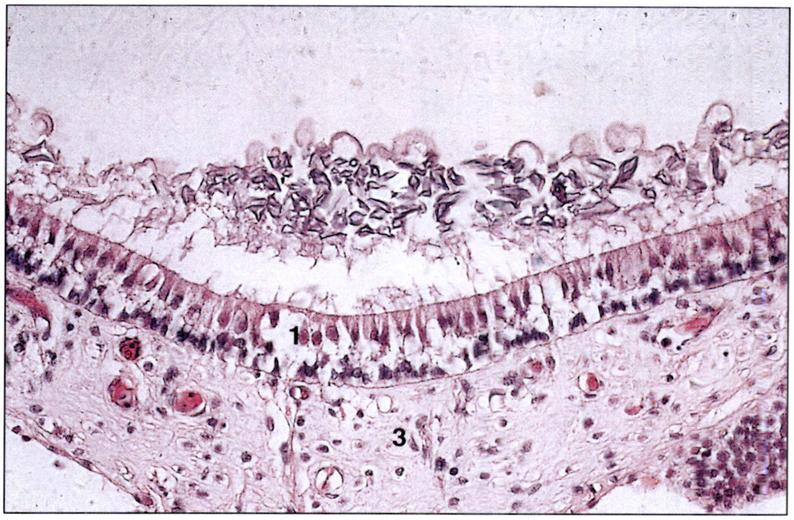

14.38 Inner ear. Macula (cat). (1) Columnar epithelium of the macula consists of neuroepithelial cells and supporting cells continuous with the lining epithelium of the vestibule. (2) Otoliths. (3) Connective tissue. H & E. ×160.

14.39

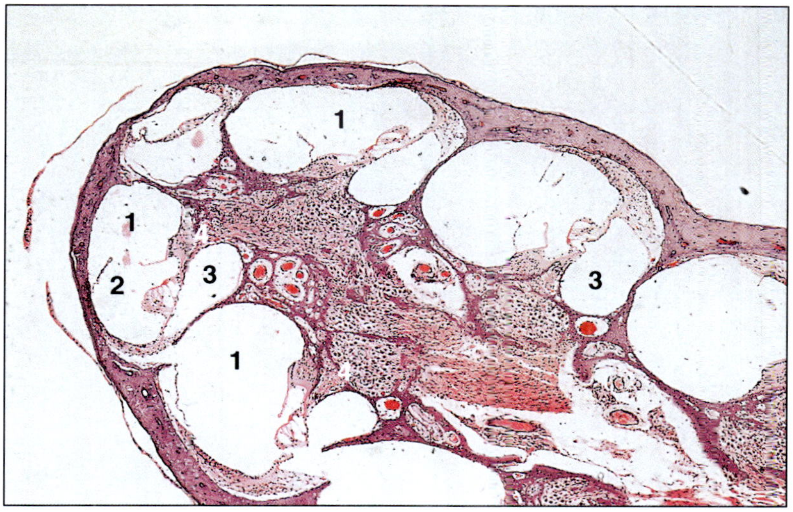

14.39 Inner ear. Cochlea (cat). (1) Dorsal scala vestibuli. (2) Middle cochlear duct. (3) Ventral scala tympani. (4) Spiral ganglion. H & E. ×7.5.

14.40

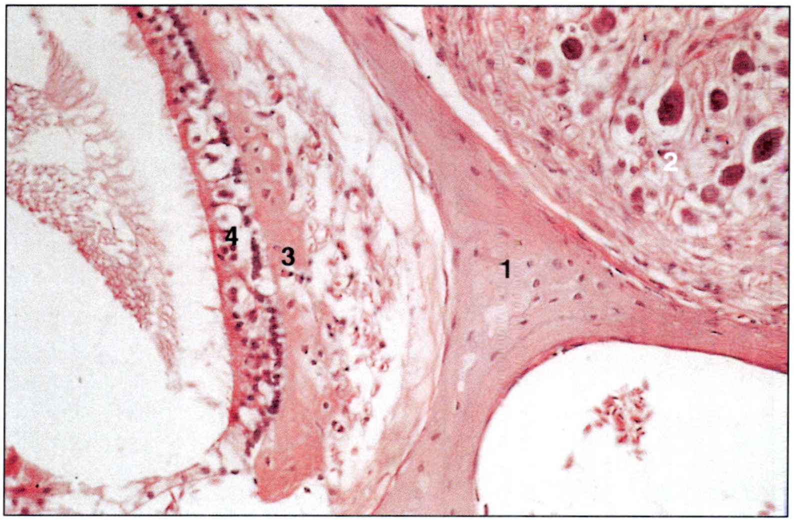

14.40 Inner ear. Spiral organ (of Corti) (cat). Located on the floor of the cochlear duct. (1) Osseous spiral. (2) Spiral ganglion. (3) Basilar membrane. (4) Sensory and supporting cells. H & E. ×160.

Clinical correlates

Diseases of the ear in domestic animals are probably not commonly investigated by pathologists, although the three broad categories otitis externa, otitis media and defects of hearing may be considered. Otitis externa (**14.41**), or inflammation of the external ear canal, may be a problem restricted to the waxy integument of this site or it may be part of a widespread skin condition. Usually only chronic cases of this very common condition, in which the severe thickening of the walls of the ear canal may raise clinical suspicion of tumour development, are submitted for histopathological examination.

14.4

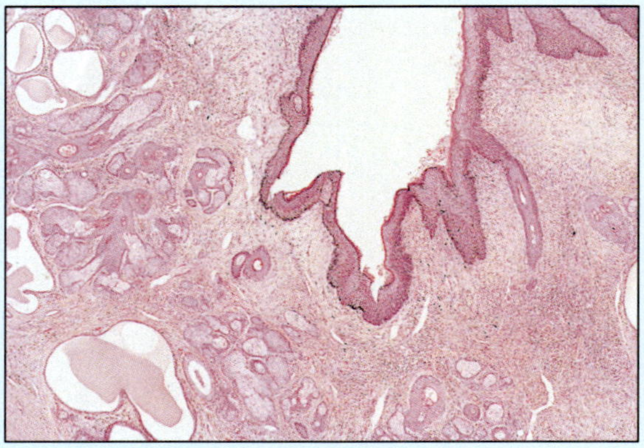

14.41 Otitis externa (dog) The surface epithelium (centre) is hyperplastic and there is dermal fibrosis. The patchy appearance of the dermis is caused by a mixed, mainly mononuclear, inflammatory infiltrate. The sebaceous glands are hyperplastic and there is cystic dilatation of the ceruminous glands, some of which are seen filled with eosinophilic cerumen. H & E. ×20.

Avian ear

The external ear lacks a pinna and ceruminous glands. The auditory ossicles are fused to form a cartilaginous rod, the columella, which extends from the tympanic membrane to the oval window. The membranous labyrinth is essentially similar to that of the mammal (**14.42**). The saccule, however, differs in that it contains two maculae. The cochlear duct also possesses a terminal expansion that is peculiar to birds, the lagena, and is separated from the dorsal scala vestibuli by the tegmentum vasculosum, a thin connective tissue membrane integrated with a highly folded vascular epithelium.

Reptilian and amphibian ears

The external pinna and ceruminous glands are absent. Some terrestrial frogs and toads that utilize audible calls in their courtship and territorial behaviour have acute hearing. Many amphibians possess external tympanic membranes; others lack them entirely. However, some aquatic amphibians have lateral line systems with which they detect water-transmitted vibratory signals and hydrostatic pressure changes (see **14.50**).

Crocodilians are capable of hearing air-transmitted sounds. They have slit-like auditory openings that can be closed when they submerge themselves.

Most lizards have ears with tympanic membranes that are located close to the integumentary surface

14.42

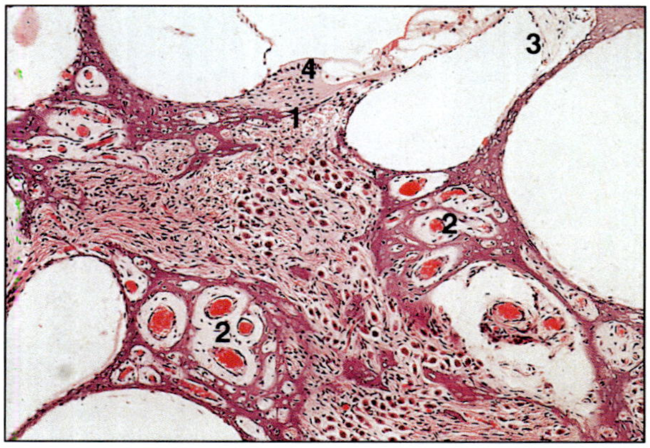

14.42 Avian inner ear. (1) Spiral ganglion. (2) Osseous labyrinth. (3) Membraneous labyrinth. (4) Neuroepithelial sensory cells. H.& E. ×125.

of the skull. In some species the tympanic membrane is flush with the skin surface. In others it lies within a shallow depression or deeper auditory meatus.

Snakes, chelonians and the tuatara lack external auditory structures. The philosophical question of whether their sense of 'hearing' is limited to substrate-transmitted vibrations is a topic of spirited debate.

The inner ear is responsible for the spacial and postural orientation of the animal within its environment. The morphological and histological features of the amphibian and reptilian inner ear are sufficently similar to the mammalian and avian ear that further discussion is not warranted here.

Organ of smell (olfactory organ)

The nose, in addition to its role in the respiratory system, also functions as the olfactory organ In the nasal cavity, brown–yellow olfactory epithelium occurs together with pinkish respiratory epithelium. It is a pseudostratified columnar epithelium with olfactory (sensory) cells, basal cells and supporting cells. Tubular mucoserous glands (Bowman's) lie in the lamina propria and secrete onto the surface through simple ducts lined with cuboidal cells (14.43 and 14.44).

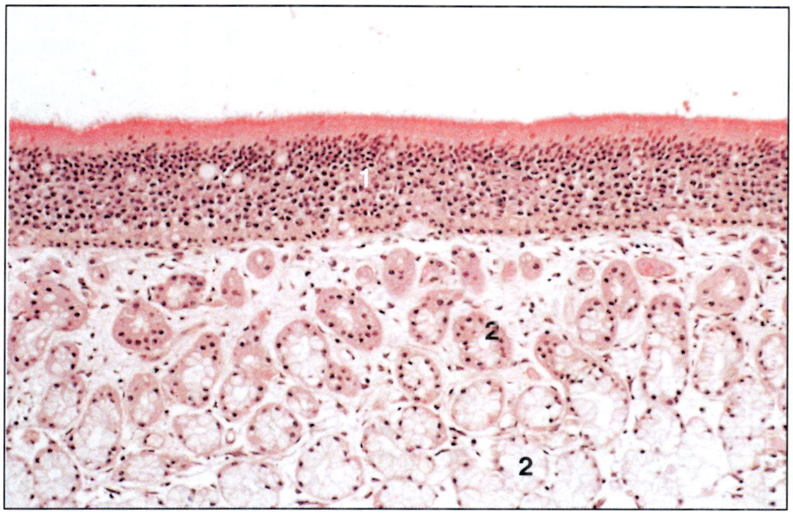

14.43

14.43 Olfactory organ (horse). (1) The olfactory epithelium is pseudostratified ciliated columnar with many rows of nuclei; the more superficial are of the sustentacular cells; the deeper nuclei are of the olfactory nerve cells. (2) Vascular connective tissue with mucous glands. H & E. ×160.

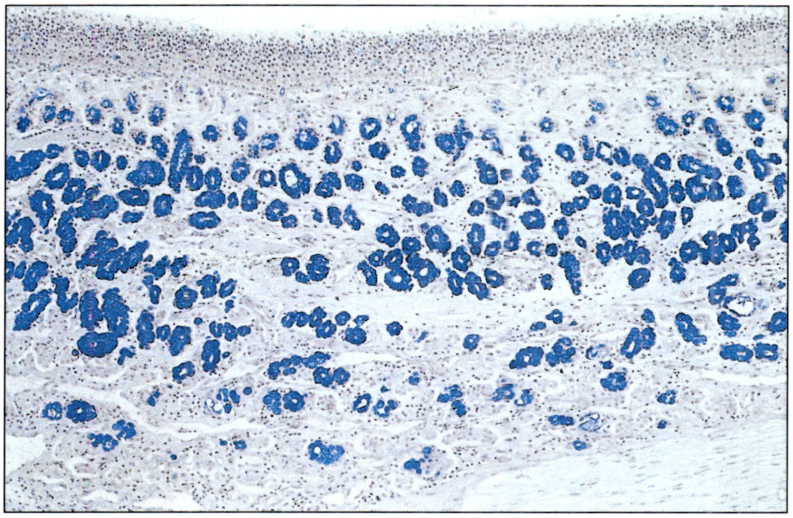

14.44

14.44 Olfactory organ (horse). The mucous cells stain deep blue. Alcian blue. ×100.

Other specialized sense organs

Besides sight, hearing, taste, touch and the perception of pain, heat and cold, many of the lower vertebrates possess highly specialized organs that augment their awareness of their external environment.

Parietal eye

In addition to their paired lateral eyes, many lizards and the primitive tuatara (*Sphenodon punctatus*) have a parietal eye. This photosensitive organ consists of a scale-like and cell-poor cornea, a cellular lens, a central chamber filled with clear fluid and a few macrophages, and a cup-shaped pigmented visual epithelium that is analagous to the retina and choroid (**14.45**). The parietal eye is partially responsible for regulating basking and other thermoregulating behavioural activities, and it can warn of the approach of potential predators whose shadows are detected by the upward directed eye-like structure.

Facial and labial pit organs

Rattlesnakes, water moccasins, copperhead snakes and other pit vipers possess paired facial pit organs (**14.46**) with which they sense very small differences in the background thermal environment. This ability to discriminate slight temperature variations aids in prey detection both before and after the prey animals have been envenomated.

Non-venomous snakes of the family Boidae (boas, pythons and anacondas that are ambush predators) possess labial pit organs (**14.47**), which help them locate warm-blooded prey. These branched pit-like depressions are lined with lightly keratinized squamous epithelium through which numerous dendritic sensory neurons penetrate.

Vomeronasal organ

Most snakes and lizards have well-developed vomeronasal (Jacobson's) organs (**14.48**), which assist in sampling and discriminating chemosensory stimulatory particles such as prey-related scent or pheromones. The vomeronasal organ consists of a mushroom-shaped rounded column with a cartilaginous core. This column is surrounded by a cup-shaped spherical cavity. The luminal surfaces of the column and cavity are covered with ciliated columnar or pseudostratified columnar epithelium through which myriad numbers of tiny dendritic nerves pass between adjacent cell membranes. These nerve endings project out into the lumen (**14.49**).

Lateral line organ

Most fish and many amphibians (particularly aquatic frogs, newts and salamanders) have lateral line systems (**14.50**) that are sensitive to slight changes in hydrostatic pressure and water-borne vibration. Tall cuboidal to fully columnar cells form vibration- and pressure-sensitive neuromasts that receive and transmit impulses from the aquatic environment to the animal's central nervous system.

14.45

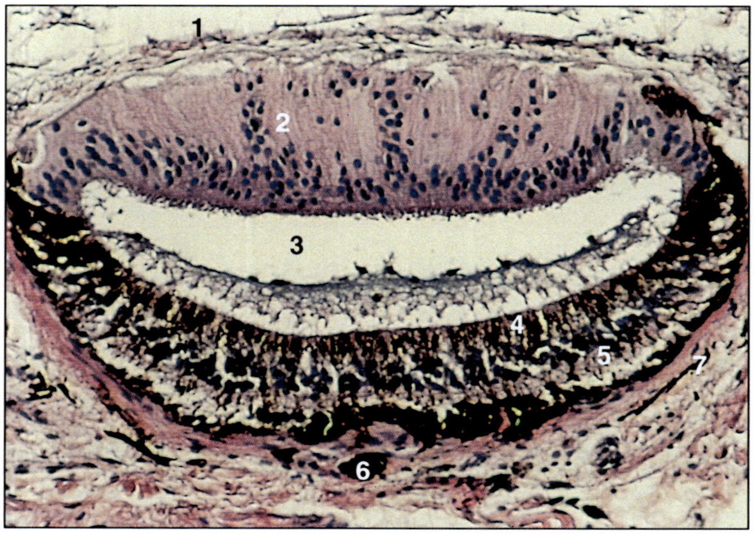

14.45 Whole mount section of the parietal eye of a green iguana (*Iguana iguana*). At the top of the image is a relatively thick, but avascular, cornea (1). A cellular lens (2), composed of tall columnar cells packed closely and parallel to each other, lies beneath the cornea. The lumen (3) of the central chamber contains clear fluid and is surrounded at the sides and back by heavily pigmented photosensitive retinal cells (4) and unpigmented ganglion cells (5). A giant melanin-packed macrophage (6) can be seen at the bottom of the capsule. The parietal nerve exits the rear of the parietal eye and courses through the parietal foramen. A thin connective tissue capsule (7) envelops the parietal eye where it is surrounded by calvarial bone. H & E. ×125.

.46

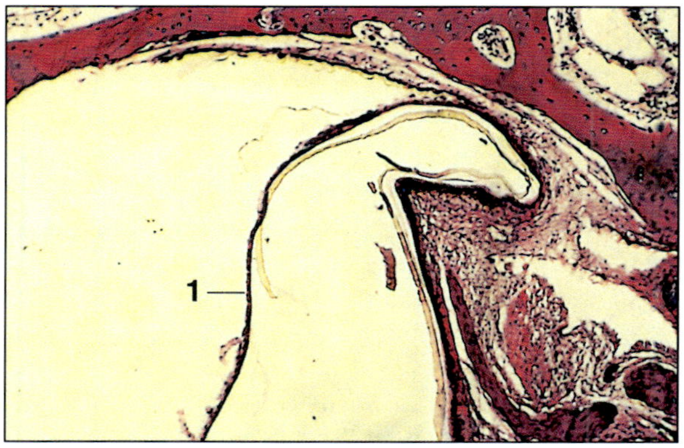

14.47

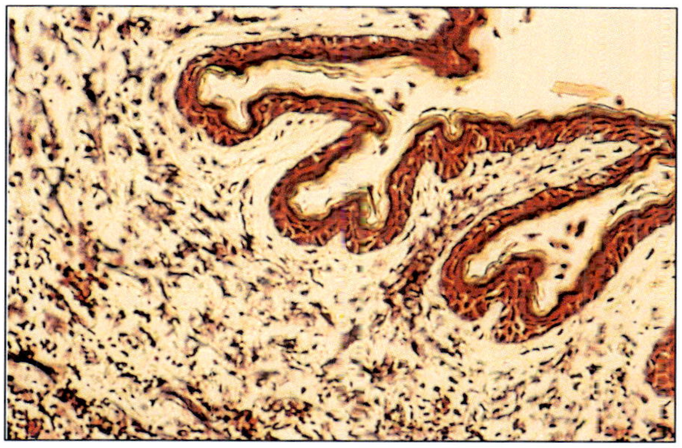

14.46 Facial pit organ of a western diamondback rattlesnake (*Crotalus atrox*) is surrounded on its inner surfaces by a cup-shaped bony depression. A thin, lightly keratinized diaphragm-like membrane (1) divides the posterior of the pit chambers into two compartments. Within the membrane are embedded numerous dendritic neuron endings. H & E. ×20.

14.47 Labial pit organ of a reticulated python (*Python reticulatus*). These infrared superficial depressions over much of the external surface of upper lips of some boas and pythons consist of parallel branched or unbranched shallow passages lined by a thin layer of lightly keratinized squamous epithelium. A rich network of dark staining, fine dendritic nerve endings penetrate to just beneath the epithelium. Bodian's silver stain. ×125.

.48

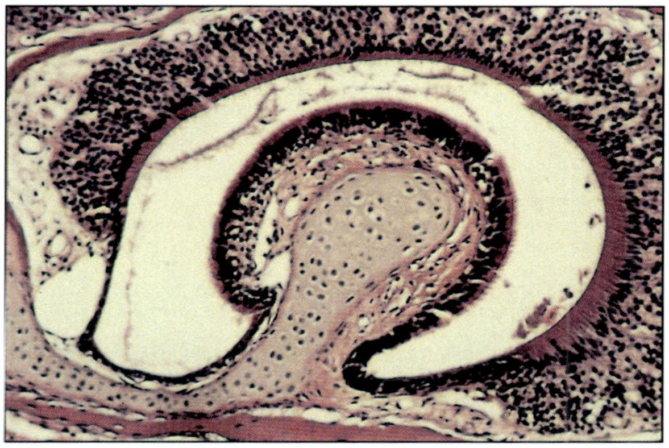

14.49

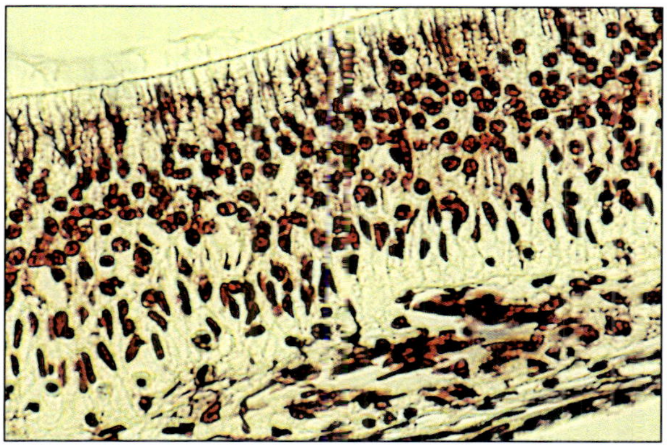

14.48 Whole mount sagittal section of the vomeronasal (Jacobson's) organ of a small skink (*Scinella lateralis*). The raised mushroom-shaped protruberance is supported by a core of hyaline cartilage and is surrounded by a narrow cavity the surfaces of which are covered on all sides by ciliated simple columnar epithelium. H & E. ×125.

14.49 Section through the superficial surface of the vomeronasal organ of a green iguana (*Iguana iguana*). Note the myriad number of thin dendritic nerve endings that course between and penetrate the epithelium to the lumenal surface. Bodian's silver stain. ×250.

14.50 Cross-section of the dermis and the pressure-sensitive lateral line of an aquatic salamander (*Amphiuma tridactyla*). The clear central cavity is lined with large, plump columnar glandular secretory cells. H & E. ×250.

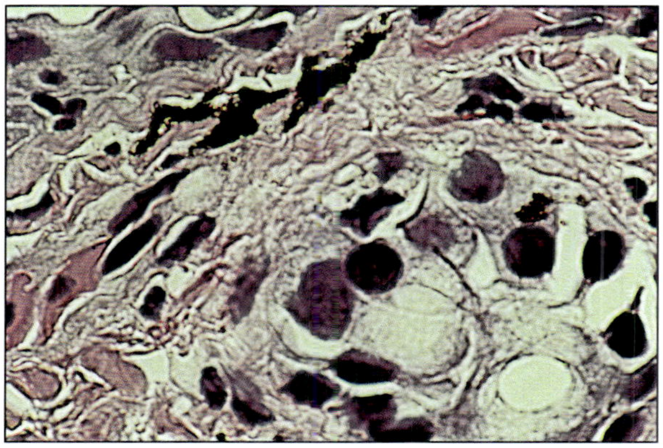

14.50

Electric organ

Some teleost fish, such as the electric eel and electric catfish [and at least one family of elasmobranch ray, such as the torpedo (*Torpedo* spp.)], possess specialized muscles arranged into discrete electric organs (electroplax) that produce and detect powerful electric impulses. Paired electric lobes on the medulla oblongata are the motor centres for the integration of electroplax activity. When these specialized muscular organs suddenly discharge their electrical potential, prey fish and predators are subjected to pulses of high amperage electrical current that can be incapacitating or fatal. Some electric eels produce pulses of direct current that measure 600 V.

Swim bladder

Most but not all teleost fish possess a specialized elongated gas- (or oil-) filled organ: the swim bladder. This is a major hydrostatic organ that helps these fish maintain their buoyancy and orientation within a column of water. In some bottom-feeding species the swim bladder is much reduced or may be absent. In fast swimming fish it is elongated and, thus, enhances streamlining. The swim bladder is formed from thin sheets of dense fibrocollagenous connective tissue laid at acute angles to each other. This arrangement aids in maintaining its shape and reducing deformation. In some fish, skeletal muscles insert into its outermost surface. In other species the swim bladder is only attached to the body wall along its dorsal surface. The swim bladder is lined by a thin, much flattened, non-keratinized squamous epithelium.

Several bacterial, viral and protozoan diseases are characterized by inflammation of the swim bladder. Thus, when performing a necropsy on a fish, it is important to examine this organ for haemorrhage(s), oedematous thickening, discolouration or other abnormality.

15. LYMPHATIC SYSTEM

The lymphatic system has a dual function: the lymphatic vessels drain interstitial tissue, returning fluid to the bloodstream; and lymphoid tissue produces phagocytes and the immunologically competent cells, which are the body's most important defence mechanism against invasion by pathogens. Lymphoid tissue is widely distributed in the body and comprises: lymph nodes and associated lymphatic vessels; spleen; thymus; local aggregations of lymphoid tissue in the mucosa of the digestive, respiratory and urogenital tracts; and any local tissue aggregation of lymphocytes.

Lymphoid tissue consists predominantly of lymphocytes. These and a variable number of plasma cells, macrophages and other cells are supported by a delicate network of reticular fibres that fill the spaces between the trabeculae. Diffuse lymphatic tissue and lymphatic nodules are the components of most lymphatic organs, and also appear in the connective tissue of the digestive, respiratory, urinary and reproductive organs, among other locations. The former is characterized by a moderate concentration of scattered lymphocytes; the latter comprises an aggregation of mostly small, densely packed lymphocytes.

Lymph nodes

A lymph node contains diffuse and nodular lymphatic tissue and lymphatic sinuses that are organized into a cortical and medullary region. A capsule of connective tissue sends fine vascular fibrous trabeculae into the substance of the node. Afferent lymphatic vessels enter the capsule and drain into the subcapsular sinus. From there the lymph drains into a labyrinth of sinuses extending along the trabeculae, eventually emptying into the efferent lymphatics in the hilus. In the cortex, circular aggregations of lymphocytes form follicles or nodules (**15.1–15.4**).

5.1

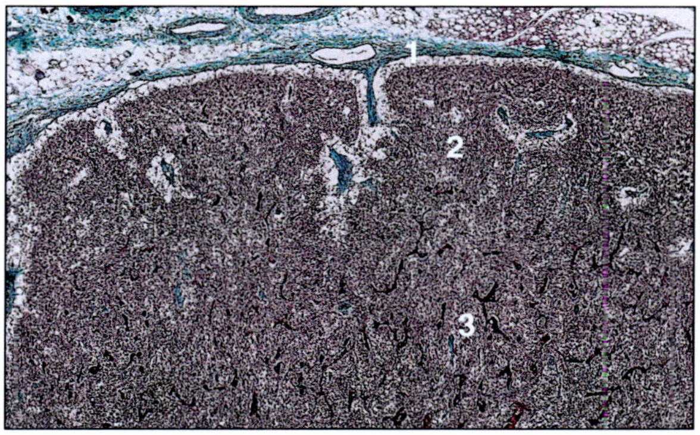

15.1 Lymph node (dog). (1) Connective tissue capsule. Cortex with (2) lymphatic follicles and (3) paracortex. Masson's trichrome. ×20.

15.2

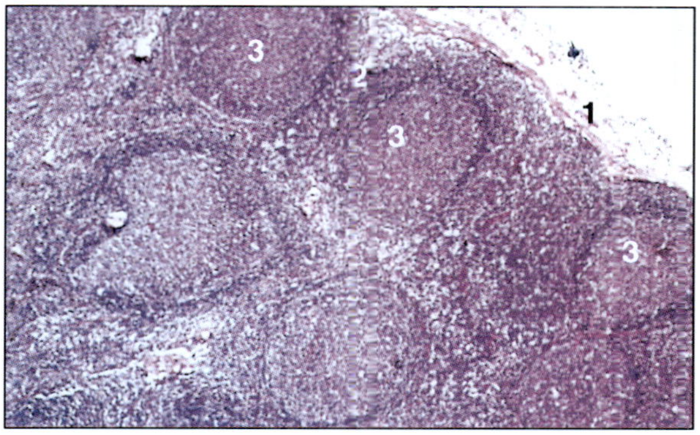

15.2 Lymph node (sheep). (1) Connective tissue capsule. (2) Connective tissue trabeculae. (3) Lymphatic tissue. H & E. ×62.5.

5.3

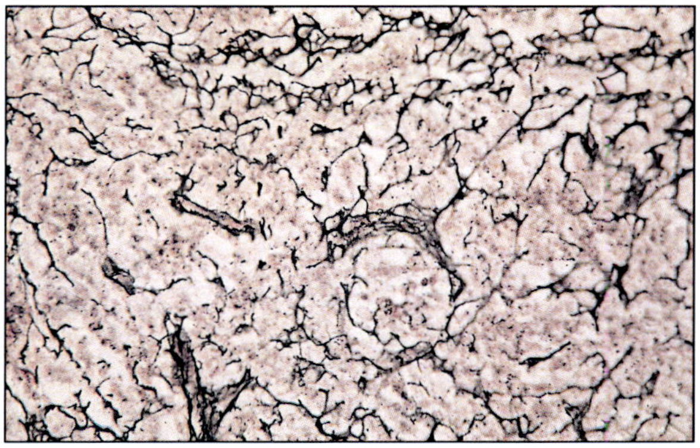

15.3 Lymph node (cat). The reticular fibres form a black network and support the cells of the lymphatic tissue. Gordon and Sweet. ×100.

15.4

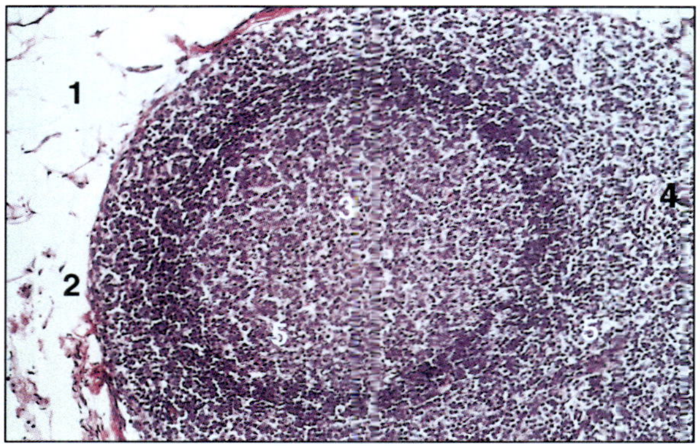

15.4 Lymph node (dog). (1) Connective tissue capsule with some fat cells. (2) Subcapsular sinus. (3) Cortical follicle. (4) Parafollicular tissue. (5) Sinusoid. H & E. ×125.

The primary follicle is a solid packed, evenly distributed mass of cells. The secondary follicle has an outer rim of densely packed small lymphocytes and a pale staining, loosely packed germinal centre, with a mixed population of lymphoblasts, dendritic reticular cells and macrophages (**15.1** and **15.4–15.6**). The secondary follicle responds actively to antigen stimulus, and B lymphocytes (originating in the bone marrow) are present, as are macrophages. Thymus-derived T lymphocytes between the follicles form the paracortex (**15.7**).

In the medulla there is a looser aggregation of cells. Sinusoidal spaces are lined with endothelial cells on a reticular framework with attached macrophages. Rosette-like clusters of lymphocytes, plasma cells, macrophages and leucocytes form the medullary cords (**15.8** and **15.9**). The sinuses are fenestrated and lymphocytes and macrophages have free access.

Monoclonal antibodies are used to identify subsets of lymphocytes and other cells in lymphoid tissue. The cell surface glycoproteins CD4 and CD8 are expressed on exclusive populations of mature T lymphocytes in the parafollicular and deep cortex of lymph nodes (**15.10–15.12**). The anti-CD21 monoclonal antibody recognizes the follicular dendritic cells and the cell processes (**15.13**). Haemolymph nodes, dark red aggregations of lymphoid tissue the function of which is unknown, are present in ruminants. The sinusoids are filled with blood instead of lymph (**15.14**).

15.5

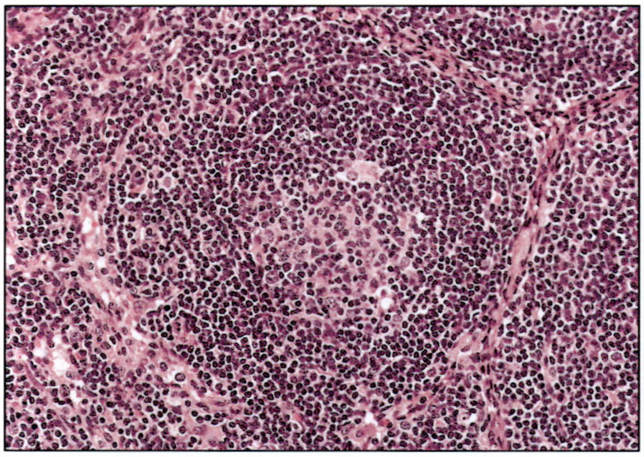

15.5 Lymph node. Cortex (dog). A single follicle is present. The central zone is the pale staining reactive germinal centre. There is an outer rim of closely packed small lymphocytes. H & E. ×125.

15.6

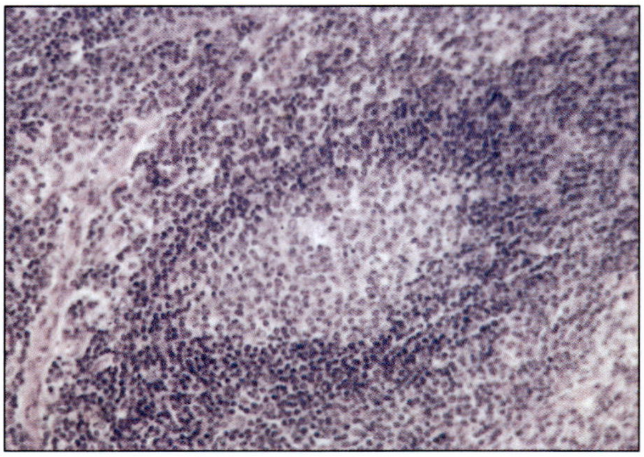

15.6 Lymph node. Cortex (dog). The germinal centre is composed of lymphoblasts, reticular cells and macrophages. H & E. ×125.

15.7

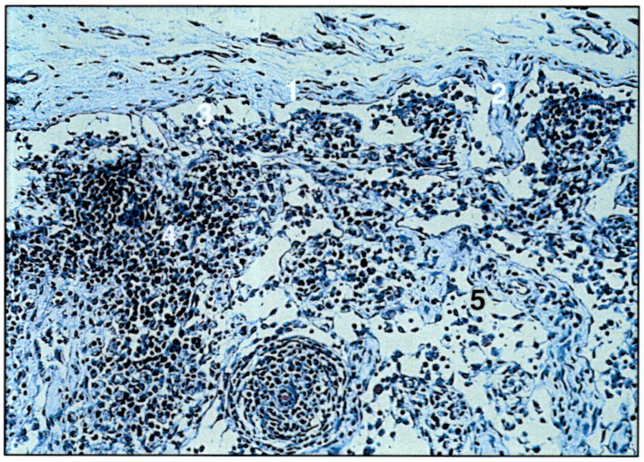

15.7 Lymph node. Paracortex (pig). (1) Connective tissue capsule. (2) Connective tissue trabeculae. (3) Subcapsular sinus. (4) Thymus-derived T lymphocytes. (5) Sinusoid. Alcian blue. ×125.

15.8

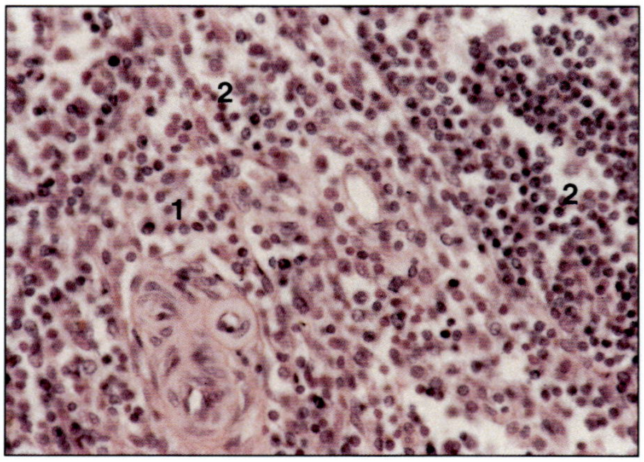

15.8 Lymph node. Medulla (dog). (1) Loose aggregation of lymphoid tissue. (2) Open meshwork of sinusoids. H & E. ×250.

5.9

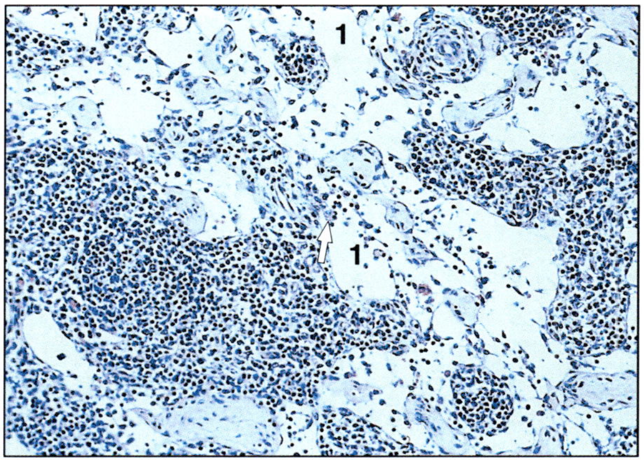

15.9 Lymph node. Medulla (dog). (1) Sinusoid lined by macrophages. Also, clusters of small lymphocytes (arrowed). Alcian blue. ×125.

15.10

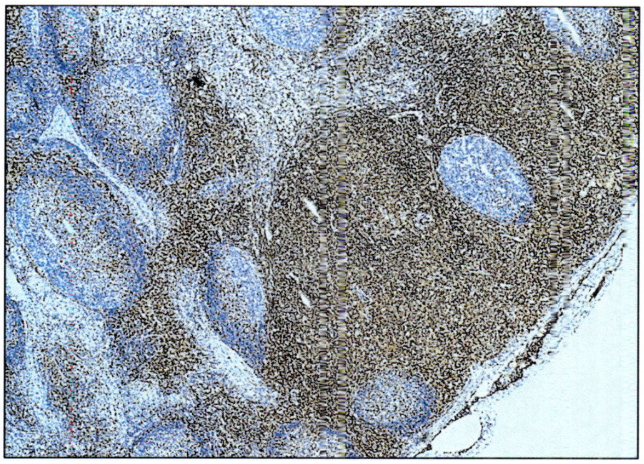

15.10 Lymph node (cat). Anti-CD4 monoclonal antibody. The avidin/biotin method detects an exclusive population of T lymphocytes in the parafollicular and deep cortex of the lymph node; brown reaction. Avidin/biotin method. ×62.5.

.11

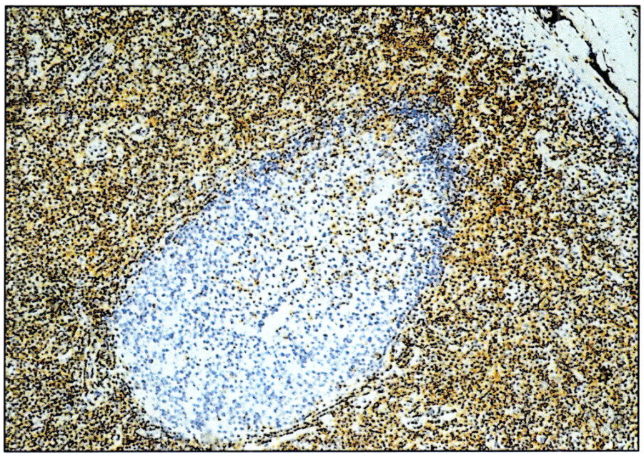

15.11 Lymph node (cat). Anti-CD4 monoclonal antibody. The avidin/biotin method detects an exclusive population of T lymphocytes in the parafollicular and deep cortex of the lymph node; brown reaction. Avidin/biotin method. ×125.

15.12

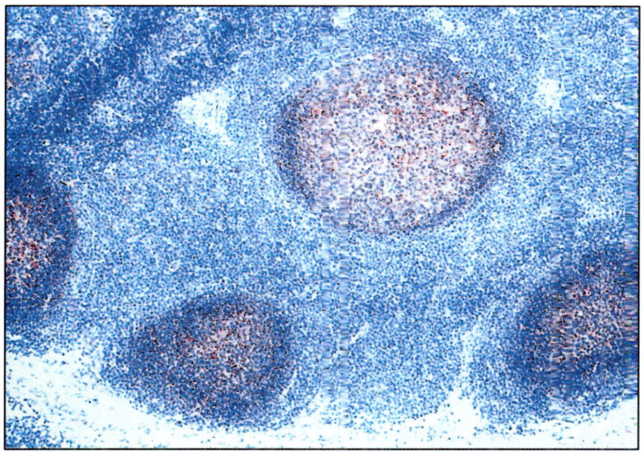

15.12 Lymph node. Cortex. Anti CD8/CD4 monoclonal antibody. This subset of positive cells are rarely present in the follicle germinal centre. Avidin/biotin method. ×100.

.13

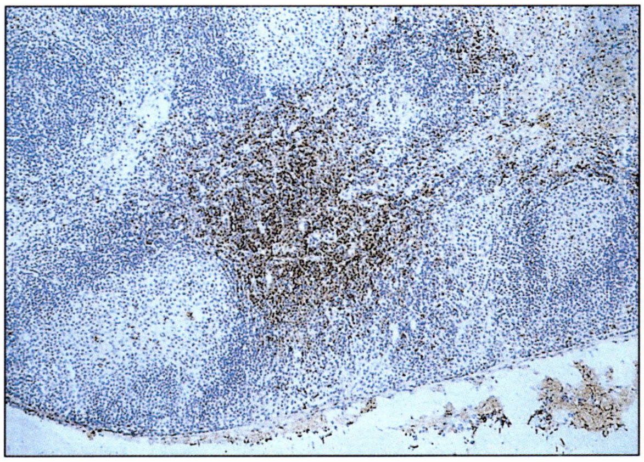

15.13 Lymph node. Cortex. Anti-C.D.21 monoclonal antibody. This method recognizes the follicular dendritic cells and the cell processes; stained red. Avidin/biotin method. ×62.5.

15.14

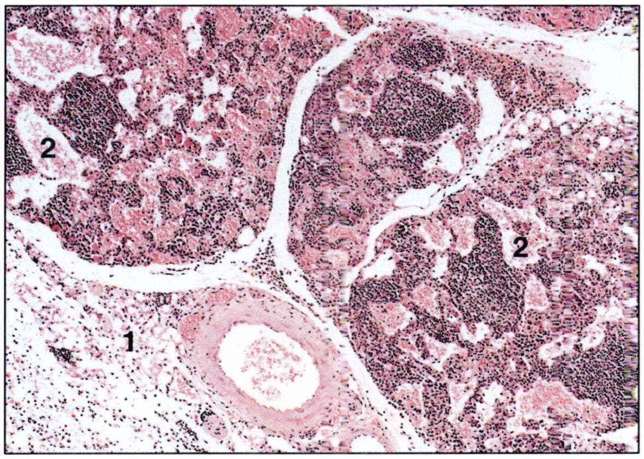

15.14 Haemal lymph node (ox). (1) Connective tissue capsule. (2) Blood filled sinusoids. H & E. ×20.

Spleen

The spleen, the largest organ in the lymphatic system, is usually situated in the cranial part of the abdominal cavity on the left of the stomach (in ruminants on the left lateral wall of the reticulum). It contains the largest collection of reticulo-endothelial cells in the body. It has no afferent lymphatics. The capsule consists of smooth muscle, collagen and elastic fibres with fibrocytes, and extends into the gland to form the supporting framework for the parenchyma, which is divided into red and white splenic pulp (**15.15**).

White pulp contains lymphatic follicles (which may be primary or secondary), together with dense accumulations of T lymphocytes arranged around arteries to form the periarterial lymphatic sheaths. Splenic corpuscles, arterioles with a cuff of T lymphocytes, occupy an eccentric position in the white pulp (**15.16** and **15.17**). The arteriolar branches leave the white pulp and enter the red pulp as straight penicilli. Some acquire a coat of reticular fibres and become ellipsoids (well developed in the cat) and empty into the splenic sinusoids of the red pulp (**15.18**). These sinusoids are wide channels lined with endothelial cells with gaps occupied by macrophages. Foreign material is recognized and removed as part of the immune response; senescent erythrocytes are also removed from the circulation (**15.19**).

Red pulp, so called because of the large number of erythrocytes it contains in the reticular framework, is a loose arrangement of blood filled, fenestrated sinusoids, opening into venules and draining into the splenic vein to leave at the hilus. The region between the red and white pulp is the marginal zone and is phagocytic (**15.20**). The spleen thus functions as part of the immune system and part of the mononuclear phagocyte system.

15.15

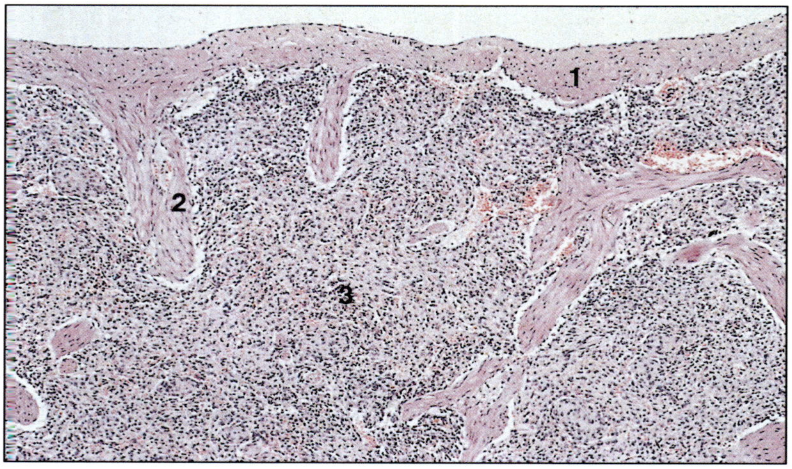

15.15 Spleen (horse). (1) Fibromuscular capsule. (2) Fibromuscular trabeculae. (3) Splenic pulp. H & E. ×12.5.

15.16

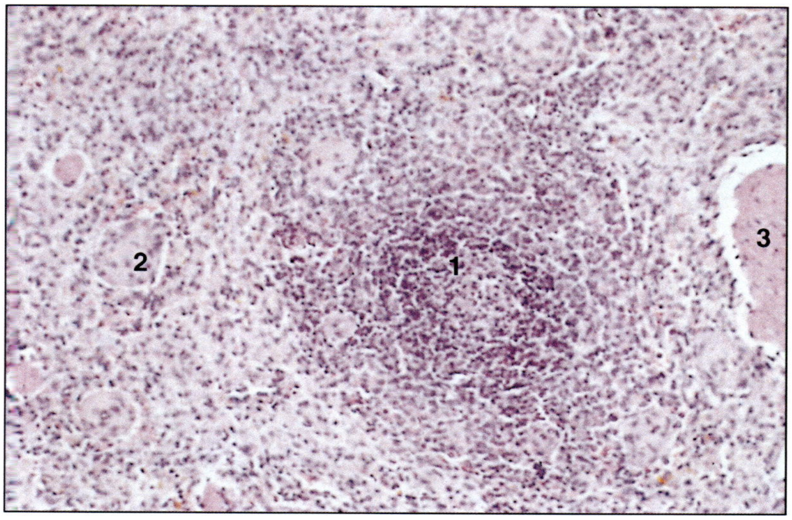

15.16 Spleen (horse). (1) White pulp. (2) Red pulp. (3) Trabecula. H & E. ×62.5.

15.17 Spleen (dog). (1) White splenic corpuscle with an eccentric arteriole (arrowed). (2) Sinusoids of the red pulp filled with erythrocytes. H & E. ×125.

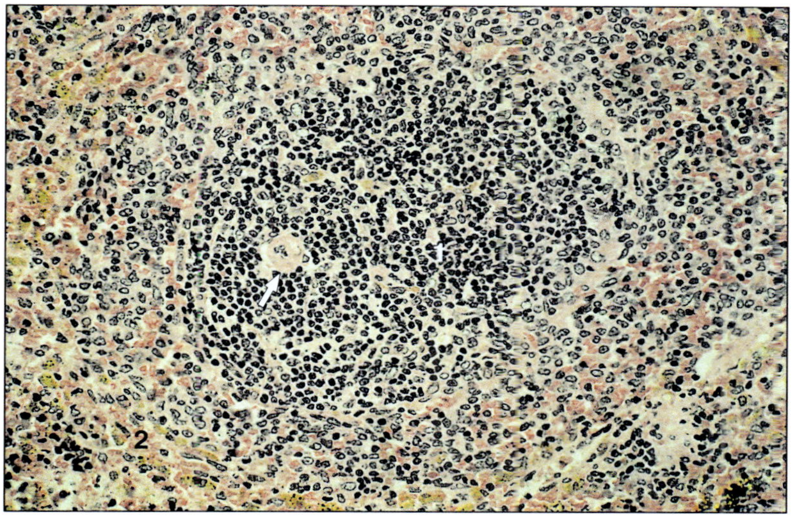

15.17

15.18 Spleen (cat). (1) Part of a trabecula. (2) Ellipsoid. (3) Blood filled sinusoids of the red pulp. H & E. ×250.

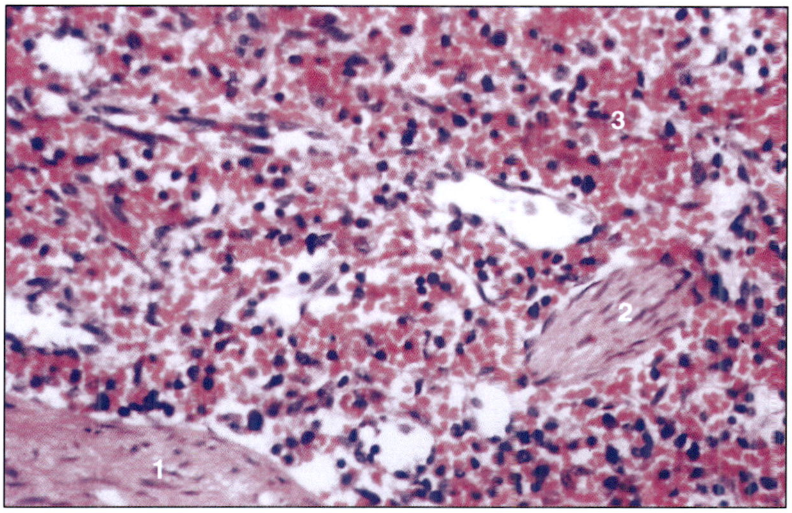

15.18

.19

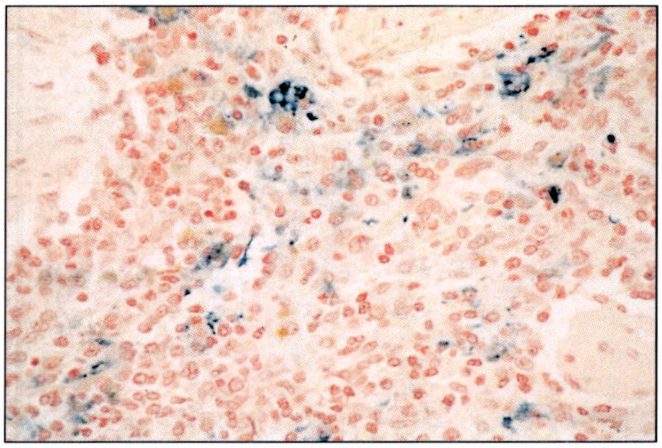

15.19 Spleen (dog). The site of iron deposits as a result of erythrocyte phagocytosis are blue. Perls' Prussian blue. ×125.

15.20

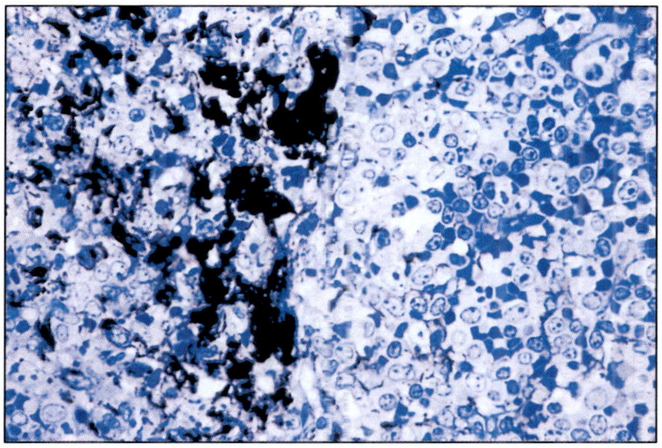

15.20 Spleen (dog). The marginal zone has a large population of macrophages. These are shown filled with phagocytosed carbon particles. Toluidine blue. ×250.

Thymus

The thymus is a central lymphoid organ exporting a specialized subpopulation of lymphocytes (T cells) to other sites, such as lymph nodes, bone marrow, spleen and tonsils. There are no lymphatic follicles and it has no phagocytic function. In the embryo a network of endodermal cells from the pharyngeal pouches is infiltrated by large numbers of lymphocytes (thymocytes) originating in the bone marrow. Whorls of these endodermal cells, often with a keratinized core, are seen in the thymus and are called thymic (Hassall's) corpuscles (**15.21**). The thymus is enclosed in a fine connective tissue capsule; trabeculae extend into the gland dividing it into lobes and lobules (**15.22**). A framework of epithelial (reticular) cells supports the thymocytes, separating them from the circulating blood by forming a blood–thymus barrier. This prevents the thymocytes differentiating into antibody-producing plasma cells. The cortex of each lobule is densely populated by small lymphocytes.

The medulla is much less dense, and the epithelial cells are more numerous (**15.23–15.25**). Spaces in the cortical area are caused by dead lymphocytes phagocytosed by local macrophages. Fat is present in the capsule and the interlobular connective tissue. The epithelial cells are also regarded as the source of thymic hormone (thymosin) that promotes the maturation of T lymphocytes, and hormone-like substances (thymosin and thymopoietin) that induce differentiation of thymocytes. The fetal thymus, after birth, is a very extensive organ, with no fat in the connective tissue capsule. Some regression occurs after birth (**15.26** and **15.27**).

15.21

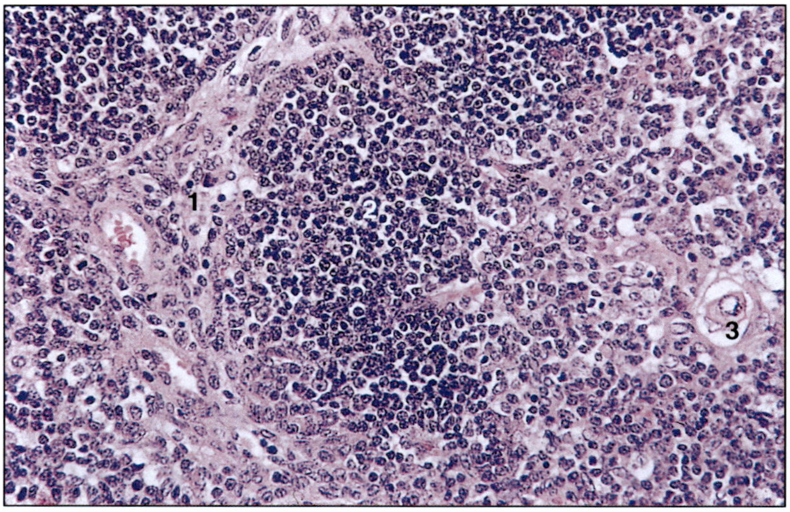

15.21 Thymus (ox). (1) The supporting epithelial cells derived from the pharyngeal endoderm. (2) Thymocytes. (3) Thymic corpuscle. H & E. ×125.

15.22

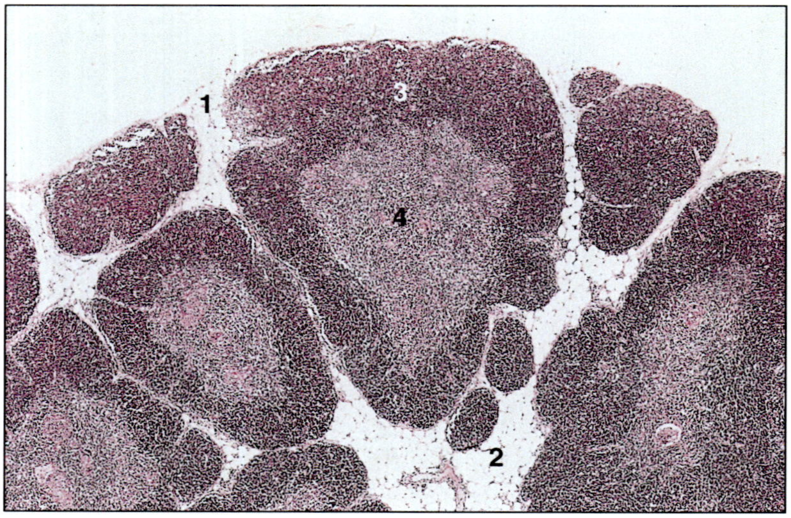

15.22 Thymus (ox). (1) Fine connective tissue capsule. (2) Fat laden interlobular connective tissue. Thymic lobule with (3) outer cortex of densely packed thymocytes, and (4) inner less cellular medulla. H & E. ×62.5.

.23

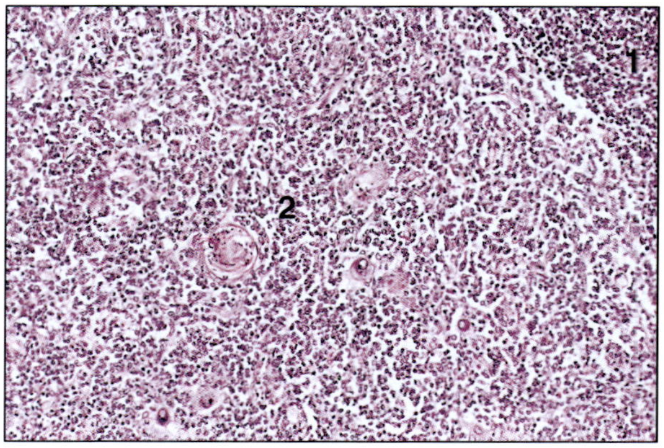

15.23 Thymus (ox). (1) Thymocytes in the cortex. (2) Medulla with epithelial cells and few thymocytes. H & E. ×125.

15.24

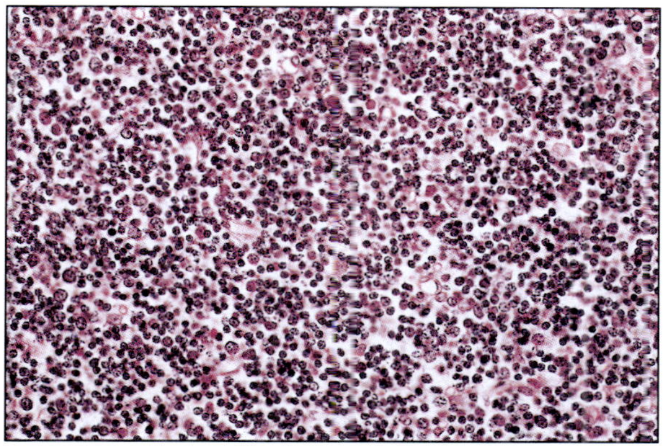

15.24 Thymus (ox). The small dark blue cells are the densely packed cortical thymocytes. H & E. ×250.

.25

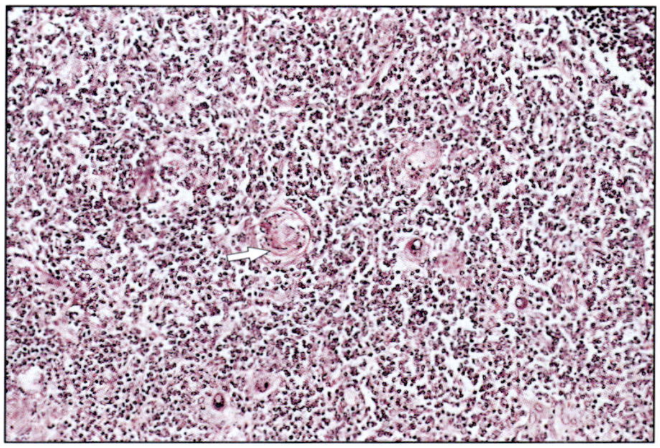

15.25 Thymus (ox). The central medullary zone is less cellular; a thymic (Hassall's) corpuscle is arrowed. H & E. ×125.

.26

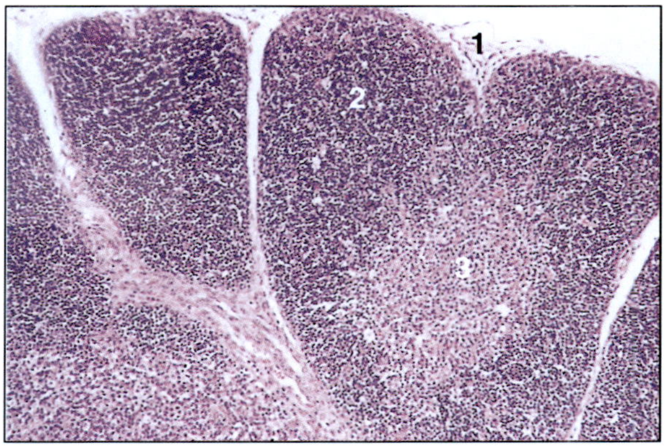

15.26 Fetal thymus (ox). (1) The connective tissue of the capsule and the supporting trabeculae; there are no fat cells. Thymic lobules with (2) cortex and (3) medulla. H & E. ×62.5.

15.27

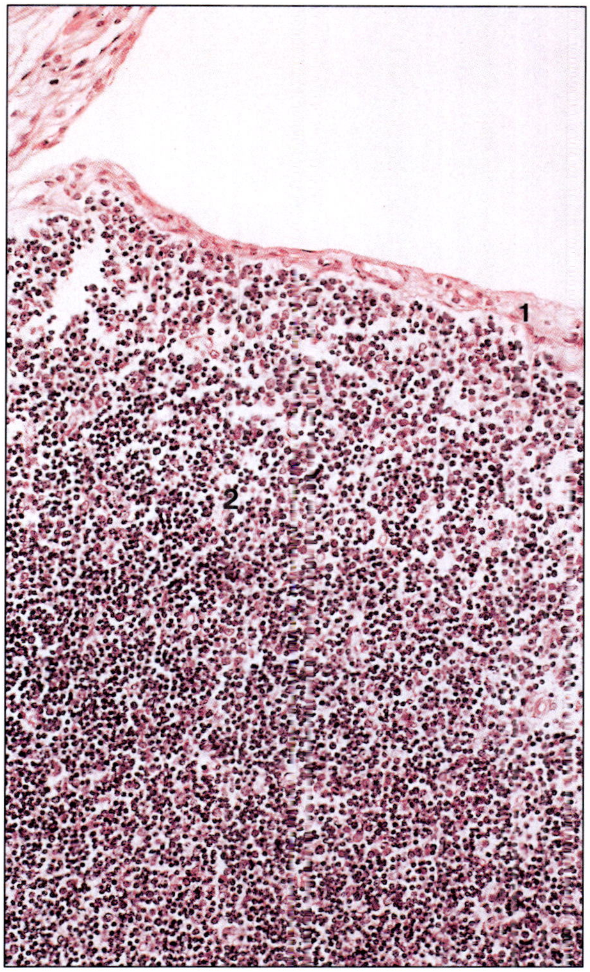

15.27 Fetal thymus (ox). (1) Connective tissue capsule. (2) Cortical zone of the thymic lobule with loosely arranged thymocytes. The intercellular supporting framework is composed of epithelial cells. H & E. ×125.

Local aggregations of lymphoid tissue

Tonsil (mucosal associated lymphoid deposits)

The palatine, lingual and pharyngeal tonsils have the same histological appearance. Stratified squamous epithelium overlies dense aggregations of lymphoid tissue in the lamina propria (**15.28**). Small lymphocytes migrate through the epithelium into the pharynx (**15.29**). Primary and secondary lymphatic follicles are present depending upon the activity of the immune response. There are no afferent lymphatics; the lymph drains into local nodes in the efferent lymphatic vessels. There are also no sinusoids.

Some tonsils contain crypts. Examples include the lingual tonsils of the horse, pig and oxen; the tubal tonsils of the pig; the paraepiglottic tonsils of the pig, sheep and goat; and the palatine tonsils of the horse, pig and ruminant. A crypt with its associated lymphatic tissue constitutes a tonsillar follicle, and several follicles form the tonsil. It is lined with stratified squamous epithelium (**15.30**). Examples of tonsils without crypts include the tubal tonsils of ruminants, the paraepiglottic tonsil of the cat and the palatine tonsils of carnivores.

15.28

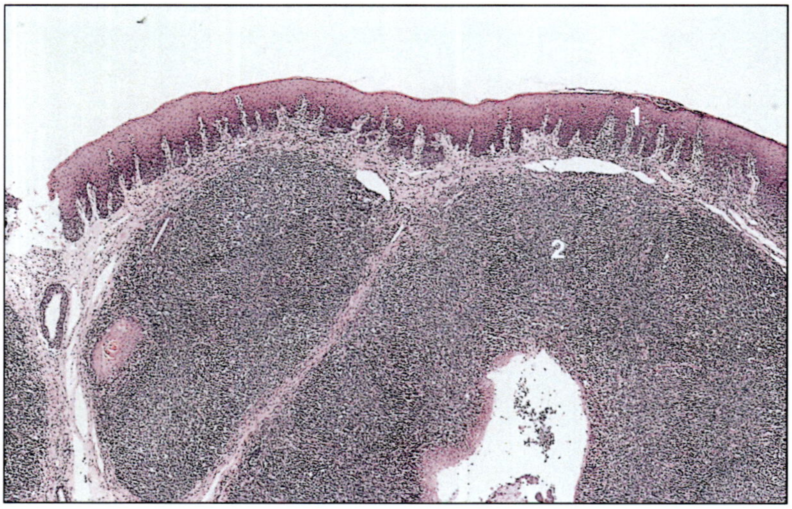

15.28 Tonsil (dog). (1) Stratified squamous epithelium. (2) Dense aggregation of lymphoid tissue in the lamina propria. H & E. ×20.

15.29

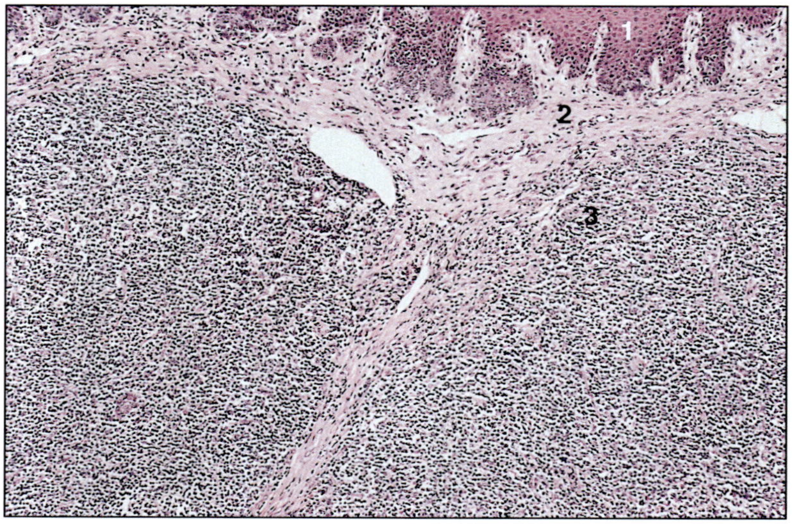

15.29 Tonsil (dog). (1) Stratified squamous epithelium. (2) Connective tissue lamina propria. (3) Lymphoid tissue. H & E. ×125.

Alimentary tract and gut-associated lymphatic tissue

Lymphoid tissue occurs in subepithelial sites in the alimentary tract as lymphatic nodules, dispersed lymphocytes and plasma cells. Many wandering lymphocytes traverse the gut epithelium and are present between the epithelial cells. Most of these lymphocytes are T cells and simple luminal antigens, and initiate the immune response. The large aggregations of lymphoid tissue may eliminate the villus in the small intestine and cause the M cells (membranous epithelial cells) to become flattened (*see* Chapter 8, **8.51**).

A microfolding of the luminal plasma membrane of the M cells turns the luminal antigens into endocytes and presents them to the intraepithelial and subepithelial lymphocytes. Large aggregations of lymphocytes often bulge through the muscularis mucosa into the submucosa (**15.31** and **15.32**). Similar local aggregations of lymphoid tissue occur in the respiratory and urinary tracts.

Lymphatic vessels begin blindly as thin endothelial lined tubes with a minimal amount of supporting connective tissue. Larger lymphatic vessels such as the thoracic duct have a few smooth muscle fibres in their walls. Numerous valves are present.

15.30

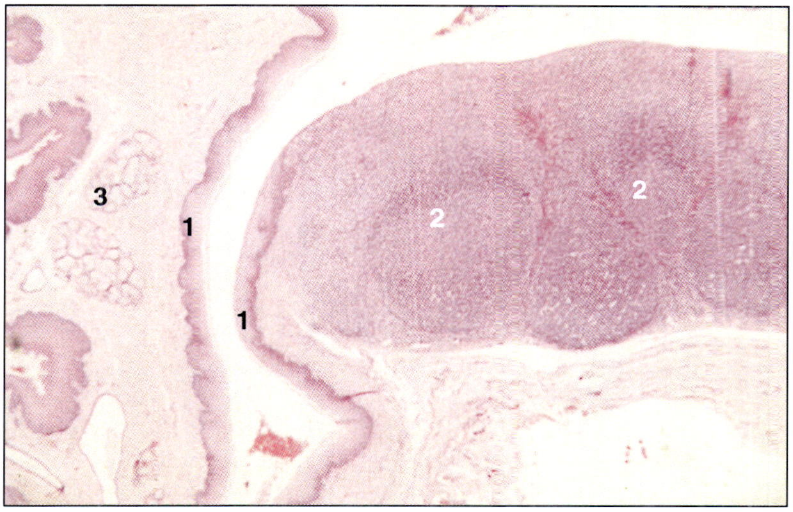

15.30 Tonsil (dog). (1) Stratified squamous epithelium lining the crypt. (2) Dense aggregations of lymphoid tissue in the lamina propria. (3) Mucus-secreting salivary glands. H & E. ×7.5.

.31

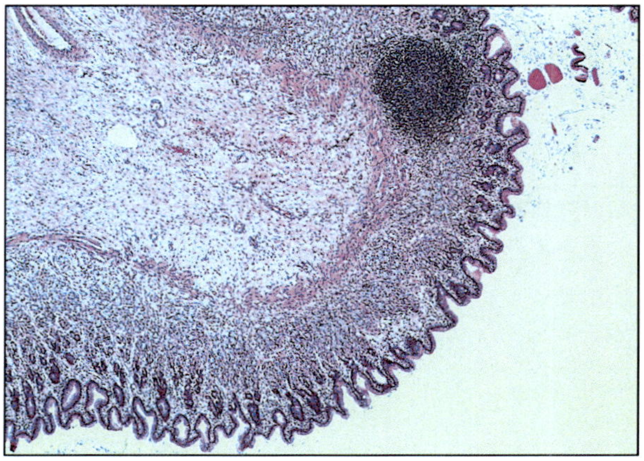

15.31 Stomach (cat). A lymph nodule is present in the mucosal/submucosal layer of the stomach. H & E. ×7.5.

15.32

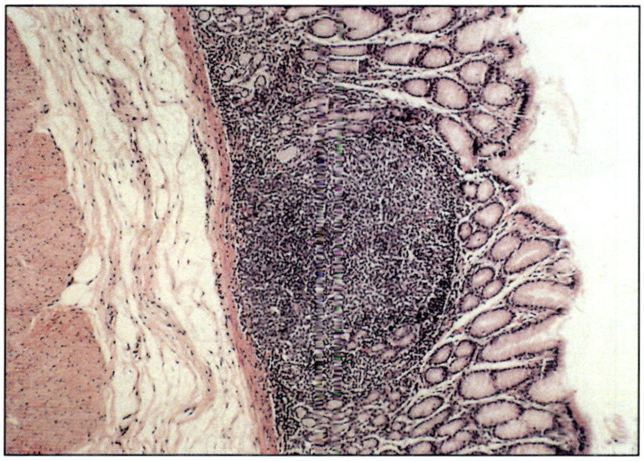

15.32 Abomasum (goat). A lymph nodule in the lamina propria of the mucosa. H & E. ×62.5.

Clinical correlates

The thymus, spleen, bone marrow and other primary and secondary lymphoid organs are common sites for inflammation because of the phagocytic activity of some of their cellular components. Primary lymphoid tumours such lymphosarcoma are relatively common in many domestic species. Leukaemia, in which abnormal cells circulate in the blood, is less common. Lymphoid tumours may affect almost any site in the body (**15.33–15.38**), from lymphoid organs (**15.33**) to visceral tissues (**15.36, 15.37**) and even skin (**15.35**). Secondary (metastatic) tumour deposits are often found in the lymphatic tissues, the nodes and ducts, draining the site of the primary neoplasm (**15.38**).

15.33

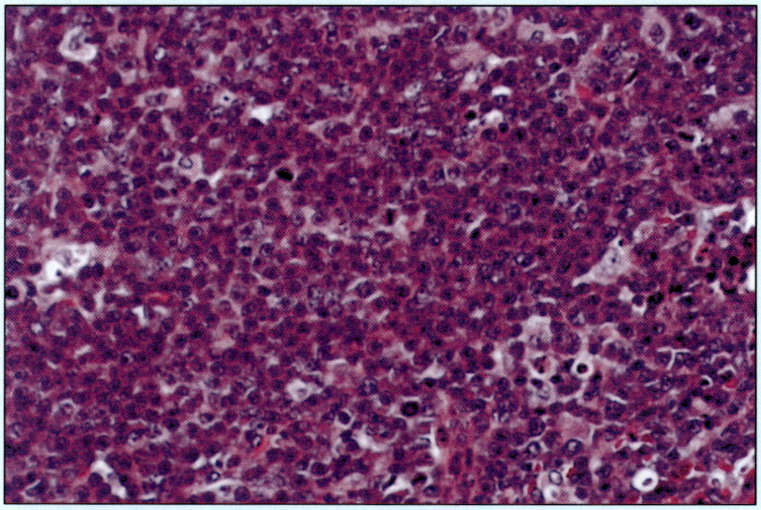

15.33 Lymphosarcoma (dog). Section of lymph node from a 4-year-old male dog showing dense sheets of large, immature lymphoid cells with round-to-irregular nuclei and prominent nucleoli. Several mitotic figures are present. H & E. ×250.

15.34

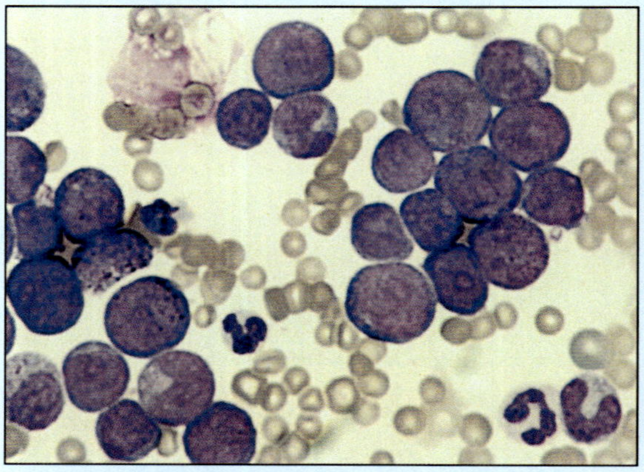

15.34 Feline prolymphocytic leukemia. Note the immaturity of these neoplastic cells, which is characterized by their large nuclei, scanty cytoplasm and prominent nucleoli. Wright's. ×250.

15.35

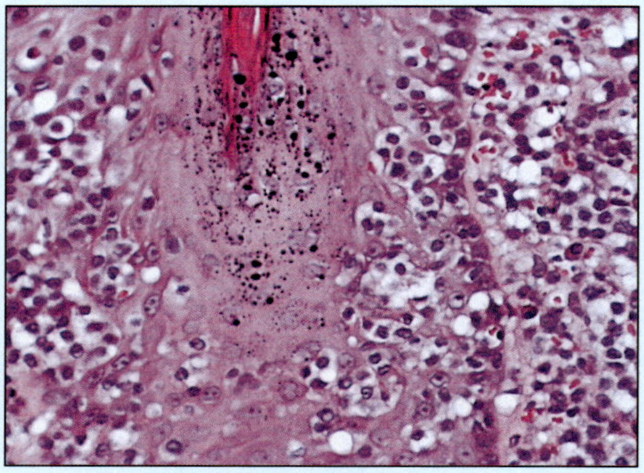

15.35 Epitheliotrophic lymphosarcoma (dog). In this skin section, taken from a 10-year-old neutered female dog the superficial dermis is occupied by sheets of monomorphic medium-sized lymphoid cells. These cells invade the epithelium in numerous clusters (Pautrier's microabscesses). H & E. ×250.

15.36

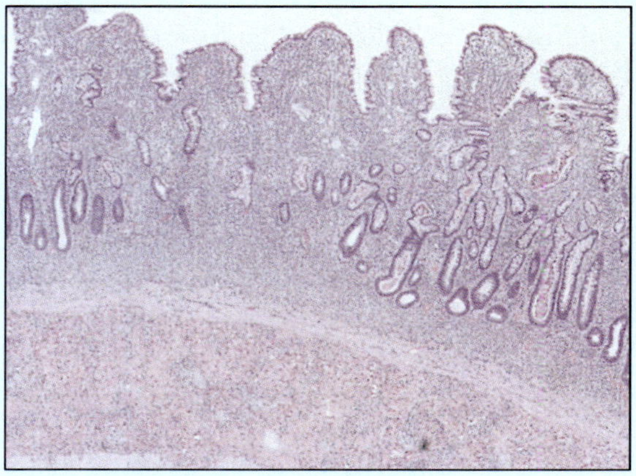

15.37

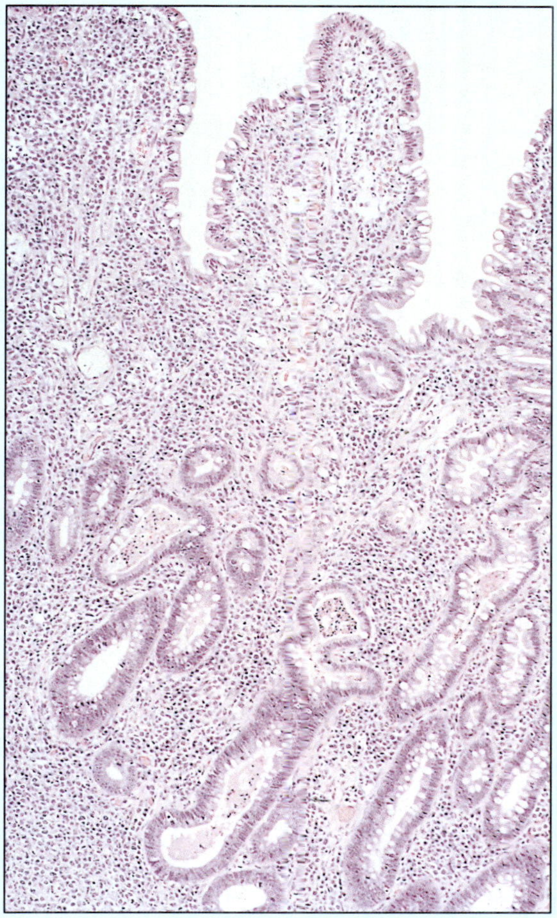

15.36, 15.37 Alimentary lymphosarcoma (dog). Sections from the small intestine of a 12-year-old Staffordshire Bull Terrier with a history of weight loss and diarrhoea. **15.36** (lower power) shows shortened villi and crypts distorted by a heavy cellular infiltrate which extends through all layers of the intestinal wall. In **15.37** the infiltrating population are large lymphoid cells. In dogs alimentary lymphosarcoma most commonly affects the small intestine and is usually primary but may be associated with multicentric lymphosarcoma. H & E. **15.36**, ×25; **15.37**, ×125.

15.38

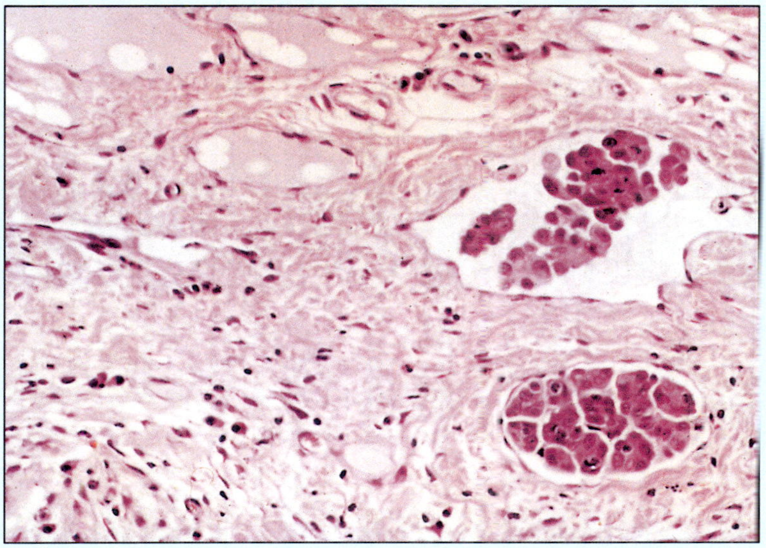

15.38 Lymphatic metastases (bitch). From an 11-year-old female Doberman with mammary carcinoma. Groups of large tumour cells with dark nuclei and eosinophilic cytoplasm within thin-walled lymphatic vessels. The other lymphatics in the section are dilated and the connective tissue is oedematous, which suggests possible lymphatic blockage by tumour deposits. H & E. ×250.

Avian lymphatic system

The lymphoid system in the bird consists of the spleen, thymus, local nodules in the wall of the lymphatic vessels and the mucosae, and the cloacal bursa (of Fabricius). There are no lymph nodes, although diffuse lymphatic tissue and lymphatic follicles are present.

Thymus

The thymus has a fine connective tissue capsule extending into the gland and dividing it into a variable number of lobes. The lobes are divided into lobules as in mammals. Each lobe has a cortex and medulla of thymocytes. These cells are the source of T lymphocytes. The reticular cells form islands of vacuolated cells, the equivalent of the mammalian thymic corpuscle.

Bursa

The cloacal bursa is an oval sacculated organ dorsal to the cloaca and communicating with it by a small opening. It is a central lymphoid organ that seeds B lymphocytes to the germinal centres of peripheral lymphoid deposits and the spleen, and is the primary site for the synthesis of immunoglobulin in the young bird before involution commences from 3–4 months. The mucosal wall is thrown into folds covered by a pseudostratified columnar epithelium continuous with that of the cloaca. The folds are subdivided by connective tissue trabeculae into lobules. Each fold consists of a densely populated outer cortex of lymphocytes and an inner sparsely populated medulla separated by a layer of undifferentiated epithelial cells (**15.39** and **15.40**). Lymphoid tissue and the overlying mucous membrane are in close apposition and lymphocytes migrate through the epithelium.

The mucosal associated lymphatic tissue is present in the tubular digestive tract. The densest aggregation is found in the narrow proximal region of the caecum, the so-called polycryptic caecal tonsil. Both T and B lymphocytes are present.

Spleen

The capsule is fibromuscular as in the mammal, but thinner. The trabeculae are poorly defined. The white pulp is lymphoid tissue sheathing an artery and the red pulp is a loose arrangement of fenestrated blood sinusoids. The function of the spleen is phagocytosis of senescent erythrocytes, lymphopoiesis and antibody production as in the mammal.

15.39

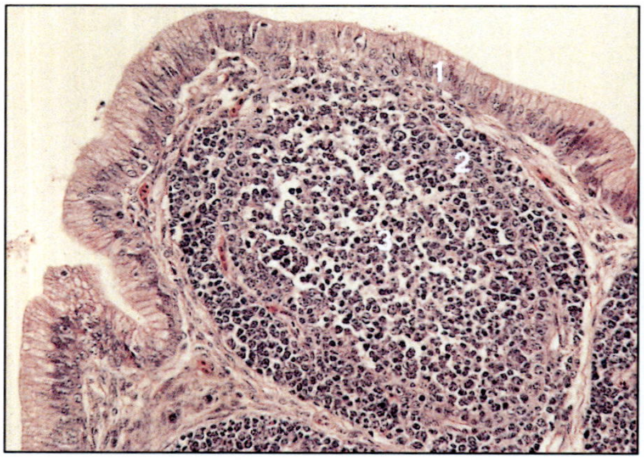

15.39 Cloacal bursa (bird). (1) Simple columnar epithelium of the cloaca. (2) Cortical area of densely packed lymphocytes. (3) Sparsely populated medulla. H & E. ×62.5.

15.40

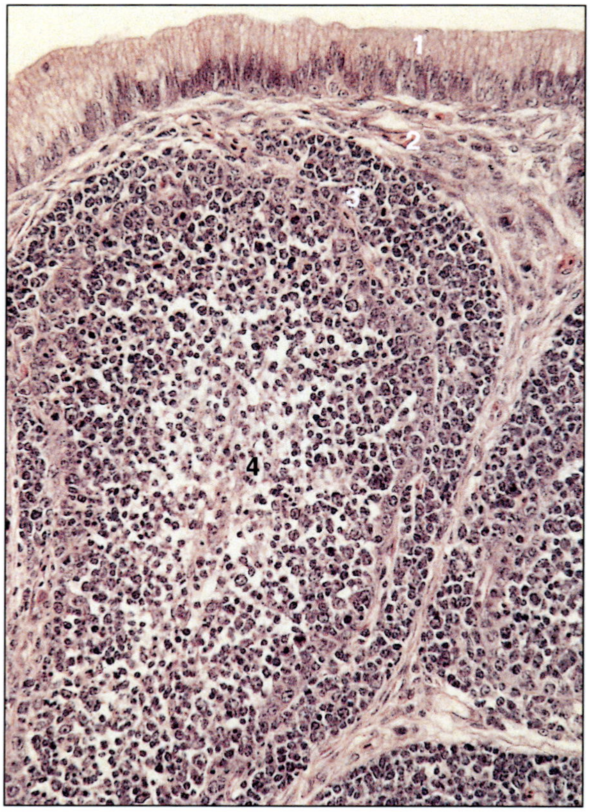

15.40 Cloacal bursa (bird). (1) Simple columnar epithelium of the cloaca. (2) Connective tissue lamina propria. (3) Cortex. (4) Medulla. H & E. ×125.

Reptilian lymphatic system

Although differences exist between various lymphoreticular and immune systems within the class Reptilia, these systems have many similarities both in form and in function. The thymus may be retained as a functional organ throughout life, or it may involute, either seasonally or because of age and become inactive. Haemopoiesis normally occurs in the bone marrow. It can occur within extramedullary sites, such as liver, spleen or kidneys, if the animal experiences acute blood loss caused by traumatic haemorrhage, chronic blood loss or anaemia. Pre-existing mature erythrocytes and even pluripotential thrombocytes can participate in the formation of erythrocytes by being recruited and transformed into erythrocytes through mitotic and amitotic division. The reptilian spleen is similar to the mammalian, and together with large bone-marrow macrophages removes senescent blood cells. During the recycling of haeme pigment from engulfed erythrocytes, reptiles produce the green degradation product biliverdin (**15.41**), instead of the bilirubin that is produced in mammals. Lymph is circulated by contractile lymph hearts, as in amphibians.

The thymus of reptiles is similar to that of mammals (**15.42**). In many reptiles, the thymus (or thymic lobes) lies adjacent to the parathyroid lobes and the ultimobranchial bodies, which are ventral and very near the internal carotid arteries, jugular veins and vagus nerves. The lymphoid structure is encapsulated by dense fibrocollagenous connective tissue. It may be lobulated by fine connective tissue trabeculae (in many snakes) or nonlobulated. If lobulated, it may be further arranged into discrete medullary and cortical regions, depending upon the family within the class Reptilia. A hollow cavity may or may not be present. The parenchyma comprises the following: small, round thymic lymphocytes or thymocytes, which predominate; epithelial ('epithelioid') cells with pale staining nuclei and prominent nucleoli; elongated, pink staining myoid cells; pearl-like, pale pink concentrically lamellated (Hassall's) corpuscles; occasional macrophages; and granulocytes, especially heterophils (**15.42**). Mucoid cysts have been described in some reptilian thymic specimens. Small blood vessels penetrate the thymus at the hilus or enter directly through the capsule and branch out into smaller arterioles, capillaries and venules before exiting in a parallel manner.

The alimentary, respiratory, cardiovascular, urogenital and integumentary systems of reptiles contain discrete aggregates of lymphoid tissue. Although reptiles lack a true bursa of Fabricius (similar to that which is present in birds), there are well-delineated lymphoid nodules located within the intestine and cloacal vent of many species.

.41

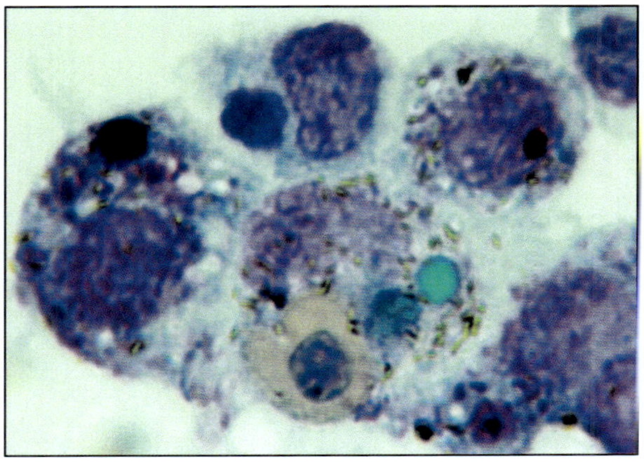

15.41 Bone marrow specimen from an iguana. This section contains several macrophages with engulfed cellular material and bacteria. Note the green inclusion within the large macrophage which contains biliverdin, the degradation product of haemoglobin in amphibians, reptiles and birds. H & E. ×250.

15.42

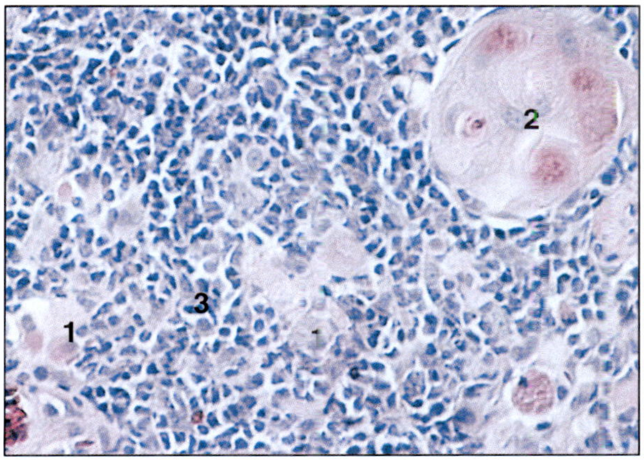

15.42 Section of cortical part of a thymic lobule from a desert tortoise (*Xerobates agassizi*). (1) Epithelial cells. (2) Concentric (Hassall's) corpuscle. (3) Thymocytes. H & E.×125.

Amphibian lymphatic system

The immune system of many amphibians is intermediate between that found in teleost fish and in some reptiles. The thymus is present but variable in size and complexity, depending upon the family of amphibian. In adult amphibians the thymus is located in the ventral cervical region, usually just cranial to the heart and great vessels. There may be a discrete spleen or, in some amphibians, a combined splenopancreas that serves as a site for lymphoreticular, haemopoietic, digestive and endocrine functions.

Multiple contractile vessels, called 'lymph hearts', circulate lymph throughout the body. Discrete lymph nodes are lacking, but lymphoid patches or aggregates are located in the walls throughout the alimentary, respiratory and urogenital systems. Küpffer cells are arranged within the hepatic sinusoids, as they are in higher vertebrates.

Amphibian leucocytes were described previously and are similar to those observed in birds and reptiles.

Fish lymphatic system

Generally, the lymphoreticular system of fish is more primitive than that of amphibians and reptiles. Lymph nodes are lacking, but aggregates of lymphoid tissue are located in the walls of the alimentary and urogenital systems. Leucocytes consist of lymphocytes, plasmacytes, large and small monocytic macrophages, heterophil-like granulocytes, eosinophils, azurophils and basophils. In some species, two types of basophilic granulocytes have been described. The spleen of fish serves as a site of haemopoiesis, although erythrocytes may mature after they have been released into the circulation. It has an immunogenic function, joining with other lymphoid organs in the production of (at least) serum neutralizing antibodies in response to antigenic challenge. It removes senescent erythrocytes from the circulating pool of red cells. Stellate (Küpffer) cells line the hepatic sinusoids. The mucus covering the integument of many fish represents the first line of defence against invasion by pathogenic micro-organisms: immunoglobulin A antibodies secreted with the mucus confer a degree of immunity specifically directed against certain antigens. Lymphatics drain erythrocyte-free blood plasma that seeps through capillary walls, and return it to the veins. Lymphatics also drain fat, as chylomicrons, from the intestinal villi.

Clinical correlates

Primary lymphoid neoplasms such as thymic lymphosarcoma (**15.43**), multicentric lymphosarcoma and lymphatic leukaemia occur in some exotic species. Secondary tumour deposits can also affect the lymphatic system. Other types of lymphatic tumours can infiltrate sites that usually do not contain a substantial lymphoreticular component (**15.44**).

15.43

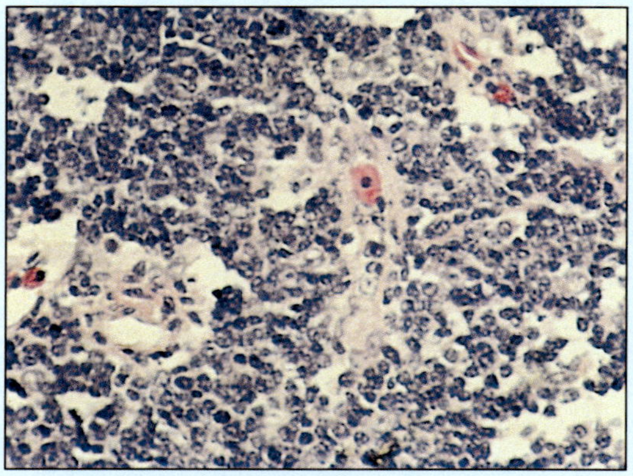

15.43 Thymic lymphosarcoma in a desert tortoise (*Xerobates agassizi*). The distinction between the cortical and medullary zones is lost as thymocytes proliferate and distort the architecture of the thymic lobule. Scattered pale-staining histiocytes, blood vessels and small smooth muscle fibres are also present. H & E. ×125.

15.44

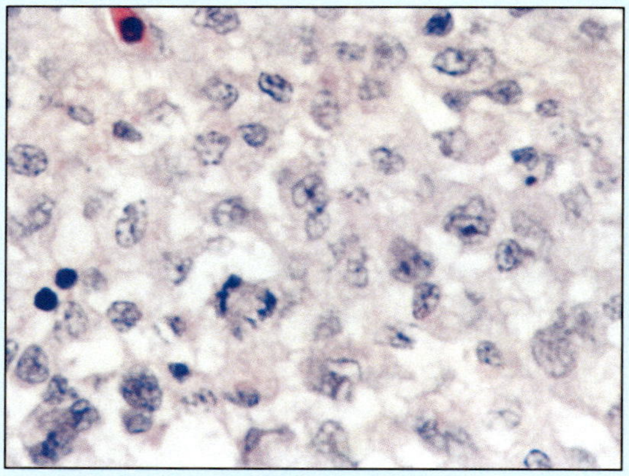

15.44 Malignant histiocytic lymphoma (lymphosarcoma) in a boa constrictor (*Boa constrictor*). This neoplasm is composed of histiocytic macrophages with vesicular nuclei, prominent nucleoli and quite abundant pale cytoplasm. The mitotic index is high. H & E. ×125.

The immune system

The primary function of the lymphatic cells in the lymph nodes, spleen, thymus and mucosal sites is the protection of the body from invasion by organisms such as bacteria and viruses, and foreign antigens. This protection, the immune response, constitutes the body's main defence mechanism, and operates in two ways: humoral response, the synthesis and release of free antibody into the blood; and cell-mediated immunity, the production of sensitized cells with antibody receptors on the surface. Both of these aspects of the immune response are carried out by lymphoid cells, the commonest being small lymphocytes. These circulate freely between the blood and the lymph, and between the lymphoid organs. They migrate into connective tissue and form diffuse cellular infiltrations.

There are two distinct populations of small lymphocytes: the T and B cells. They are morphologically identical but functionally distinct and are identified by using special markers. Both cells first appear in the yolk sac of the embryo, migrating via the blood to the liver in the mammal, and the spleen both in birds and in mammals. From there they migrate to the bone marrow. In the final migration, the T stem cells migrate to the developing thymus and the B stem cells to the cloacal bursa and equivalent gut epithelial related sites in the mammal.

T cells

The T cells are thymus-dependent and differentiate in the cortical zone of this primary lymphoid organ, probably under the influence of thymic hormone. They are protected from antigenic challenge at this stage by the blood–thymus barrier. The differentiated T cells enter the circulation and leave the thymus to form the majority of the circulating pool of small lymphocytes. Local populations are found in the paracortical areas of lymph nodes and the periarterial lymphatic sheaths in the spleen (see **15.10–15.12, 15.16** and **15.17**).

On coming into contact with an antigen, the differentiated T cell is activated, transformed into a lymphoblast and undergoes clonal expansion. This is the primary response and the resultant population of small sensitized lymphocytes enters the recirculating pool of cells until contact is made with the specific antigen. This constitutes cell-mediated immunity. Target cells are destroyed by direct contact with the killer cells, natural killer and T-cytotoxic lymphocytes. Other activated T lymphocytes, T helpers and T suppressors, secrete lymphokines. These modulate the immune reaction or macrophage function by attracting mononuclear phagocytes to the area, or by transferring sensitivity to uncommitted lymphocytes locally. Some sensitized T cells persist in the recirculating pool for months or years, acting as memory cells and able to provide instant and rapid response to the antigen, constituting the secondary response.

B cells

B cells differentiate in the bone marrow in the mammal and the cloacal bursa in the bird, enter the circulation and settle in the germinal centres of lymphatic follicles. Antigenic stimulation of these cells results in rapid division into lymphoblasts, with enlargement of the germinal centre: an activated nodule (see **15.1** and **15.4–15.6**). The activated B lymphocytes have immunoglobulin on the cell surface. They migrate down the medullary cords and develop into plasma cells, synthesizing and secreting antibody: the primary response. Some B cells are retained in the lymph nodule as memory cells and are able to respond rapidly to a second challenge: the secondary response. T and B lymphocytes act together in the immune response and stimulate and cooperate with macrophages, whether they are of blood or of tissue origin. They cannot be considered in isolation.

Macrophages

Macrophages are long lived, actively phagocytic cells widely distributed throughout the body. They form that part of the body defences called the mononuclear phagocyte system and they originate in the bone marrow. A committed stem cell matures into a monocyte, is released into the circulation, leaves the blood and migrates into the tissues. There it increases in size, in lysosomal enzyme content and endocytotic activity to become a macrophage capable of phagocytosis. Macrophages may be free or fixed. Free macrophages are scattered in the connective tissue as histiocytes (**15.45**), in body cavities, in pulmonary alveoli as dust cells, and in the spleen and lymph nodes (see **15.8** and **15.9**). Fixed macrophages line the blood and lymph sinusoids of the bone marrow, liver (**15.46**), spleen (see **15.18**) and lymph nodes, where they are supported by a fine network of reticular fibres (previously known as the reticuloendothelial system). As the blood or lymph moves slowly along the sinusoids, the lining macrophages recognize non-self (foreign protein, bacteria) and altered self (senescent erythrocytes) materials and ingest and degrade them. Macrophages participate positively in the immune response by processing and presenting antibody on the cell surface to T lymphocytes, thus triggering activation and proliferation of these cells. This part of the host response is important in that the T lymphocytes secrete lymphokines, substances that attract more macrophages to the site by chemotaxis, thus increasing the numbers. This can have a deleterious effect, as over-reaction of the host response can cause an allergic reaction and, at worst, anaphylactic shock.

15.45

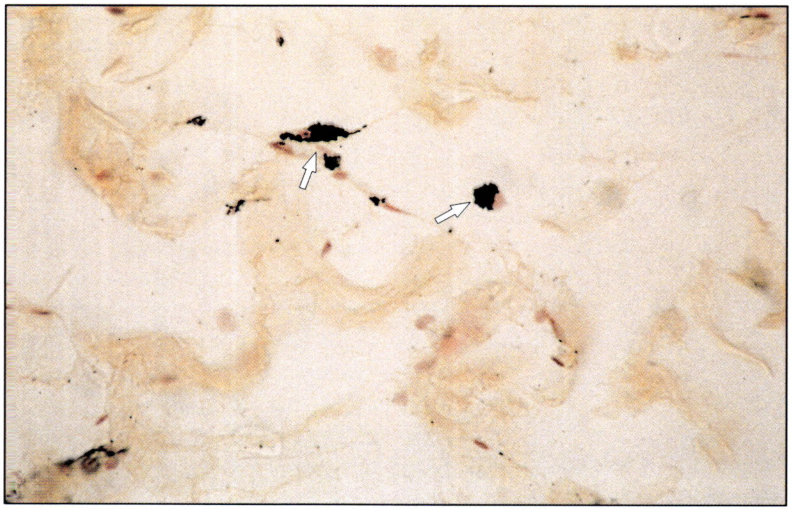

15.45 Loose connective tissue (dog). The histiocytes have phagocytosed the injected carbon particles (arrowed). ×250.

15.46

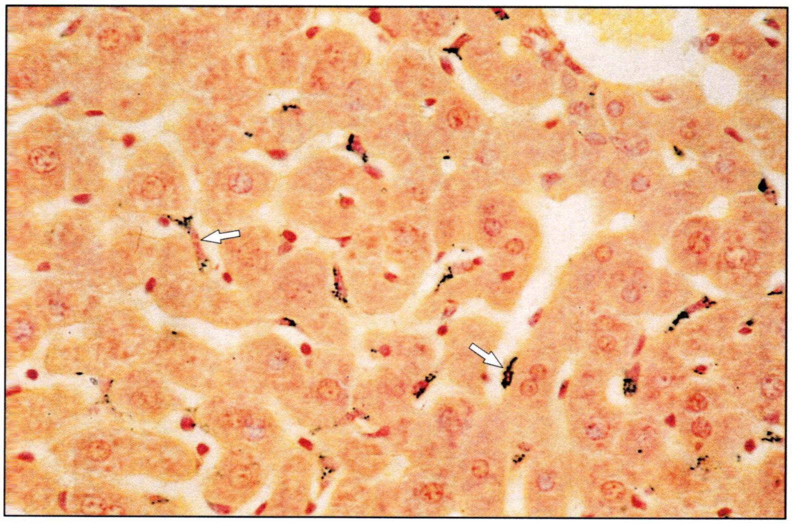

15.46 Liver (sheep). The macrophages lining the sinusoids have phagocytosed the injected carbon particles (arrowed). Safranin/haematoxylin. ×250.

16. INTEGUMENTARY SYSTEM

The integument includes the skin and its derivatives. Skin, the largest organ in the body, consists of an epidermis, a specialized epithelium derived from ectoderm, and a dermis, vascular dense connective tissue derived from mesoderm. Irregular projections of the dermis, papillae, interdigitate with evaginations of the epidermis, the dermal ridges. Beneath the dermis is the hypodermis (subcutis), a layer of loose connective tissue containing a variable amount of fat, which connects the skin to the underlying tissues. The dermis and hypodermis contain the blood vessels, lymphatic vessels and nerves supplying the skin. Sweat, sebaceous and mammary glands, as well as hair and feather follicles, are epidermal structures located in the dermis and hypodermis.

Skin

Skin is classified as thick or thin. Thick skin occurs in areas of wear and tear such as the footpad (**16.1**), and thin skin covers the rest of the body (**16.2**). The epithelium of the epidermis is stratified squamous, and contains keratinizing epithelial cells: keratinocytes. The number of cell layers varies considerably from two to four in thin skin (**16.2**) to 12–20 in thick skin (**16.1** and **16.3**). The epithelium is keratinized in areas of wear such as the footpad (**16.1** and **16.4**). In less exposed areas the surface cells are dead squames and are sloughed off to be replaced from the basal layer. The skin of the nose of the horse is thin, with fine hairs, sebaceous and sweat glands, and

6.1

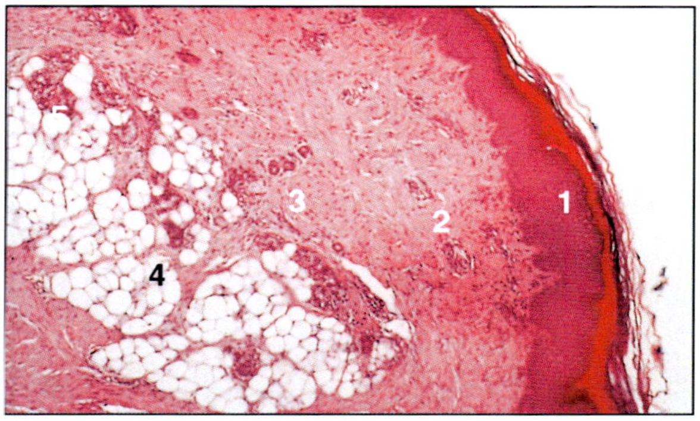

16.1 Digital pad (cat). (1) Epidermis: stratified squamous keratinized epithelium. (2) Dermis: connective tissue. (3) Hypodermis: loose connective tissue. (4) Adipose tissue. (5) Sweat glands. H & E. ×20.

16.2

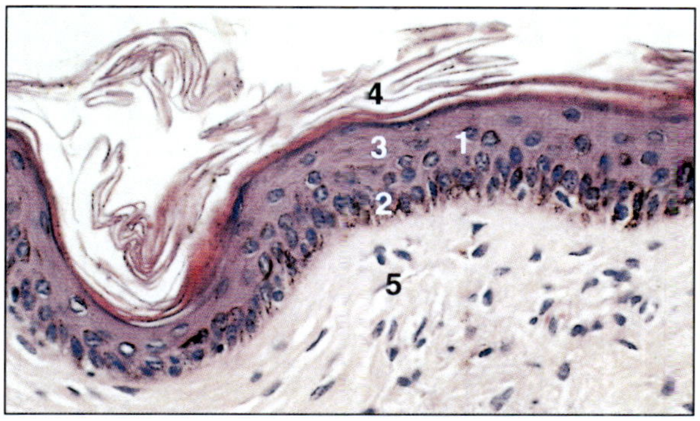

16.2 Thin hairless skin (horse). (1) The epidermis is three layers deep. The basal germinal layer (2) has melanocytes and clear cells; the middle layer (3) is hexagonal keratocytes; and the surface layer (4) is dead squames in the process of being shed. (5) Dermis: vascular connective tissue. H & E. ×125.

6.3

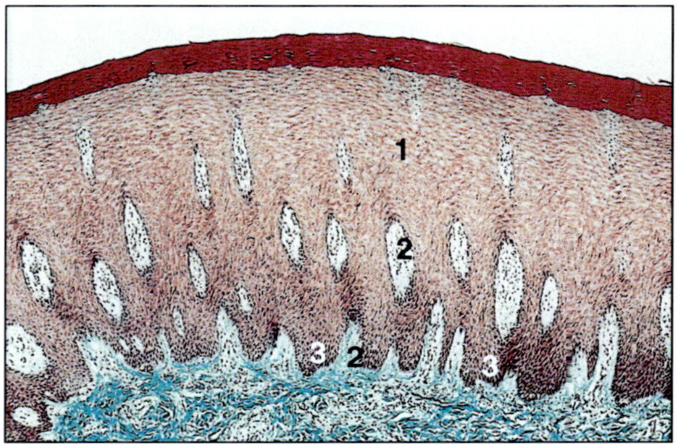

16.3 Dental pad – thick skin (ox). (1) The epidermis is at least 20 cells deep. (2) Dermal papillae project into the epidermis, necessary for the nutrition of the epidermal cells. (3) Equivalent epidermal pegs. Masson's trichrome. ×62.5.

16.4

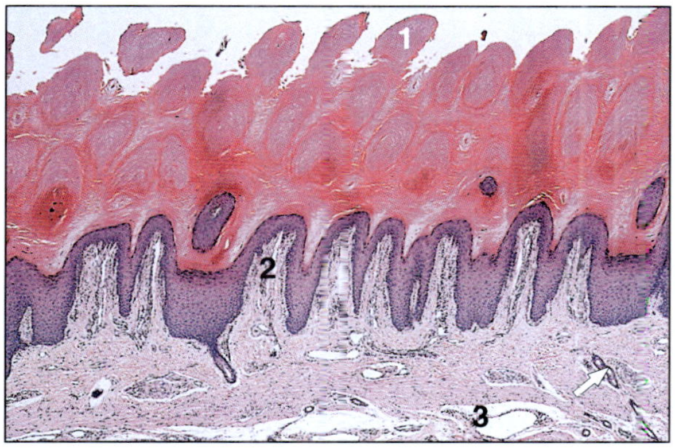

16.4 Digital pad – thick skin (dog). (1) The epidermis is heavily keratinized. (2) Dermal papillae project into the epidermis. (3) Hypodermis: loose connective tissue with sweat glands (arrowed). H & E. ×62.5.

occasional sinus hairs. The planum of the nose of the other domestic mammals is covered by a thick, highly keratinized epidermis (**16.5**).

Epidermis

The cell layers are clearly defined in the epidermis of thick skin as follows.

- The basal or germinal layer (stratum basale, stratum germinativum) consists of a mitotically active layer of columnar or cuboidal keratinocytes on a basement membrane adjacent to the dermis (**16.6**).
- In the spinous layer (stratum spinosum) the keratinocytes are cuboidal, polygonal or flattened. These cells have delicate radiating processes, tonofilaments, that connect with similar cells; this is also known as the prickle cell layer (**16.7**).
- The granular layer (stratum granulosum) is formed by cells migrating towards the surface and accumulating basophilic granules of keratohyalin in the cytoplasm (**16.8**). These granules are a keratin precursor.
- In the clear layer (stratum lucidum), as each cell nears the surface its nucleus dies. The cell loses its clear-cut outline and becomes homogeneous and translucent (**16.9**). It is in the epidermis of the planum nasale of several species, the footpads of carnivores and the thick skin of the teat.
- The cornified layer (stratum corneum) is the outer layer, consisting of cells that are non-nucleated, keratinized and desquamating (**16.1**, **16.3** and **16.4**).

In structures composed of hard keratin, such as hooves and claws, both the granular and clear layers are absent. The epidermis of thin skin is composed of relatively few cells, but the number varies with the location. It lacks a clear layer and the granular layer is now always evident (**16.2** and **16.10**).

Skin colour is determined by the presence or absence of pigment cells, or melanocytes, in the basal layer (**16.11**). These cells originate from the neural crest. Langerhans cells are mainly in the stratum spinosum of the epidermis. These are specialized clear dendritic epithelial cells that resemble and are involved in the processing of antigens (**16.6**). Also present in the basal layer are Merkel's cells, which are similar in appearance to the Langerhans cells, but may have a few granules. They are members of the amine–precursor–uptake–decarboxylation neuroendocrine system.

16.5

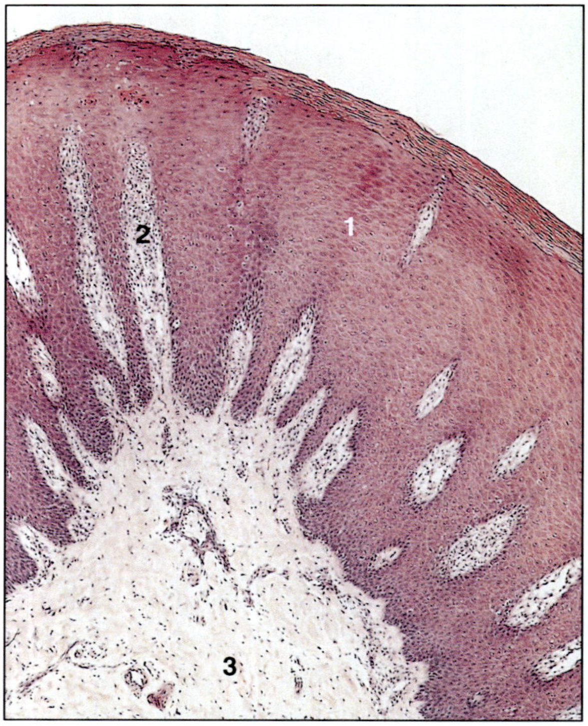

16.5 Planum nasale – thick skin (ox). (1) The epidermis is at least 20 layers of cells; the surface cells are keratinized. (2) Deep vascular dermal papillae project into the epidermis. (3) Hypodermis. H & E. ×62.5.

16.6

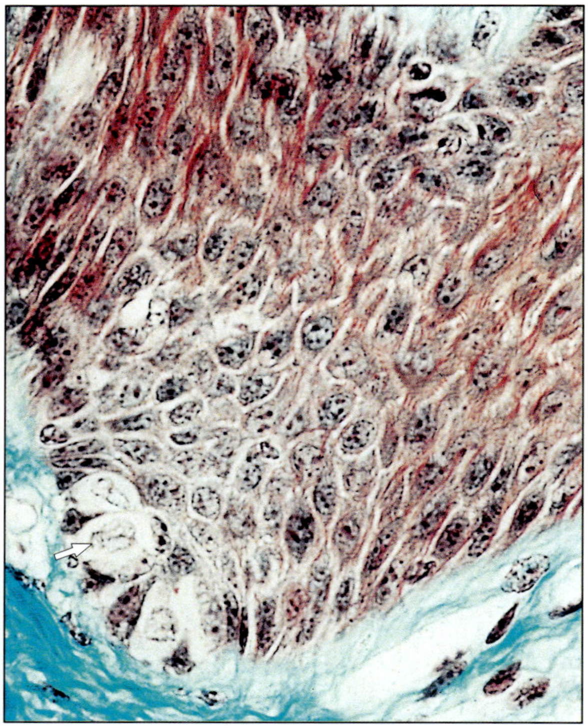

16.6 Epidermis – stratum germinativum (basale; ox). Clear cells (arrowed) lie in the basal germinal layer of columnar keratocytes. Masson's trichrome. ×250.

6.7

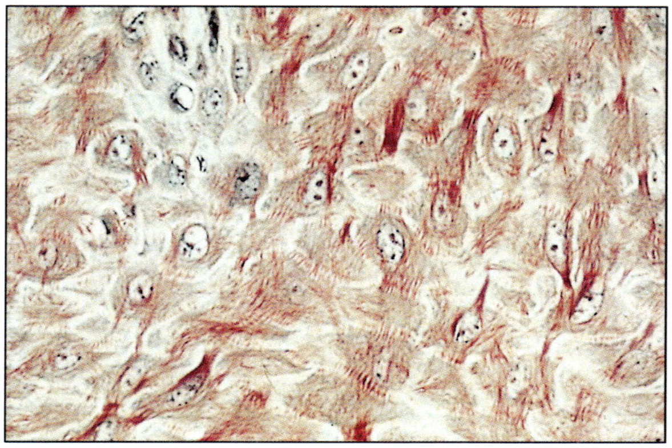

16.7 Epidermis – stratum spinosum (prickle cell layer; ox). The hexagonal keratocytes have a large clear nucleus. The cytoplasm has extensive spines or prickles around the circumference. Masson's trichrome. ×250.

16.8

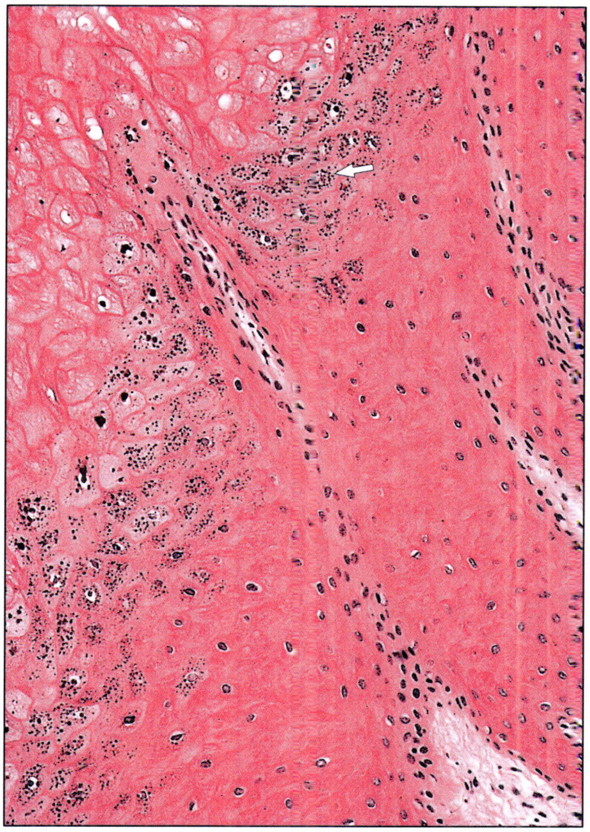

16.8 Epidermis – stratum granulosum. Hoof (horse). The keratocytes have distinctive deep blue granules in the cytoplasm (arrowed). H & E. ×125.

6.9

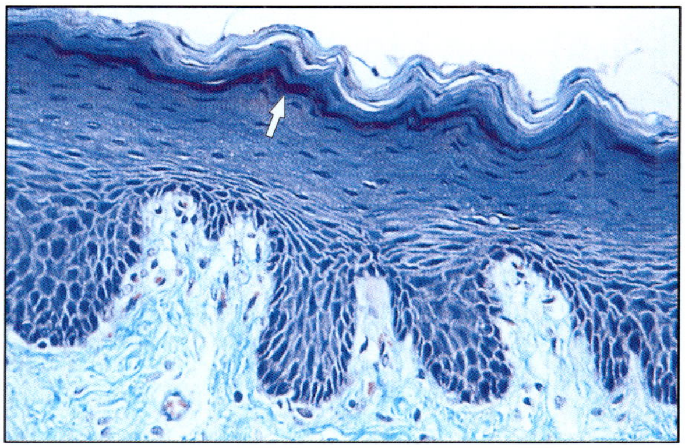

16.9 Epidermis – stratum lucidum (dog). Digital pad. The bright thin line (arrowed) marks the clear layer of thick skin. Gomori's trichrome. ×100.

.10

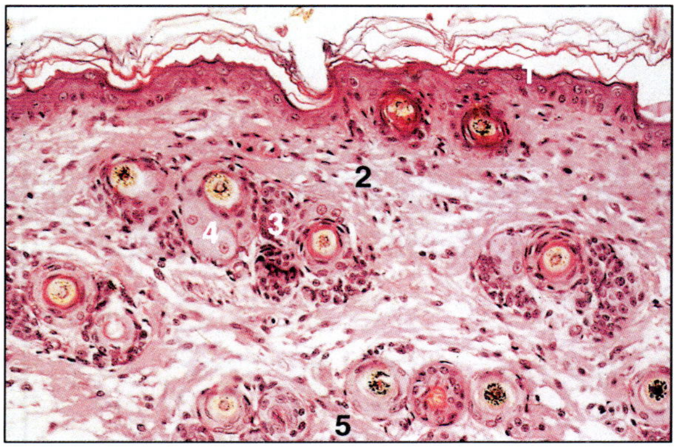

16.10 Thin skin (cat). (1) Epidermis with two layers of keratocytes. The free surface shows desquamating dead cornified cells. (2) Dermis. (3) Groups of hair follicles. (4) Sebaceous glands. (5) Smooth muscle. H & E. ×62.5.

16.11

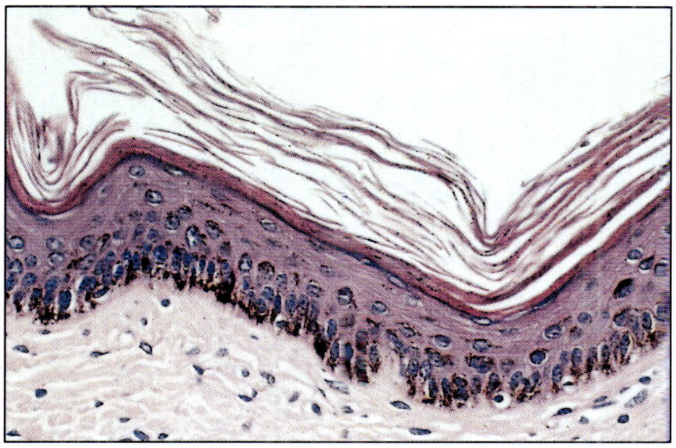

16.11 Pigmented skin (cat). The epidermis is four cells thick; melanocytes with brown pigment granules are present in the basal layer, the stratum germinativum. H & E. ×125.

Dermis

The dermis consists of loose and dense irregular connective tissue. In thick skin the superficial, loose tissue of the dermis, the papillary layer, forms projections: the dermal papillae at the dermal–epidermal junction. This increases the surface area for nutrition and may cause surface ridges in the skin. Equivalent epidermal pegs interdigitate with these and anchor the skin. The deep layer of dense irregular tissue is called the reticular layer. Dermal papillae are reduced or absent in thin skin.

Hypodermis

The hypodermis consists of loose areolar connective tissue with deposits of fat. This may be deposited in well-nourished animals as a continuous layer beneath the skin, the panniculus adiposus, or be confined to places such as the footpad to absorb pressure (see **16.1**, **16.12** and **16.13**).

16.12

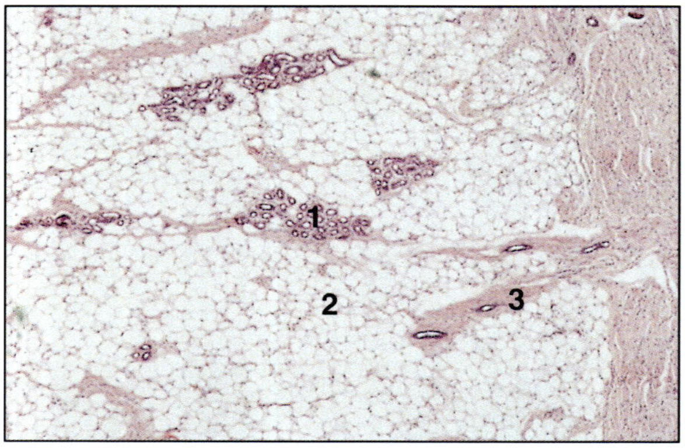

16.12 Digital pad – hypodermis (dog). (1) Sweat glands. (2) Fat cells. (3) Connective tissue. H & E. ×62.5.

Sebaceous and sweat glands

Sebaceous glands are associated with the hair follicles and secrete sebum, an oily substance. The basal layer of each gland is squamous or cuboidal epithelium. As the cells divide, some are pushed towards the surface away from the basement membrane. Vacuolated secretory cells synthesize lipid; the mature secretory cells degenerate, forming sebum. This is a form of holocrine secretion (**16.14–16.17**). The smooth muscle of the hair follicle, the arrector pili, contracts and helps to express the sebum onto the skin surface. Sebaceous glands may open directly onto the surface of the skin in the absence of hair follicles in sites such as the tarsal gland of the eyelid (**16.18**).

Sweat glands may be winding and highly coiled, or tubular and sac-like. There are two types: apocrine and merocrine.

Apocrine gland

The apocrine gland, which is more common, is situated in the dermis. The simple columnar epithelium has surface blebs of cytoplasm. These pinch off into the lumen, forming a mucoserous secretion. Their function is not completely understood, but may involve the secretion of pheromones. Contractile myoepithelial cells lie between the secretory cells and the basement membrane (**16.19**).

Merocrine gland

The merocrine (eccrine) sweat gland is situated in the dermis or the hypodermis. The epithelium is cuboidal and the secretion traverses the luminal cytoplasm without rupturing the membrane. There are few myoepithelial cells (**16.12** and **16.13**). The excretory ducts of both types of glands open into a hair follicle or directly onto the skin surface.

16.13

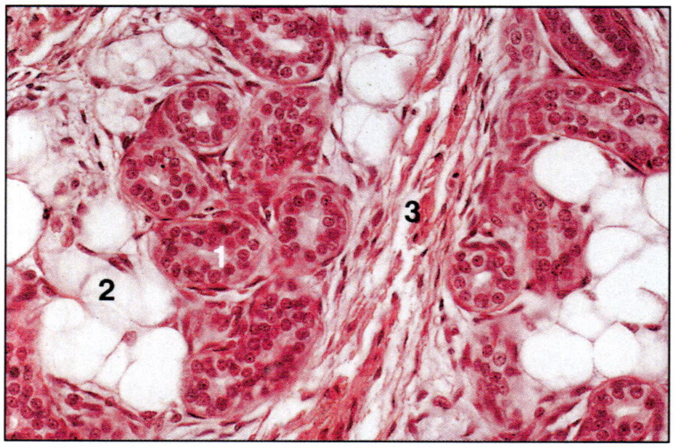

16.13 Digital pad – hypodermis (cat). (1) Sweat glands. (2) Fat cells. (3) Connective tissue with blood vessels. H & E. ×125.

16.1

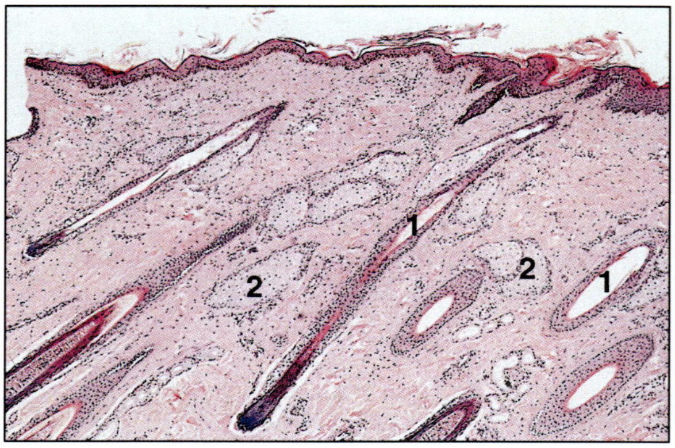

16.14 Skin (horse). (1) Single hair follicles are present in the dermis. (2) Sebaceous glands. H & E. ×62.5.

.15

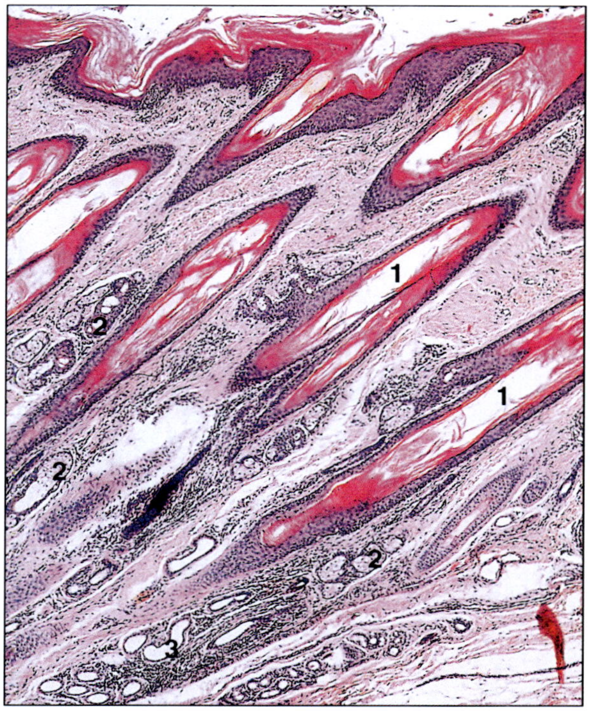

16.15 Skin (dog). (1) Single hair follicles are present in the dermis of the digital pad. (2) Sebaceous glands. (3) Sweat glands. H & E. ×125.

16.16

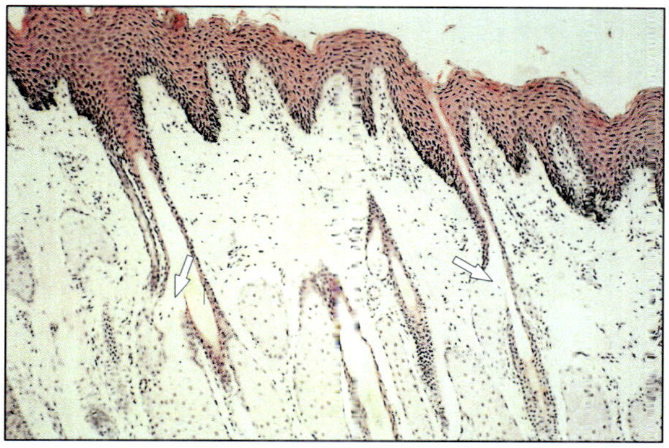

16.16 Flank skin (horse). The sebaceous glands are numerous, associated with the hair follicles, often opening directly into the follicle (arrowed). H & E. ×25.

16.17

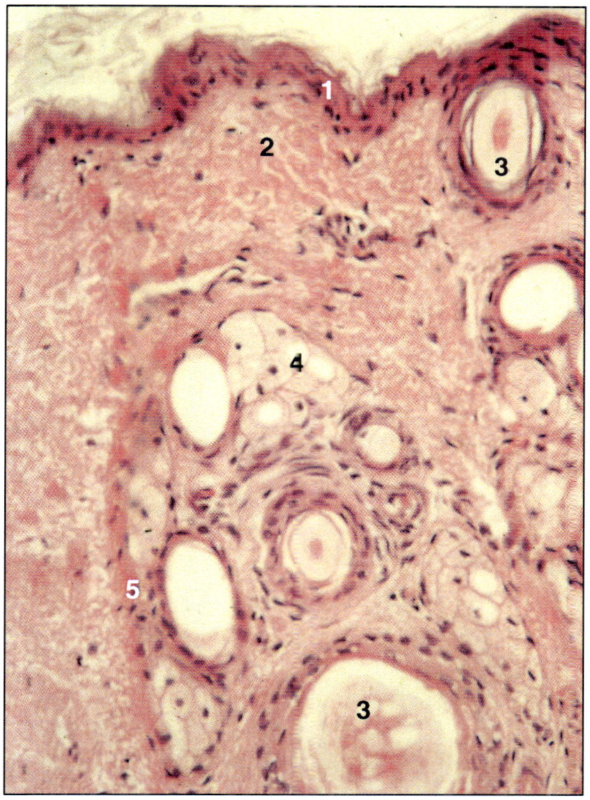

16.17 Skin (sheep). (1) Epidermis. (2) Dermis. (3) Hair follicle. (4) Sebaceous glands. (5) Arrector pili muscle; contraction assists expression of the sebum. H & E. ×160.

.18

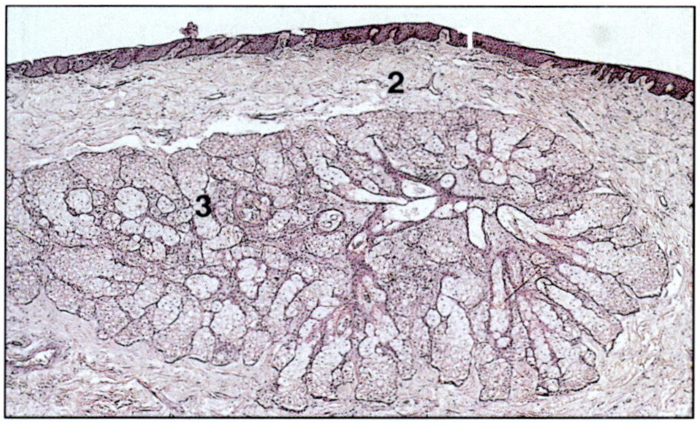

16.18 Eyelid (horse). (1) Epidermis. (2) Dermis. (3) Tarsal gland, sebaceous secretion. H & E. ×62.5.

.19

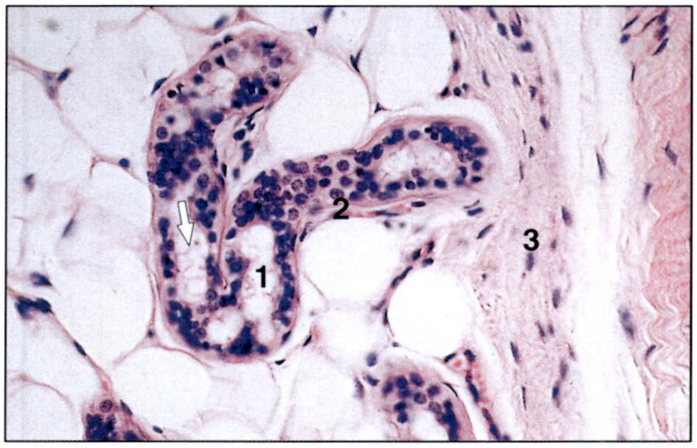

16.19 Apocrine sweat gland (dog). (1) Gland tubule lined by a simple columnar epithelium; secretory blebs are arrowed. (2) The myoepithelial cells lie between the secretory cell and the basement membrane. (3) Dermal connective tissue. H & E. ×160.

Clinical correlates

In veterinary practice, especially small animal practice, skin disease is one of the most common problems encountered. Horses and production animals also suffer from skin diseases with a relatively high frequency. Genetic factors are important within particular breeds, and environmental factors are responsible in many cases.

Inflammation of the skin is termed dermatitis (**16.20**). The skin has a fairly limited range of possible response patterns to inflammation; when an area of skin is pruritic the animal tends to traumatize it, producing secondary changes such as thickening of the epidermis. Over time, hyperpigmentation and scarring of the dermis can develop.

Infection by microorganisms including bacteria, fungi, viruses and parasites can cause skin disease. In some cases the development of disease may result from a defect in immunity or a breakdown in the host–parasite relationship. In canine demodicosis (**16.21**), *Demodex canis* mites (also found in low numbers in the hair follicles of normal dogs) pass from dam to pups during suckling, and proliferate to cause disease. Species-specific demodex mites are widespread in many species, including humans.

The integument is also a common site of neoplasms. In some tumours, such as squamous cell carcinoma (**16.22**; see **2.30**) and cutaneous haemangioma and haemangiosarcoma, chronic exposure to solar radiation is a known predisposing factor. Lightly pigmented areas are particularly vulnerable to actinic, or sunlight induced, lesions. A high incidence of neoplasia, both benign and malignant, is recognized in the dog and a few examples (**16.23–16.26**) are shown here.

16.20

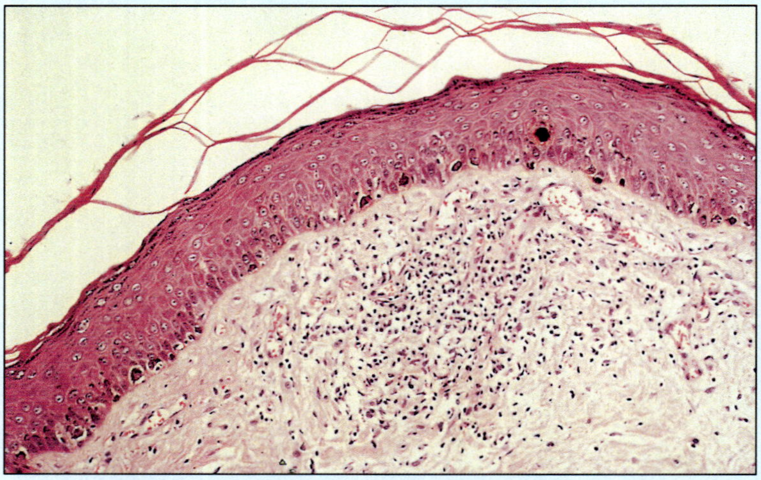

16.20 Dermatitis (dog). In this section of skin from a dog with dermatitis, there is epidermal hyperplasia with an increased thickness of stratum spinosum (acanthosis) and a mild increase in the depth of the stratum corneum (hyperkeratosis) where the keratin is arranged in a loose, woven pattern. There is slight dermal congestion and oedema and a heavy, mostly perivascular, dermal inflammatory infiltrate of neutrophils. Epithelial pigmentation is quite prominent. H & E. ×62.5.

16.21

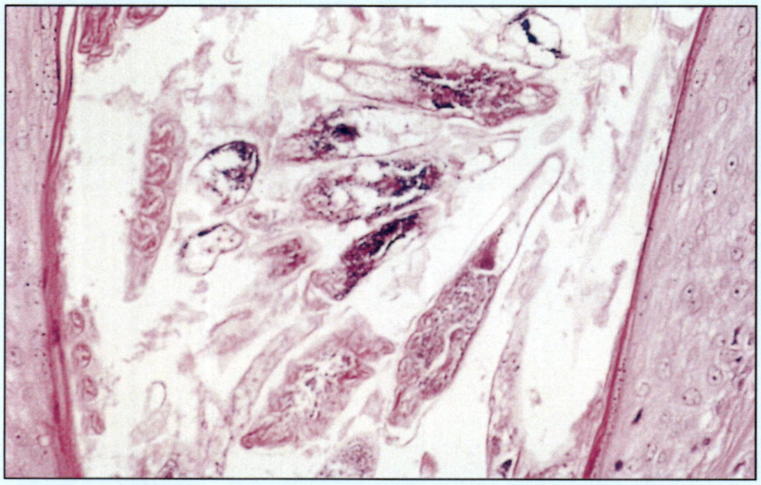

16.21 Demodicosis (dog). This high-power micrograph shows a canine hair follicle packed with demodex mites. The mites have elongated, cigar-shaped bodies with four pairs of legs at the head end. H & E. ×250.

.22

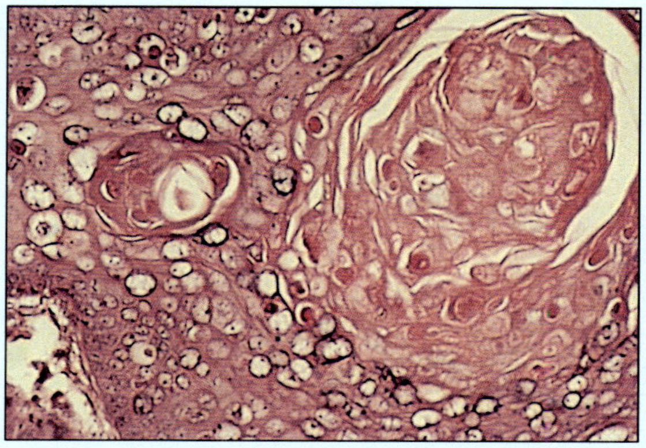

16.22 Squamous cell carcinoma of the foot of an Indian hedgehog (*Hemiechinus hemiechinus*). Note the marked cellular atypia, squamous metaplasia and keratin 'pearls.' H & E. ×125.

16 23

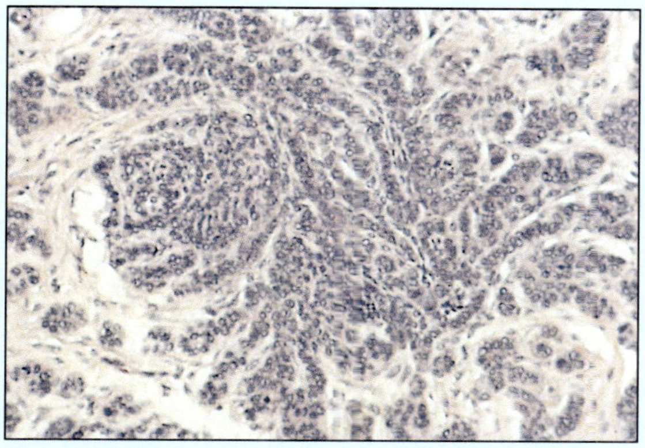

16.23 Basal cell tumour (dog). The basaloid epithelial cells of this tumour adopt a mixed lobular-to-adenoid and spiral-like 'Medusa-head' pattern. Some of these lesions are locally infiltrative, but complete excision is usually curative. H & E. ×62.5.

.24

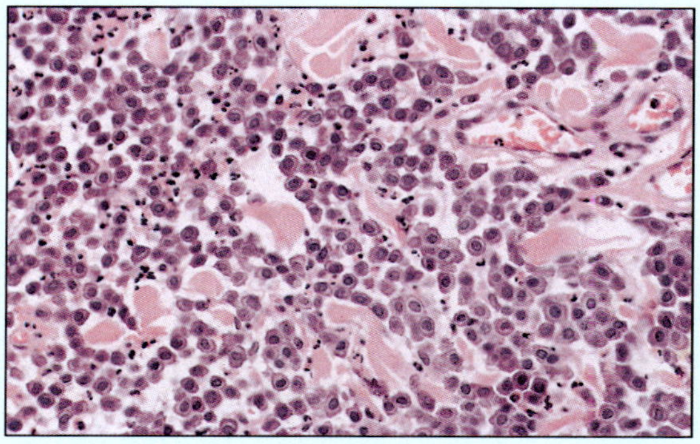

16.24 Mast cell tumour (dog). From a 5-year-old Boxer. This breed suffers from a high incidence of these, and other, skin tumours. Irregular sheets and clusters of round cells with round nuclei and well-defined, noticeably granular cytoplasm extend through the connective tissue, accompanied by numerous eosinophils. H & E. ×250.

16.25

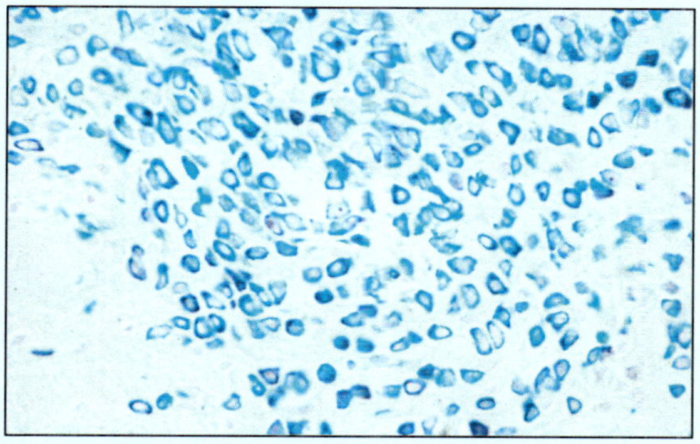

16.25 Mast cell tumour (dog). In this example of a canine mast cell tumour, the granular cytoplasm of the mast cells are highlighted a blue colour by a special stain. Astra blue. ×125.

16.26

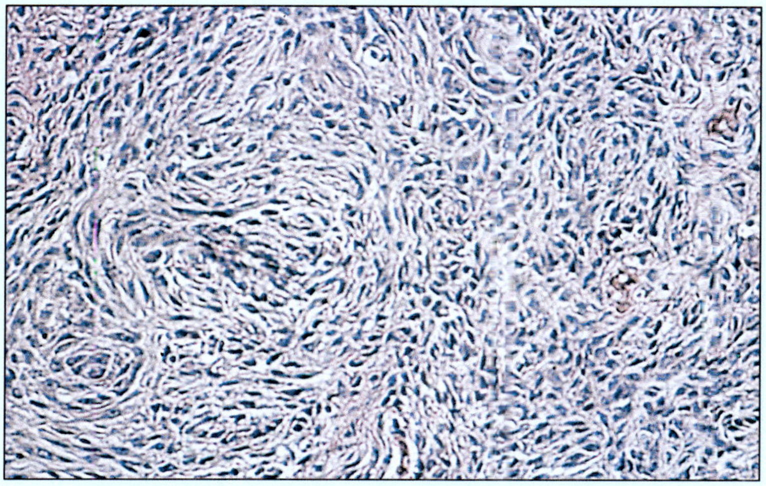

16.26 Canine malignant haemangiopericytoma. This tumour is unusual because it metastasized widely to several visceral organs. The anaplastic and pleomorphic cells form whorl-like structures centred around small blood vessels. H & E. ×125.

Avian skin

Avian skin consists of an epidermis, which is generally thinner than that of mammals, and a dermis, which in feathered skin lacks papillae and is non-glandular (**16.27**).

Feathers are keratinized epidermal derivatives. During initial development a dermal–epidermal papilla is formed. This sinks beneath the surface and becomes a follicle as in the mammal (**16.28**). The epidermal cells proliferate to form a cylinder. This becomes the quill, whereas the upper part becomes ridged to form the vane.

Combs and wattles are skin appendages. The dermis contains an extensive network of sinus capillaries and abundant mucous connective tissue. They are epidermal target organs, highly developed in the male, and are responsive to the sex hormones.

The uropygial (preen) gland is the only skin gland in birds and is found at the base of the tail. The bilobed gland, which produces an oily secretion, is bound by a connective tissue capsule and drained by lobar ducts (**16.29**). Each tubule is divided into a sebaceous zone, fatty zone and a glycogen zone; the glycogen zone stains selectively with periodic acid–Schiff. They are lined with a multilayered epithelium that is very similar to that of the mammalian sebaceous gland. The basal cells multiply, accumulate a fatty secretion in the cytoplasm and degenerate. The secretion is passed through each duct to the isthmus and then to the papilla, which opens onto the surface (**16.30** and **16.31**).

Reptilian skin

Depending upon the family within the class Reptilia, there are enormous differences in the integument of snakes, lizards, chelonians, crocodilians and the tuatara. Snakes and lizards possess skin covered by scales, rounded tubercles or other epidermal extensions (**16.32–16.34**). Rattlesnakes

16.27

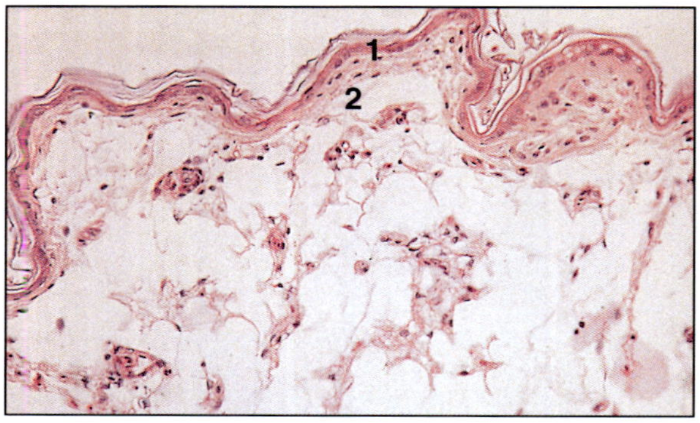

16.27 Skin (bird). (1) Epidermis. (2) Dermis. H & E. ×25.

16.28

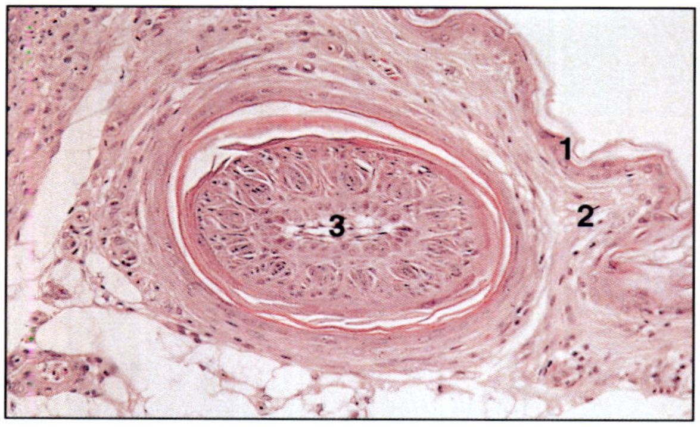

16.28 Skin (bird). (1) Epidermis. (2) Dermis. (3) Developing feather follicle. H & E. ×62.5.

16.2

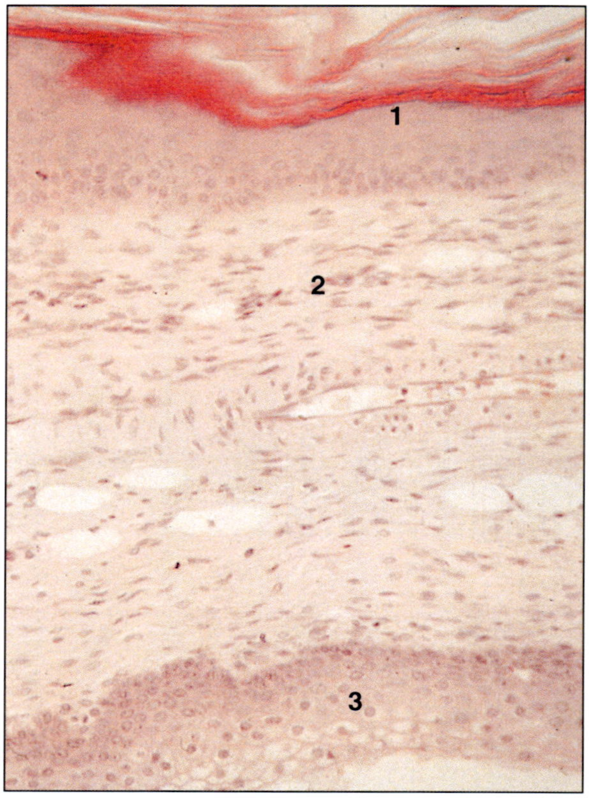

16.29 Uropygial gland (bird). (1) Epidermis. (2) Dermis. (3) Lobar duct lined by stratified epithelium. H & E. ×62.5.

.30

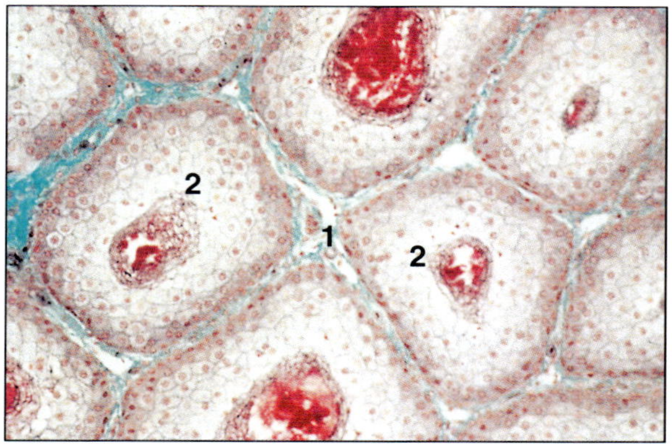

16.31

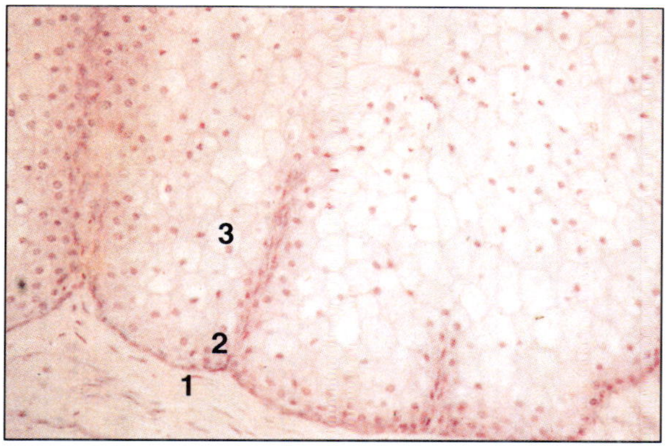

16.30 Uropygial gland (bird). (1) Connective tissue. (2) Secretory glands units. Masson's trichrome. ×100.

16.31 Uropygial gland (bird). (1) Connective tissue. (2) Basal layer of the secretory epithelium. (3) Superficial layers of fat filled cells. H & E. ×250.

16.32

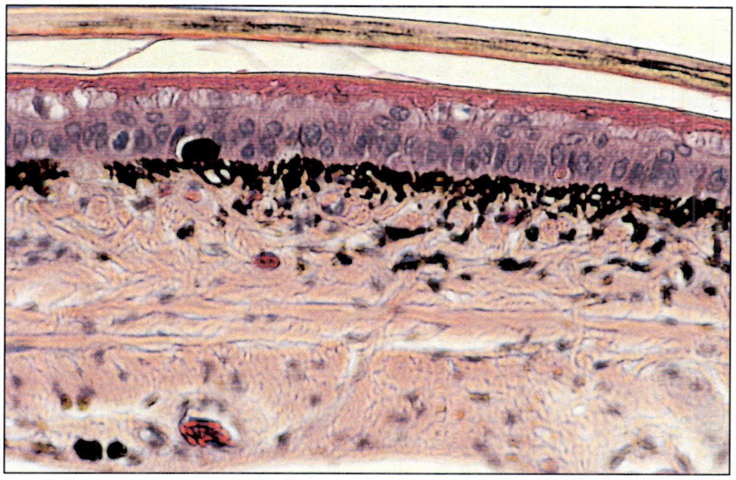

16.32 Section of pre-ecdysis integument of a mountain kingsnake (*Lampropeltis zonata*). The uppermost keratinized, lightly pigmented, pale pink layer is disengaged from the lightly cornified eosinophilic epithelium that lies immediately above the stratified squamous layer. Numerous black melanophages are present in the upper dermis. H & E. ×125.

.33

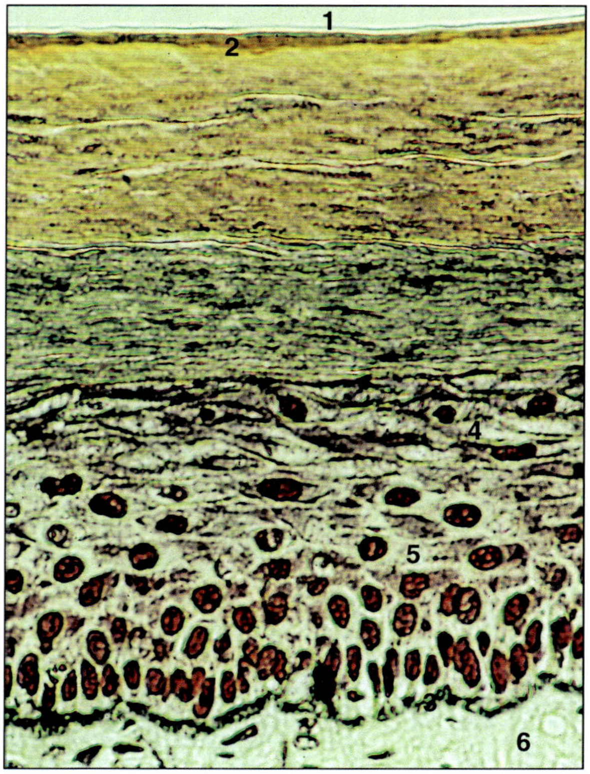

16.34

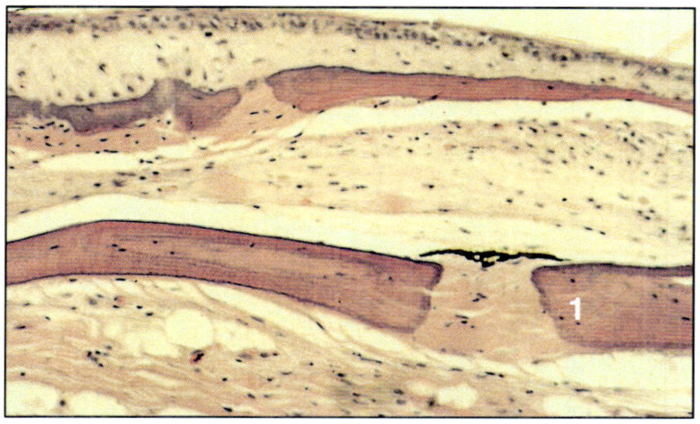

16.34 The integuments of some reptiles, particularly crocodilians and some lizards, contain multiple bony plaques called osteoderms (1). This section of a blue-tongued skink (*Tiliqua scincoides*) contains several of these ossified flat structures that are attached at their ends by fibrous connective tissue. These hinge-like connections permit flexibility. H & E. ×12.5.

16.33 Immediately beneath the squamous epithelium of the section in **16.33** are dendritic neurons that, when treated with silver-containing dyes, stain black. (1) Senescent stratum corneum. (2) Current stratum corneum. (3) Stratum basale. (4) Stratum granulosum. (5) Stratum spinosum. (6) Dermis. Bodian's silver. ×125.

have an epidermally derived, loosely segmented, hollow rattle that vibrates when the tail tip is moved rapidly (**16.35**). A new button-like segment is added each time the rattlesnake moults its skin. Embedded osteoderms are present in the skin of many reptiles: for example, on the dorsal and lateral surfaces of crocodilians and on the limbs of some tortoises. The bony box-like shells of most chelonians are covered with keratinous plates (**16.36** and **16.37**). Even the soft and leathery shells of soft-shelled turtles are covered with lightly keratinized squamous epithelium. Snakes shed their senescent epidermis periodically as inverted tubes of (usually) unbroken old skin from which they crawl. Lizards, crocodilians, the tuatara and chelonians moult their old epidermis piecemeal. Aquatic turtles shed one or more of their hard outermost layers of shell plates periodically. Many tortoises merely add more keratin concentrically to their plates (or scutes) as they grow throughout life.

Reptiles lack sweat glands. However, some lizards have a few sebaceous glands. In some species, modified sebaceous glands secrete holocrine, pheromone-rich waxy substances that are important inducers or releasers of sexual or territorial behaviour (**16.38–16.40**). Other scent-producing secretions are elaborated by cloacal and hemipenial sheath glandular structures (*see* Chapter 11, **11.41**) and by the sexual-segment granularity observed in the distal convoluted tubules of some male lizards and snakes (see Chapter 9, **9.21**).

16.35

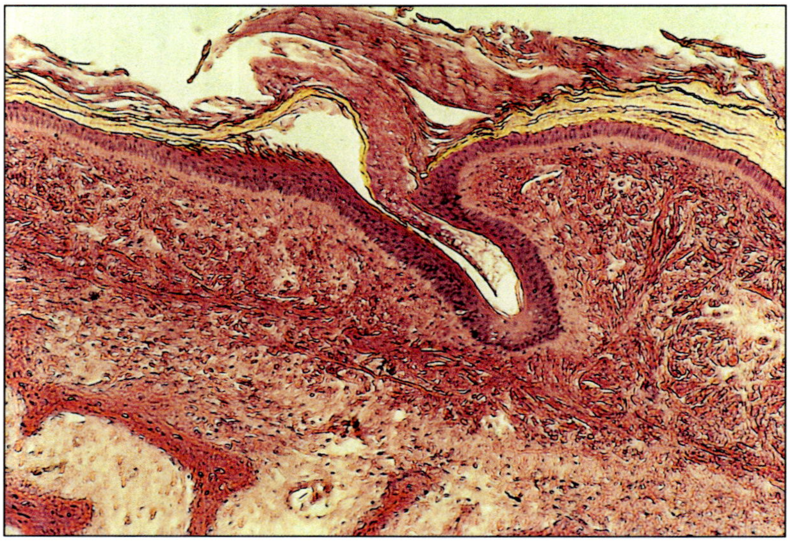

16.35 Rattle of a small Mexican rattlesnake (*Crotalus enyo*). This keratinized structure forms as a button-like protruberance to which a loosely interlocking segment is added each time the snake moults its integument. The most cranial segment retains a living core of dermis, whereas the tissues of the distal segments are no longer living. H & E. ×12.5.

16.36

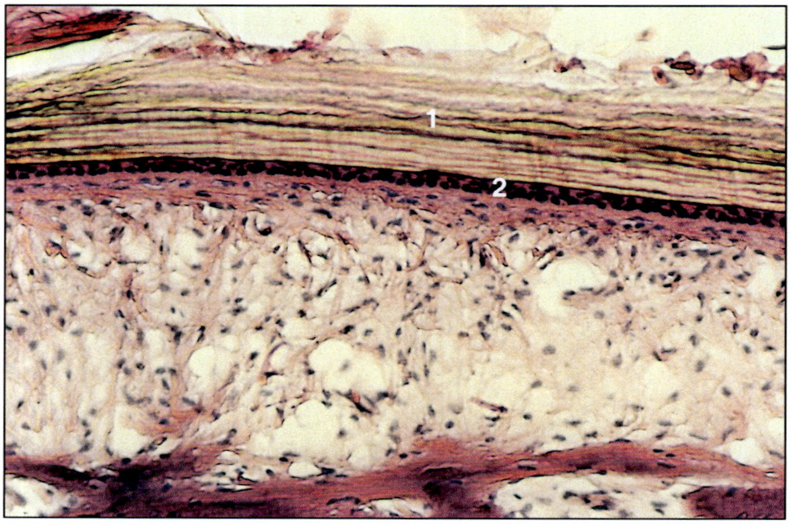

16.36 The carapacial shell of a red-eared slider turtle (*Trachemys scripta elegans*), is covered by a layer of horn-like keratin (1) and a variable thickness of stratified squamous epithelium (2). The dermis is variable in thickness, depending upon the size and species of the turtle. It covers multiple layers of membranous compact and cancellous bone in which bone marrow fills the cancellous spaces. H & E. ×62.5.

.37

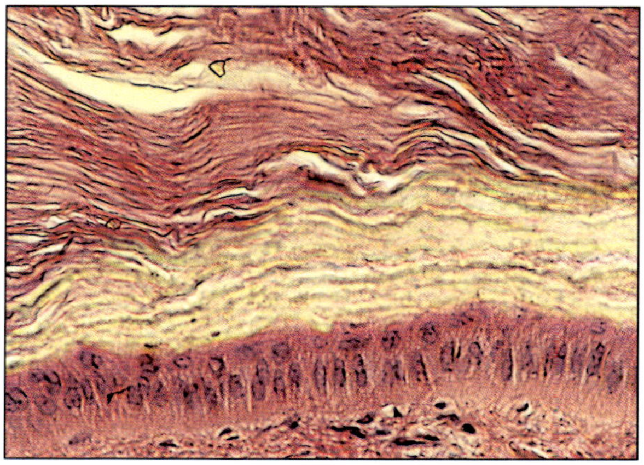

16.38

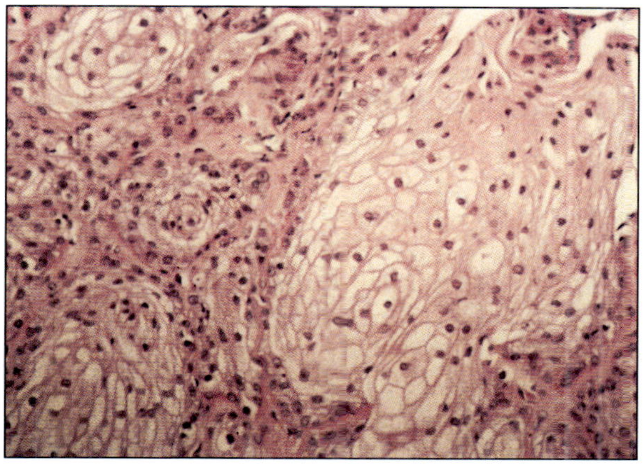

16.37 Section of the most superficial layers of the keratinized carapace of a terrestrial tortoise (*Xerobates agassizi*). Most terrestrial tortoises possess a much thicker carapacial and plastral shell than aquatic turtles or terrapins of the same size. H & E. ×100.

16.38 Mental gland from a desert tortoise. This modified sebaceous glandular structure is believed to produce a pheromone-rich secretion that initiates and at least partly mediates premating courtship behaviour. H & E. ×100.

16.39 A cross-section of the skin of the ventral thigh of a sexually mature male green iguana (*Iguana iguana*), containing two femoral pores (1). The eosinophilic holocrine secretion from these glands is exuded as a waxy substance. H & E. ×12.5.

16.39

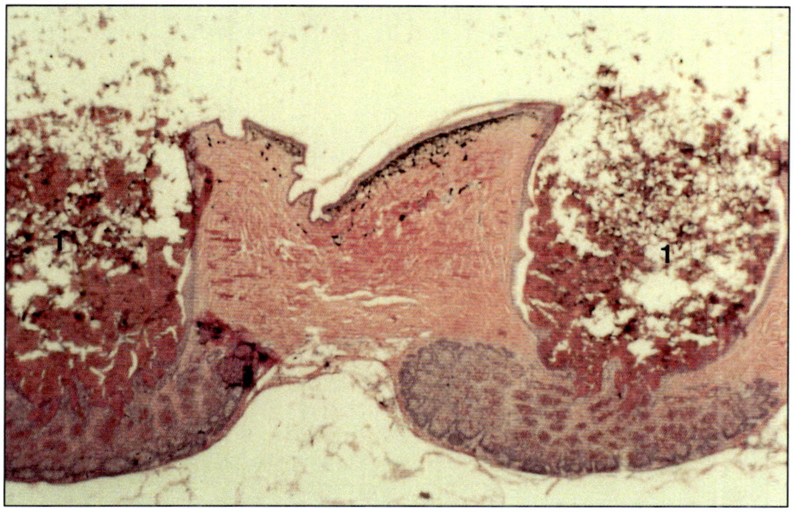

16.40 Medium-power magnification of a femoral pore from a male iguana. Note the eosinophilic secretion and cellular debris being extruded into the ductal system that empties its contents onto the epidermal surface (arrow). H & E. ×100.

16.40

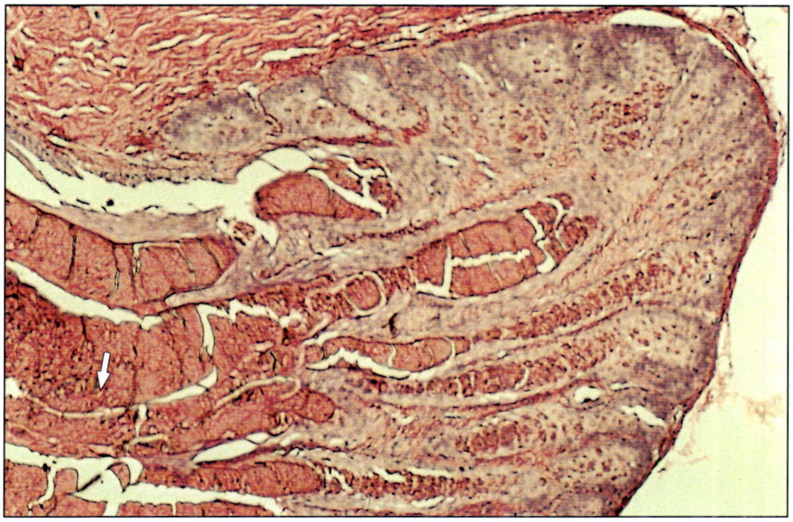

Amphibian skin

Amphibian skin is either smooth or warty, lacks scales and is kept variably moist by secretions that are produced by skin glands (**16.41**). When the skin secretions of many anuran and some caudate amphibians come into contact with a predator's (or human's) mucous membranes or are swallowed or injected, a lethally toxic reaction may result. Recently, investigations have shown that the skin secretions of some amphibians possess potent antimicrobial properties that are effective against a diverse group of pathogens.

16.41

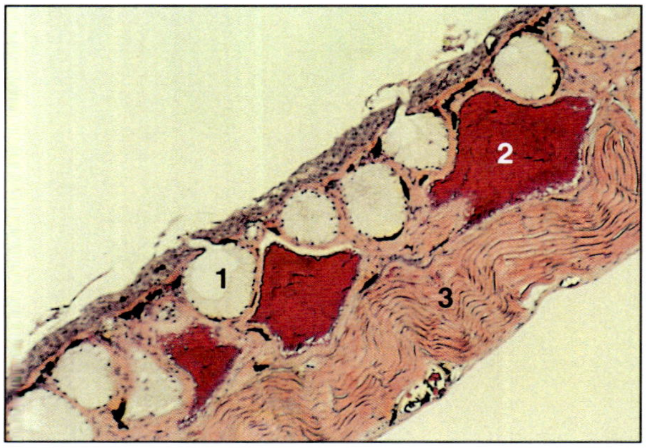

16.41 Full thickness section of the skin of an African clawed frog (*Xenopus laevis*). The integument contains two types of glandular structures: (1) clear-staining mucus-secreting glands and (2) highly eosinophilic poison glands. The secretory products of both are carried to the skin surface via short ducts. (3) Much of the thickness of the subepithelial tissue is comprised of skeletal muscle fibres. H & E. ×12.5.

Fish skin

Fish possess a varied spectrum of skin. The integument of many elasmobranchs, particularly sharks and rays, is characterized by the presence of embedded tooth-like denticles. Other elasmobranchs lack these mineralized structures. Teleost fish may be either scaled or scaleless, but most of them have integument containing mucous glands that secrete lubricative products onto the skin and fin surfaces. These mucoid secretions often contain immunoglobulin A antibodies, which provide a protective defence against infection. The mucous glands may be alveolar structures with short epithelium-lined ducts, or groups of scattered goblet cells with mucopolysaccharide-rich secretions that flow over and cover the skin. Various barbels or other appendages aid in sensory or visual camouflage, species-specific territorial or courtship recognition, and defence functions.

Clinical correlates

For a general discussion of clinical correlates, see the domestic animals section. Inflammation can be superficial or it can be extensive and involve deeper structures that are located beneath the epidermis and dermis (**16.42**). Snakes of the genus *Pituophis* exhibit a high incidence of pigment cell integumentary tumours (chromatophoromata).

16.42

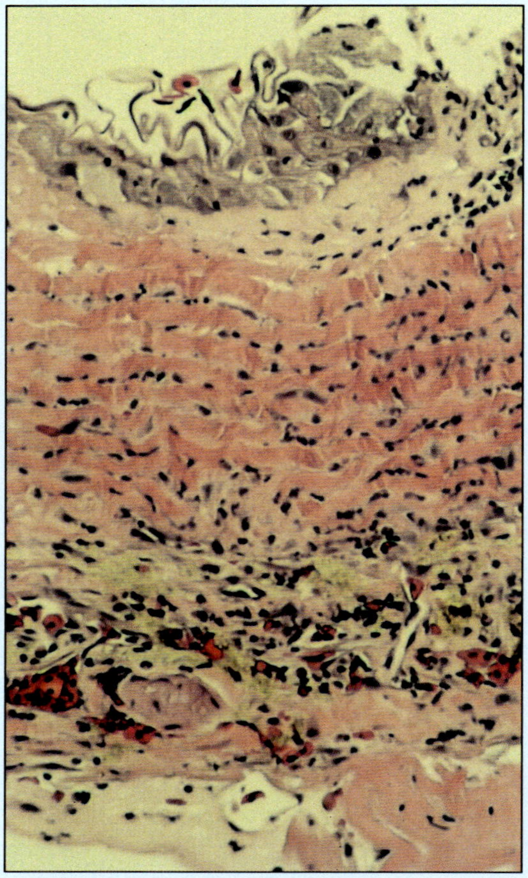

16.42 Non-suppurative dermatitis, dermal ulceration and superficial myositis in the skin of a clawed frog (*Xenopus laevis*). The epidermis is disrupted, and the dermis and skeletal muscular tissues are infiltrated by mixed mononuclear leucocytes. H & E. ×125.

Specialized integumentary structures

Special skin glands (adnexae)

Anal glands

These are modified tubulosaccular sweat glands opening into the anus. They are present in the dog, cat and pig (**16.43**).

Anal sacs

These are present in carnivores and are located between the internal and external anal sphincters. The walls are lined with sebaceous and apocrine glands in dogs and cats (**16.44** and **16.45**).

Perianal (circumanal) glands

These are modified sebaceous glands found in the skin around the anus of dogs, consisting of non-patent masses of polygonal cells.

.43

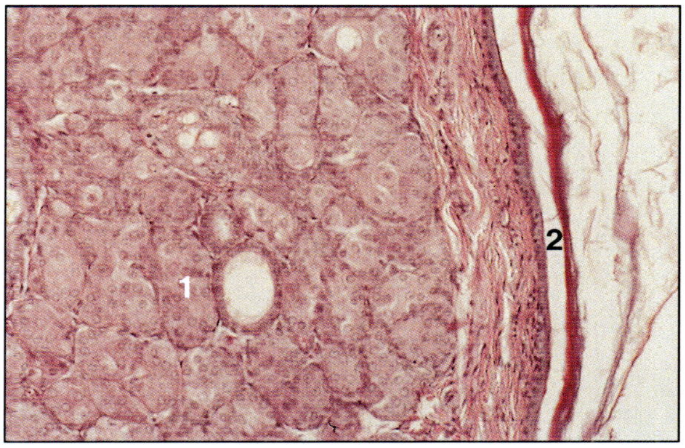

16.44

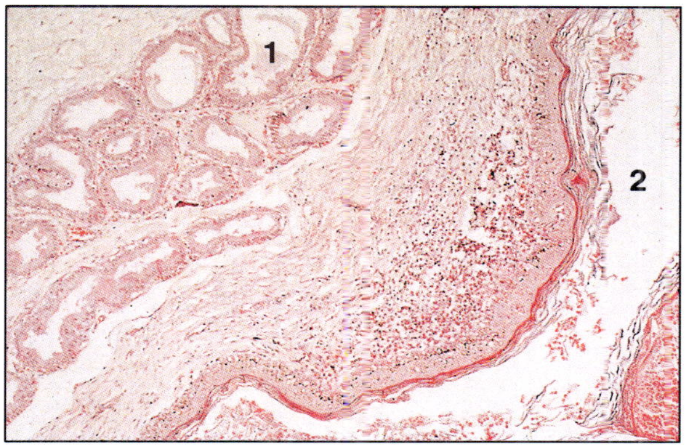

16.43 Anal gland (cat). (1) Tubular, saccular sweat glands in the circumanal connective tissue. (2) Anus lined by stratified squamous keratinized epithelium. H & E. ×100.

16.44 Anal sac (dog). (1) Apocrine tubular glands. (2) Anal sac. H & E. ×62.5.

16.45 Perianal sinus (dog). (1) The glands are a mixture of sebaceous and sweat glands. (2) Hair follicle. (3) Dermal connective tissue. H & E. ×125.

16.45

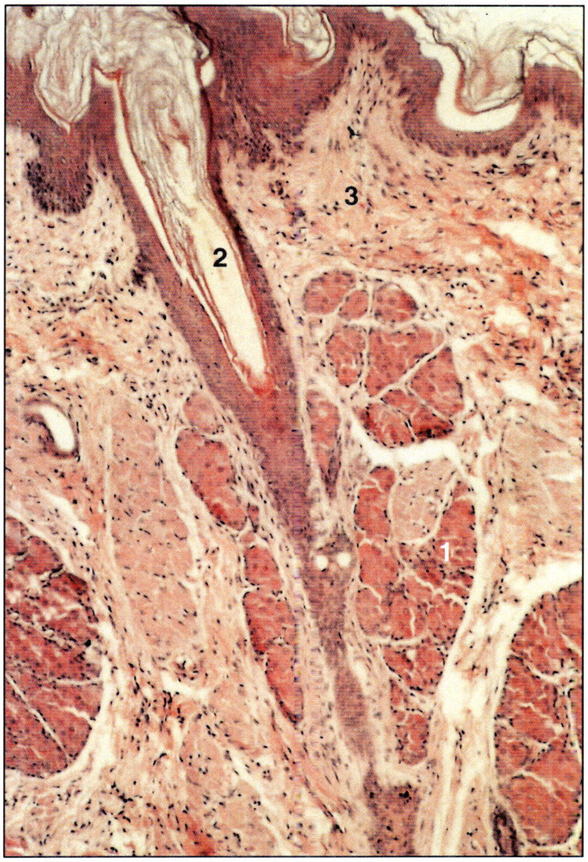

Supracaudal or tail glands

These are local concentrations of sebaceous glands in the dog and cat. The secretion is used in grooming (16.46 and 16.47). A similar function in birds is served by the uropygial or preen gland (see 16.29–16.31).

Other glands

There are many other small collections of glands serving a variety of purposes. These include porcine carpal glands (16.48 and 16.49); merocrine; the sebaceous scent or horn gland of the goat; the submental sebaceous gland of the cat; and the interdigital glands of the sheep, a mixture of sebaceous and sweat glands (16.50 and 16.51).

Specialized glands in reptiles and amphibians

Several specialized glands exist in amphibians and reptiles. Many amphibians, especially frogs and toads, possess both mucus-secreting dermal glands and highly toxic poison glands that secrete complex alkaloid and amine-rich venom-like substances. Crocodilians and some chelonians possess paired modified sebaceous mental glands located on the underside of the front of their mandibles (see 16.39). These structures are larger in males than in females. Some lizards have femoral pores or anal pores (see 16.40 and 16.41) with waxy holocrine secretions that are believed to contain pheromones.

16.46

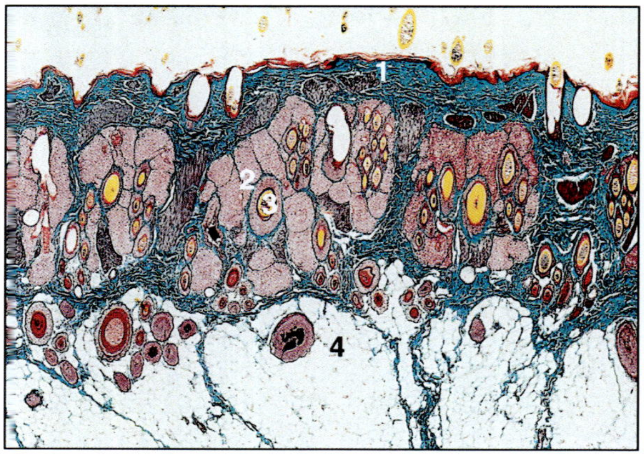

16.46 Supracaudal organ (cat). The supracaudal organ or tail gland is an area of sebaceous secretory units in the tail region; the secretion is used in grooming. (1) Epidermis. (2) Sebaceous glands. (3) Hair follicles. (4) Hypodermis. Sacpic staining method. ×12.5.

16.4

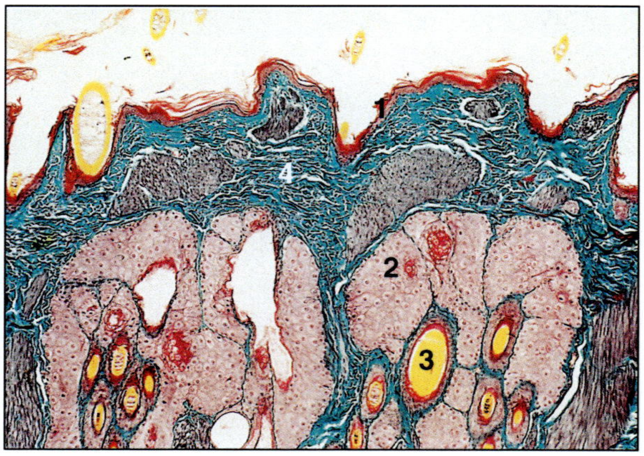

16.47 Supracaudal organ (cat). (1) Epidermis. (2) Sebaceous glands. (3) Hair follicles. (4) Dermis. Sacpic staining method. ×100.

16.48

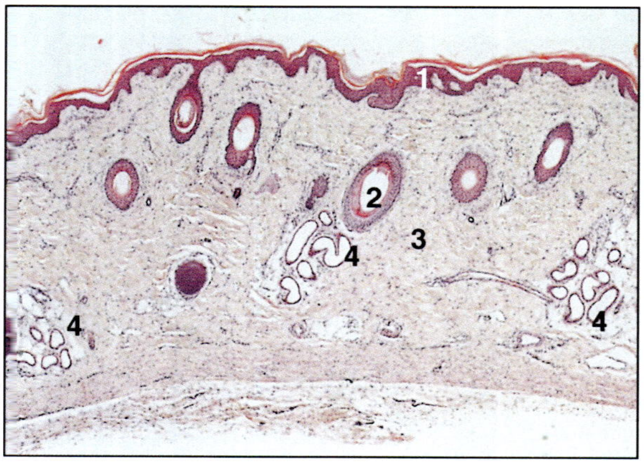

16.48 Carpal skin (pig). (1) Epidermis. (2) Hair follicles are distributed singly. (3) Dermis. (4) Merocrine carpal sweat glands. H & E. ×12.5.

16.4

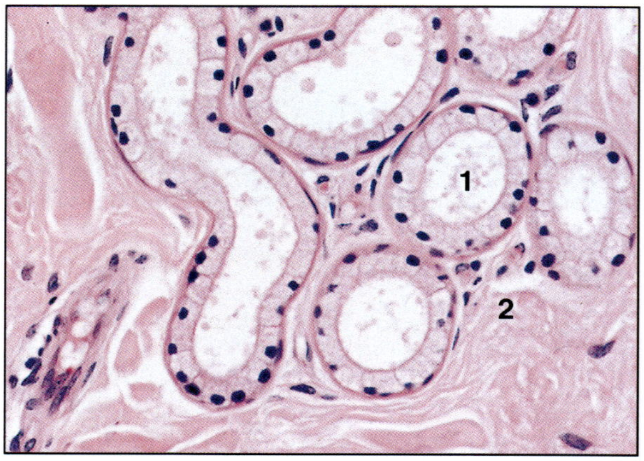

16.49 Carpal skin (pig). (1) Merocrine sweat glands are lined by a cuboidal epithelium. (2) Dermis. H & E. ×125.

The femoral-pore secretions of some desert-dwelling lizards are highly fluorescent when exposed to ultraviolet illumination. These species are able to see these secretions in reflected ultraviolet light. The femoral and anal pores are more highly developed in male lizards than in female lizards.

.50

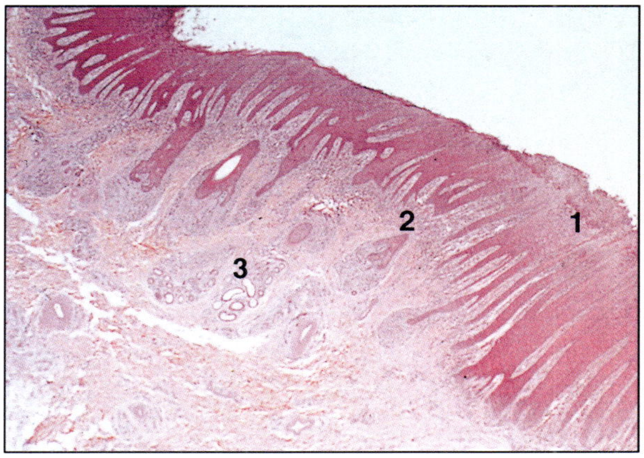

16.50 Interdigital skin (sheep). (1) Epidermis. (2) Dermis. (3) Sebaceous and sweat glands. H & E. ×12.5.

16.51

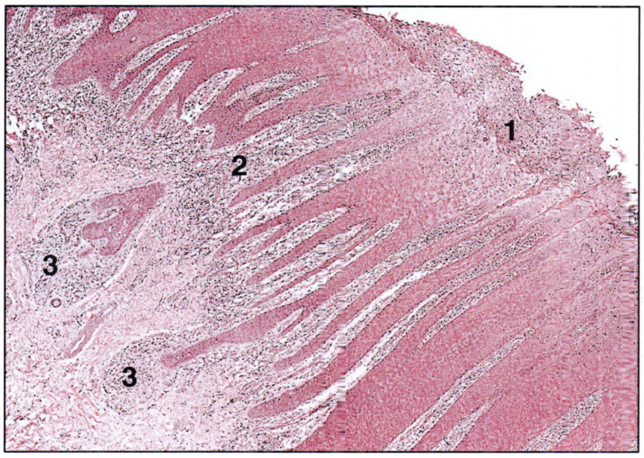

16.51 Interdigital skin (sheep). (1) Epidermis with epidermal pegs. (2) Dermis with deep dermal papillae. (3) Glandular region of the dermis. H & E. ×125.

Hair

Hair follicles develop in the embryo as localized proliferations of the epidermal epithelium, growing down into the underlying mesenchyme to form a cylinder with an expanded distal end or bulb (16.52). The bulb is invaginated by a vascular papilla of dermal connective tissue; the germinal (matrix) cells of the bulb proliferate to form the hair. A hair near its origin consists of a central medulla of cuboidal cells, a cortex of flattened cells orientated parallel to the long axis of the hair, and an outer cuticle. The germinal cells also form the inner root sheath. This grows from the papilla of the hair bulb to the opening of the sebaceous gland, where the hair becomes a cuticle. The hair cuticle consists of scale-like cells that partially overlap so that their free edges are directed upward. The cells of the sheath cuticle are directed downwards so that the hair and the sheath interlock. The peripheral outer root sheath represents a downward continuation of the epidermis. A dermal sheath abuts the basement membrane of the external root sheath, surrounds the follicle and blends with the rest of the dermal connective tissue. The arrector pili muscle attaches to the connective tissue sheath

16.52

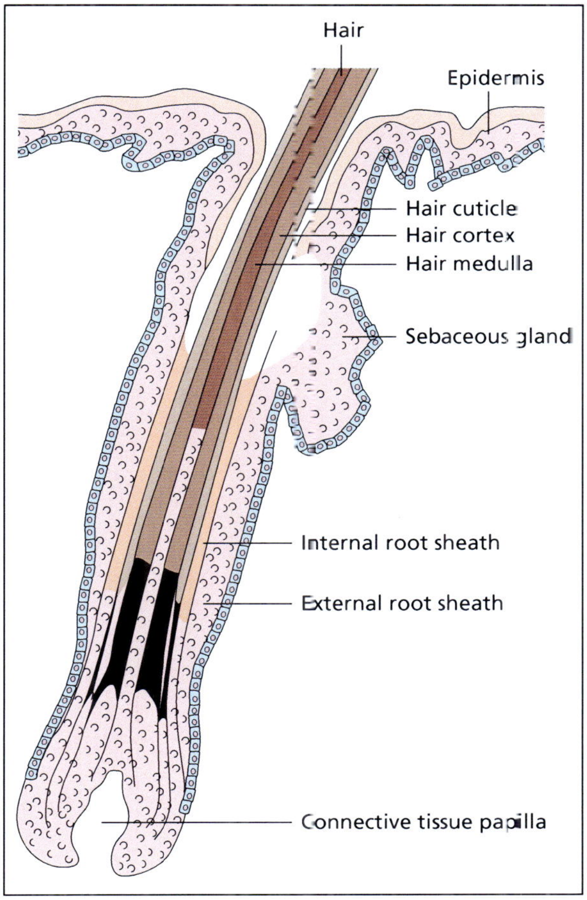

16.52 Hair follicle.

of the follicle and the superficial layer of the dermis (**16.53–16.58**). As the hair approaches the surface, both the medullary and the cortical cells shrink and become keratinized, lose their nucleus and acquire air bubbles (see **16.11** and **16.14–16.17**). Hair colour is determined by the relative proportions of pigment granules and air bubbles. Dark hair has more pigment and fewer bubbles (**16.55** and **16.56**).

Hair follicles are evenly and singly arranged in the horse and ox (see **16.14** and **16.57**), but occur in groups of three in the pig and as compound follicles in the dog and cat (**16.58**). Hair follicles are set obliquely in the skin except in sheep, where they are vertical (see **16.17** and **16.59**). Compound follicles consist of a large cover hair and a variable number of fine wool hairs. Hairs are replaced at regular intervals, with the large coarse hairs of the mane and tail lasting throughout life.

16.53

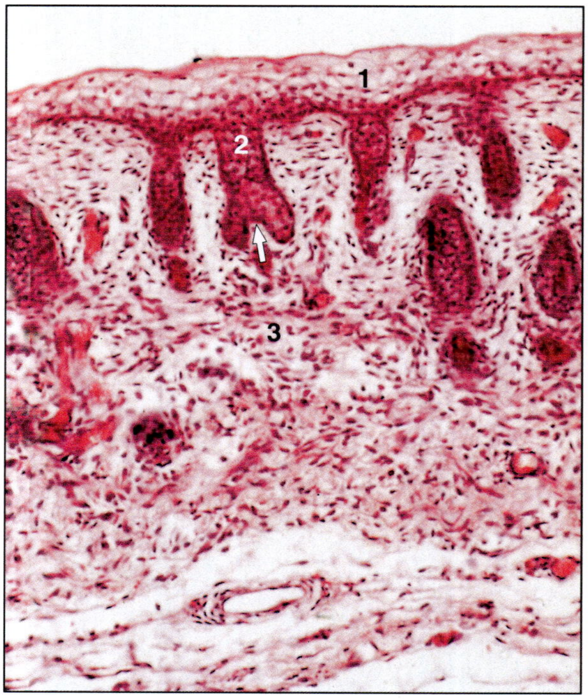

16.53 Skin. Cat embryo. (1) Ectoderm. (2) The ectodermal cylinder with the invaginated papilla (arrowed) forms the primordium of the hair follicle. (3) Mesoderm. H & E. ×125.

16.5

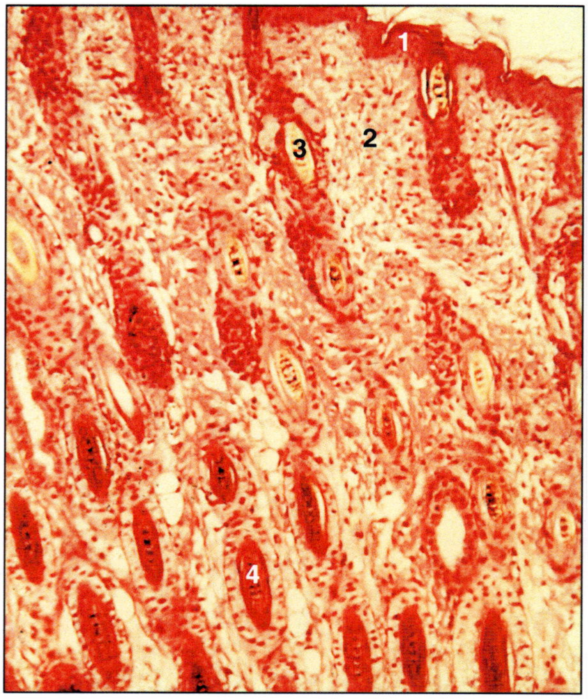

16.54 Neonatal skin (cat). (1) Epidermis. (2) Dermis. (3) Hair shaft. (4) Root sheath. H & E. ×125.

16.55

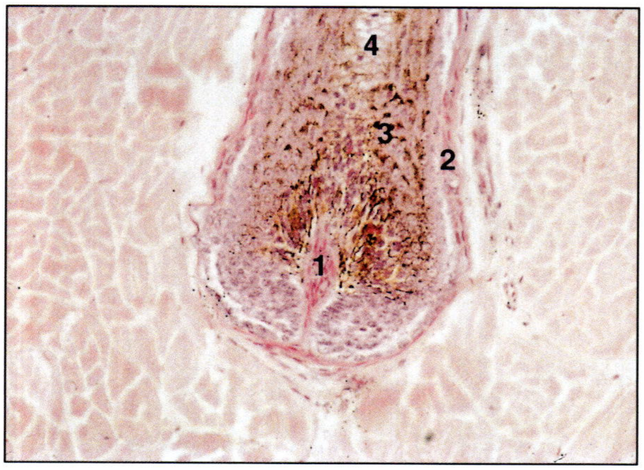

16.55 Bulb region of the hair follicle. Horse (skin). (1) Dermal papilla. (2) Dermal root sheath. (3) Epidermal root sheath: (a) outer sheath, (b) inner sheath. (4) Hair. Note the melanin pigment in the epidermal sheath. H & E. ×125.

16.56

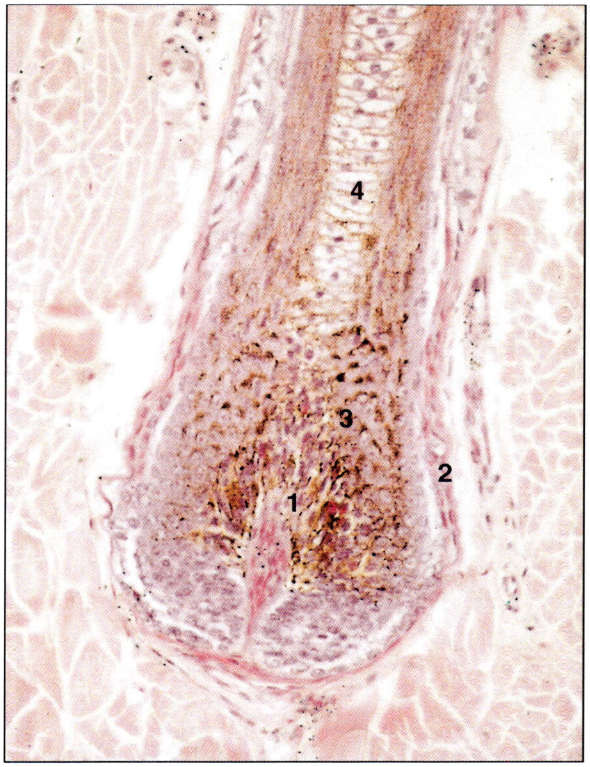

16.56 Hair follicle. Skin (horse). (1) Dermal papilla. (2) Dermal root sheath. (3) Epidermal root sheath with (a) outer sheath and (b) inner sheath. (4) Hair. Note pigmentation. H & E. ×250.

16.57

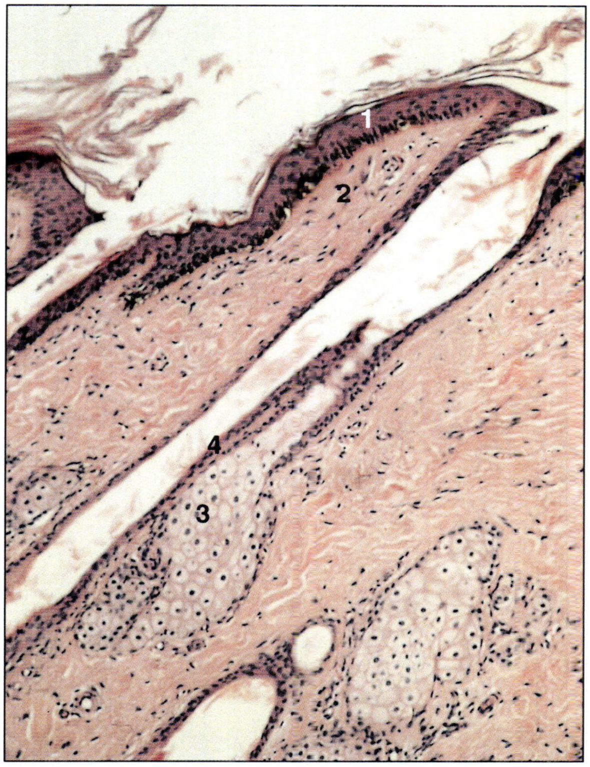

16.57 Skin (horse). (1) Epidermis. (2) Dermis. (3) Sebaceous gland opening into the hair follicle. (4) Epidermal root sheath is reduced to two layers of cells; the inner layer is thin horny scales. Note the oblique set of the hair follicle. H & E. ×125.

16.58

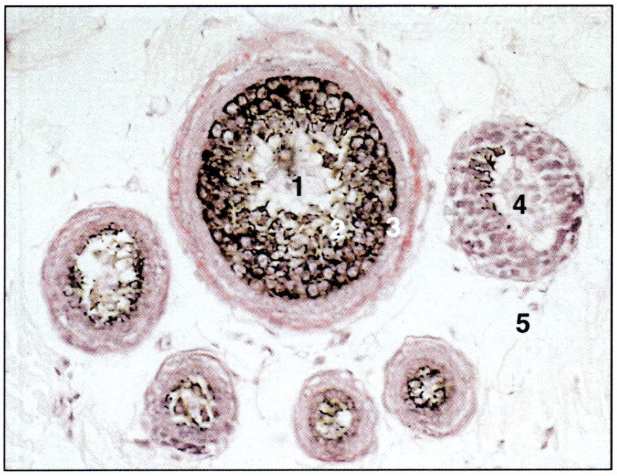

16.58 Skin. Compound hair follicles (cat). (1) Large cover hair cut in cross-section: (2) epidermal sheath and (3) hair. (4) Fine wool/lanugo hairs. (5) Dermis. H & E. ×25.

16.59

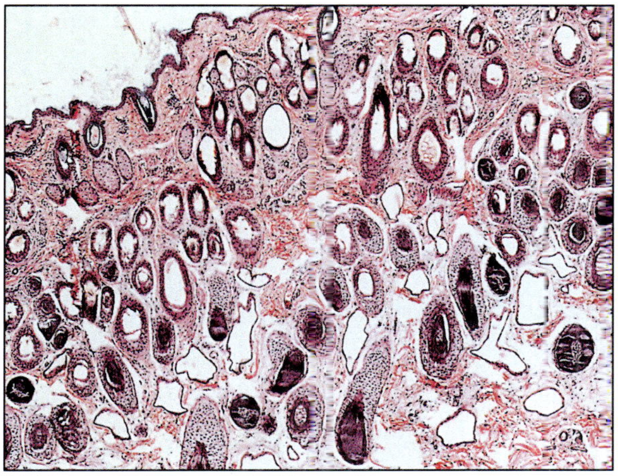

16.59 Woolly skin. Flank (sheep). The hair follicles are all of the smaller wool/lanugo type, set individually in the dermis and lying vertically. H & E. ×12.5.

Sinus (tactile) hairs (vibrissae)

Tactile hairs are limited to the facial region. The dermal sheath is highly developed and split by a blood sinus into inner and outer layers. In horses, pigs and ruminants the sinus is trabeculated throughout its length. In carnivores the upper region is non-trabeculated, forming an annular sinus. Free sensory nerve endings are associated with the epidermal cells of the hair and the dermal sheath (**16.60** and **16.61**).

Hooves, horns and claws

Hooves, horns and claws are highly specialized derivatives of the epidermis. The dermis is very vascular and develops deep papillae, which are often sufficient to raise macroscopic ridges. It merges with the periosteum where present. The hypodermis is absent where the skin covers bone, but forms a deep layer at the 'frog' (a pad of soft horn between the bars on the sole of a horse's hoof), the bulb (swollen part of the wall behind the frog) and the digital pad where extensive fat deposits form shock-absorbing cushions.

Where the papillae are regular, the overlying epidermis gives rise to a hair-like structure: the horn tubule. Cells at the tip of the papilla form a core or medulla and grow towards the surface. They then shrink and disappear to leave a hollow tube surrounded by columns of cells equivalent to the hair cortex. The cells of the basal layer at the tip of the epidermal peg also grow towards the surface to form intertubular horn (**16.62** and **16.63**).

The epidermis is markedly keratinized and this forms the hard outer surface of the hoof, horn and claw (**16.64–16.66**).

16.60

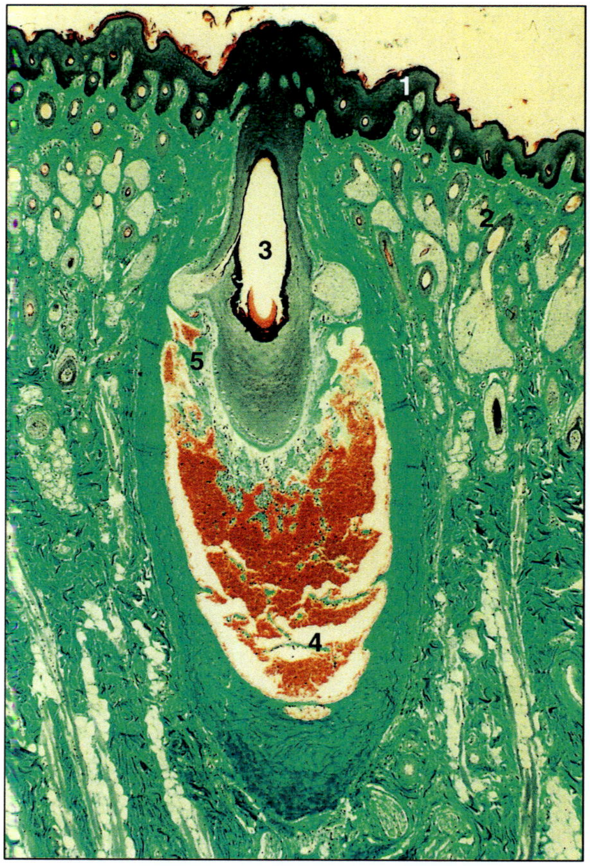

16.60 Sinus/tactile hair (horse). (1) Epidermis. (2) Dermis. (3) Hair follicle. (4) Blood sinus in the dermal sheath. (5) Connective tissue trabeculae of the dermal sheath. Masson's trichrome. ×12.5.

16.6

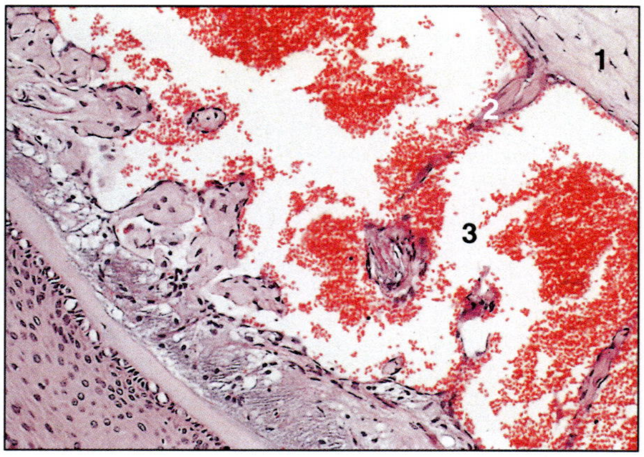

16.61 Sinus/tactile hair (horse). (1) Dermal sheath. (2) Connective tissue trabeculae of the dermal sheath. (3) Blood sinus. H & E. ×125.

.62

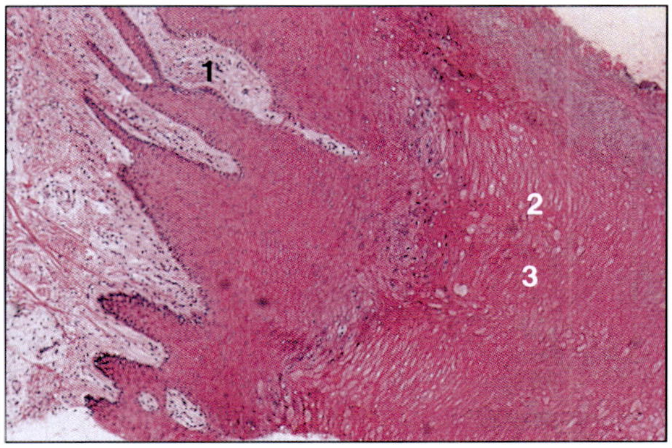

16.62 Hoof (calf). (1) Deep dermal papillae. Stratified squamous epithelium with (2) tubular and (3) intertubular horn. H & E. ×12.5.

16.63

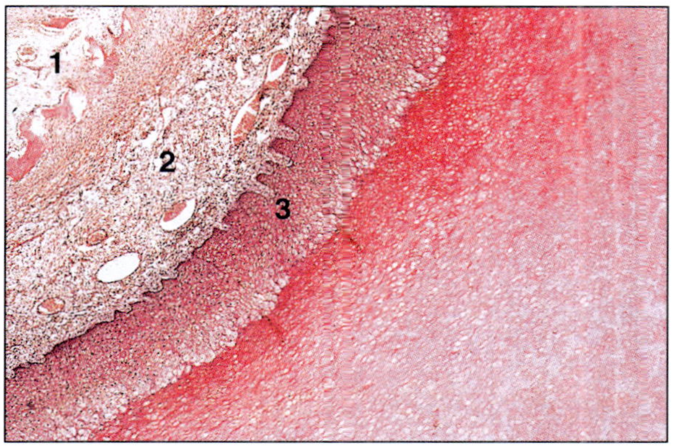

16.63 Hoof (foal). (1) Developing bone. (2) Vascular dermis. (3) Stratified squamous epithelium. H & E. ×12.5.

.64

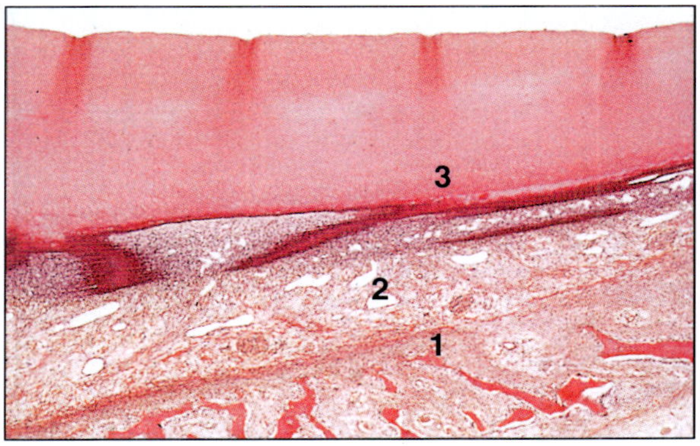

16.64 Hoof (foal). (1) Phalangeal bone. (2) Vascular dermis. (3) Epidermis with a thick stratum corneum. H & E. ×12.5.

16.65

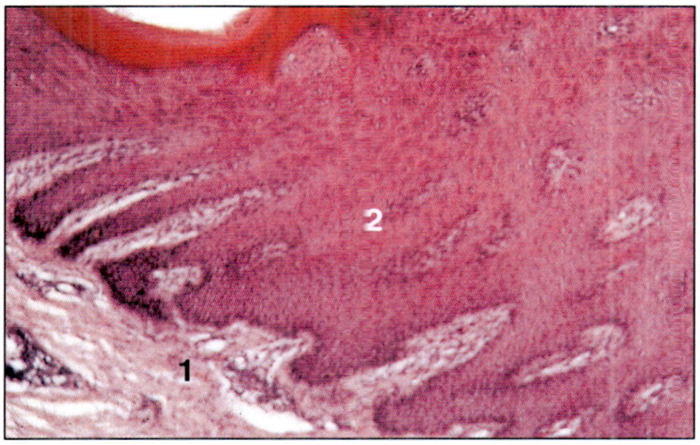

16.65 Hoof (goat). (1) Dermis (2) Stratified squamous epidermal epithelium, with a thick stratum corneum. H & E. ×125.

16.66 Hoof (goat). The epidermis clearly shows all the layers of a stratified squamous epithelium; note the stratum corneum. H & E. ×250.

16.66

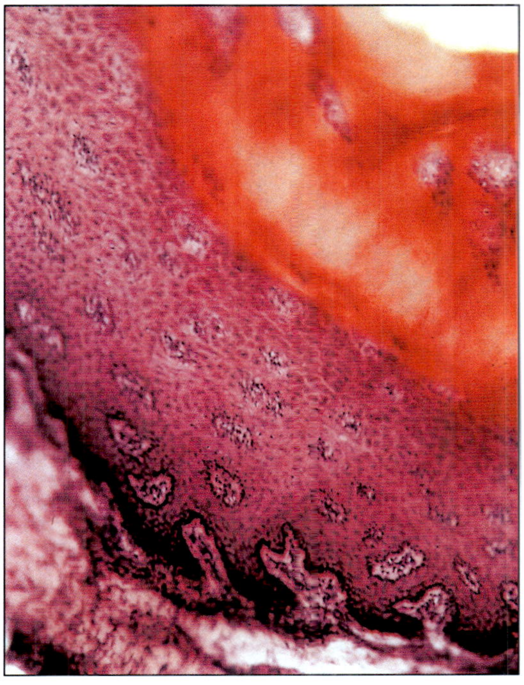

Claws are horny plates forming a protective covering on the dorsal surface of the terminal phalanges in the carnivore. The skin is reflected around the third phalanx to form a fold: the bed of the claw. The basal layers of the epidermis form the germinal matrix and grow to become the horny claw (16.67–16.69). The cavity of the cornual process forms the core of the horn and is lined with respiratory mucosa. A reflection of skin covers the cornual process, and the epidermis proliferates to become the horn sheath composed of tubular and intertubular horn (**16.70** and **16.71**).

The chestnut and ergot are genetically determined areas of tubular and intertubular horn, and are free from hair and glands. A thick pad of adipose tissue lies beneath the ergot.

16.67

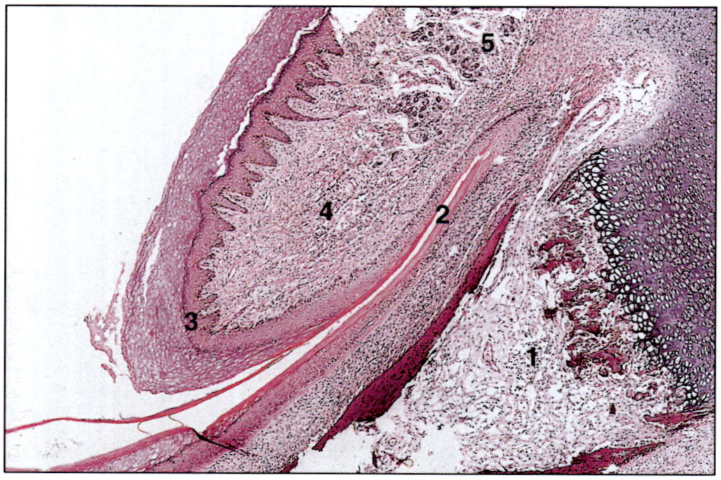

16.67 Claw (dog). (1) Third phalanx. (2) Claw fold. (3) Stratified squamous epithelium. (4) Dermis. (5) Digital pad. H & E. ×12.5.

16.68

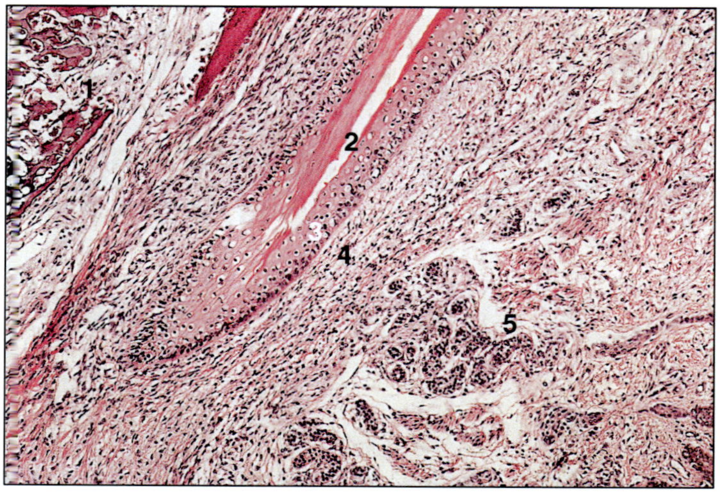

16.68 Claw (dog). (1) Third phalanx. (2) Claw fold. (3) Stratified squamous epithelium. (4) Dermis. (5) Digital pad. H & E. ×62.5.

16.69 Claw (dog). The superficial clear area of the stratified squamous epithelium is the developing claw (equivalent to the human nail). H & E. ×125.

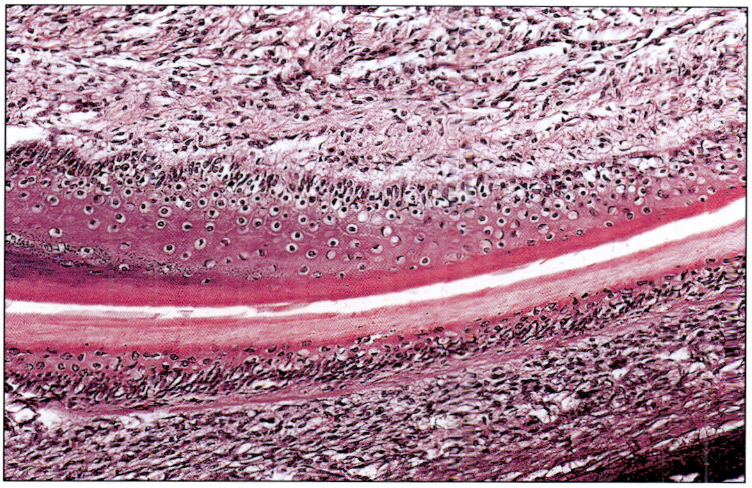

16.69

16.70 Horn (goat). The deep dermal papillae are stained green and surrounded by epidermal cells in columns, the horn tubules. Masson's trichrome. ×250.

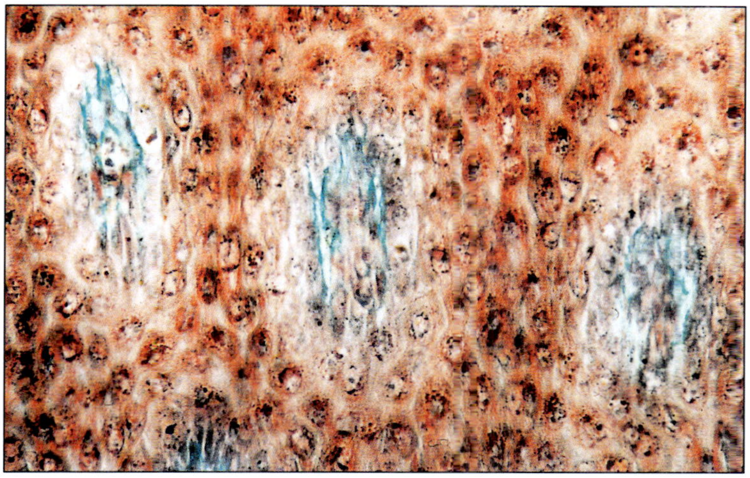

16.70

16.71 Horn (goat). The undulating effect is caused by the alternating tubular and intertubular arrangement of the developing horn. Masson's trichrome. ×250.

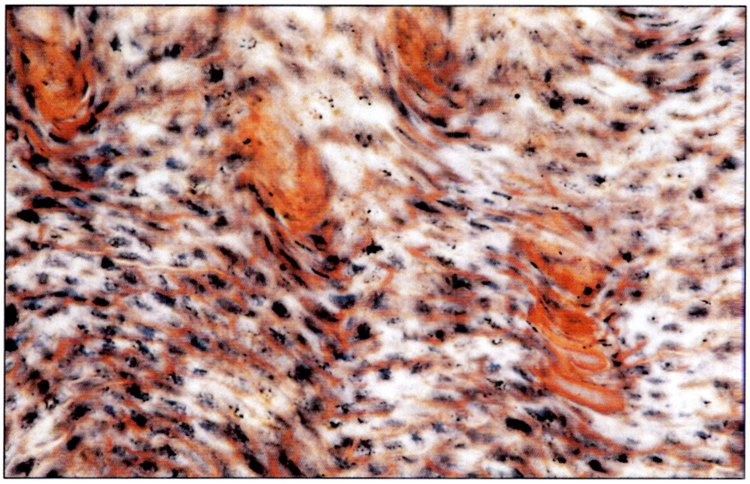

16.71

APPENDICES

Appendix Table 1 (see page 9)
Derivatives of the three germ layers

Ectoderm	Mesoderm	Endoderm

Central nervous system and eye
Central nervous system and ear
Hypophysis cerebri
Epiphysis cerebri
Chromaffin tissue
Epidermis, hair, nails, skin glands
Epithelium of
  oral and nasal cavity
  glands
  tooth enamel
	Muscle
	Connective tissue
	Blood, bone marrow
	Lymphoid tissue
	Kidney
	Gonad and genital ducts
	Suprarenal cortex
	Epithelium of
	  blood vessels
	  lymphatic vessels
	  body cavities
		Epithelium of
		  pharynx
		  auditory tube
		  thyroid, parathyroid, thymus
		  larynx, trachea, lungs
		  digestive tube, liver and pancreas
		  bladder
		  caudal vagina, vestibule
		  urethra

Appendix Table 2 (see page 51)
Differential white cell count: proportion of white blood cells in the domestic animals, species variation

Species	Polymorphonuclear leucocytes (neutrophils) (%)	Eosinophils (%)	Basophils (%)	Lymphocytes (%)	Monocytes (%)
Horse	35–75	2–12	0–3	15–50	2–10
Cattle	15–45	2–20	0–2	45–75	2–7
Sheep	10–50	1–10	0–3	40–75	1–6
Pig	28–45	1–11	0–2	39–62	2–10
Dog	60–77	2–10	Rare	12–30	3–10
Cat	35–75	2–12	Rare	20–50	1–4
Chicken	10–33	1–4	1–3	48–82	1–6
Size	12–15µm	10–15µm	10–15µm	Small, 6–9µm Large, 9–15µm	12–18µm

Kidneys

A1–A7 illustrate the structure of the kidneys (see page 137).

A1

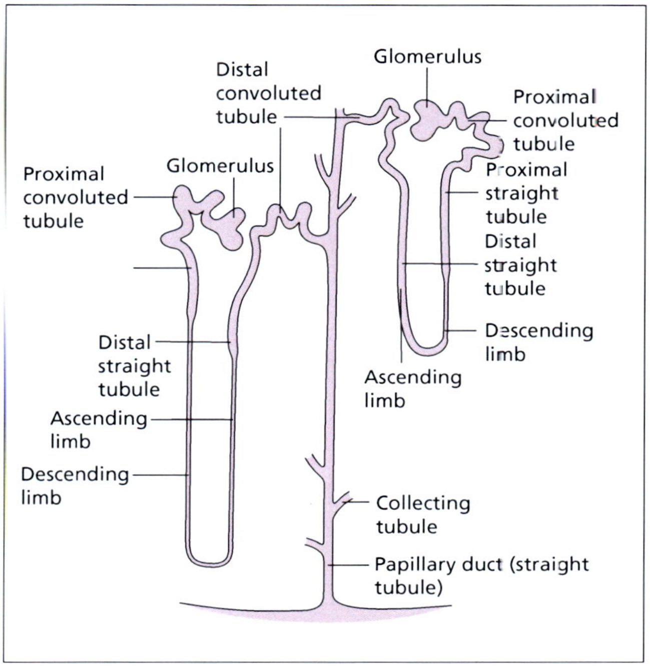

A1 Two cortical nephrons. On the left is a juxtamedullary nephron with a long loop of the nephron. On the right is an outer cortical glomerulus with a short loop of the nephron.

A2

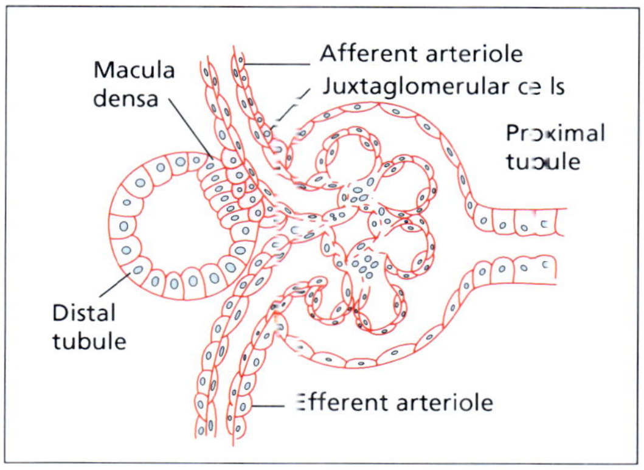

A2 Glomerulus and related structures.

A3

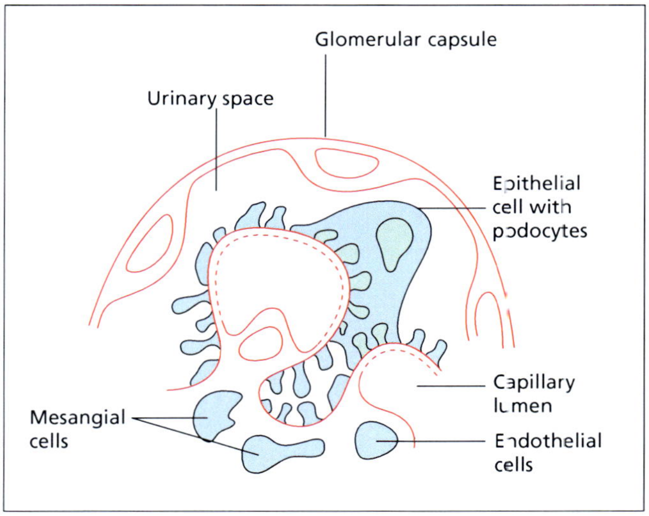

A3 Renal glomerulus.

A4

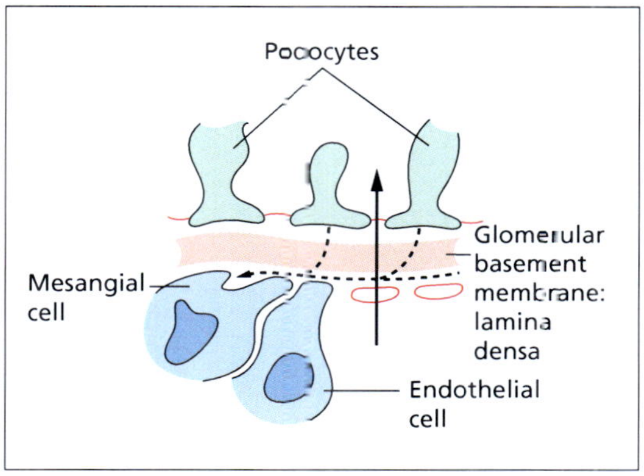

A4 Glomerular filter. The straight vertical arrow indicates the direction of ultrafiltration. The dashed lines show the flow of basement membrane in the perpendicular direction into the lamina rara interna and mesangium.

A5

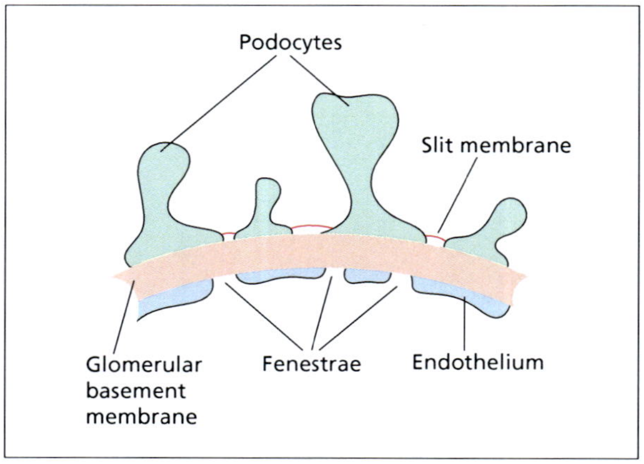

A5 Glomerular capillary wall.

A6

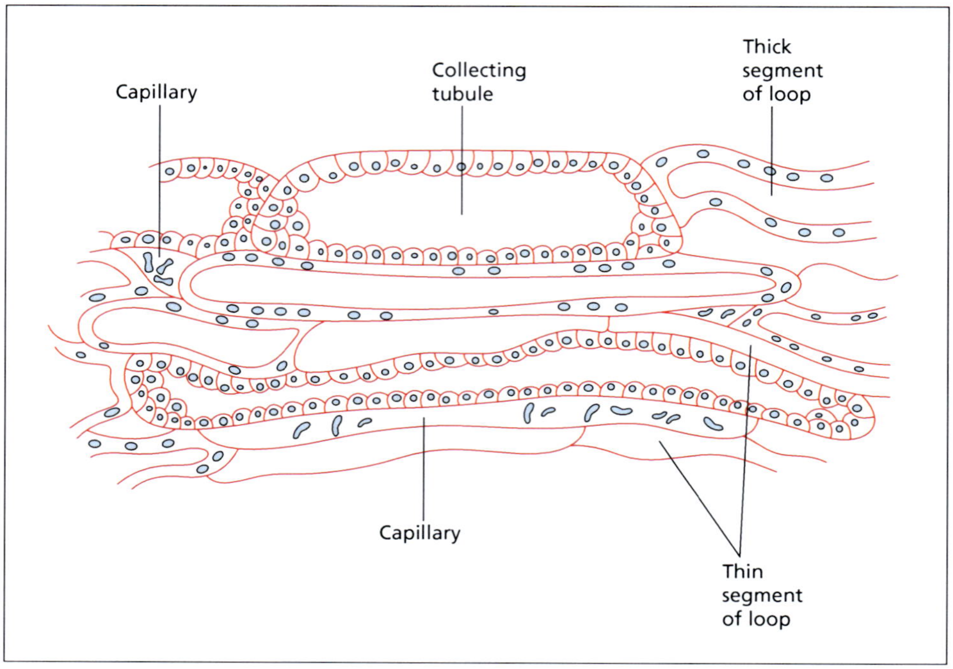

A6 Medulla, longitudinal section.

A7

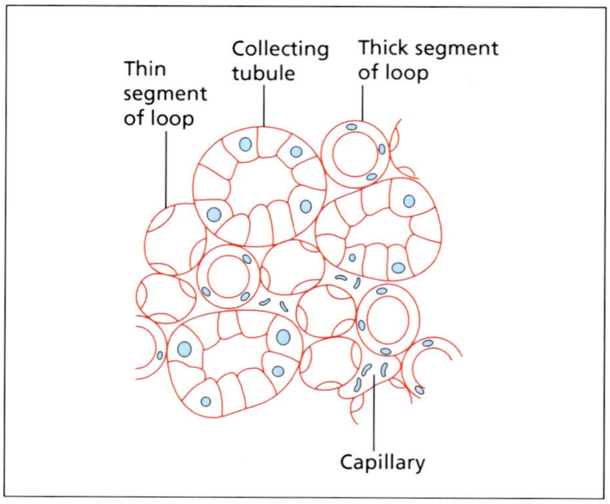

A7 Medulla, transverse section.

Appendix Table 3
Placentation

Definition	Placentation	The intimate apposition of the fetal membranes and parental tissue for the purpose of physiological exchange
Classification	Choriovitelline placenta chorioallantoic placenta	In the majority of mammals the chorioallantoic placenta is the definitive one
		The vascular allantoic mesoderm fuses with the chorion and forms the fetal vascular bed apposed to the maternal vascular bed in the endometrium
		The choriovitelline placenta is transitory
		In the mare and domestic carnivore, the yolk sac precedes the allantois in fusing with the chorion, vascularizing and forming the early fetal bed; this is a choriovitelline placenta and remnants may persist until term in the umbilical chord and form the umbilical vesicle (see 12.39–12.44)
External configuration	Diffuse placenta	Involves the whole chorionic surface, separation at term is simple with no loss of maternal tissue, non-deciduate (e.g. sow and mare)
	Cotyledonary placenta	Chorionic villi are restricted to the maternal curuncle, and the two together form a placentome, the unit of the ruminant placenta; no loss of maternal tissue at term, non-deciduate (e.g. cow, sheep and goat)
	Zonary placenta	Invasive zone is confined to a girdle-like band; loss of maternal tissue occurs at term, deciduate (e.g. carnivores)
	Discoidal placenta	Invasive zone is restricted to a single or bilateral disc-shaped area; loss of maternal tissue occurs at term, deciduate (rodents, primates)

Appendix Table A3 continues on p. 288.

Appendix Table 3 (cont) Placentation		
Definition	Placentation	The intimate apposition of the fetal membranes and parental tissue for the purpose of physiological exchange
Histological classification	See 12.44	
Synchoral fusion	Chorionic sacs of adjacent fetuses may fuse in up to 90% of multiple pregnancies	
	Vascular anastomosis between circulations	Rare, except in the cow

INDEX

Abomasum, 108
Accessory glands, male reproductive system, 174–5
Acidophils, pituitary gland, 151
Acinus
  liver, 124–5
  pancreas, 129
Addison's disease, 158
Adenocarcinoma, 146, 206
Adenohypophysis, 150–51, 161
  pars distalis, 150
  pars intermedia, 152
  pars nervosa, 152
  pars tuberalis, 152
Adenoma, 123
  ovarian, 206
  pulmonary, 30
  renal, 148
  ultimobranchial body, 166
Adipose tissue, 40
Adrenal gland, 156–9
  adrenal cortex, 156
  adrenal medulla, 156
  amphibians, 163
  birds, 160
  fish, 163
  reptiles, 163
Adrenalin, 156
Agranulocytes, 53–4
Air sacs, 95
Albumen, 209, 210
Alcian blue, 16
Allantois, 196, 203
Alveolar cell, 90
Alveoli
  lungs, 88, 90
  mammary glands, 194
Amnion, 196
Amphibians
  blood cells, 57–8
  bone, 64
  bone marrow, 64
  digestive system, 117–18, 120, 122
  endocrine system, 161–5
  heart, 69
  hypervitaminosis D, 80
Amphibians (*cont.*)
  lymphatic system, 80, 259–60
  metamorphosis, 117
  reproductive system
    female, 212
    male, 180
  respiratory system, 95, 96
  sense organs
    ear, 242–3
    eye, 236–8
    lateral line, 244, 246
  skin, 274
  specialized glands, 276
  urinary system, 145
Ampulla
  ear, 240
  female reproductive system, 188
  male reproductive system, 170, 174
Anaemia, 61
Anal canal, 116
Anal glands, 275
Anal pores, 276
Anal sacs, 116, 275
Anal sphincter, 116
Androgens, 156
Anisocytosis, 61
Antibodies, 260, 261, 274
Antidiuretic hormone, 153
Anus, 116
Apocrine glands, 266
Arachnoid, 219
Areolae, placenta, 198, 200
Artefacts, 18
Arteries, 71–2
Arterioles, 72
Arteriovenous anastomoses, 78
Arthritis, 50
Astrocytes, 220–2
Atria, parabronchi, 94
Atrioventricular node, 68
Auditory canal, 239
Auditory tube, 84
Auricle, 239
Aves, *see* birds
Axon, 215–16
Azurophils, 58

B lymphocytes, 60, 248, 258, 261
Basilar membrane, 239, 240
Basophils, 53, 151
  amphibians, 57
  birds, 56
  reptiles, 57
Bidder's organ, 182
Bile, 124–5, 128
Bile duct, 124–5, 128
Biliverdin, 259
Birds
  blood cells, 56
  bone, 63
  digestive system, 132–6, 143
  endocrine system, 160
  lymphatic system, 258
  reproductive system
    female, 208–10
    male, 178–9
  respiratory system, 93–5
  sense organs
  ear, 242
  eye, 236–7
  skin, 270–1
  urinary system, 143
Bladder, *see* urinary bladder
Blood, 51
  smear preparation, 51
Blood cells, 51–8
  amphibians, 57–8
  birds, 56
  reptiles, 57–8
  see also erythrocytes; leucocytes; platelets
Blood–brain barrier, 222
Bone, 44–9
  amphibians, 64
  birds, 63
  endochondral ossification, 47–8
  growth of long bone, 48–9
  intramembranous ossification, 49

Bone (*cont.*)
  reptiles, 64
  spiculated bone, 63
Bone marrow, 59–60, 262
  amphibians, 64
  reptiles, 64
Bovine spongiform
    encephalopathy, 226
Bowman's capsule, 138
Bowman's glands, 243
Bowman's membrane, 230, 236
Brain, 219
Bronchiolar–alveolar carcinoma,
    92
Bronchioles, 88–90
Bronchus, 87, 88, 94
Bulbourethral glands, 175
Bursa (of Fabricius), 258

Caecum, 116, 134
Calcitonin, 160, 166
Cancellous bone, 44
Capillaries, 74
Carcinoma, 123
  adenocarcinoma, 146, 206
  bronchiolar–alveolar, 92
  renal, 146
  squamous cell, 30, 122, 236,
    268
Cardia, stomach, 111
Cardiac muscle, 68–9
Cardiovascular system, 71–8
  see also heart
Carpal glands, 276
Cartilage, 40–2
  elastic cartilage, 42
  fibrocartilage, 42
  hyaline cartilage, 40
Caruncles, uterus, 191, 200
Cell structure, 21
Cementum, 102
Cervix, 191
Chief cells, 112, 120, 155
Cholangitis, 128
Choleliths, 128
Cholesteatoma, 226
Chondrocytes, 40
Chorion, 196
Choroid, 232–4, 236, 238
Chromaffin system, 156, 160,
    163
Chromatophoromata, 274
Chromophils, 151
Chromophobes, 150, 161
Chromosomes, 21
Circumanal glands, 275
Circumvallate papilla, 97–8
Cirrhosis, liver, 124, 127
Clara cells, 90
Claws, 264, 280–2
Clitoris, 194
Cloaca
  amphibians, 180
  birds, 136, 143, 210
    bursa, 258
  reptiles, 144, 181
Cochlea, 240
Collagen fibres, 32
Colon, 116
  sacculated, 119
Columella, 242
Columnar epithelium, 22
Comb, 270
Compact bone, 44
Conjunctiva, 227
Connective tissue, 31–40
  cell types, 34–8
  dense connective tissue, 38–9
  embryonal connective tissue, 31
  loose areolar connective tissue,
    38
  mesenchyme connective tissue,
    31
  mucoid connective tissue, 31
  special types of, 40
Cornea, 228, 230
  birds, 236
  reptiles, 237, 244
Corpora albicans, 186, 212
Corpora arenacea, 159
Corpora atretans, 212
Corpora cavernosa, 172, 173
Corporus luteum, 186, 192, 199,
    212
Corpus spongiosum urethrae,
    172
Cortical cells, 163
Cryptorchidism, 178
Crypts
  of Lieberkühn, 114
  tonsils, 254
Cuboidal epithelium, 22
Cushing's disease, 153
Cystic ovarian disease, 205
Cytoplasm, 21
Demodicosis, 268
Dendrites, 215–16
Denticles, 274
Dentine, 102
Dermatitis, 268
Dermis, 266, 268, 270, 280
Dermoids, 236
Descemet's membrane, 230
Diabetes mellitus, 132, 149
Digestive system, 97–136
  amphibians, 117–18, 120, 122
  birds, 132–6
  lymphatic tissue, 255
  reptiles, 117–23
Distal convoluted tubule
    (DCT), 140
  birds, 143
  reptiles, 144
Duodenum, 114
Dura mater, 219
Duvernoy's glands, 118
Dysgerminoma, 206, 214

Ear, 239–43
  amphibians, 242–3
  birds, 242
  external ear, 239, 242
  inner ear, 240
  middle ear, 239
  reptiles, 242–3
Egg shell, birds, 209–10
Elastic cartilage, 42
Elastic fibres, 32
Elastic tissue, 40
Electric organs, 246
Embryonal connective tissue, 31
Enamel, 102
Endocardium, 78
Endocrine glands, 30, 149
Endocrine pancreas, 130, 149
Endocrine system, 149–66
  amphibians, 161–5
  birds, 160
  reptiles, 161–6
Endolymphatic systems, 80
Endometrial glands, 189–91
Endometrium, 189–91, 199
Endomysium, 67
Endoneurium, 217
Endothelial cells, 38
Enteritis, 122
Eosin, 15

Eosinophils, 38, 53
amphibians, 57
birds, 56
reptiles, 57
Ependyma, 219
Epicardium, 78
Epidermis, 263, 264–5, 270, 280
Epididymis, 170, 180
Epiglottis, 84
Epimysium, 66
Epineurium, 216
Epiphysis cerebri, 159
Epithelium, 22–7
columnar, 22
cuboidal, 22
myoepithelium, 27
olfactory, 243
pseudostratified, 24
respiratory, 82
squamous
simple, 22–4
stratified, 25–7
transitional, 26
see also specific organs
Ergot, 284
Erythrocytes, 51–3
amphibians, 57
birds, 56
fish, 260
production of, 60, 259, 260
removal of, 250, 259
reptiles, 57
Erythropoietin, 137
Eustachian tube, 239
Exocrine glands, 28
Exocrine pancreas, 129, 136
External ear, 239, 242
Eye, 227–38
amphibians, 237–8
birds, 236–7
development of, 228
fish, 237–8
parietal eye, 244
reptiles, 237–8, 244
structure of, 230–4
Eyelids, 227–8

Facial pit organs, 244
Fallopian tubes, *see* oviducts
Fangs, reptiles, 118
Fat cells, 36
Feathers, 270
Feline parvovirus, 226
Femoral pores, 276
Fibroblasts, 34
Fibrocartilage, 42
Fibrosis
liver, 126–7
pancreas, 132
Fish
electric organs, 246
endocrine system, 163, 164
haemopoiesis, 64
heart, 69
liver, 124–5
lymphatic system, 260
pancreas, 131
reproductive system
female, 212
male, 180
respiratory system, 95
sense organs
eye, 237–8
lateral line organ, 244
skin, 274
swim bladder, 246
urinary system, 145
Fixation, 10
Foliate papilla, 97–8
Follicle-stimulating hormone, 184
Forestomach, 107
Freemartinism, 205
Freezing, 12
consequences of freezing unfixed tissues, 12–14
Fundus, stomach, 111
Fungiform papilla, 97–8

Gall bladder, 128
reptiles, 128
Ganglia, 216, 218
Gastric glands, 108–12
Gastritis, 122
Gills
amphibians, 95
fish, 95, 145
Gingivitis, 105
Gizzard, 133
Glands, 28–30
endocrine glands, 30, 149
exocrine glands, 28
see also specific glands
Glands of Möll, 227
Glands of Zeiss, 227
Glomerular capsule, 138
Glomerulonephritis, 146
Glomerulus, 138
fish, 145
Glossitis, 122
Glucagon, 130
Glucocorticoids, 156
Goblet cells
digestive system, 116, 122
gall bladder, 128
female reproductive system, 191, 192
integumentary system, 274
respiratory system, 82, 94
Goitre, 155, 165
Gonadotrophic hormone, 199
Graafian follicle, 184
Granulocytes, 53, 259, 260
production of, 60
Granulosa, 206, 214
Granulosa cells, 184, 186
Guttural pouch, 84

Haemangioma, 268
Haemangiosarcoma, 80, 268
Haematoxylin and eosin (H & E) stain, 15
Haemolytic anaemia, 61
Haemopoiesis, 59–60, 64, 145, 259, 260
Hair, 277–80
sinus hairs, 280
Hair follicles, 277–8
Hard palate, 100
Harderian gland, 228, 236
Head kidney, 145
Heart, 78
amphibians, 69
fish, 69
reptiles, 69
see also cardiovascular system
Hemipenes, 181
Hepatic artery, 124
Hepatic lipidosis, 126
Hepatic portal vein, 124
Hepatitis, 126
Hepatopancreas, 125, 131
Hermaphroditism, 182
Herring bodies, 152
Heterophils, 53

Heterophils (*cont.*)
amphibians, 57
birds, 56
reptiles, 57
Hilus
kidney, 137
ovary, 183
Histological sections
artefacts, 18
preparation of, 10–14
blood smear preparation, 51
fixation, 10
freezing, 12–14
paraffin embedding, 10–12
staining, 14–16
Hooves, 264, 280
Horns, 280–2
Hyaline cartilage, 40
trachea, 87, 93
Hydrocephalus, 226
Hyperadrenocorticism, 158
Hypercalcaemia, 70, 166
Hyperparathyroidism, 165
Hyperthyroidism, 155, 165
Hypervitaminosis D, 80, 127
Hypoadrenocorticism, 158
Hypodermis, 266, 280
Hypoparathyroidism, 165
Hypophyseal pouch, 150
Hypophyseal stalk, 152
Hypophysis, 150–53
adenohypophysis, 150–51, 161
amphibians, 161
birds, 160
cerebri, 150
neoplasms, 153
neurohypophysis, 152, 161
reptiles, 161
Hypothyroidism, 162, 165

Ileum, 114
Immune system, 261–2
amphibians, 260
fish, 260
Immune-mediated anaemia, 61
Incus, 239
Infundibulum, 188, 209, 212
Inner ear, 240
Insulin, 130
Integumentary system, 263–84
see also skin
Interdigital glands, 276
Interstitial cell tumour, testicular, 177
Intestine
large, 116
small, 114–16
Intussusception, 122
Iris, 230, 234
Islets of Langerhans, 130, 131, 136
Isthmus, 188, 209

Jacobson's organ, 244
Jejunum, 114
Juxtaglomerular apparatus, kidney, 140, 143

Keratin, 264, 272
Keratinocytes, 263, 264
Keratitis, 236
Kidneys, 137–41, 145
amphibians, 145
birds, 143
collecting tubule, 140
fish, 145
renal corpuscle, 138
renal tubule, 140
tumours, 146
uriniferous tubule, 138
Küpffer cells, 260

Labia, 194
Labial pit organs, 244
Lacrimal apparatus, 228
Lactiferous ducts, 194
Lagena, 242
Lamellae, of bone, 44–6
Langerhans cells, 264
Large intestine, 116
birds, 136
Larynx, 86
Lateral line systems, 242, 244
Leiomyoma, 123
Leiomyosarcoma, 123
Lens, 228, 230, 236, 238
parietal eye, 244
Leucocytes, 53–4
amphibians, 57
birds, 56
fish, 260
production of, 60
Leucocytes (*cont.*)
reptiles, 57
Leukaemia, 62, 256, 260
Leukoplakia, preneoplastic, 122
Leydig cells, 167
Light microscopy, 18
Lingual sheath, 118
Lingual tonsil, 99, 254
Liver, 124–7
amphibians, 124–5, 127
fish, 124–5
reptiles, 124–5, 127
Loop of Henle, 140, 143
Lungs, 88–90
amphibians, 95, 96
tumours, 92
Lymph hearts, 259, 260
Lymph nodes, 247–8
Lymphatic system, 247–62
amphibians, 260
birds, 258
fish, 260
reptiles, 259
Lymphatic vessels, 80
Lymphocytes, 38, 54, 247–9, 255, 261
production of, 60
see also B lymphocytes; T lymphocytes
Lymphokines, 261, 262
Lymphosarcoma, 236, 256, 260

M cells, 255
Macrophages, 34, 54, 248, 250, 252, 262
Macula densa, kidney, 140
Maculae, 240
Malignant catarrhal fever (MCF), 236
Malleus, 239
Mammary glands, 194, 204
tumours, 204
Masson's trichrome, 16
Mast cells, 35
Mastitis, 204
Megakaryocytic myelosis, 62
Meibomian gland tumours, 236
Meissner's nerve plexus, 112, 116
Melanin, 96, 125
Melanocytes, 264
Melanoma, 236

Melatonin, 159
Membranous labyrinth, 240, 242
Merkel's cells, 264
Merocrine glands, 266, 276
Mesenchyme connective tissue, 31
Metamorphosis, amphibians, 117, 145
Metamyelocytes, 60
Metarubricytes, 60
Microglia, 222
Microscopy, 18
Middle ear, 239
Mineralocorticoids, 156
Mitral valve dysplasia, 80
Monocytes, 38, 54, 262
Mordant, 14
Motor endplate, 67
Mucoid connective tissue, 31
Mucosa
  digestive tract, 105, 107, 120
  oviducts, 209
  ureter, 141
  urethra, 142
  uterus, 210
  vagina, 192
  vas deferens, 170–1
Mucus cells, 100
Mucus-secreting glands
  amphibians, 276
  fish, 274
  gall bladder, 128
  gastric, 112
  lacrimal glands, 228
  oesophagus, 106
  oropharynx, 104
  reptiles, 119, 181
  small intestine, 114
  ureter, 141
Muscle, 65–70
  cardiac muscle, 68–9
  smooth muscle, 65
  striated (skeletal) muscle, 66–7
Muscle spindles, 67
Muscularis externa
  digestive system, 105, 106, 112, 116
  birds, 132, 134
  ureter, 141
Muscularis mucosa, 105, 108, 112, 116
Myasthenic conditions, 70
Myeloblasts, 60
Myelocytes, 60
Myocardium, 68–9, 78
  degeneration, 80
Myoepithelium, 27
Myometrium, 191
Myopathies, 70
Myositis, 70

Nasal cavity, 243
Nephroblastoma, 146
Nephron, 140
Nephrotic syndrome, 146
Nerves, 216
Nervous system, 215–26
  central nervous system, 220, 226
  peripheral nervous system, 216
Neural crest, 215, 216
Neural tube, 215
Neurilemma, 216
Neuroglial cells, 216, 220
Neurohypophysis, 152, 161
Neurons, 215–16
Neuropathies, 70
Neurosecretory bodies, 152
Neutrophils, 36, 61
Nictitating membrane, 227–8, 237
Nissl's granules, 215
Node of Ranvier, 216
Nucleus, 21
Nurse cells, 184

Oesophagitis, 122
  birds, 132
Oesophagus, 106, 119
Oestradiol, 184, 186
Olfactory organ, 243
Oligodendrocytes, 216, 220
Omasum, 108
Oocytes, 184, 186
  amphibians, 212
  birds, 208, 209
  fish, 212
  reptiles, 212
Oral cavity, birds, 132
Organ of Corti, 239, 240
Oropharynx, 104, 119
Os penis, 173
Osmic acid, 15
Osseous labyrinth, 240
Ossicles, auditory, 239, 242
Ossification
  endochondral, 47–8
  intramembranous, 49
Osteoblasts, 46
Osteoclasts, 46
Osteoderms, 272
Osteopenia, 66
Osteosarcoma, 49
Otitis externa, 242
Otoliths, 240
Ovaries, 183–4
  amphibians, 212
  birds, 208
  cortex, 183, 208
  fish, 212
  follicular development, 184
  medulla, 184
  reptiles, 212
  tumours, 205–6
Oviducts, 188
  birds, 209–10
  reptiles, 212–13
Ovulation, 186
Oxyphil cells, 155
Oxytocin, 152, 153

Palate, 100
Palatine tonsil, 254
Pancreas, 129–32, 149
  amphibians, 131
  birds, 136
  fish, 131
  reptiles, 131–2
Pancreatic polypeptide, 130
Pancreatitis, 132
Paneth cells, 115
Parabronchus, 94
Paraffin embedding, 10–12
Parathyroid gland, 155, 165
  amphibians, 163
  birds, 160
  reptiles, 163
Parietal cells, 112
Parietal eye, 244
Pars ciliaris retinae, 232, 234
Pars iridica retinae, 234
Penis, 171, 172–3
  reptiles, 181
Peptic ulceration, 113
Perianal glands, 275

Perianal sinuses, 275
Perichondrium, 82, 86
Pericytes, 38, 74
Perilymphatic systems, 80
Perimetrium, 191
Perimysium, 67
Perineurium, 217
Periodic acid Schiff (PAS) stain, 15–16
Periosteum, 44
Phaeochromocytoma, 158
Phallodeum, 180
Pharyngeal tonsil, 254
Pharyngitis, 122
Pharynx, 84
Pia mater, 219, 220
Pigment cells, 36
Pineal gland, 159, 165
  amphibians, 164
  fish, 164
  reptiles, 164
Pinealocytes, 159
Pinealoma, 165
Pinna, 239, 242
Pituitary gland, *see* hypophysis cerebri
Placentation, 196–202
  carnivores, 202
  mare, 199
  reptiles, 212
  ruminants, 200
  sow, 198
Placentome, 200
Plasma cells, 34–5, 105, 194, 255
Plasmalemma, 21
Platelets, 55
Pneumocytes, 90
Pneumonia, 92
Podocytes, 138
Poison glands, 276
Polycryptic caecal tonsil, 258
Polymorphonuclear leucocytes (PMLs), 53
Preen gland, 270–1
Pregnancy, mammary glands and, 194
  see also placentation
Prepuce, 173
Progesterone, 186, 192
Promyelocytes, 60
Prorubricytes, 60
Prostate glands, 174, 177
Prostate glands (*cont.*)
  hyperplasia, 177
Proventriculus, 133
Proximal convoluted tubule (PCT), 140, 143
Pseudobranch, 95
Pseudostratified epithelium, 24
Pulmonary adenoma, 30
Pupil, 234, 237
Purkinje's fibres, 68
Pyloric glands, 112
Pylorus, stomach, 111

Ramithecae, 120
Rathke's pouch, 150
Rectal canal, 116
Rectum, 116
Reissner's membrane, 240
Renal corpuscle, 138, 143
Renal failure, 146
Renal pelvis, 141
Renal tubule, 140
Reproductive system
  female, 183–214
    amphibians, 212
    birds, 208–10
    fish, 212
    reptiles, 212–13
  male, 167–84
    amphibians, 180
    birds, 178–9
    fish, 180
    reptiles, 180–1
  tumours, 177
Reptiles
  blood cells, 57–8
  bone, 64
  bone marrow, 64
  digestive system, 117–23, 124, 127, 128, 131–2
  endocrine system, 161–6
  heart, 69
  hypervitaminosis D, 80
  lymphatic system, 259
    vessels, 80
  reproductive system
    female, 212–13
    male, 180–1
  sense organs, 244
    ear, 242–3
    eye, 237–8
    parietal eye, 244
Reptiles (*cont.*)
  skin, 270–2
  specialized glands, 276
  urinary system, 144
Respiratory epithelium, 82
Respiratory system, 82–96
  amphibians, 95
  birds, 93–5
  fish, 95
Rete ovarii, 184
Rete testis, 169
Reticular tissue, 40
Reticulocytes, 60
Reticulum, 107, 108
Retina, 228, 230, 234, 236, 238
Rhabdomyoma, 70
Rhabdomyosarcoma, 70
Rubriblasts, 60
Rubricytes, 60
Rumen, 107, 108

Saccule, 240, 242
Salivary glands, 100–1
  amphibians, 120
  reptiles, 120
    modified (Duvenoy's), 118
Salt-secreting glands, 120
Sarcolemma, 65
Sarcoplasm, 65
Scales, 274
Scanning electron microscopy, 18
Schwann cells, 216
Sclera, 230–2
  birds, 236
Scrapie, 226
Sebaceous glands, 266–7, 274, 276
Sections, histological, *see* histological sections
Semicircular canals, 240
Seminal vesicles, 175
Seminiferous tubules, 167
  birds, 178–9
  lower vertebrates, 180
Seminoma, 177
Seromucous glands, 82, 106, 116
Serosa, 105, 116, 188
  reptiles, 120
Serotonin, 159
Serous cells, 100, 228

Sexual segment, reptilian kidney, 144
Shell gland, 210
Silver impregnation, 16
Sinoatrial node, 68
Sinus hairs, 280
Sinusoids, 74
Skeletal muscle, 66–7
Skin, 263–74
 amphibians, 274
 birds, 270–1
 fish, 274
 reptiles, 270–2
Small intestine, 114
 birds, 134
Smooth muscle, 65
Soft palate, 100
Somatostatin, 130
Spermathecae, 180, 212
Spermatocytes, 168
Spermatogonium, 168
Spermatophore, 180
Spermatozoa
 amphibians, 180
 birds, 178
 fish, 180
 production of, 167, 168, 180
 reptiles, 180
 structure of, 169
Spherocytes, 61
Spinal cord, 219
Spleen, 250
 amphibians, 260
 birds, 258
 fish, 260
Splenopancreas, 132, 260
Squamous cell carcinoma, 30, 122, 236, 268
Squamous epithelium
 simple, 22
 stratified, 25–6
Staining, 14–16
Stapes, 239
Stilling cells, 163
Stomach, 107–12
 birds, 133–4
 reptiles, 119–20
Striated muscle, 66–7
Submucosa, digestive tract, 105, 133, 134
Supracaudal glands, 276
Sustentacular cells, 168, 180
 tumours, 177
Sweat glands, 266–7
Swim bladder, 246
Synapses, 215

T lymphocytes, 60, 248–50, 252, 255, 258, 261, 262
Tactile hairs, 280
Taenia coli, 116
Tail glands, 276
Tail kidney, 145
Tapetum cellulosum, 234
Tapetum fibrosum, 234
Tapetum lucidum, 232–4
Taste buds, 84, 97–8
Teat, 194
Tectorial membrane, 240
Teeth, 102–4
 amphibians, 118
 reptiles, 118
  fangs, 118
Tela choroidea, 219
Teratoma, 206, 214
Testicles, retained, 176
Testis, 167, 182
 birds, 178–9
 fish, 180
 rete testis, 169
 tumours, 182
Testosterone, 167
Thecal cell tumours, 206, 214
Thoracic duct, 80
Thrombocytes, 55
 amphibians, 58
 birds, 56
 fish, 58
 reptiles, 58
Thymocytes, 252, 258
Thymus, 252, 261
 amphibians, 260
 birds, 258
 reptiles, 259
Thyrocalcitonin, 154
Thyroid gland, 154–5, 165
 amphibians, 162
 birds, 160
 reptiles, 162
Thyrotrophin, 154
Thyroxine, 154
Tissue sections, *see* histological sections
Tongue, 97–8
 birds, 132
Tongue (*cont.*)
 reptiles, 118
Tonsils, 99, 132
 lymphoid tissue, 254
Trachea, 86
 birds, 93–4
Tracheobronchial syrinx, 94
Transitional epithelium, 26
Transmissible spongiform encephalopathies, 226
Transmission electron microscopy, 18
Tri-iodothyronine, 154
Trophoblast cells, 198
Tubuli recti, 169
Tunica adventitia, 72, 74, 76
Tunica albuginea
 female reproductive system, 183, 184, 208
 male reproductive system, 167, 172, 178
Tunica intima, 71, 74, 76
Tunica media, 71–2, 76
 mineralization, 80
Tunica vaginalis, 167
Tunica vasculosa, 167
Tympanic membrane, 239, 242, 243

Ulcerative stomatitis, 122
Ultimobranchial body, 160, 163, 164, 166, 259
Umbilical cord, 203
Units, of histological measurement, 18
Ureters, 141
 amphibians, 145
 birds, 143
 reptiles, 144
Urethelium, 26, 141, 142
Urethra, 142
 male reproductive system, 171–2, 174
Urinary bladder, 142
 amphibians, 145
 reptiles, 144
Urinary system, 137–48
 amphibians, 145
 birds, 143
 fish, 145
 reptiles, 144
Uriniferous tubule, 138

Urodeum, 179, 210
Urolithiasis, 166
Uropygial gland, 270–1
Uterine tubes, *see* oviducts
Uterus, 188, 189–91, 206
  birds, 210
  cervix, 191
  endometrium, 189–91, 199
  myometrium, 191
  perimetrium, 191
  reptiles, 212
Utricle, 240

Vagina, 192, 210
Vas deferens, 170–1, 179, 180
Vasopressin, 152
Veins, 76
Venom glands, reptiles, 118
Ventriculus, 133
Venules, 74
Vestibule
  ear, 240
  nasal cavity, birds, 93
  vulva, 194
Vibrissae, 280
Villi, intestinal, 114–16
Visceral pleura, 88
Vocal cords, 86
Vomeronasal organ, 244
Vulva, 194

Wattles, 270

Yolk sac, 196, 203

Zona pellucida, 184, 186, 212